Bruce & Borg's

Psychosocial Frames of Reference

Theories, Models, and Approaches
for Occupation-Based Practice

FOURTH EDITION

Bruce & Borg's

Psychosocial Frames of Reference

Theories, Models, and Approaches
for Occupation-Based Practice

FOURTH EDITION

Terry Krupa, PhD, OT Reg (Ont), FCAOT
Professor
School of Rehabilitation Therapy
Queen's University
Kingston, Ontario, Canada

Bonnie Kirsh, PhD, OT Reg (Ont)
Associate Professor
Department of Occupational Science and Occupational Therapy
Rehabilitation Sciences Institute
University of Toronto
Toronto, Ontario, Canada

Deborah Pitts, PhD, OTR/L, BCMH, CPRP
Assistant Professor of Clinical Occupational Therapy
USC Chan Division of Occupational Science and Occupational Therapy
University of Southern California
Los Angeles, California

Ellie Fossey, PhD, MSc, DipCOT (UK)
Professor of Occupational Therapy
Department of Occupational Therapy
Monash University
Frankston, Victoria, Australia

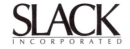

SLACK
INCORPORATED

www.Healio.com/books

ISBN: 978-1-61711-622-3

Copyright © 2016 by SLACK Incorporated

Bruce and Borg's Psychosocial Frames of Reference: Theories, Models, and Approaches for Occupation Based Practice, Fourth Edition includes ancillary materials specifically available for faculty use. Included are PowerPoint slides. Please visit www.efacultylounge.com to obtain access.

The procedures and practices described in this publication should be implemented in a manner consistent with the professional standards set for the circumstances that apply in each specific situation. Every effort has been made to confirm the accuracy of the information presented and to correctly relate generally accepted practices. The authors, editors, and publisher cannot accept responsibility for errors or exclusions or for the outcome of the material presented herein. There is no expressed or implied warranty of this book or information imparted by it. Care has been taken to ensure that drug selection and dosages are in accordance with currently accepted/recommended practice. Off-label uses of drugs may be discussed. Due to continuing research, changes in government policy and regulations, and various effects of drug reactions and interactions, it is recommended that the reader carefully review all materials and literature provided for each drug, especially those that are new or not frequently used. Some drugs or devices in this publication have clearance for use in a restricted research setting by the Food and Drug and Administration or FDA. Each professional should determine the FDA status of any drug or device prior to use in their practice.

Any review or mention of specific companies or products is not intended as an endorsement by the author or publisher.

SLACK Incorporated uses a review process to evaluate submitted material. Prior to publication, educators or clinicians provide important feedback on the content that we publish. We welcome feedback on this work.

Published by: SLACK Incorporated
6900 Grove Road
Thorofare, NJ 08086 USA
Telephone: 856-848-1000
Fax: 856-848-6091
www.Healio.com/books

Contact SLACK Incorporated for more information about other books in this field or about the availability of our books from distributors outside the United States.

Library of Congress Cataloging-in-Publication Data

Krupa, Terry, 1956- , author.
  Bruce & Borg's psychosocial frames of reference : theories, models, and approaches for occupation-based practice / Terry Krupa, Bonnie Kirsh. -- Fourth edition.
      p. ; cm.
  Bruce and Borg's psychosocial frames of reference
  Psychosocial frames of reference
  Preceded by Psychosocial frames of reference / Mary Ann Giroux Bruce, Barbara A. Borg. 3rd ed. 2002.
  Includes bibliographical references and index.
  ISBN 978-1-61711-622-3 (alk. paper)
  I. Kirsh, Bonnie, 1955- , author. II. Bruce, Mary Ann. Psychosocial frames of reference. Preceded by (work) III. Title. IV. Title: Bruce and Borg's psychosocial frames of reference. V. Title: Psychosocial frames of reference.
  [DNLM: 1. Occupational Therapy--methods. 2. Mental Disorders--rehabilitation. WM 450.5.O2]
  RC487
  616.89'165--dc23
                              2015030661

Printed in the United States of America.

Last digit is print number: 10 9 8 7 6 5 4 3 2 1

Dedication

This book is dedicated to all of the people who have personal experience with mental illness and have taught us so much and continue to inspire us.

Contents

Bruce and Borg's Psychosocial Frames of Reference: Theories, Models, and Approaches for Occupation Based Practice, Fourth Edition includes ancillary materials specifically available for faculty use. Included are PowerPoint slides. Please visit www.efacultylounge.com to obtain access.

Acknowledgments

We extend our thanks to Andrea Mihaly and Anne Holley-Hime, who contributed to the development of this text.

We thank our family, friends, and colleagues who supported and encouraged us throughout this project.

About the Editors

Terry Krupa, PhD, OT Reg (Ont), FCAOT is a Professor in the Occupational Therapy Program of the School of Rehabilitation Therapy at Queen's University, Canada. She holds cross appointments in the Department of Psychiatry and the School of Nursing. She has practiced in the mental health field for over 30 years, as a clinician, educator, and researcher/scholar. Terry has been involved in the development and evaluation of a range of services and intervention approaches focused on improving the health, well-being, and full community participation of people living with mental illness. Terry has been the recipient of the Canadian Association of Occupational Therapist's Muriel Driver and Leadership Awards. She was the inaugural recipient of the Pioneer Award for Recovery Research presented by Psychosocial Rehabilitation Canada.

Bonnie Kirsh, PhD, OT Reg (Ont) is an Associate Professor in the Department of Occupational Science and Occupational Therapy, with cross appointments to the Rehabilitation Sciences Institute and the Department of Psychiatry at the University of Toronto. Prior to becoming an academic, she was a clinician and an administrator in the field of occupational therapy and mental health. Her work focuses on community engagement for people experiencing mental illnesses, with a focus on systems, services, and interventions that enable people to obtain and maintain meaningful and productive roles. Bonnie was appointed to the Mental Health Commission of Canada and has participated on boards of community mental health agencies. She has also been the recipient of the Canadian Association of Occupational Therapist's Muriel Driver Award.

Deborah Pitts, PhD, OTR/L, BCMH, CPRP is an Assistant Professor of Clinical Occupational Therapy in the USC Chan Division of Occupational Science and Occupational Therapy. She has developed an expertise in the philosophy and practice of psychiatric rehabilitation with a particular interest in how occupation influences the "lived experience" of recovery for persons labeled with psychiatric disabilities. Deborah has served as an occupational therapy clinician, educator, scholar, and consultant, and as a surveyor for behavioral health facilities in the United States. Deborah has worked actively to advance the mental health knowledge and practice in occupational therapy, through her leadership in the American Occupational Therapy Association (AOTA) Mental Health Special Interest Section and in the development of the competencies for AOTA Board Certification in Mental Health. She was the 2011 recipient of Occupational Therapy Association of California's Annual Practice Award in acknowledgment of her long-standing commitment to advocating for the role of occupational therapy in mental health

Ellie Fossey, PhD, MSc, DipCOT (UK) has conducted occupational therapy research and taught in occupational therapy undergraduate and postgraduate programs at La Trobe University in Melbourne for over 20 years, as well as in Singapore, and previous positions in South Australia and Coventry, England. Ellie is a member of La Trobe University's Living with Disability Research Centre and an Honorary Fellow in the Department of Psychiatry, The University of Melbourne. Her research and teaching focus on frameworks for understanding people's everyday lives and occupations, the ways in which these may be affected by health conditions and changing life circumstances, and on occupation-focused practices. Ellie's research has predominantly attended to time use, education, and work-related issues faced by people whose lives are disrupted by mental health issues. She is widely published in occupational therapy, disability, and mental health journals and has particular interests in using qualitative and collaborative approaches to research within these fields.

Contributing Authors

Lynn Cockburn, PhD, MEd, MSPH, OT Reg (Ont), OT(C) (Chapter 2)
Assistant Professor
Department of Occupational Science and Occupational Therapy
International Centre for Disability and Rehabilitation
University of Toronto
Toronto, Ontario, Canada

Larry Davidson, PhD (Chapter 5)
Professor of Psychology
Program for Recovery and Community Health
Department of Psychiatry
Yale University, School of Medicine
New Haven, Connecticut

Rebecca Gewurtz, PhD, OT Reg (Ont) (Chapter 16)
Assistant Professor, Occupational Therapy
School of Rehabilitation Science
McMaster University
Hamilton, Ontario Canada

Erin McIntyre, OTD (Chapters 3, 13, 15)
Senior Occupational Therapist
South London and Maudsley NHS Foundation Trust
London, United Kingdom

Patricia Rigby, PhD, OT Reg (Ont) (Chapter 7)
Associate Professor
Department of Occupational Science and Occupational Therapy
Rehabilitation Sciences Institute
University of Toronto
Toronto, Ontario, Canada

Introduction

Welcome to the fourth edition of Bruce & Borg's text on psychosocial occupation-based practice. We hope that you will find that this work, like the previous versions, presents models and practice approaches that are useful in enabling occupational therapists to address psychosocial concerns relevant to human occupation. In this edition, we maintained many features of previous versions, but you will also find many important differences.

This book is largely edited and written by four occupational therapists who are located in different countries. The decision to expand the editorial and authorship base was purposeful and reflects our effort to offer a broader (although by no means comprehensive) range of international applications of knowledge and practice developments in the psychosocial arena. In addition, the text has been developed with complementary instructional materials to support teachers in educational settings.

Similar to earlier versions, the book examines psychosocial models of practice and their applications across a wide range of practice areas in occupational therapy, and not only to practice focused on the needs of people living with identified mental illnesses. That said, in some chapters, efforts are made to highlight the relevance of specific models to practice with people with mental illnesses, particularly where the issues experienced by this group have historically been poorly addressed.

Many of the seminal psychosocial practice models featured in earlier versions of the text are offered and updated; however, there are several notable differences. We have organized models and practice approaches according to the level at which they intervene to create change: occupation, person, environment, and transdisciplinary. The occupational models or approaches that are presented in this text have, as their central domain of concern, a focus on "what people do" in their daily lives. We explore the elements of these models that are relevant to and inform psychosocial occupational therapy practice. A second group of models reflect those that intervene at the level of the person. That is they understand strengths and problems in occupation as evolving largely from features or qualities of the individual, and the therapeutic processes suggested are directed to changing or building upon these features. These person-level models have largely been the focus of previous versions of this text. A third group of models and approaches focus on the psychosocial context and environment to elicit and enable a positive change in occupation. In some cases, these environmental models fall outside narrow definitions of "clinical" practice, to encourage occupational therapists to engage in population level practices. Finally, we offer a small group of models of practice that we label as transdisciplinary. Transdisciplinary models provide ways to develop conceptualizations of psychosocial practice issues, practice language, and approaches that are shared across disciplinary boundaries.

Psychosocial health is a fundamental element of all human health and well-being, and we know that the occupational lives of people served by occupational therapists both influence and are influenced by psychological, emotional, and social factors. Occupational therapists practicing in contemporary health and social sectors require the knowledge, attitudes, and skills to identify and address these psychosocial factors. We hope that the information, resources, and practice examples offered in this book will contribute to this competency base.

Introduction to Psychosocial Occupational Therapy

This book was written for occupational therapy students and practitioners, as well as other health professionals who want to advance their knowledge of psychosocial factors related to occupations. It explores the psychological, emotional, and social experiences of humans carried out in context and their connections to occupational engagement and well-being. An understanding of the psychoemotional determinants of occupation enables the development and implementation of effective occupational therapy interventions and the construction of environments and opportunities that promote the expression of strengths and growth, both of which are core to the mission of occupational therapy practice. Section I of this book (Chapters 1 and 2) introduces the core concepts, values, and philosophy that form the basis of this work and provides a historical trajectory of occupational therapy.

Chapter 1 examines what is meant by the term *psychosocial* and sets out the multileveled approach used in this text—it moves beyond the individual to include physical, social, political, and institutional environments. The chapter sets out a framework that is carried throughout the text, which enables an occupational lens to be applied to the study of psychosocial practice. At the core of the framework is occupation, the central domain of the profession. The concept of occupation as we use it has both performance and experience components to it, in recognition not only of the actions and behaviors necessary to human occupation, but also of the rich and subjective experiences that accompany them. Motivation and meaning are given high importance because these factors provide an understanding of why and how people engage in occupations, as well as what occupations satisfy their needs. Within this framework, human occupation influences and is influenced by the context within which it occurs, so environments and opportunities play an important part of the discussions that follow. Family relationships, policy contexts, organizational cultures, access to resources, and personal life experiences are all recognized as important influences on the psychological, emotional, and social elements of occupation. In addition, the chapter highlights the important role that occupational therapists and others can play in creating the opportunity for participation in occupations; participation that will contribute to health and well-being.

Chapter 2 provides a picture of how psychosocial practice in occupational therapy has developed over the years, to fully appreciate how we have come to hold our current beliefs and practices, as well as how the relationship between health and occupation evolved. The tensions that have been faced in psychosocial occupational therapy theory and practice, and the directions that have been pursued as a result, reveal a great deal about the centrality of occupation. The chapter demonstrates how the application of this value to the psychological, emotional, and social health of people has developed into the area of practice addressed by this book, psychosocial occupational therapy. The historical perspective also helps us appreciate how deeply ingrained occupation is as an essential core of all occupational therapy practice. The chapter not only helps us reflect back on our roots and our development, it also inspires us to look forward as a profession. It sets the tone for subsequent discussions in this text that examine emerging arenas and promising practices that the field may wish to take up, discuss, and evaluate.

Together, the chapters in this section pave the way for the reader to appreciate the psychological, emotional, and social dimensions of occupation, how they developed, and how they may be understood and applied in current and future psychosocial practice.

Defining Psychosocial Practice in Occupational Therapy

Terry Krupa, PhD, OT Reg (Ont), FCAOT

Individuals are referred to occupational therapy when they have experienced a disruption in their ability to take part in necessary and valued occupations. This disruption often elicits emotional and psychological responses, including denial, anger, fear, hopelessness, resistance to treatment, loneliness, sadness, grief, anxiety, and other responses. These issues transcend a specific diagnosis or practice setting and may not be the primary reason for the referral but must be understood and addressed if client-centered, meaningful, occupation-based outcomes are to be developed and met. Whether the individual is a teen with a bipolar disorder, a child with cerebral palsy, an adult with a spinal cord injury, or an elder with arthritis, psychosocial factors must be considered. (American Occupational Therapy. Association, 2004, p. 670)

OBJECTIVES

The objectives of this chapter are as follows:

» Define *psychosocial* in occupational therapy theory and practice.

» Discuss the relationship between psychosocial and mental health practice.

» Distinguish between mental health and mental illness.

» Introduce a framework for psychosocial occupational therapy practice.

» Consider a life-span perspective for psychosocial factors.

Krupa, T., Kirsh, B., Pitts, D., & Fossey, E. *Bruce & Borg's
Psychosocial Frames of Reference: Theories, Models, and Approaches for
Occupation-Based Practice, Fourth Edition* (pp 3-16).
© 2016 SLACK Incorporated.

DEFINING PSYCHOSOCIAL OCCUPATIONAL THERAPY PRACTICE

Occupational therapists are concerned with human occupation; it is the profession's central domain of concern. The most recent edition of *Willard & Spackman's Occupational Therapy* (Boyt Schell, Gillen, & Scaffa 2014), defines occupation as

> ...the things that people do that occupy their time and attention; meaningful, purposeful activity; the personal activities that individuals choose or need to engage in and the ways in which each individual actually experiences them. (p. 1237)

This definition captures the complexity of occupation, suggesting that occupation has both performance and experience elements, and that humans engage in occupations within broader social contexts. With occupation as its core domain, contemporary occupational therapy practice has at least three widely recognized foci, which follow:

1. Enabling successful and satisfying engagement in meaningful occupations

2. Promoting health through occupation

3. Enabling an occupationally just society, so that all people can maximize their potential through occupation (Townsend & Polatajko, 2007)

Conceptual models in occupational therapy capture how these outcomes result from a complex interplay of factors. In this book, we hope to advance the reader's knowledge and understanding of psychosocial factors related to occupation and occupational therapy interventions. The concept of psychosocial in this book refers to human psychological, emotional, and social function and experience that occurs within daily occupations carried out in context. These psychological, emotional, and social factors are typically thought of as person-level factors; those that are internal to the individual. Although the idea that psychological and emotional factors are internal factors may be fairly obvious, it may be less clear how social factors are internal. Yet, the beliefs, values, attitudes, morals, standards, etc. that humans hold are internalized factors underlying human occupation, occurring through a process of socialization. In this way, they are highly influenced by individual variations, expressions, modifications, and adjustments.

The psychological, emotional, and social factors underlying human occupation are influenced by occupations and by the environmental contexts within which occupations occur. It is in this regard that we can speak of occupations that are psychologically demanding and socially complex, and of environmental conditions that enable or challenge psychological, emotional, and social capacities and well-being. In this book, we hope to show that these psychosocial factors are integrally linked to occupations and the environments within which occupation occurs. We advocate for a practice that is directed to creating conditions and contexts that support psychological, emotional, and social health and well-being, and enable successful and satisfying engagement in occupation.

COMPARING PSYCHOSOCIAL WELL-BEING AND MENTAL HEALTH

Psychosocial well-being is often considered synonymous with mental health and the terms are frequently used interchangeably. That said, the link between psychosocial well-being and mental health warrants further consideration.

The definitions of mental health are as follows:

- ...a state of well-being in which the individual realizes his or her own potential, can cope with the normal stresses of life, can work productively and fruitfully, and is able to make a contribution to her or his own community (World Health Organization [WHO], 2001)

- ...a state of successful performance of mental functioning resulting in productive activities, fulfilling relationships with other people and the ability to adapt to change and cope with adversity (United States Department of Health and Human Services, 2000)

- ...the capacity of the individual, the group, and the environment to interact with one another in ways that promote subjective well-being, the optimal development and use of mental abilities (cognitive, affective and relational), the achievement of individual and collective goals consistent with justice, and the attainment and preservation of conditions of fundamental equality (Health and Welfare Canada, 1988, pp. 7–8)

These definitions combine several related but distinct elements of mental health. On one hand, the definitions imply that, at its core, mental health includes engagement in activities that are personally and socially rewarding, effective, and constructive. In this way, the definitions of mental health are closely aligned with core values and assumptions of occupational therapy: engagement in meaningful occupation is a determining factor in health (including mental health) and well-being.

The second element of these definitions refers to particular psychosocial features of human function as central to mental health. The definitions suggest that the "mental" in mental health includes psychological, emotional, and social functions. They also suggest that the process of achieving health through engagement in daily activities requires a personal response that applies psychological, emotional, and social capacities to meet demands, challenges, and even hardships.

Finally, one of the definitions of mental health, from Health and Welfare Canada, explicitly defines the concept as both an individual and social phenomenon. This definition suggests that social and environmental conditions create the context for both positive societal engagement and personal experiences of flourishing and well-being. Real world examples where such conditions are compromised appear daily in global news reports. They include, for example, poor mental health associated with high levels of unemployment, economic decline, human rights violations, and natural disasters. Real world examples of opportunities and contexts that promote positive human occupation, mental health, and well-being are also common and include the sense of freedom that individuals experience in countries that respect and promote diverse religions, cultures, and sexual orientations; and the well-being of workers employed in organizations that have policies to promote work-life balance.

For the purposes of this book, because there are so many points of convergence between these ideas, we embrace the link between psychosocial and mental health practice, and we will use the terms interchangeably. We go beyond the person-level to consider how occupational and environmental level conditions are integral to psychosocial health, well-being, and potential.

Indeed, a core value guiding this text is that enabling healthy occupation of individuals by creating and nurturing real opportunities for the expression and growth of human strengths and capacities is infinitely more valuable than treating, in isolation, perceived psychological, emotional, and social weaknesses of individuals.

DISTINGUISHING BETWEEN MENTAL HEALTH AND MENTAL ILLNESS

In addition to understanding the concepts and terms *psychosocial* and *mental health*, it is important to distinguish between mental health and mental illness. Problems in mental health do not necessarily equate with mental illness. Variations and deviations in mental health are a central experience of the human condition and of course these variations will be expressed in the domain of occupation. Mental illness, or disorder, on the other hand, is specifically defined as a health condition that can be diagnosed by specific health professionals, such as physicians and psychologists. Like all illnesses, these health professionals use recognized and standardized classifications to identify and define mental illness. The *Diagnostic and Statistical Manual of Mental Disorders* is perhaps the most widely used clinical diagnostic tool, with version 5 the most recent revision of the manual (American Psychiatric Association, 2013). The *International Classification of Diseases*, published by WHO (2013), has also been adopted by many countries.

Mental illness diagnoses are determined according to symptom and impairment patterns (based largely on self-report and observable behaviors) that are psychological, emotional, and social in nature, but consideration is also given to the presence of disability and the duration of functional issues. There is therefore an effort to distinguish between everyday variations in human experience and illness. For example, it is not uncommon for people to say that they feel down, defeated, or even depressed. We recognize this as a fairly typical human experience, even while we might acknowledge that a tendency toward pessimism and feeling blue can be fairly stable individual qualities. However, these feelings of depression can only be identified as a mental illness if there is evidence of a set of factors (outlined in detail within the *Diagnostic Statistical Manual of Mental Disorders* and *International Classification of Diseases* classification systems): sustained depressed mood, weight loss/gain, sleep disturbances, extreme feelings of worthlessness, etc. Like all illnesses, mental illnesses are treated by a range of medical, rehabilitation, and support interventions and approaches.

It is important to note that individuals can be diagnosed with a mental illness and still enjoy positive mental health. It is not unusual, for example, for people to experience mental illness as episodic, with significant periods during which symptoms do not interfere or cause distress. Even people who experience persistent symptoms of mental illness may come to manage these while enjoying many elements of a fulfilling and healthy lifestyle. It is likely that in our daily lives we meet (often unknowingly) people with diagnosed mental illness who are enjoying the benefits of participating in productive and social activities, contributing to their communities, coping with daily demands and adversities, and dreaming about the potential of future occupational opportunities. Our growing access to personal accounts of people living with mental illness provides the opportunity to hear about these stories and transform how we see and think about mental illness, occupations, and occupational justice with respect to occupational opportunities. They are reminders that satisfying occupations are essential to health and well-being for all people, including those living with mental illnesses.

Many countries are currently increasing the attention paid to mental health and mental illness among their citizens. There are many reasons for this, but a few prevalent reasons are presented below:

- There is a growing recognition that the rates of mortality associated with problems of mental health and mental illness are unacceptably high. Suicide rates are considered a public health issue worldwide (Nock, Borges, & Ono, 2012) and the rates of suicide and suicide attempts among young people are particularly concerning (Kokkevi, Rotsika, Arapaki, & Richardson, 2012). There is evidence that problems of mental health and mental illness are experienced by a significant percentage of people, either directly, or in the context of their important social relationships (United States Centers for Disease Control and Prevention, 2011).

- In countries where market economies have become increasingly knowledge-based (as opposed to focused on manufacturing), problems of mental health appear to be particularly prevalent, likely related to the considerable pressures placed on mental functioning. Simply put, these high mental (i.e., cognitive, psychological, affective, and relational) demands can lead to mental injury, just as heavy and poorly protected physical labor can lead to physical injury (Dewa, Lesage, Goering, & Caveen, 2004).

- Mental disorders are a major contributor to the burden of disease experienced by children and youth with mental illness. The mental health of young people is particularly worrisome given the importance of these early years in laying a foundation for adult autonomy, achievement, well-being, and pro-social community participation (Patel, Flisher, Hetrick, & McGorry, 2007).

- The social and economic costs associated with disabilities connected to mental illness are now recognized as very high, accounting for a significant and rising percentage of disability-adjusted life years (defined as the sum of years of life lost [YLLs] and years lived with disability [Murray et al., 2012]). Mental health–related issues now account for over 30% of short- and long-term workplace disability claims (Dewa et al., 2004).

- The stigma associated with mental health problems and mental illness has received wide recognition as a factor that contributes to the unwillingness of people to seek help or to disclose their health issues, even where disclosure might bring them support and legally sanctioned accommodations. This stigma goes beyond personal attitudes of individuals; it is embedded in the fabric of societal structures. For example, the inclination toward sensationalism with the media results in representations of social problems associated with mental illness, far beyond their actual impact (Whitley & Berry, 2013). Likewise, legislation and policies have traditionally been poorly designed or implemented to protect people with problems of mental health or mental illness from discrimination (Corrigan, Markowitz, & Watson, 2004).

The increased interest in addressing the mental health of citizens has taken many forms in response to the complex, endemic and entrenched nature of the problem. Examples of these efforts are as follows:

- Increased attention to international conventions that protect the right of people with disabilities, including those with poor mental health or mental illness, to participate in meaningful work and leisure and respectful, equitable social interactions (see, for example, United Nations, 2006)

- The development and implementation of national mental health strategies; all G8 countries now have mental health strategies

- The development of workplace guidelines and standards for psychological safety (Mental Health Commission of Canada, 2013); still in its infancy, these standards have yet to be widely disseminated and implemented.

- The development of online professional development resources to advance knowledge and skills related to evidence-based service delivery for people who experience problems of mental health (see for example, www.mhpod.gov.au).

- The development of a range of focused anti-stigma strategies, including powerful media promotions; messages from respected and high profile advocates; advocacy organizations fueled by the passions and energies of people with lived experience; and targeted education initiatives that increase awareness and understanding and promote and sustain grass-root change. For example, the Time to Change initiative in the UK (www.time-to-change.org.uk/) and the Like Minds Like Mine initiative in New Zealand (www.likeminds.org.nz/) are national and publicly funded campaigns to reduce stigma and discrimination related to mental health and mental illness.

Another focus has been to increase awareness of mental health by increasing the mental health literacy of the public. Mental health literacy can be defined as "the knowledge and skills that enable people to access, understand and apply information for mental health" (Canadian Alliance on Mental Illness and Mental Health, 2012). Literacy activities can be directed to the general public with a view to improving understanding and awareness and to create the means for shared discussion and dialogue. Mental health literacy, similar to general health promotion and public health literacy, places more of an emphasis on empowerment for health (Jorm, 2011). Literacy activities can also be directed to people who experience mental illness and problems of mental health, with the goal of empowering them to understand and exercise their rights and responsibilities in important social roles. The overall goal is to break down the "us and them" thinking that underlies stigma and discrimination (including the disposition toward self-stigma or shame) so that dialogue about mental health can reflect an attitude of "it's about us—all of us."

Unfortunately, the context within which occupational therapists practice is often structured in such a way that these mental health, or psychosocial elements, of well-being can be poorly addressed. For example, occupational therapists who largely (but not exclusively) practice within health service systems work in settings that are highly specialized or narrowly focused. So, for example, occupational therapists who work in settings focused primarily on health conditions considered physical in nature, may find themselves restricted in their capacity to address (or even evaluate) psychosocial factors integrally associated with occupation. This is troublesome given that many of the most common health conditions that occupational therapists encounter (i.e., cardiac conditions, stroke, Parkinson's disease, chronic back pain) have all been linked to significant problems in psychological, emotional, and social health and well-being. Of course, the situation is similar for occupational therapists practicing within the mental health or behavioral health system. They may find themselves restricted in their ability to address occupational concerns related to physical function and well-being.

KEY DEVELOPERS

While defining occupation as a means to enable mental health and well-being is a core purpose of this book, readers are reminded that this has been a focus of occupational therapy theory and practice since its inception. In this regard, the information presented in this text should be considered complementary to seminal texts and scholarship on this topic.

Within occupational therapy, much of the knowledge base related to psychosocial practice has emerged within the context of mental health practice because occupational therapists have a long history of working within the mental health system. Specific evolutionary points and key leaders are outlined in detail in Chapter 2, and key developers of the field are identified in each of the chapters, linked to particular frames of reference, models, and practice approaches.

The profession has always looked to knowledge and scholarship beyond its own boundaries to inform its understanding of occupation. In the realm of psychosocial practice this has included knowledge advanced in the fields of psychology, education, sociology, anthropology, human ecology, and even philosophy. Psychology in particular provides foundational knowledge for understanding the distinct person-level, psychological, emotional, and social dimensions that underlie human occupation. Among the range of theories and frameworks available in psychology, one that is akin to the concerns of this book is the framework of positive psychology (Duckworth, Steen, & Seligman, 2005; Keyes & Lopez, 2005). Positive psychology focuses on the personal dimensions of psychological and social well-being that lead to continual growth and development, productivity, and fulfilling social relations and overall flourishing as opposed to states of languishing or floundering (Keyes, 2002, 2005). Positive psychology and the field of psychology generally have enhanced our understanding of the nature and measurement of personal dimensions of mental health and well-being and of the processes of healing in these realms.

Similarly, human ecology, which focuses on the interactions of humans with their environments, has been important to the profession's understanding of the occupation and environmental conditions and processes that enable human occupation. The work of Bronfenbrenner (1977) for example, has been instrumental in understanding how human potentials are realized within broader environmental structures. Contemporary applications of ecological perspectives provide frameworks for the understanding of multiple intersections between the individual and the social environment in the creation of health and well-being (see for example, Krieger, 2001, or Levins & Lopez, 1999). These ecosocial frameworks are complicated, but highly relevant to occupational therapy practice in their effort to construct holistic and dynamic views of health and well-being.

A FRAMEWORK FOR THE PSYCHOSOCIAL ELEMENTS OF OCCUPATION

A specific goal of this text was to advance the development of a framework for the psychosocial elements of occupation that would facilitate understanding, discussion, and ultimately be applied in practice. This framework is not meant to replace the conceptual models of occupation that are currently available, but rather, the intent is to complement these with a theoretical, but practical, representation of a broad range of psychosocial factors underlying occupation.

SETTING THE STAGE: AN OCCUPATIONAL ANALYSIS FOCUSING ON PSYCHOSOCIAL ELEMENTS

Introducing the framework using an occupational analysis exercise serves two purposes. First, theoretical frameworks, no matter how well constructed, run the risk of drawing attention away from the central domain of focus to a reductionist view of the distinct components of the framework. Introducing the framework by means of an occupational analysis can help to link the concepts to practical applications of human occupation by interpreting and evaluating psychosocial elements in relation to what people need to do, want to do, and are expected to do. Second, the exercise provides the opportunity to consider the

---

Box 1-1. Vignette: Sarah

Sarah is attending a party held by a friend from high school. She really wants to attend the party and has invested a fair bit of energy in dressing and grooming herself. She knows that her friend has invited a group known as the popular clique at school. They have never been friendly with Sarah, and in fact, she experiences the group as "putting her down." Sarah arrives at the party and is greeted warmly by many friends. When she passes the clique, they appear to look her way then they carry on talking and laughing among themselves. Sarah starts to think about going home.

---

framework in relation to occupations that engage a range of psychological, emotional and social features.

> Imagine this scenario, one that is likely familiar: You have received an invitation to a party. The party starts at 8 p.m. on Saturday. It is now Saturday at 6:30 p.m. and you are just getting ready. How do you decide what to wear? What happens if you get this wrong?

Perhaps you will start by considering some basic but important information. You might consider the weather and try and imagine the environmental conditions for the party (Will the party be inside/outside; will there be blasting air conditioning?). Maybe you will look for evidence of a particular party theme that can help you decide (Ah, it's a formal/semi-formal, pool party, or maybe a costume party?). You might use your familiarity with the hosts and guests to make a best estimate about dress. Perhaps there are gender-based considerations related to this task (Will the other men be wearing tuxedos or suits?). What you wear might be dictated on some level by your personal beliefs and values and your connections to your family's cultural background. Maybe you want to blend these family cultural considerations with the norms of this other social group. If you are feeling emotionally low, you might be disposed to wear something somber that matches your mood, just as if you are feeling bright and happy you might feel that you might be inclined to wear bright colors and clothing with a bit of flair. You might try on a few items of clothing with a view to evaluating how they show particular features of your body (These slacks hide my flaws/accentuate my good features). Maybe you will consider the meaning that the party holds for you (I'm looking forward to the chance to relax and let loose with some good friends), or if there is a particular outcome you would like to see transpire (i.e., attracting the attention of a particular person or networking for a potential job).

What happens if you get it wrong and your clothing decisions are notably out of sync with the context? Maybe you can imagine feeling some discomfort and (depending on how wrong) some level of distress. Maybe it will affect your mood at the party, or leave you a little more reserved or cautious in conversations with others, or about attending such functions in the future. Perhaps you will stay with

the people who know you best for a source of support and a sense of acceptance. Perhaps you will draw on your sense of humor to get you through, or chalk this event up as a good story to tell at future social events.

The example provides a fairly simple, everyday occupation—getting dressed for a social gathering—that, upon analysis presents a complex set of psychological, emotional, and social demands and responses—self-concept, mood, self-confidence, body image, autonomy, meaning, sense of belonging, and social interpretations. The difficulties encountered engender examples of coping, perhaps with a view to getting through the event, and perhaps even overcoming the situation to experience some measure of enjoyment.

For most of us, the example is evaluated as fairly mundane and harmless. Yet for people who, for a range of reasons, experience disruptions in their psychological, emotional, and social capacities, the scenario can be potentially threatening to their personal sense of well-being and mental health. Consider the vignettes of Sarah, Robert, and Ian in Boxes 1-1, 1-2, and 1-3.

Sarah is highly invested in the party and it appears to hold great meaning in relation to her sense of desired identity. The vignette suggests that her decisions are highly influenced by her perception of the standards held by her peers, a threatening situation in that her sense of belonging in the situation is shaky. While the social situation may actually be less than welcoming and accepting, in the end, this combination of factors contributes to her negative interpretation of the social exchange, and her inability to respond in a positive social manner. Sarah is likely a teenager or young adult, a developmental period during which the capacity to negotiate issues of autonomy, social acceptance, personal identity, and coping abilities in the face of adversity can be fragile and likely to affect her experience of her occupations.

Robert's party presents him with several difficult psychological, emotional, and social issues to negotiate. The party offers a potential opportunity to reclaim the identity of family member if he can navigate a complicated social situation where he perceives that others associate his primary identity with mental illness. The opportunity is an important one, in that in his day-to-day life he may have few naturally occurring opportunities to engage with

---

BOX 1-2. VIGNETTE: ROBERT

Robert, a 45-year-old man, has been invited to his brother's wedding. Robert has been estranged from his family for several years. He lives alone in a public housing unit and is supported by a disability pension. He experiences his family relationship as stressful. He believes he failed his family and their expectations of him when he was diagnosed with schizophrenia. He thinks that most people who attend the wedding will know that he has a mental illness and has been hospitalized. He's anxious about the wedding. He desperately wants to "fit in." He has been working with his occupational therapist for several months to plan for the event. The day before the wedding, he makes his way to the emergency department of a local hospital complaining of symptoms of his mental illness.

BOX 1-3. VIGNETTE: IAN

Ian is preparing to attend his first party since his motorcycle accident 7 months ago that resulted in the loss of his right arm above the elbow. The party is a barbecue/pool party that some of his friends are hosting to celebrate his 23rd birthday. Lately, Ian has been irritable around his parents and girlfriend, at times bordering on verbally abusive. He has been unwilling to plan for this party with any of these people who have been so important to him.

---

people in society's major integrating activities. Given his long history of paranoid symptoms, he is at risk of having his interpretation of his outsider status invalidated by others (including service providers meant to provide him with support), even though his interpretations may be quite accurate. Reclaiming his identity and finding a measure of belonging and acceptance in the party context means fitting in, and his clothing and overall physical demeanor are an integral part of this. However, Robert is poor, and he finds the task of saving and shopping for clothing both anxiety provoking and depressing. The increase in his symptoms is real, but they also present a way to bow out of attending. In the end, his mental health is both preserved (his anxiety and other symptoms decrease) and compromised (a missed opportunity to show caring toward significant others, to realize respect and acceptance in spite of differences, to build identity, and to hope for the possibility of more opportunities).

Ian's party is meant to be a public celebration for him; a celebration marking several important events (his birthday, the fact that he lived through a serious accident, a recognition of his recovery, and a welcome back to his social network). Yet the event appears to be holding alternate, less positive and conflicted meanings for him. Perhaps it aggravates his concerns related to his body image (made worse by the fact that it is a pool party requiring some form of sparse beachwear?) and represents the first social event where he must negotiate his injuries and disabilities in public. While the party is a demonstration of love and respect by others, it may rouse his own poorly reconciled issues related to self-acceptance and identity. For example, the loss of a limb in the accident may have compromised

his sense of personal strength, beauty, and independence. Unable to name, express, and deal with these issues, he may be at risk for negative emotional displays toward the people he loves. Interestingly, if he does attend the party, it presents an important opportunity to cope, adjust, and generally move ahead.

A FRAMEWORK OF PSYCHOSOCIAL FACTORS

The framework is represented visually in Figure 1-1.

The Core Domain: Occupation as Performance and Experience

At the center of the framework is occupation, the core domain of the profession. Positive human occupation is represented by two interactions: performance and experience. The focus on occupation as performance has been somewhat of a trademark of the profession. Performance suggests a focus on observed behaviors in the tasks and activities that comprise human occupation, and on function evaluated in relation to particular standards considered to be desirable, normative, or necessary. Psychological, emotional, and social functions underlying human behavior are essential elements of performance in occupation.

Occupational performance considered alone compromises the ability to attend directly to the rich lived and subjective experience of occupation. The idea of experience

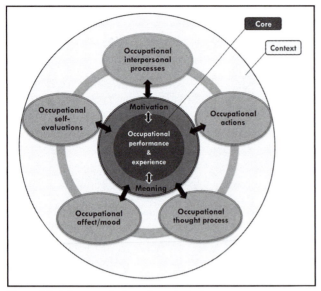

Figure 1-1. A framework of psychosocial factors.

in occupation has received some attention in occupational therapy, but generally explanations of the concept have been largely relegated to notions of personal satisfaction and the experience of meaning and spirituality, all necessary but insufficient as full descriptions of experience. Understandings of fundamental psychological, emotional, and social dimensions of occupation provide the opportunity for a fuller definition of experience, including such elements as self-agency, the sense of belonging and contributing, personal integrity, pleasure, investment, and overall a sense of well-being. These subjective experiences can result in developing and sustaining dispositions toward futures characterized by further occupational engagement and active participation, and ultimately adaptation and growth.

The concept of *flow*, which emerged in the psychology literature in the 1980s, is highly relevant to the experience of occupation. Csikszentmihalyi (1993) described flow as the experience of being totally involved in an activity to the point where there is an altered sense of time and loss of self-consciousness, a state of mind that is associated with strength and satisfaction. Occupational therapists have highlighted the importance of creating occupational opportunities and conditions that would be likely to lead to experiences of flow (Emerson, 1998; Jonsson & Persson, 2006; Rebeiro-Gruhl & Polgar, 1999).

Both performance and experience are highlighted in our occupational analysis exercise. In each of our vignettes, dressing for the party activates a series of performance-related concerns and the potential for an array of experiences that have the potential to affect future occupational engagement.

THE CONTEXT OF OCCUPATION

In this model, human occupation is embedded within a context. Blesedell Crepeau and colleagues (2014) highlight that a distinguishing feature of occupational therapy is its perspective that any individual's occupations must be understood within his or her specific context. The specific context of any occupation will, to some extent, establish standards and govern the processes of doing while positioning these within local and broad social settings and relations. Social standards governing relations will vary in their formality, but almost always provide opportunity for personal expression. Our example of dressing for a party sets the occupation in a specific context where details, if not known, can be pursued or reasoned and there is considerable room for personal preferences and decisions.

Identifying the occupational context is not always a given for occupational therapy. Often the focus is on creating occupational opportunities that, at present, do not exist. In this case, the therapist becomes engaged in "imagining" the specific details of occupational opportunities that match the performance and experience wants and needs of any individual, or even a group of individuals. For example, the occupational therapist working with Robert might consider with Robert, "What other occupational opportunities might be developed, to reclaim the role of family member? How might these opportunities be created to match both performance capacities and resources, and the need for belonging, respect, and contributing,?" Yet, imagining potential opportunities still requires being attuned to social settings and relations and their implications for the individual.

THE FOUNDATION OF OCCUPATIONAL ENGAGEMENT: MOTIVATION AND MEANING

In this framework, motivation and meaning are ascribed the highest order of importance in determining engagement in occupations, and the performance and experiences that result. Together, motivation and meaning provide an overarching understanding of why individuals engage in occupations, what occupations they engage in, and how they go about this involvement.

Motivation is a commonly used term typically referring to the impetus for human behaviors. Motivation is actually an exceptionally complicated construct that belies our usage of the term in daily conversation. In this book, we borrow Wlodkowski's (1999) definition of motivation as purposeful, "…a natural human process for directing energy to accomplish a goal" (p. 2). Consideration of motivation leads us to attend to how energy is directed toward goals. Wlodkowski, for example, describes motivated behavior patterns as being aroused, having direction, demonstrating a preference, and persisting. In this regard, we might be concerned about motivation if an individual shows a lack of drive or interest for occupations, if occupational patterns appear haphazard or lacking in consistency, or if there is a pattern of not following through with plans or goals.

Meaning in occupation is closely connected to motivation in that it relates to the purpose that individuals give to occupations, but it extends this idea by providing some shape and definition to these meanings. The meanings associated with occupation are those that are experienced by the individual as having significance. Descriptions of meanings typically include language such as *important* and *valued*. Although the meanings ascribed to occupation are highly individual, they are not completely idiosyncratic. Indeed, commonalities in meaning can be defined, and from an occupational therapy perspective this means that practice that is sensitive to personal meaning has an available and ordered knowledge base. Hasselkus (2002) stresses that although meaning can only be understood at the level of the person, meanings ascribed to occupation are socially created and organized. She cites Berman (1993), who suggests that meaning reflects the interplay between two forces, "our search for uniqueness and self-hood with our search for community and belonging" (p. 3). This dynamic interplay extends to the occupational therapist's reasoning processes in psychosocial practice.

Taken together, motivation and meaning are conceptualized as foundational drivers for occupation. They also mediate the outcomes associated with occupation. They increase the likelihood that engagement in occupations will lead to both improvements in performance and enhance the individual's experience of the occupation. In this way actions directed to human occupation evolve from motivations and meaning, and they, in turn, influence motivation and meaning.

The vignettes suggest meanings that are remarkably similar. While a party, by definition, is a social activity, and can be expected to hold meanings associated with connecting with others, for these three people in our vignettes, the party is rife with concerns about acceptance (both of the self and by others) and belonging. It is both the promise of this meaning and the potential for failure in achieving these meanings that transfers emotion to the event and its associated activities.

PSYCHOLOGICAL, EMOTIONAL, AND SOCIAL ELEMENTS OF OCCUPATION

Although a broad range of specific psychological, emotional, and social functions that underlie human functioning have been defined, they have not been subject to much systematic development in relation to human occupation. In the profession's broad models of occupation, these discrete functions tend to be recognized as individual performance components, but are generally dealt with in a more superficial way. So, for example, in the Canadian Model of Occupational Performance and Engagement (Townsend & Polatajko, 2007), the Ecology of Human Performance model (Dunn, McClain, Brown & Youngstrom, 2003), and the Person-Environment-Occupational Performance model (Baum & Christiensen, 2005), they are positioned within the person-level affective components and psychosocial skills.

So far in this chapter, a range of specific psychological, emotional, and social elements of occupation have been identified. The framework provides organization of these discrete functions within specific dimensions, and links these explicitly to occupation. Although the list of functions described here is fairly comprehensive, it should not be considered complete. Rather, it offers a way to think and talk about these psychosocial elements of human occupation.

Self-Perceptions That Enable and Are Enabled by Occupation

This refers to the range of functions related to human perceptions of the self. The notion of *self-perception* suggests that individuals hold insights, awareness, views, evaluations, and judgements about themselves that contribute to their participation in occupation. These self-perceptions as evaluative can be quite general as suggested by the concept of *self-esteem*, or quite specific, as in the case of *body image*. Similarly, self-efficacy refers to an individual's perceptions of his or her own capacity for achieving specific goals or demands. The concept of *self-compassion* suggests a personal disposition to be kind and forgiving in self-judgements, whereas the concept of *self-identity* suggests a sense of the self as a unique and integrated whole, and *locus of control* implies a sense of the self as having the agency, and the capacity, to be self-determining.

Our vignettes provide evidence of self-evaluations in operation. We can assume, for example, that all three individuals are dealing with issues of fragile self-perceptions that affect their decisions and actions in relation to their party invitations. As mentioned, Sarah's tenuous sense of self-esteem is typical of adolescence, and even more so for adolescent women (Robbins & Trzesniewski, 2005). Ian's self-perception issues appear to have initiated fairly recently, in relation to an accident that resulted in significant losses of the "self" including disturbances in his body image. Robert's self-perceptions appear to have been constructed over time as his personal and social self became more and more tied to the constraints of the identity of mental illness and patient.

At the same time, participation in the activity has the potential to positively bolster their self-perceptions, building a condition for future participation. Theories have been developed to explain sustained investment and engagement based on personal capacities and self-perceptions. For example, activities that pose challenges that use and stretch personal capacities are likely to sustain engagement, whereas those that are perceived as overwhelming are likely to compromise self-perceptions, a sense of personal control, and lead to anxiety and other uncomfortable emotional experiences (Csikszentmihalyi, 1993).

Affect/Mood That Enables and Is Enabled by Occupation

Mood and affect refer to the broad range of human emotions experienced in the context of occupation. They can include emotions typically experienced as pleasurable, such as happiness, satisfaction, love, joy, awe, contentment, or those experienced as unpleasant, such as anxiety, fear, anger, hate, sadness, grief, unhappiness, and discontent. Emotions experienced in the context of occupation are perhaps most closely associated with what Russell and Barchard (2002) refer to as *attributed affect*, or emotion that is tied to an event, person, or thing.

We know that the relationship between human occupation and affect is complicated. It makes intuitive sense to think that positive emotions will be associated with occupations that are ascribed value. Yet unpleasant emotions play an important part in our occupational engagement. Some amount of anxiety, for example, can be the emotional impetus for people to invest attention in their level of involvement. So, in our example, some level of anxiety or worry about the party will likely lead us to spend more time and effort in tending to how we dress and prepare for a party. Too much anxiety, however, can be problematic in that it can lead to feeling overwhelmed, helpless, and vulnerable and ultimately in a compromised position to tackle situations. This is certainly the case suggested by our vignettes.

Grief is another important and complex emotion. Both grief and anxiety are unpleasant but fundamental to psychosocial health. Grief, a response to loss, is an emotional validation of the importance of aspects of one's life. At the same time, grief needs to be reconciled for people to move on, to participate and benefit from their occupations. The study of Ian suggests someone who is grieving the sudden, unanticipated, and permanent loss associated with his physical body.

A body of research is evolving that demonstrates the potential positive impact of participation in a range of activities on mood and affect. These have included, for example, studies of the impact of participation in physical activities (Bossman, Kanning, Koudela-Hamila, Hey, & Ebner-Priemer, 2013), social participation (Murray et al., 2007), arts and cultural activities (Australian Expert Group, 2004), and leisure activities (Pressman et al., 2009).

Thought Processes That Enable and Are Enabled by Occupation

This refers to the content and form of thoughts (the "what and how") and the relationship of these to their participation in occupations. They include, for example, an individual's perceptions and interpretations of situations, the flexibility of these thoughts, their logic, coherence, and reasoning. How we think about people, events, situations, etc. affects our participation. Our interpretations and reasoning around how to dress for the party are examples of thought processes. Sarah is profoundly affected by her thought processes in that she is disposed to interpret the situation as subjecting her to negative valuations by others. Robert's concern that others at the party will know about his mental illness is suspect because his illness is associated with disordered thought processes, even though his interpretation of the situation might be quite valid. In both cases, their behaviors in relation to the activity are highly influenced by their thinking.

The process of engaging in activities can provide the conditions for revising thoughts, distracting from troublesome thought patterns, or refining the meanings given to particular thoughts. For example, if he attended the party, Robert might receive feedback to suggest that even though others know about his mental illness, he is still largely treated with respect and dignity, and perhaps even that a few people appear genuinely pleased to see him.

Interpersonal Processes That Enable and Are Enabled by Occupation

Interpersonal processes refer to those functions that support human relationships and interactions. They include, for example, receiving and responding to social information, the capacity to understand and appreciate the feelings and needs of others, respecting differences, trusting others, and social enactment behaviors. Each of our vignettes suggests individuals who have the capacity to establish and maintain human relationships, although issues of trust and particular social skills do emerge. Engagement in activities, in turn, creates the conditions to challenge and develop these capacities, and ultimately to experience the multiple benefits associated with connecting with others.

Coping Processes That Enable and Are Enabled by Occupation

Finally, actions that enable and are enabled by occupation refer to the broad range of functions associated with coping. They include, for example, regulating emotions and impulses, adapting to change, responding to frustrations and stresses, monitoring personal responses, etc. Occupation-enabling actions help people to engage in occupations in a successful and satisfying manner, even when internal or external issues or barriers arise. In the party example, a range of potential actions is presented in response to challenges. Our vignettes of Sarah, Robert, and Ian, however, suggest difficulties with coping, demonstrated by avoidance of the situation, an exacerbation of acute mental instability, and problems with emotional regulation. While these difficulties may have few long-term consequences, they do rob each individual of the range of benefits that might be experienced by successfully negotiating the challenges. Participation in the activity provides the opportunity to develop and practice coping and adaptive strategies.

THE CONTEXT OF OCCUPATION

Just as there is a context for specific occupations, people engaging in these occupations operate within a broader context that can enable or interfere with psychological, emotional, and social aspects of human occupation. Access to resources and economic status, family relations and the person's broader social network, sociocultural influences, and life experiences are all examples of important influences. We can expect, for example, that Sarah's ability to act in ways that reflect a healthy sense of self will be infinitely more likely if she has a supportive and affirming family. Robert's situation suggests that his poverty places him at a disadvantage in many social relations. Ian may be in a good position to overcome his issues related to loss and grief if he has access to good role models who will help him to envision possibilities.

Although the framework provides an organizing framework, many psychosocial elements of human occupation reflect multi-dimensional constructs that combine dimensions that are both internal and external to the individual. *Empowerment*, for example, is frequently cited as a powerful psychosocial construct, and in its idealized form suggests people who are marginalized and vulnerable overcoming adversity to find justice. However, definitions of empowerment used in the health and social sectors can vary widely. Some definitions highlight empowerment as located in the individual and reflect a process of developing control and agency, and the sense of having a meaningful voice in society. Other definitions stress that empowerment is essentially a social construct that refers to the objective community conditions that ensure equitable access to resources and ensure meaningful participation (Clark & Krupa, 2002). In these cases, application of the framework depends on the ability to recognize and integrate ideas across the distinct elements of the framework.

DEVELOPMENTAL CONSIDERATIONS

Any understanding of psychosocial dimensions of human occupation would be incomplete without a full consideration of development of these dimensions over the lifespan. Theories of psychological, emotional, and social development help therapists to evaluate the extent to which particular occupational behaviors and experiences are likely or to be expected. Consider the brief examples provided in Box 1-4. The examples focus on one particular occupation-related scenario that requires emotional regulation and behavioral control in response to a frustration. Each of the scenarios will likely trigger a slightly different interpretation. The cases of the youngster and the adolescent might be interpreted as responses that reflect efforts to negotiate the independence that is the hallmark of these periods where emotional maturity is still under development. Perhaps the adolescent who puts a hole in the wall draws a different interpretation; negotiating independence that includes damaging property might be perceived as pushing acceptable limits of behavior. With a 30 year old, we might expect a better controlled response, particularly given the expectation of emotional maturity and role differentiation from his family of origin. Whereas this expectation is perhaps no different for the second 30 year old, the information that he has a brain injury leads to re-evaluating his challenges related to emotional regulation emerging from the injury and the extent to which typical development milestones have been compromised. Finally, the older adult may be understood as experiencing a very high level of despair and frustration in the context of negotiating adjustment to personal decline in aging.

Occupational therapists draw heavily on developmental theories of occupation to understand these kinds of situations. Drawing from developmental theories from the field of psychology, occupational therapists interpret experiences and behaviors related to specific psychological, emotional, and social dimensions of human function. For example, Erikson's psychosocial theory (1959) informs understanding of critical psychosocial tasks associated with specific life stages from birth to death, and Kohlberg's theory of moral development (2008) proposes stages in the

BOX 1-4. BRIEF VIGNETTES OF EMOTIONAL REGULATION

Tommy wants to use the car. He is not allowed. He becomes angry and slams his fist against the wall.

Tommy is 4 years old and is verbally hostile against his parents for not letting him play with his car. He hits the wall with his fist.

Tommy is 17 years old and is verbally hostile toward his parents who will not lend him the family car for an evening.

Tommy is 17 years old and is verbally hostile toward his parents who will not lend him the family car for an evening; he slams his fist through the wall.

Tommy is 30 years old and is verbally hostile toward his parents for refusing to loan him their car for an evening, becomes angry, and slams his fist against the wall.

Tommy is 30 years old and is verbally hostile toward his parents who will not loan him their car for an evening. He becomes angry and slams his fist against the wall. Tommy has a brain injury as a result of a motor vehicle accident.

Tommy is 89 years old. The occupational therapy driving evaluation has suggested that he is not competent to drive. His driving licence has been formally revoked. He becomes angry with and verbally hostile toward his son who has removed his car keys and slams his fist against the wall.

development that see the increasing capacity of internal controls on behavior in relation to social standards.

CONCLUSION

The framework provided in this chapter provides a way of thinking about and organizing the psychosocial elements of occupation. The chapters in this book are closely aligned with the components of the framework and provide additional background information and explanations for particular factors. They also offer an introduction as to how the ideas presented in this framework can be linked to practice. For example, the following chapter in this section demonstrates how the ideas presented in the framework evolved over time. Section II presents two transdisciplinary models influencing psychosocial practice in occupational therapy. Section III in the book presents well-known conceptual models of occupation that have advanced our understanding and practice in the psychosocial arena. Section IV considers specific psychological, emotional and social factors as they present at the level of the "person" and links these to well-known evidence-informed approaches. Finally, Section V of the book offers examples of occupational therapy approaches and interventions to address psychosocial factors at the level of the occupational context and/or broader environment.

LEARNING ACTIVITIES/ DISCUSSION QUESTIONS

1. Select one of the following psychological functions and use scholarly resources to trace its development across the lifespan: self-esteem, body image, or self-identity.

2. Use the scholarly resources available to you to investigate why depression is common among people who experience stroke, Parkinson disease, or chronic pain.

3. Consider one of the following occupations: nursing in an emergency department, police work, enlisted military personnel, taxi driver, or real estate agent. Conduct an occupational analysis of this work, with a focus on psychological, emotional, and social demands.

REFERENCES

American Occupational Therapy Association. (2004). Psychosocial aspects of occupational therapy. *American Journal of Occupational Therapy, 58,* 669-672.

American Psychiatric Association. (2013). *Diagnostic and statistics manual of mental disorders (DSM 5).* Arlington, VA: American Psychiatric Association.

Australian Expert Group. (2004). *Participation in the arts and cultural activity: Stage 2 report. Evidence, Issues and Recommendations.* Canberra, Australia: Statistics Working Group Secretariat.

Baum, C. M., & Christiansen, C. H. (2005). Person-environment-occupational performance model. In C. H. Christiensen & C. M. Baum (Eds.), *Occupational Therapy, Performance, Participation and Well-Being* (pp. 242-267). Thorofare, NJ: SLACK, Incorporated.

Berman, H. J. (1993). The tree and the vine: Existential meaning and Olmstead's personal journal of retirement. *Journal of Aging Studies, 7,* 81-92.

Blesedell Crepeau, E. Boyt Schell, B. A., Gillen, G., & Scaffa, M. E. (2014). Analyzing occupations and activity. In B. A. Boyt Schell, G. Gillen, & M. E. Scaffa (Eds.), *Willard & Spackman's occupational therapy,* 12th Edition (pp. 234-264). Philadelphia: Lippincott, Williams & Wilkins.

Bossman, T., Kanning, M., Koudela-Hamila, S., Hey, S., & Ebner-Priemer, U. (2013). The association between short periods of everyday life activities and affective states: a replication study using ambulatory assessment. *Frontiers in Psychology, 4,* 1-7.

Boyt Schell, B. A., Gillen, G., & Scaffa, M. E. (Eds). (2014). *Willard & Spackman's occupational therapy,* 12th Edition, Philadelphia: Lippincott, Williams & Wilkins.

Bronfenbrenner, U. (1977). Toward an experimental ecology of human development. *American Psychologist, 32,* 513-531.

Canadian Alliance on Mental Illness and Mental Health. (2012). *Mental Health Literacy.* Ottawa: CAMIMH.

Clark, C., & Krupa, T. (2002). Empowerment in community mental health: Giving shape to an elusive ideal. *Psychiatric Rehabilitation Journal, 25*(4), 341-349.

Corrigan, P., Markowitz, F. E., & Watson, A. C. (2004). Structural levels of mental illness stigma and discrimination. *Schizophrenia Bulletin, 30,* 481-491.

Csikszentmihalyi, M. (1993). *The evolving self: A psychology for the third millennium.* New York: HarperCollins.

Dewa, C., Lesage, A., Goering, P., & Caveen, M. (2004). Nature and prevalence of mental illness in the workplace. *Healthcare Papers, 5*(2), 12-25.

Duckworth, A. L., Steen, T. A., & Seligman, M. E. P. (2005). Positive psychology in clinical practice. *Annual Review of Clinical Psychology, 1,* 629-651.

Dunn, W., McClain, L. H., Brown, C., & Youngstrom, M. J. (2003). The ecology of human performance. In E. B. Crepeau, E. S. Cohn, & B. A. B. Schell (Eds.), *Willard & Spackman's occupational therapy,* 10th edition (pp. 223-227). Philadelphia: Lippincott, Williams & Wilkins.

Emerson, H. (1998). Flow and occupation: A review of the literature. *Canadian Journal of Occupational Therapy, 65,* 37-44.

Erikson, E. (1959). *Identity and the life cycle.* New York: W. W. Norton & Co.

Hasselkus, B. R. (2002). *The meaning of everyday occupation.* Thorofare, NJ: SLACK, Incorporated.

Health and Welfare Canada. (1988). *Striking a balance: Mental health for Canadians.* Ottawa: Ministry of Supply and Services.

Jonsson, H., & Persson, D. (2006). Towards an experiential model of occupational balance: An alternative perspective on flow theory analysis. *Journal of Occupational Science, 13*(1), 62-73.

Jorm, A. (2011). Mental health literacy: Empowering the community to take action for better mental health. *American Psychologist,* doi: 10.1037/a0025957.

Keyes, C. L. (2002). The mental health continuum: From languishing to flourishing in life. *Journal of Health and Social Research, 43,* 207-222.

Keyes, C. L. (2005). Mental illness and/or mental health? Investigating axioms of the complete state model of health. *Journal of Consulting and Clinical Psychology, 73*(3), 539-548.

Keyes, C. L., & Lopez, S. J. (2005). Toward a science of mental health: Positive directions in diagnosis and interventions. In C. R. Snyder & S. J. Lopez (Eds.), *Handbook of positive psychology* (pp. 45-59). New York: Oxford University Press.

Kohlberg, L. (2008). The development of children's orientation towards a moral order: I. Sequence in the development of moral thought. *Human Development, 51,* 8-20.

Kokkevi, A., Rotsika, V., Arapaki, A., & Richardson, C. (2012). Adolescents' self-reported suicide attempts, self-harm thoughts and their correlates across 17 European countries. *Journal of Child Psychology and Psychiatry, 53*(4), 381-389.

Krieger, N. (2001). Theories for social epidemiology in the 21st century: An ecosocial perspective. *International Journal of Epidemiology, 30,* 668-677.

Levins, R., & Lopez, C. (1999). Toward an ecosocial view of health. *International Journal of Health Services, 29,* 261-293.

Mental Health Commission of Canada. (2013). *Psychological health and safety in the workplace—Prevention, promotion, and guidance to staged implementation.* Retrieved from http://shop.csa.ca/en/canada/occupational-health-and-safety management.

Murray, C. J., Vos, T., Lozano, R., Naghavi, M., Flaxman, A. D., Michaud, C.,…Shibuya, K. (2012). Disability-adjusted life years (DALYs) for 291 diseases and injuries in 21 regions, 1990–2010: a systematic analysis for the Global Burden of Disease Study 2010. *The Lancet, 380,* 2197-2223.

Murray, G., Judd, F., Jackson, H., Fraser, C., Komiti, A., Pattison, P., Wearing, A., & Robins, G. (2007). Ceremonies of the whole: Does social participation moderate the mood consequences of neuroticism? *Social Psychiatry & Psychiatric Epidemiology, 42,* 173-180.

Nock, M. K., Borges, G., & Ono, Y. (2012). *Suicide: Global perspectives from the WHO World Mental Health Surveys.* New York: Cambridge University Press.

Patel, V., Flisher, A. J., Hetrick, S., & McGorry, P. (2007). Mental health of young people: A global public-health challenge. *The Lancet, 369,* 1302-1313.

Pressman, S. D., Matthews, K. A., Cohen, S., Martire, L. M., Scheier, M., Baum, A., & Schulz, R. (2009). Association of enjoyable leisure activities with psychological and physical well-being. *Psychosomatic Medicine, 71,* 725-732.

Rebeiro-Gruhl, K. L., & Polgar, J. M. (1999). Enabling occupational performance: Optimal experiences in therapy. *Canadian Journal of Occupational Therapy, 66*, 14-22.

Robbins, R. W., & Trzesniewski, K. H. (2005). Self-esteem development across the lifespan. *Current Directions in Psychological Science. 14*(3), 158-162.

Russell, J. A., & Barchard, K. A. (2002). Toward a shared language for emotion. In L. F. Barrett & P. Salovey (Eds.), *The wisdom in feeling: Psychological processes in emotional intelligence* (pp. 363-382). New York: The Guilford Press.

Townsend, E. A., & Polatajko, H. J. (2007). *Enabling occupation II: Advancing an occupational therapy vision for health, well-being & justice through occupation.* Ottawa: Canadian Association of Occupational Therapists.

United Nations. (2006). Convention on the rights of persons with disabilities. Retrieved from www.un.org/disabilities/default.asp?id=150.

United States Centers for Disease Control and Prevention. (2011). *Burden of mental illness.* Retrieved from www.cdc.gov/mentalhealth/basics/burden.htm.

United States Department of Health and Human Services. (2000). *Healthy people 2010: Understanding and improving health.* Washington, DC: Government Printing Office.

Whitley, R., & Berry, S. (2013). Trends in newspaper coverage of mental illness in Canada: 2005–2010. *Canadian Journal of Psychiatry, 58*(2), 107-112.

Wlodkowski, R. (1999). *Enhancing adult motivation to learn.* San Francisco: Jossey-Bass.

World Health Organization. (2001). *World Health Report 2001—Mental health: New understanding, new hope.* Retrieved from www.who.int/whr/2001/en/.

World Health Organization. (2013*). International Classification of Diseases.* Retrieved from www.who.int/classifications/icd/en/.

2

Evolution of Psychosocial Practice in Occupational Therapy

Lynn Cockburn, PhD, MEd, MSPH, OT Reg (Ont), OT(C)

I have also taught occupational therapy's history and application to university students, who challenged my views about the meaning of history in today's practice environment. Skillfully, students argued that occupational therapy's past practice was obsolete in light of today's standards. Their arguments cite important new technological advances, but overlook how occupational therapists made professional advances in the context of their own times. Lessons, I believe, can be learned from history. Understanding how opportunities are gained and lost is an important history lesson when applied to today's professional dilemmas. These discussions and experiences gave me opportunities to question my own views. Grasping for a deeper understanding and recapturing occupational therapy's past brings meaning to the present. (Peters, 2011, p. 216)

OBJECTIVES

The objectives of this chapter are as follows:
  - » Describe the evolution of concepts related to health through occupation.
  - » Discuss the evolution of psychosocial occupational therapy with a particular focus on North America, the United Kingdom, Australia, and New Zealand.
  - » Describe historical tensions of competing paradigms in psychosocial occupational therapy practice.
  - » Describe the influence of evidence-based practice on psychosocial occupational therapy.
  - » Describe the influence of employment and payment structures, the profile of occupation health in service systems, trauma and violence, stigma and discrimination, knowledge from diverse sources, and interprofessional practice.
  - » Describe emerging arenas for practice in psychosocial occupational therapy practice.

Krupa, T., Kirsh, B., Pitts, D., & Fossey, E. *Bruce & Borg's Psychosocial Frames of Reference: Theories, Models, and Approaches for Occupation-Based Practice, Fourth Edition* (pp 17-33).
© 2016 SLACK Incorporated.

EVOLUTION OF CONCEPTS RELATED TO HEALTH THROUGH OCCUPATION

Occupational therapists believe that people need to have meaningful engagement in everyday activities and occupations to achieve and maintain optimal health and well-being, including psychosocial health. The idea that engaging in everyday activities could help one to resume a normal life after illness or injury was a core belief in the beginning of the profession. During what has come to be known as the Progressive Era, the 1890s to 1920s, the profession's founders believed that it was not enough to have confidence in the therapeutic power of occupation; it was also vital to take collective action to organize and name this work as unique from other professions (Gutman, 1997; Harley & Schwartz, 2013; Schwartz, 2009). Occupational therapy associations, such as the American Occupational Therapy Association (AOTA), were founded by social leaders who held deep convictions about the importance of occupation and the need to more firmly establish support for the inclusion of occupation as a key component of health, medical, educational, and vocational systems. Similar beliefs were held by founders in Australia (Anderson, Bell, & New South Wales Association of Occupational Therapy, 1988), Britain (Wilcock, 2002), Canada (Friedland & Brumer, 2007), and New Zealand (New Zealand Association of Occupational Therapy, 2006). Three social movements, each embracing occupation in unique ways, were particularly influential in the development of the profession: the mental hygiene movement, the arts and crafts movement, and the settlement house movement (Friedland, 2011).

The mental hygiene movement (beginning in the late 19th century and gaining momentum around 1908) focused on improving hospital care and preventing mental illness. A lack of meaningful occupations was associated with poor mental health, whereas their provision was seen to promote health and prevent further illness. Many of the early supporters of occupational therapy, such as Eleanor Clarke Slagle and Goldwin Howland, were involved in this movement and in the emergence of mental hygiene associations in the early 1900s (Friedland & Brumer, 2007). These associations continue today in the form of mental health associations.

The Arts and Crafts movement advocated traditional craftsmanship, beauty in design, and simple forms in goods produced, as well as economic and social reform. Emerging in the second part of the 19th century, the movement was a response to industrial transformations, which often created deplorable working conditions and poor quality goods. William Morris, a leader in this movement, believed that engagement in art and craft occupations to create everyday goods was vital to developing a more humane society. While the movement was focused on health and illness directly, it was also considered to lay the groundwork to socialize populations who had been largely excluded, such as those with disabilities, mental illness, and the impoverished (Schemm, 1994, as cited by Friedland, 1998).

The third influential movement, the settlement house movement, emerging in the late 19th century, advanced settlement houses as places where impoverished and immigrant populations could learn skills that would help them to better manage their lives. Run by social reformers who believed it was not enough for the middle classes to simply provide money (alms) to the poor, settlement houses engaged reformers actively in community endeavors. The settlement house movement contributed a social justice foundation to occupational therapy, as many of the social reformers who worked in these communities went on to become pioneer occupational therapists. These foundational philosophies continue to be referenced in current professional literature (e.g., Frank, 2013; Table 2-1).

THE EVOLUTION OF PSYCHOSOCIAL OCCUPATIONAL THERAPY

The history of the profession of occupational therapy is grounded in theories related to mental illness and how people return to mental health after emotional disruptions (Friedland, 2011; Quiroga, 1995; Sedgewick, Cockburn, & Trentham, 2007; Wilcock, 2001, 2002). Many of the profession's founders worked in the field of psychiatry and believed that the whole person—mind, body, and spirit—needed to be treated for recovery to occur. They drew from humanitarian and humanistic philosophies and cared deeply about social change and development. Humanitarianism refers to a concern for the human condition; a belief that society has an obligation to help people, including those who are ill or disabled, and a belief in the value and dignity of each person. Also evident in the philosophical foundation of occupational therapy is a philosophy of humanism. In many respects humanism overlaps with the concept of the humanitarian, but they are not identical. To have a humanistic orientation implies not only a humanitarian concern for the human condition, but also the belief that each person lives and makes choices based upon his or her unique, personal perspective. A humanistic orientation supports the belief that people can and do take responsibility for shaping their own lives through the actions they take. The humanistic philosophy is most explicit today in the priority given to establishing client-centered therapeutic relationships where the occupational therapy service recipient's desires drive therapeutic goals.

Humanitarian and humanistic ideologies were apparent in both North America and Europe during the 18th and 19th centuries, when well-intentioned community leaders looked for ways to take care of people who were having psychological and emotional problems. Innovative, but often

TABLE 2-1
FOUNDERS AND PIONEERS OF PSYCHOSOCIAL OCCUPATIONAL THERAPY PRACTICE
Susan Tracy emphasized the importance of using activities that would be of interest and were meaningful to the patient (1912).
Adolph Meyer addressed the complex biological and psychological interactions of persons that influence their social performance in daily life and saw problems of mental health and mental illness as a breakdown in normal living habits (1922).
Eleanor Clarke Slagle recommended the use of purposeful activity to develop a person's habits, which in turn would support health and well-being (1922).
William Rush Dunton focused on the formation of habits to help the patient work and socialize in the community; his writing brought many early moral treatment concepts into occupational therapy (1915, 1919, 1922).
Louis J. Haas wrote about the importance of helping the person achieve competence and a sense of pride from activities completed in the workshop (1925).
Bryan and Marsh used industrial therapy to help patients continue to be productive (Keilhofner & Burke, 1977).
Philip King Brown, founder and director of the Arequiopa Sanatorium from 1910 to 1928, used occupation to both treat illness and to address social inequality (Harley & Schwartz, 2013).
Thomas Bessell Kidner, in the early part of the 20th century, believed in the power of the use of one's hands and in manual education for the promotion of health (Friedland, 2011).
Goldwin Howland, from the 1920s through the 1940s, was a strong advocate for occupational therapy as a key component in health care (Friedland, 2011).
Helen LeVesconte (1935) believed in the importance of the relationship between the therapist and the client, and that the client should have increasing control in the process of occupational therapy as therapy progressed (Friedland, 2011).

large, institutions were created, separated from local communities. Re-engaging in what were seen as normal activities was believed to be a way for these patients to regain control over their illnesses and their own lives. Those enacting this moral treatment believed that people became mentally ill because they had "succumbed to external pressures," developed faulty habits, and became disengaged from society (Kielhofner, 1992, p. 17). Once the new profession of occupation therapy was established in the 1920s and 1930s, many of these institutions employed occupational therapists. Because they were originally intended to be places of safety, rest, recovery, and healing, these institutions were known as *asylums*: residents were given asylum from the harsh realities of living in communities in which they were not accepted. People who were not mentally ill, but did not fit into society's ideals, such as those who were poor or had developmental disabilities, were also placed in asylums. Over time, asylums became places that were not seen as places of refuge, but rather as places that removed people from their communities for long periods (sometimes entire lifetimes) and the term *asylum* took on negative connotations.

As occupational therapy became established, the profession focused on strengthening educational and clinical programs to respond to the needs of society. By the middle and latter part of the 20th century, the profession was well established in many countries, and emerging in others. The profession was addressing a range of client populations, was aware that the medical field was becoming firmly grounded in science, and was trying to cope with the high rates of attrition due to marriage (an important issue at a time where women's ability to work was socially constrained). In the United States, occupational therapy leaders began to see the need for a new kind of legitimacy. Using detailed and personal accounts of what it was like to be part of these contentious years, Peters (2011) provided a fascinating description of the discussions and conflicts that emerged as American occupational therapy leaders grappled with the tensions between philosophy and science in attempts to become a more established health profession, while retaining core values.

The evolution of a scientific perspective had implications for the profession. One negative outcome of the scientific movement was that it categorized patients and activities in a way that attempted to match a particular activity with the treatment of a particular diagnosis or to relieve specific symptoms. Matching symptom with activity tended to eliminate the personalization of intervention and the appreciation of the interpersonal and cultural contexts in which activities occurred. Changes specific to the field of mental health became evident. With the advent of more scientific approaches that included medical and pharmaceutical products that could treat mental illness, along with public discussions about the need to re-examine the restrictions of institutional living, new movements began that advocated for the reintegration of people living with mental illnesses into mainstream society.

The dismantling of asylums was a slow and uneven process. It was not until the 1960s, when what is now known as *the deinstitutionalization movement* started, that alternatives to institutional care became more commonly available. Italy was a forerunner in this process, and developed a comprehensive community-based system (Tansella, 1986). In 1963, the U.S. Congress passed the Community Mental Health Act, which supported community integration and mandated that treatment of adults with mental illness be provided in the least restrictive setting (Ray & Finley, 1994). This Act was the impetus for the closure of large state and private mental health facilities, and patients were released to community settings where it was expected that they would receive supportive services (Gutman, 2011; Sharfstein, 2000). Similar efforts were underway in other places, such as Britain (Turner, 2004) and Canada (Nelson, Lord, & Ochocka, 2001). Unfortunately, the process of moving people into communities was not initially matched with new models of service delivery, the creation of welcoming communities, or adequate funding for affordable housing. As a result, many former patients became socially marginalized within communities (Accordino, Porter, & Morse, 2001; Gostin, 2008; Gutman, 2011).

The transitioning of people from institutions to communities had significant effects on service providers, including occupational therapists, since the change required both a change in focus for service delivery and a restructuring of the service structure itself. In many jurisdictions, such as Canada, the United Kingdom, New Zealand, and Australia, occupational therapy continued to have a significant profile in mental health service provision and development, even though their employment contexts shifted considerably. In the United States, however, the move to community based care saw the loss of occupational therapy positions and indeed, the loss of involvement of the profession in the mental health field at all levels; efforts are now being made to reverse this trend (Gutman, 2011, 2012).

In the 1960s and 1970s, mental health occupational therapists were particularly influenced by psychodynamic and behavioral theories, both of which reflected a scientific approach to explaining behavior. Many occupational therapists viewed this scientific movement as a negation of humanism, a loss of holism, and a shift from the original philosophical base of the profession. However, there was also recognition that, within psychosocial occupational therapy, there could be benefits from drawing upon the psychological sciences. For example, the increased understanding of psychodynamics and the principles of interpersonal relations contributed to the profession's understanding of the therapeutic relationship, strengthened the appreciation of the meaning of activities, and provided a way to understand and respond to confused, chaotic, and otherwise nonproductive behavior. This knowledge also increased awareness of the critical role and importance of social and interpersonal communication and group process. The foundation was laid for the application of psychosocial occupational therapy within a therapeutic group setting or therapeutic milieu (Fidler & Fidler, 1963).

Beginning in the 1980s, the discipline of occupational science added diverse voices to discussions about health through occupation. Occupational science, coming from social and behavioral science, is focused on the study of humans as complex occupational beings. This growing body of work contributes to the articulation of theoretical assumptions underlying the concept of health through occupation, and to the evidence supporting those understandings (e.g., Backman, 2004; Christiansen & Townsend, 2010; Jonsson, 2008; Rebeiro, 1998; Yerxa, 1990, 1998a, 1998b; Zemke & Clark, 1996).

THE TENSIONS OF COMPETING PARADIGMS IN PSYCHOSOCIAL PRACTICE

Biomedical Model

In psychosocial practice, the biomedical model conceptualizes psychological, emotional, and social problems and mental illnesses as disease or disorder states. Biomedical perspectives lead to interventions that focus on parts of a person, to treat or manage the disorder. The biomedical perspectives of health have been consistently present in occupational therapy, although the emphasis varies depending on the social context, the perspectives of the occupational therapist, the practice setting, and the population. Given the dominance of the biomedical model, embracing this paradigm assisted occupational therapy to develop into a recognized health profession. This biomedical, scientific approach was *reductionistic*; observable phenomena were reduced into measurable units whose relationship to each other could be described (Kielhofner, 1992, p. 35). Using this paradigm, occupational therapists working in psychosocial areas of practice carefully observed and measured their clients' mood, motivation and drive, attention and other cognitive functions, emotional stability, and other characteristics, and used improvements in these areas as indications that therapy was successful. The model was particularly prevalent in in-patient units of hospitals, where access to natural occupations was limited and where individuals were more likely to present with acute forms of mental illnesses requiring more intensive forms of treatment and care.

Rehabilitation Model

Beginning in the 1940s, there were increasing references to rehabilitation, reflecting a shift in how occupational therapy named its work. The 1950s and 1960s saw the emergence of new medical specialties in rehabilitation medicine, primarily focused on physical rehabilitation. While the aims of occupational therapy in its early days were social integration and health, the aim of rehabilitation was to eliminate illness and its symptoms or impairments or do away with disability (Friedland, 1998). In the later part of the 20th century, definitions of rehabilitation began to broaden to recognize other factors, such as the role of environments, and desired outcomes expanded to include goals such as return to work and social participation.

In the field of mental health, two terms—*psychiatric rehabilitation* and *psychosocial rehabilitation* (PSR)—emerged in the 1970s as new approaches to mental health work. These approaches were much needed because the negative consequences of the deinstitutionalization movement were evident with the large numbers of people who experienced exclusion in their communities. PSR aimed to find ways to reduce the stigma and discrimination related to mental illness, to link non-medical concepts with interventions, and to improve community living and citizenship opportunities for people living with mental health-related disabilities. It valued client involvement in the treatment process and placed emphasis on client autonomy, self-determination, decision making, and empowerment. William Anthony, one of its key developers, highlighted similarities between physical and psychosocial rehabilitation (Anthony, 1992). Both approaches emphasized that although symptoms and impairments might be treated medically, it was a rehabilitation approach that was necessary to promote functioning and community life. Today, PSR is widely applied, has a strong interdisciplinary base, and is supported by research and training centers such as the Center for Psychiatric Rehabilitation at Boston University. Many occupational therapists have found PSR a compatible approach to the profession's philosophies and models of practice, and have made significant contributions to its development (e.g., Bullock & Bannigan, 2011; Krupa, Fossey, Anthony, Brown, & Pitts, 2009).

The values and principles of the psychiatric rehabilitation approach were translated into a broad range of community-based programs, including for example, the Clubhouse, which supported employment, education and housing, and Assertive Community Treatment. Occupational therapists have been involved in delivering services within all of these programs.

Recovery

The concept of recovery has become a guiding framework in mental health service delivery and reform. Developed initially from the perspectives of those with lived experience of mental illness (Deegan, 1997), service providers, and academics (Jacobson, 2003; Jacobson & Greenley, 2001), recovery describes the processes by which individuals with the lived experience of mental illnesses and/or substance use undergo a journey to health and the achievement of their full potential. Recovery in mental health is linked to the recovery models and processes used in treatment for substance use and abuse (Substance Abuse and Mental Health Services, 2012). A key part of recovery focuses on the person's identity: rather than seeing oneself as being primarily a person with a significant mental illness, the person develops a sense of self that incorporates health, personal responsibility, hope, and participation in meaningful occupations. This recovery framework is compatible with both humanistic and occupational perspectives. The recovery approach is covered more fully in Chapter 3 of this book.

Empowerment Models

The empowerment paradigm emerged in the 1980s and 1990s. Nelson and colleagues (2001) identified three common elements in this paradigm. First, empowerment includes a personal dimension of both perceived and actual power, including the power to make choices in one's life and to have control over life events. Second, empowerment is a process involving "self in community." As persons with mental health–related disabilities become more integrated into their communities, and power relations shift, they establish a more positive identity, learn valued social roles, and participate in community life. Third, empowerment includes access to valued resources, particularly material resources such as housing, and many other resources necessary for daily life. This focus on the material and structural conditions of people's lives is a hallmark of an empowerment perspective.

As part of both the recovery and empowerment, there has been an increase in support and action for people with lived experience to be involved actively in occupational therapy and other programs and services in a variety of roles such as peer support workers, peer specialists, and co-researchers (International Association of Peer Supporters, 2013; Nelson et al., 2001). Peer specialists have emerged as an important component of practice teams. Occupational therapists now collaborate with peer specialists in service programs and in community settings. Embracing the values of the empowerment paradigm, therapists around the world also take active roles in social justice movements, and national and state organizations that advocate for better policies, and improved access to housing, education, and employment.

This focus on the value of lived experience has extended to the inclusion of the voices and perspectives of persons with lived experience of mental health problems and illnesses as part of the profession's evidence base. This has included people with lived experience as partners in research studies, promoting client perspectives in the development of occupational therapy professional practices (Cockburn & Trentham, 2002; Hammell, 2007; Lorenzo & Joubert, 2011; Restall, 2013). It has also included occupational therapy efforts to support research centers directed by people with mental health issues to provide the context for the exploration of research questions that capture things that are most meaningful in their lives (see for example, Rebeiro, Day, Semeniuk, O'Brien, & Wilson, 2001).

Population and Public Health Approaches

Population health and public health perspectives address the needs and experiences of large groups of people. Viewing mental health with a population lens allows us to see how occupations engaged in by groups of people are perceived to be health promoting (or not), are similar or different between groups, and how the similarities and differences are shaped by the environments in which people live (Mallinson, Fischer, Rogers, Ehrlich-Jones, & Chang, 2009). Social determinants of health models argue that health is the result of a number of social factors that influence or determine the health status of populations. Social determinants of health include peace, shelter, education, food, income, a stable ecosystem, sustainable resources, social justice, and equity (WHO, 1986); all of these factors have occupational components and fit with recovery and empowerment paradigms. These are not simply present or absent, but rather affect people in a variety of ways in gradients in a given context (Commission on Social Determinants of Health, 2008).

Health, including mental health, outcomes are not simply the result of individual lifestyle factors; they are the result of a number of social enablers and barriers evident in each person's specific context. Therefore, occupational engagement and meaning are not only individual constructs, but are socially constructed, affected by the contexts in which people live. For example, a diagnosis of depression can be both the result of and affected by levels of safety and security, housing policies and the availability of housing, access to food and water, access to a secure income, as well as social policies addressing service provision and human rights.

Language About Service Recipients: A Reflection of Paradigmatic Tensions

As the discussion about biomedical, rehabilitation, recovery, and empowerment paradigms makes evident, there are multiple words and definitions for describing the people who receive occupational therapy services. The terms are influenced by the philosophical beliefs of the profession, the theoretical models specific to populations, and the environments of practice. It is crucial that psychosocial occupational therapists have an understanding of these terms so that they can participate in related discussions both within, and external to, the profession.

When occupational therapy began, recipients of services were typically seen in hospital settings and were referred to as patients. Over time, many mental health professionals believed that the term *patient* reinforced the sick role and supported the idea of pathology or illness and the individual's need to be taken care of by health professionals. Wishing to emphasize wellness, the term *client* was used to focus on problems of living, not illness, and to encourage personal responsibility for health. Likewise, people who live in communities are *citizens* or *residents*.

As part of the movement for disability rights, person-first language emerged as a way to emphasize that a person is a person first; someone who lives with an impairment or disadvantage has the disability as only one of many other characteristics, and not their primary feature (Morin, 2013). From this perspective, a person previously known as a schizophrenic would be referred to as a person with schizophrenia or a person living with schizophrenia. Some occupational therapists are aligning with disability activists who advocate for the term *disabled person* (Hammell, 2011).

FACTORS INFLUENCING PSYCHOSOCIAL OCCUPATIONAL THERAPY

The Return to Occupation

With the evolution of the scientific approach, the occupational therapy profession was faced with challenges to its foundational beliefs, values, and goals. Yerxa wrote that being professional and committing to developing science was not incompatible with a concern for the client as a human being (1967, p. 1). She urged therapists to realize that the outcome of therapy could not be fully understood or reduced to bits and pieces of observable phenomena; rather, meaningful therapy, like a meaningful life, is composed of occupations that must be understood in their context and from the client's point of view. Yerxa's writing led the way for reflection regarding the art of occupational therapy, including the importance of the therapist's ability to communicate concern and empathic understanding to the patient or client. At the same time, Reilly (1962, 1966) called for a return to the roots of the profession and a reaffirmation of the importance of occupation to one's health and well-being.

Beginning in the late 1970s, a concern for occupation has been reaffirmed as the core domain of the profession (Christiansen, 1999; Hammell, 2009a; Peters, 2011). Practitioners have increasingly emphasized occupationally based and client-centered practice (i.e., what is important in the client's home, school, work, or community environments). With this reaffirmation came concepts and ideas related to occupation that were debated and subject to further development and revision. For example, the notion that occupation consists of self-care, leisure, and productivity activities has been subject to debate, and new conceptualizations of occupational patterns are emerging (Hammell, 2009b; Jonsson, 2008; Stamm, Cieza, Machold, Smolen, & Stucki, 2006). There is also more discussion and awareness that not all occupations are positive. For example, forced participation in occupations and occupations driven by addictions are examples of occupational experiences that may have negative outcomes on personal health and well-being. The personal significance attached to engagement in an occupation is not always observable, and this significance cannot be assumed to be positive. The feeling elicited by engaging in occupations can include frustration, boredom, or humiliation (Hammell, 2009).

Influence of Evidence-Based Practice on Psychosocial Occupational Therapy

Occupational therapists engage in their work to create positive change in the lives of individuals, populations, and societies. The results of these change processes are referred to as outcomes. The concept of *outcome*, while routinely accepted in current practice, has also gone through an evolutionary process in occupational therapy. When the profession was established, health and return to work were often the identified outcomes that therapists were hoping to achieve, although the actual word *outcome* may not have been used. With the rise of the rehabilitation framework, function (in terms of being able to carry out everyday occupations) and independence were identified as valued outcomes. With time, work and employment, social

relationships, and community membership and participation, also emerged as important outcomes.

In psychosocial occupational therapy, the influence of competing paradigms, the re-emergence of occupation as the core of the profession, and the pressures to engage in evidence-based practice have underscored the complexity of determining the most important outcomes, and sparked professional discussions and debates. Authors such as Tickle-Degnen remind occupational therapists that occupational therapy outcomes are "often theoretical constructs (occupational performance, quality of life) as opposed to direct observables (death/life, range of motion) and are continuous, rather than interval or ratio types of data" (Tickle-Degnen, 2011, sl.3). This also means that they can be more difficult to accurately measure than the outcomes that are directly observable or easy to count. There has been ongoing discussion about other important outcomes such as quality of life, well-being, and happiness, and these types of outcomes have also been researched as having important relationships to the process of engagement in everyday occupations. Along with occupational therapy, the fields of psychology, public health, medicine, economics, and many others are also debating what outcomes should be used and these fields are also making contributions to understandings of the relationships between occupational engagement, health, and well-being.

Evidence-based practice (EBP) is now well established in the lexicon of psychosocial occupational therapy practice across many countries. In principle it is based on the use of the best evidence available to promote health and provide care. For example, EBP is clearly articulated in the Centennial Vision of the American Occupational Therapy Association (AOTA, 2007). With EBP, each therapist must find ways to sort out and evaluate research data and other evidence to keep up to date with the ever-expanding body of information. Professional expertise is critical to EBP and psychosocial occupational therapists are expected to be able to critique and understand quantitative, qualitative, and mixed methods studies, knowing which types of questions to ask of research to evaluate rigour, applicability, and potential benefit to clients. They are expected to think deeply about the relevance of evidence for their practices. In many cases evidence relevant to occupational therapy is found in non-health care fields such as economics, political science, and justice studies. Reliable research findings of many kinds must be combined with client values and needs, and practitioners' expertise and clinical judgement.

Employment and Payment Structures

In the early days of the profession, occupational therapists were paid primarily through health systems. Often working in hospitals or in programs for veterans, payment came from government or private sources. As the discipline

<hr>

BOX 2-1. VIGNETTE: ANNETTE

Annette is an American therapist who has been practicing in the field of mental health for about 25 years. She grew up in the 1960s and 1970s in a home and community that embraced the changes that were coming with the civil rights and feminist movements of the time; she still feels the optimism that she learned during those years about the possibilities for a more inclusive society. She was drawn to occupational therapy for many reasons, including its emphasis on the therapeutic use of creativity, seeing the client as a whole person, and the importance of occupations in everyday life. During her career in the 1980s and 1990s, she was actively involved in the new field of psychosocial rehabilitation, and worked with colleagues to develop strategies to assist clients to live in their communities and advocate for themselves. Recently, she has been watching what is happening with the introduction of the Patient Protection and Affordable Health Care Act (ACA, 2010) and wondering if it might be a good time to consider a new type of psychosocial occupational therapy work, both to contribute to the new health care landscape, and to broaden her professional abilities.

<hr>

evolved into an established, organized profession, new employment positions were launched and new avenues for payment appeared. There have been several factors influencing employment and payment structures of occupational therapists in the mental health arena. First, the movement from institutional to community practice has impacted payment sources and structures. For example, occupational therapists working in community mental health practice found job evaluation processes and pay scales were different, and typically less generous, than those in hospital settings. Second, the profession has witnessed an increase in private practice, including psychosocial practice. Finally, employment structures and payment schemes are highly related to the sociopolitical context of practice. For example, in the United States, positions for psychosocial occupational therapists in hospitals, including psychiatric hospitals, were historically common. Private insurers paid for psychiatric care only to a limited extent (Peters, 1984). During the 1980s and 1990s, reimbursement issues continued to develop. State and federal reimbursing agencies such as Medicare and Medicaid, feeling the economic crunch, demanded more careful accountability in the use of state and federal institutions (Foto, 1988a, 1988b; Hanft, 1988). Today, therapists in the United States are faced with more federal transformations in health care payment and need to be familiar with the Patient Protection and Affordable Health Care Act (ACA, 2010) as it comes into force. The ACA service provision framework includes a range of rehabilitation, mental health, and substance use services for covered persons who have behavioral health issues (Braveman & Metzler, 2012; Stoffel, 2013; Box 2-1).

Occupational therapists globally are identifying opportunities for new funding structures that come along with new roles and practice contexts, such as becoming members of primary care teams, increased involvement in prevention and wellness programs, increased roles in habilitation and rehabilitation, and expanded behavioral health services. Changes in the health care landscape can provide more

opportunities for occupational therapists to be involved in innovative programs and advocacy initiatives to ensure that the contributions and cost-effectiveness of the professional are fully recognized (Goodman, 2013; Hinojosa, 2013).

Spirituality in Psychosocial Practice

A discussion about the evolution of perspectives of mental health and psychosocial occupational therapy would not be complete without acknowledging the role of spirituality and religion in the field. Spirituality as part of the therapeutic process is a theme that has been woven through the profession since its beginnings and continues to be explored (Barnitt & Mayers, 1993; Egan & Delaat, 1994; Kirsh, 1996; Kroeker, 1997; Townsend & Polatajko, 2007). Although the mind-body-spirit paradigm is an area that deserves much more attention than what we can cover here, two considerations regarding spirituality should be kept in mind; the influence of the personal spiritual and religious beliefs of therapists on their practices, and second, the inclusion of spirituality in the theories, conceptualizations, and practices in psychosocial occupational therapy. An example of the latter was illustrated by research conducted by Wilding, May, and Muir-Cochrane (2005), which found that people with mental illness discovered that spirituality could motivate and sustain their engagement with occupations.

Trauma, Violence, War, and Disaster

The impacts of trauma, war, violence, and disasters have been woven into the history of psychosocial occupational therapy practice (Eldar & Jelic, 2003). Occupational therapy had spurts of growth during both World War I and World War II, and other wars and upheavals have also influenced its development (Friedland, 2011; Gutman, 1997). Occupational therapy can play a significant role in the recovery process for those who have experienced violence in home situations (Javaherian, Underwood, &

DeLany, 2007), in community situations (Precin, 2011a; Simo-Algado, Mehta, Kronenberg, Cockburn, & Kirsh, 2002), or with veterans returning to civilian life (Amaker, Woods, & Gerardi, 2009).

Occupational therapists come into contact with abuse and violence in homes and communities in many ways—physical, financial and economic, emotional and psychological, sexual, and interpersonal/relational. Victims of abuse can be men or women, and come from all parts of society. Sometimes the occupational therapist is working directly with a survivor of violence or with communities that have a history of violence and trauma in their homes and networks (AOTA, 2012; Gorde, Helfrich, & Finlayson, 2004; Helfrich, Aviles, Badiani, Walens, & Sabol, 2006; Watson & Swartz, 2004). A therapist may learn about or suspect violence in the course of working with a client on other issues; survivors will be present in all practice settings. Many survivors of trauma and abuse are isolated from family and friends, with limited access to information and support, and may be reluctant to disclose their experiences.

Occupational therapists work with these clients as they rebuild their lives, using the full range of strategies and tools that are available to identify issues, to treat physical and emotional wounds, and to assist in the development of coping strategies to recover, compensate, or adapt to the challenges arising from the violent experiences, including post-traumatic stress disorder (Amaker et al, 2009; Eldar & Jelic, 2003; Montz, Gonzales, Bash, Carney, & Bramlett, 2008; Newton, 2007). Therapists must remember that there are professional and ethical responsibilities to promote the health and safety of these individuals and to act according to legal requirements.

Occupational therapy can play a significant role in the prevention of violence in community settings (Robbins, 2001). For example, Rai (2002) suggested that occupational therapists can contribute to creating a person-environment-occupation match with a view to reducing workplace violence. Occupational therapists may also work with people who have been the perpetrators of abuse and violence, and who want to make changes in their lives to be less abusive and live more peacefully; usually this type of work is done with other professionals such as social workers or police, as part of larger programs. Occupational therapy interventions can include life review and planning, training in social skills, assertiveness, preparing for and maintaining productivity roles, anger management, parenting, and spiritual exploration as related to daily occupations (AOTA, 2012; Buchanan & Higson-Smith, 2004).

Occupational therapists have also worked with national emergency committees to include psychosocial support for emergency preparedness and to enable access to safe and supportive services when disasters occur. These programs can be targeted for people affected by the disaster who have no prior mental health concerns, as well as those who have a previous experience of mental illness (Precin, 2011b). Services can include improving coping skills and resilience, dealing with trauma and loss, addressing psychological trauma, and promotion of recovery and resilience. Health and humanitarian workers also need to receive services and support during and following emergencies and occupational therapy can contribute to these programs (WHO, 2013).

Deepening Understandings of Discrimination and Stigma

Social reform movements that aim to decrease discrimination and marginalization in society have come in waves globally. At the time that occupational therapy was being established in North America and Britain, poverty was widespread in both cities and rural areas. In the early 1900s, large numbers of immigrants were arriving in North America from Europe. Many encountered difficulties and faced discrimination in finding ways to become included in established social structures or to find work that was lucrative or meaningful. Large factories and mechanization were having an impact on how people worked—often for long hours under difficult conditions. Only those who were of sound mind and body could sustain these efforts; those who were deemed weak were looked down on. In many places systemic racism was also prevalent. During these times mental health issues and mental illnesses were not to be discussed. Likewise, although the field of psychiatry was growing, it was often seen to be a less important field of medicine and received fewer financial and other resources. People who were experiencing poor mental health and mental illnesses found that they were marginalized and segregated in their communities. There have been social movements to decrease stigma and exclusion, and to promote civil rights, women's rights, disability rights, workers' rights, and rights related to sexuality and sexual orientation. All of these movements have links to mental health and illness; lack of opportunity and living in oppressive situations have a negative effect on mental health. The best evidence currently suggests that an effective way to reduce stigma is to facilitate contact between the public and people who are subject to stigma, and this contact should show them in pro-social roles and activities (Corrigan, Morris, Michaels, Rafacz, & Rüsch, 2012). Subsequently, enabling highly stigmatized groups, like those with lived experience of mental illness, to participate in socially meaningful occupations can be a powerful anti-stigma strategy, in that it can provide a foundation for positive social contacts. Krupa (2010) highlighted the importance of identifying and addressing sources of this stigma within the profession of occupational therapy. For example, the ongoing separation of physical and psychosocial practice within the field likely develops conditions for sustaining stigma.

Integrating Diverse and Traditional Knowledge Into Practice

Issues related to power, decision making, and sex within the profession have always been evident. For example, the first occupational therapists were women only, a deliberate strategy by the male physician founders of the occupational therapy associations. Beginning in the 1970s, there have been examinations of the impacts of this sex imbalance: Reese examined sex in occupational therapy texts (Reese, 1987); Frank (1992) and Hamlin (1992) called for more work on feminist histories. There is now increasing awareness that sex considerations need to be included in understanding the profession, and in service provision.

Remembering that the roots of the profession lay with the recruitment of proper middle-class, white, "young ladies," who would maintain the worthy and privileged values espoused by the early founders, it is important that discussions of discrimination and social justice continue (Denshire, 2013). Perhaps unintended, these potentially biased roots also promoted a White occupational therapy, limiting racial and class diversity among occupational therapists and leaders (Peters, 2011, p. 206). Scholars and practitioners have begun to delve into the complexity of the links between social and professional oppressions, how occupations can be used to combat these, and the role of therapists in creating social and political change—with the aim of eliminating stigma and discrimination, and of promoting inclusion and full social participation for all people. For some women, including many female occupational therapists, being politically active and speaking out from a critical perspective, does not feel comfortable, and creates a professional culture that holds the profession back from reaching its potential (Cardwell, 1966; Clark, 2011; Maxwell & Maxwell, 1978; Whalley Hammell, 2013).

Internationally, psychosocial occupational therapy is also learning and growing philosophically and practically from engaging with indigenous peoples. As understandings of social marginalization, inclusion, and diversity have increased in the profession and in the broader society, therapists have become more aware of the need to integrate indigenous ways of knowing. Only a few examples of this work are provided here to illustrate the breadth of contributions available. Traditional Chinese medicine and Ayurveda call for attention to occupational balance and management to obtain good health and quality of life. Ayurveda is an Eastern system of health and medicine that has been practiced for over 5000 years and incorporates occupation as a fundamental aspect. The term *Ayurveda* is

from the Sanskrit words meaning daily living and knowing. Occupational therapists in India have been incorporating Ayurvedic principles for decades (Mailoo, 2007). Occupational therapists in Australia and New Zealand have explored indigenous ways of knowing, and provide lessons for respecting and integrating these perspectives into occupational therapy practices (e.g., Nelson, 2007; Nelson et al., 2011; Stedman, & Thomas, 2011; Thomas, Gray, & McGinty, 2011; Waugh & Mackenzie, 2011).

Interprofessional Practice

Attention to interprofessional practice has arisen from shifts in understanding about the needs of clients and patients, particularly in relation to quality of service and safety concerns, and for the need for more efficient systems (Canadian Interprofessional Health Collaborative, 2003; National Research Council, 2003). Improved professional collaboration and teamwork is now often termed *interprofessional practice* or *care*. This interest in interprofessional practice has also led to an increase in interprofessional education (WHO, 2010; National Research Council, 2003) based on the understanding that professionals need to learn collaboratively in their formative years to be able to practice collaboratively.

The interprofessional perspective is not new in occupational therapy—it was also recognized, in fact, lived out, by the early founders. Doctors, nurses, and other founders such as Eleanor Clark Slagle believed in the power of collaboration between professional groups. Attention to interprofessional work continued through the subsequent decades as therapists considered how their unique perspectives, and in some situations their occupational therapy contributions, were not valued. Occupational therapists, including mental health occupational therapists, have been strong contributors to what is now seen as an emerging field.

EVOLVING ARENAS FOR PSYCHOSOCIAL PRACTICE AND NEW PRACTICE CONTEXTS

As occupational therapy grows, new areas of practice emerge. Many occupational therapists are developing innovative programs for populations and groups, as well as opening opportunities in sectors that are new to the field.

Health and Wellness

The public appears to be increasingly aware of the importance of health-promoting activities, including mental health. Popular media has highlighted the importance of considering how daily life is conducted, the choices that

BOX 2-2. VIGNETTE: CHRIS

Chris is an occupational therapist who has been practicing in the field of mental health for about 5 years. He came as an 8-year-old immigrant to North America. He grew up in a home and community that tried to balance the need for financial security with optimism, that new lives were possible; his parents promoted the importance of a good job with social status. He was drawn to occupational therapy for many reasons, including that it is part of the health care system, the emphasis on the therapeutic use of arts and creativity, seeing the client as a whole person, and the importance of occupations in everyday life. During his career so far, he has had several positions both as an occupational therapist on an in-patient psychiatric unit in a general hospital, and in an outpatient mental health service that provided occupational therapy services. Recently he accepted a job as an occupational therapist working on a primary health care team. His position focuses primarily on those experiencing mental health–related concerns. He is typically asked to follow-up with people who are having difficulty managing their work and home lives in response to depression and anxiety and general stress concerns. He also offers groups in collaboration with the psychologist on staff. The groups use occupation-based and cognitive behavioral approaches to help people deal with stress. Knowing that people with serious mental illness have a lifespan estimate that is 25 years below the general population, he is spearheading a working group in the service that is looking at how they might collaborate with a local assertive community treatment team to provide primary care services to people with serious mental illness.

are made about physical activity and social interaction, and the need for more attention to holistic approaches to health. As in past centuries, society values doing, and understands that some occupations, such as preparing and eating a meal of fresh foods, or enjoying a card game with friends, more clearly promote good health, while engagement in others, such as overworking, smoking, or fast driving, can lead to reduced health outcomes and social problems.

The evidence for occupational therapy's potential to address these concerns in health promotion, wellness, and community development has been developing. Determined and innovative therapists are developing related intervention approaches. Examples include the Well Elderly study (Clark, Jackson, & Carlson, 2004), working with people who are homeless (Gorde et al., 2004; Helfrich et al., 2006), and refugees (Bishop & Purcell, 2013; Suleman & Whiteford, 2013), and the development of population-focused active living guides (Moll, Gewurtz, Krupa, & Law, 2013). There are also examples of innovative ways in which psychosocial occupational therapists are engaged with new technologies. Internet sites, blogs, and social networking tools are some of the new ways of addressing mental health issues.

Primary Care

Over the years, occupational therapists have been involved in primary health care and primary care. There are calls for primary care systems, which largely fund primary care or family physician services, to be transitioned to primary health care systems that include interprofessional teams designed to meet both the medical and broader health needs of the population (Letts, 2011). Changes to primary health care systems provide new opportunities for occupational therapists, including those focusing on

psychosocial health and well-being (Letts, 2011; Muir, 2012; Stoffel, 2013; Box 2-2).

Work and Workplaces

Increasingly, attention is being given to mental health and mental illness issues related to work and workplaces (WHO, 2005, 2013). Occupational therapists have a long history of working in the area of vocational rehabilitation and are continuing their involvement as the area of work and mental health expands. There are at least three areas of focus for occupational therapy practice and research in this area. The first is occupational therapy involvement in practices designed to enable sustained employment or return to work for employees whose work participation has been impacted by mental health problems or mental illness. A recent example is the development of cognitive work hardening as a means to bolster a range of work-related disabilities experienced by people who are on leave from depression with a view to improving return-to-work outcomes (Wisenthal & Krupa, 2013). A second example is the involvement of occupational therapists in the development of a range of interventions to improve the employment of people with serious and persistent mental illness who have a history of marginalization from the community workforce. This has included evidence-based supported employment, the development of social enterprises, and the creation of employment positions for people with mental illness within the mental health care system (Henry, Nicholson, Phillips, Stier, & Clayfield, 2002; Kirsh, Cockburn, & Gewurtz, 2005, 2009; Krupa, Lagarde, & Carmichael, 2003; Moll, Holmes, Geronimo, & Sherman, 2009; Williams, Fossey, & Harvey, 2010). Third, occupational therapists have participated in identifying and developing features of workplaces that promote good mental health and well-being among employees and subsequently enhance the person-environment fit to enhance productivity (Kirsh, 2000; Moll & Clements, 2008). Occupational therapists can take on a variety of roles related to work: they might engage directly with employees to assess their work situation and assist them to stay in the job, provide recommendations for accommodations to enable return to work, provide group programming for health promotion or injury prevention in workplaces, conduct research related to workplaces and mental health, or contribute to policy and program development to improve workplace health and safety (Arbesman & Logsdon, 2011; Braveman & Page, 2012; Gibson, D'Amico, Jaffe, & Arbesman, 2011; Shaw et al., 2013).

The inclusion of psychosocial factors in work and return-to-work assessments, regardless of the person's diagnosis or health condition, can be an important step in the process of finding and maintaining good work, and one that has grown over the past few decades (Arbesman & Logsdon, 2011; Braveman & Page, 2012). The Worker Role Interview is one example of an occupational therapy assessment that is used internationally to identify psychosocial and environmental factors that could influence return to work for both short-term and long-term illness or disability. For example, it is now used in Sweden as part of the comprehensive assessment process for all workers undertaking a return-to-work process (Braveman & Page, 2012; Ekbladh, Thorell, & Haglund, 2010).

Psychosocial Occupational Therapy With Children and Adolescents

Children with mental health concerns have benefited from occupational therapy since the early days of the profession. As specialized hospitals and mental health clinics were organized and operated across North America, some of the clients were children (Montgomery, 1935). Over the years, there have been many examples of how occupational therapy has made a difference in the lives of children and adolescents with a variety of psychosocial issues (Blezard, 1955; Christiansen & Davidson, 1974; Cruickshank, 1947; Davidson, 1995; George, Braun, & Walker, 1982; Quake-Rapp, Miller, Ananthan, & Chiu, 2008; Willoughby, Polatajko, Currado, Harris, & King, 2000).

Occupational therapists work with children who have mental health issues and can also address the mental health issues of those who are primarily seen for other conditions, such as mobility impairments, cognitive disabilities, or occupational impairments such as developmental coordination disorder, or difficulty with handwriting. Mental health occupational therapists work in schools and education systems provide counselling, or might be involved in the development of environmental modifications and programs to increase inclusion in classroom settings.

In many jurisdictions, children can receive psychosocial occupational therapy services through publicly funded health organizations, schools, and private practice organizations. Currently in the United States, federal legislation mandates services, including occupational therapy, for some children with disabilities, and this can include mental health, behavioral, and psychosocial needs (Bazyk & Arbesman, 2013). Another evolving area for occupational therapy is in the area of early intervention services in mental health. These early intervention services have developed to prevent significant disability and social marginalization of young people who experience mental illnesses that may have a persistent or prolonged course (Lloyd et al., 2008).

Conclusion

This chapter has provided a brief overview of the history of the profession related to psychosocial practice. The history reflects a strong commitment to the blending of theory and evidence, while aiming toward the improvement of quality of life for the people with whom occupational therapists work. From the beginning, the profession's commitment to psychosocial practice has been resilient and innovative, and it continues to adapt to new challenges with exciting developments in practice, education, social policy, and research.

We learn from reflecting on the past and about how current aspirations are similar and different than those who have gone before. Most important is that we continue to strive to find ways to use evidence, knowledge, and tools to improve mental health, quality of life, health, social participation, peace, and equity in our global community.

Learning Activities/ Discussion Questions

1. Use the Internet to identify, and then learn about, an early psychosocial occupational therapist (you could also start with the names provided in Table 2-1 or from articles in the reference list). Develop a written description of what this individual's working day might have been like, and what kinds of occupations the person would have used in practice.

2. Look for stories or videos about historical accounts of psychosocial occupational therapy available through the Internet or your library. Notice your reactions (emotional and intellectual) to the perspectives shown, and how you think current practice is different. Discuss these reactions with others.

3. Develop a concept map of ideas and events (with approximate dates and locations) in an area of mental health occupational therapy in which you are interested in (e.g., children, work, community practice, schizophrenia). For example, if you are interested in workplace mental health, create a map about where concepts, practices, and legislation related to psychiatric disability, work integration, and return to work have come from; who has promoted change in workplaces; and what key events are recognized as milestones in this field of practice.

4. Arrange to interview or talk with an occupational therapist who has been working in mental health for more than 25 years or more to learn firsthand about how practice has changed and what has remained consistent.

5. The profession of occupational therapy, including psychosocial occupational therapy, has been strongly influenced by wars and conflicts. Discuss with others in the profession how an understanding of these influences assist present-day occupational therapists and others to further develop the profession.

6. Imagine that you and your colleagues in the profession could talk with Eleanor Clarke Slagle. Discuss what you would ask her.

REFERENCES

ACA Patient Protection and Affordable Care Act, Pub. L. No. 111-148, § 3502, 124 Stat. 119, 124 (2010). Retrieved from www.healthcare.gov/law/full/index.html.

Accordino, M. P., Porter, D. F., & Morse, T. (2001). Deinstitutionalization of persons with severe mental illness: context and consequences. *Journal of Rehabilitation, 67*(2), 16-21.

Amaker, R. J., Woods, Y., & Gerardi, S. M. (2009). AOTA's societal statement on combat-related posttraumatic stress. *American Journal of Occupational Therapy, 63,* 845-846.

American Occupational Therapy Association. (2007). AOTA's Centennial Vision and executive summary. *American Journal of Occupational Therapy.* 6, 613-614.

American Occupational Therapy Association. (2014). Official documents available from the American Occupational Therapy Association. *American Journal of Occupational Therapy,* November/December 2014, vol. 68, S1-S2. doi: 10.5014/ajot.2014.686S01.

American Psychiatric Association. (2012). *DSM: History of the manual.* Retrieved from www.psychiatry.org/practice/dsm/dsm-history-of-the-manual.

American Psychiatric Association. (2013). *DSM-5 Development.* Retrieved from www.dsm5.org.

Anderson, B., Bell, J., & New South Wales Association of Occupational Therapists. (1988). Occupational therapy: Its place in Australia's history. *New South Wales Association of Occupational Therapists.*

Anthony, W. A. (1992). Psychiatric rehabilitation: Key issues and future policy. *Health Affairs, 11*(3), 164-171.

Arbesman, M., & Logsdon, D. W. (2011). Occupational therapy interventions for employment and education for adults with serious mental illness: A systematic review. *American Journal of Occupational Therapy, 65,* 238-246. doi: 10.5014/ajot.2011.001289.

Backman, C. L.. (2004). Occupational balance: Exploring the relationships among daily occupations and their influence on well-being. *The Canadian Journal of Occupational Therapy, 71*(4), 202-9.

Barnes, M., & Schwartzberg, S. L. (2009). Functional group model: Theoretical case study. In G. Kielhofner, (Ed.), *Conceptual foundations in occupational therapy,* 4th ed. Philadelphia: F. A. Davis.

Barnitt, R., & Mayers, C. (1993). Can occupational therapist be both humanists and Christians? A study of two conflicting frames of reference. *British Journal of Occupational Therapy, 56*(3), 84-88.

Bazyk, S., & Arbesman, M. (2013). *Occupational therapy practice guidelines for mental health promotion, prevention, and intervention for children & youth.* Bethesda, MD: AOTA Press.

Bishop, R., & Purcell, E. (2013). The value of an allotment group for refugees. *The British Journal of Occupational Therapy, 76*(6), 264-269. doi: 10.4276/030802213X13706169932824.

Blezard, R. (1955). Occupational therapy visits in the mental health clinic. *The Canadian Journal of Occupational Therapy, 22*(4), 139-44.

Braveman, B., & Metzler, C. A. (2012). Health care reform implementation and occupational therapy. *American Journal of Occupational Therapy, 66,* 11-14.

Braveman, B., & Page, J. J. (2011). *Work: Promoting participation & productivity through occupational therapy.* Philadelphia, PA: FA Davis.

Brown, C. (2012). *Occupational therapy practice guidelines for adults with serious mental illness.* Bethesda: MD: AOTA.

Buchanan, H., & Higson-Smith, C. (2004). Trauma, violence and occupation. In R. Watson & L. Swartz (Eds.), *Transformation through occupation.* London: Whurr Publishers.

Bullock, A., & Bannigan, K. (2011). Effectiveness of activity-based group work in community mental health: A systematic review. *American Journal of Occupational Therapy, 65,* 257-266. doi: 10.5014/ajot.2011.001305.

Canadian Interprofessional Health Collaborative. (2003). *A national interprofessional competency framework.* Retrieved from www.cihc.ca/files/CIHC_IPCompetencies_Feb1210.pdf.

Cardwell, T. (1966). President's address. *Canadian Journal of Occupational Therapy, 33*, 139-140.

Christiansen, C. H. (1999). The 1999 Eleanor Clarke Slagle Lecture. Defining lives: occupation as identity: an essay on competence, coherence, and the creation of meaning. *American Journal of Occupational Therapy, 53*, 547-558.

Christiansen, C. H., & Davidson, D. A. (1974). A community health program with low achieving adolescents. *American Journal of Occupational Therapy, 28*, 346-350.

Christiansen, C. H., & Townsend, E. A. (Eds.). (2010). *An introduction to occupation: The art and science of living*, 2nd Ed. Upper Saddle River, NJ: Pearson.

Clark, F. A., Jackson, J. M., & Carlson, M. E. (2004). Occupational science, occupational therapy and evidence-based practice: What the Well Elderly Study has taught us. In M. Molineux (Ed.), *Occupation for occupational therapists* (pp. 200-218). Oxford, UK: Blackwell Publishing.

Clark, F. P. (2011). High-definition occupational therapy's competitive edge: Personal excellence is the key. *American Journal of Occupational Therapy, 65*, 616-622.

Cockburn, L., & Trentham, B. (2002). Participatory action research: integrating community occupational therapy practice and research. *Canadian Journal of Occupational Therapy, 69*, 20-30.

Commission on Social Determinants of Health. (2008). *Closing the gap in a generation: health equity through action on the social determinants of health*. Final Report of the Commission on Social Determinants of Health. Geneva, World Health Organization. Retrieved from www.who.int/social_determinants/thecommission/finalreport/en/index.html.

Corrigan, P. W.., Morris, S. B., Michaels, P. J., Rafacz, J.D., & Rüsch, N. (2012). Challenging the public stigma of mental illness: A meta-analysis of outcome studies. *Psychiatric Services, 63*(10), 963-973.

Cruickshank, W. M. (1947). The mental hygiene approach to the handicapped child. *The American Journal of Occupational Therapy, 1*, 215-221.

Davidson, D. A. (1995). Physical abuse of preschoolers: identification and intervention through occupational therapy. *American Journal of Occupational Therapy, 49*, 235-243.

Deegan, P. E. (1997). Recovery and empowerment for people with psychiatric disabilities. *Social Work in Health Care, 25*, 11-24.

Denshire, S. (2013). Re-inscribing the white, classed, gendered beginnings of occupational therapy in Australia. Paper presented to the International Research Symposium: "Therapy and Empowerment – Coercion and Punishment: Historical and Contemporary Perspectives on Labour and Occupational Therapy" 26-27 June 2013, St. Anne's College, Oxford. Retrieved from www.pulse-project.org/node/561.

Egan, M., & Delaat, M. D. (1994). Considering spirituality in occupational therapy practice. *Canadian Journal of Occupational Therapy, 61*, 95-101.

Ekbladh, E., Thorell, L-H., & Haglund, L. (2010). Return to work: the predictive value of the Worker Role Interview (WRI) over two years. *Work: A Journal of Prevention, Assessment and Rehabilitation, 35*(2), 163-172.

Eldar, R., & Jelic, M. (2003). The association of rehabilitation and war. *Disability and Rehabilitation, 25*, 1019-1023.

Fidler, G. S., & Fidler, J. W. (1963). *Occupational therapy: A communication process in psychiatry*. New York: Macmillan.

Foto, M. (1988a). Nationally speaking-managing changes in reimbursement patterns, part 1. *American Journal of Occupational Therapy, 42*, 563-565.

Foto, M. (1988b). Nationally Speaking-Managing changes in reimbursement patterns, Part 2. *American Journal of Occupational Therapy, 42*, 629-631.

Frank, G. (1992). Opening feminist histories of occupational therapy. *American Journal of Occupational Therapy, 46*, 989-999. doi:10.5014/ajot.46.11.989.

Frank, G. (2013). Twenty-first century pragmatism and social justice: problematic situations and occupational reconstructions in post-civil war Guatemala. In M. P. Cutchin & V. A. Dickie, (Eds.), *Transactional perspectives on occupation*. New York: Springer.

Friedland, J. (1998). Occupational therapy and rehabilitation: an awkward alliance. *American Journal of Occupational Therapy, 52*, 373-380. doi:10.5014/ajot.52.5.373

Friedland, J. (2011). *Restoring the spirit: the beginnings of occupational therapy in Canada, 1890-1930*. Montreal, Quebec: McGill-Queen's University.

Friedland, J., & Brumer, N. (2007). From education to occupation: the story of Thomas Bessell Kidner. *Canadian Journal of Occupational Therapy, 74*, 27-37.

George, N. M., Braun, B. A., & Walker, J. M. (1982). A prevention and early intervention mental health program for disadvantaged pre-school children. *American Journal of Occupational Therapy, 36*, 99-106.

Gibson, R. W., D'Amico M., Jaffe L., & Arbesman M. (2011). Occupational therapy interventions for recovery in the areas of community integration and normative life roles for adults with serious mental illness: A systematic review. *American Journal of Occupational Therapy 65*:247-256. doi: 10.5014/ajot.2011.001297.

Goodman, G. (2013). Information overload: Strategies to maintain competence in a changing world. *OTJR Occupational Therapy Journal of Research, 33*, 67.

Gorde, M. W., Helfrich, C. A., & Finlayson, M. L. (2004). Trauma symptoms and life skill needs of domestic violence victims. *Journal of Interpersonal Violence, 19.6*, 691-708.

Gostin, L. O. (2008). "Old" and "new" institutions for persons with mental illness: Treatment, punishment or preventive confinement? *Public Health, 122*, 906-913.

Gutman, S. A. (1997). Occupational therapy's link to vocational re-education, 1910-1925. *American Journal of Occupational Therapy, 51*, 907-915.

Gutman, S. A. (2011). Special issue: Effectiveness of occupational therapy services in mental health practice. *American Journal of Occupational Therapy, 65*, 235-237.

Gutman, S. A. (2012). State of mental health research in the American Journal of Occupational Therapy, 2008-2011. *American Journal of Occupational Therapy, 66*, e30-e33.

Hamlin, R. B. (1992). Embracing our past, informing our future: A feminist re-vision of health care. *American Journal of Occupational Therapy, 46*, 1028-1035.

Hammell, K. W. (2007). Reflections on…a disability methodology for the client-centred practice of occupational therapy research. *Canadian Journal of Occupational Therapy, 74,* 365-369.

Hammell, K. W. (2009a). Sacred texts: A sceptical exploration of the assumptions underpinning theories of occupation. *Canadian Journal of Occupational Therapy, 76,* 6-13.

Hammell, K. W. (2009b). Self-care, productivity, and leisure, or dimensions of occupational experience? Rethinking occupational "categories." *The Canadian Journal of Occupational Therapy, 26*(2), 107-14.

Hammell, K. W. (2011). Resisting theoretical imperialism in the disciplines of occupational science and occupational therapy. *British Journal of Occupational Therapy, 74*(1), 27-33.

Hanft, B. (1988). The changing environment of early intervention services: implications for practice. *American Journal of Occupational Therapy, 42,* 724-731.

Harley, L., & Schwartz, K. B. (2013). Philip King Brown and Arequipa Sanatorium: Early occupational therapy as medical and social experiment. *American Journal of Occupational Therapy, 67,* e11-e17.

Helfrich, C. A., Aviles, A. M., Badiani, C., Walens, D., & Sabol, P. (2006). Life skill interventions with homeless youth, domestic violence victims and adults with mental illness. *Occupational Therapy in Health Care, 20*(3-4), 189-207.

Henry, A. D., Nicholson, J., Phillips, S., Stier, L., & Clayfield, J. (2002). Creating job opportunities for people with psychiatric disabilities at a university-based research centre. *Psychiatric Rehabilitation Journal, 26*(2), 181-191.

Hinojosa, J. (2012). Personal strategic plan development: Getting ready for changes in our professional and personal lives. *American Journal of Occupational Therapy, 66*(3), e34-e38.

Hinojosa, J. (2013). The evidence-based paradox. *American Journal of Occupational Therapy, 67,* e18-e23.

International Association of Peer Supporters. (2013). Retrieved from http://na4ps.wordpress.com/.

Jacobs, K. (2012). PromOTing occupational therapy: Words, images, and actions. *American Journal of Occupational Therapy, 66,* 652.

Jacobson, N. (2003). Defining recovery: an interactionist analysis of mental health policy development, Wisconsin 1996-1999. *Qualitative Health Research, 13,* 378-393.

Jacobson, N., & Greenley, D. (2001). What is recovery? A conceptual model and explication. *Psychiatric Services, 52,* 482-485.

Javaherian, H. A., Underwood, R. T., & DeLany, J. V. (2007). Occupational therapy services for individuals who have experienced domestic violence (statement). *American Journal of Occupational Therapy, 61,* 704-709.

Jonsson, H. (2008). A new direction in the conceptualization and categorization of occupation. *Journal of Occupational Science, 15,* 3.

Kielhofner, G. (1992). *Conceptual foundations of practice.* Philadelphia: FA Davis.

Kirsh, B. (1996). A narrative approach to addressing spirituality in occupational therapy: Exploring personal meaning and purpose. *Canadian Journal of Occupational Therapy, 63,* 55-61.

Kirsh, B. (2000). Organizational culture, climate and person-environment fit: relationships with employment outcomes for mental health consumers, *Work, 14,* 109-122.

Kirsh, B., Cockburn, L., & Gewurtz, R. (2005). Best practice in occupational therapy: Program characteristics that influence vocational outcomes for people with serious mental illnesses. *Canadian Journal of Community Mental Health, 72,* 265-279.

Kirsh, B., Stergiou Kita, M., Gewurtz, R., Dawson, D., Krupa, T., Lysaght, R., & Shaw, L. (2009). From margins to mainstream: What do we know about work integration for persons with brain injury, mental illness and intellectual disability? *Work, 32,* 391-405.

Kroeker, P. T. (1997). Spirituality and occupational therapy in a secular culture. *Canadian Journal of Occupational Therapy, 64,* 122-126.

Kronenberg, F., Algado, S., & Pollard, N. (2005). *Occupational therapy without borders: Learning from the spirit of survivors.* Edinburgh, UK: Elsevier, Churchill Livingstone.

Krupa, T., Fossey, E., Anthony, W. A., Brown, C., & Pitts, D. B. (2009). Doing daily life: How occupational therapy can inform psychiatric rehabilitation practice. *Psychiatric Rehabilitation Journal, 32*(3), 155-161.

Krupa ,T., Lagarde, M., & Carmichael, K. (2003). Transforming sheltered workshops into affirmative businesses: An evaluation of outcomes. *Psychiatric Rehabilitation Journal, 26,* 359-367.

Letts, L. J. (2011). Optimal positioning of occupational therapy. *Canadian Journal of Occupational Therapy. 78*(4):209-19.

Lloyd, C., Waghorn, G., Lee Williams, P., Harris, M. G., & Capra, C. (2008). Early psychosis: Treatment issues and the role of occupational therapy. *British Journal of Occupational Therapy, 71,* 297-304.

Lorenzo, T., & Joubert, R. (2011). Reciprocal capacity building for collaborative disability research between disabled people's organizations, communities and higher education institutions. *Scandinavian Journal of Occupational Therapy, 18,* 254-264.

Mailoo, V. J. (2007). The Ayurvedic model of human occupation. *Asian Journal of Occupational Therapy, 6,* 1-13.

Mallinson, T., Fischer, H., Rogers, J. C., Ehrlich-Jones, L., & Chang, R. (2009). Human occupation for public health promotion: new directions for occupational therapy practice with persons with arthritis. *American Journal of Occupational Therapy, 63*(2), 220-226.

Maxwell, J. D., & Maxwell, M. P. (1978). *Occupational therapy: The diffident profession.* Kingston, ON: Queen's University Press.

McLean, A. (2003a), Recovering consumers and a broken mental health system in the United States: Ongoing challenges for consumers/survivors and the New Freedom Commission on Mental Health. Part I: Legitimization of the consumer movement and obstacles to it. *International Journal of Psychosocial Rehabilitation, 8,* 47-57.

Moll, S., & Clements, E. P.. (2008). Workplace mental health: developing an employer resource through partnerships in knowledge translation. *Occupational Therapy Now, 10*(5), 17-19.

Moll, S., Gewurtz, R., Krupa, T., & Law, M. (2013). Promoting an occupational perspective in public health. *Canadian Journal of Occupational Therapy, 80*, 111-119.

Moll, S., Holmes, J., Geronimo, J., & Sherman, D. (2009). Work transitions for peer support providers in traditional mental health programs: Unique challenges and opportunities. *Work, 33*, 449-458.

Montgomery, R. C. (1935). Occupational therapy in the mental health clinic. *Canadian Journal of Occupational Therapy, 2*, 110-114.

Montz, R., Gonzales, F., Jr., Bash, D. S., Carney, A., & Bramlett, D. (2008). Occupational therapy role on the battlefield: an overview of combat and operational stress and upper extremity rehabilitation. *The Journal of Hand Therapy, 21*, 130-135.

Morin, D., Rivard, M., Crocker, A. G., Boursier, C. P., & Caron, J. (2013). Public attitudes towards intellectual disability: a multidimensional perspective. *Journal of Intellectual Disability Research, 57*, 279-292.

Muir, S. (2012). Occupational therapy in primary health care: we should be there. *American Journal of Occupational Therapy, 66*, 506-510.

National Research Council. (2003). *Health professions education: A bridge to quality.* Washington, DC: The National Academies Press.

Nelson, A. (2007). Seeing white: A critical exploration of occupational therapy with Indigenous Australian people. *Occupational Therapy International, 14*(4), 237-255.

Nelson, A., Gray, M., Jensen, H., Thomas, Y., McIntosh, K.,... Oke, L. (2011). Closing the gap: Supporting occupational therapists to partner effectively with First Australians. *Australian Occupational Therapy Journal, 58*, 17-24.

Nelson, G. B., Lord, J., & Ochocka, J. (2001). Shifting the paradigm in community mental health: Towards empowerment and community. University of Toronto Press.

Newton, S. (2007). The growth of the profession of occupational therapy. *U.S. Army Medical Department Journal*, 51-58.

New Zealand Association of Occupational Therapy. (2006). History of the Association. Retrieved from www.otnz.co.nz/public/about-us/history-of-otnz/

Peters, C. O. (2011). Powerful occupational therapists: A community of professionals, 1950 to 1980. *Occupational Therapy in Mental Health, 27*, 199-410.

Peters, M. E. (1984). Reimbursement for psychiatric occupational therapy services. *American Journal of Occupational Therapy, 28*(5), 307-312. doi: 10.5014/ajot.38.5.307.

Precin, P. (2011a). Return to work after 9/11. *Work, 38*, 3-11.

Precin, P. (2011b). Occupation as therapy for trauma recovery: A case study. *Work, 38*, 77-81.

Quake-Rapp, C., Miller, B., Ananthan, G., & Chiu, E. C. (2008). Direct observation as a means of assessing frequency of maladaptive behavior in youths with severe emotional and behavioral disorder. *American Journal of Occupational Therapy, 62*, 206-211.

Quiroga, V. (1995). *Occupational therapy: The first 30 years 1900 to 1930.* Bethesda, MD: American Occupational Therapy Association.

Rai, S. (2002). Preventing workplace aggression and violence—A role for occupational therapy. *Work, 1*(18), 15-22.

Ray, C. G., & Finley, J. K. (1994). Did CMHCs fail or succeed? Analysis of the expectations and outcomes of the community mental health movement. *Administration and Policy in Mental Health and Mental Health Services Research, 21*, 283-293.

Rebeiro, K. L. (1998). Occupation-as-means to mental health: A review of literature, and a call for research. *Canadian Journal of Occupational Therapy, 65*, 12-19.

Rebeiro, K. L., Day, D. G., Semeniuk, B., O'Brien, M. C., & Wilson, B. (2001). NISA: An occupation-based, mental health program. *American Journal of Occupational Therapy, 55*, 493-500.

Reese, C. C. (1987). Gender bias in an occupational therapy text. *American Journal of Occupational Therapy. 41*(6), 393-396.

Reilly, M. (1962). Occupational therapy can be one of the great ideas of 20th century medicine. *American Journal of Occupational Therapy, 16*, 1-9.

Reilly, M. (1966). A psychiatric occupational therapy program as a teaching model. *American Journal of Occupational Therapy, 20*, 61-67.

Restall, G. (2013). Conceptualizing the outcomes of involving people who use mental health services in policy development. *Health Expectations.* doi: 10.1111/hex.12091

Robbins, J. E. (2001). Violence prevention in the schools: Implications for occupational therapy. *Work, 17*, 75-82.

Schultz-Krohn, W., & Cara, E. (2000). Occupational therapy in early intervention: applying concepts from infant mental health. *American Journal of Occupational Therapy, 54*, 550-554.

Schwartz, K. B. (2009). Reclaiming our heritage: Connecting the founding vision with the Centennial Vision (Eleanor Clarke Slagle Lecture). *American Journal of Occupational Therapy, 63*, 681-690.

Sedgewick, A., Cockburn, L., & Trentham, B. (2007). Occupational therapy and mental health in Canada 1930-1950: Emergence of a profession. *Canadian Occupational Therapy Journal, 74*(6), 407-417.

Sharfstein, S. S. (2000). What happened to community mental health. *Psychiatric Services, 51*, 616-620.

Shaw, L., Kollee, A., Ren, H., Lofgren, K., Saarloos, S., Slaven, K., & Bossers, A. (2013). Advancing occupational therapy in workplace health and wellbeing: A scoping review. School of Occupational Therapy Evidence Based Practice Conference 2013. London, Ontario, Canada. March 2013.

Simo-Algado, S., Mehta, N., Kronenberg, F., Cockburn, L., & Kirsh, B. (2002). Occupational therapy intervention with children survivors of war. *Canadian Journal of Occupational Therapy, 69*, 205-217.

Stamm, T. A., Cieza, A., Machold, K., Smolen, J. S., & Stucki, G. (2006). Exploration of the link between conceptual occupational therapy models and the International Classification of Functioning, Disability and Health. *Australian Occupational Therapy Journal, 53*, 9-17.

Stedman, A., & Thomas, Y. (2011). Reflecting on our effectiveness: Occupational therapy interventions with Indigenous clients. *Australian Occupational Therapy Journal, 58*, 43-49.

Stoffel, V. (2013). Opportunities for Occupational Therapy behavioral health: A call to action. *American Journal of Occupational Therapy, 67*(2), 140-145.

Substance Abuse and Mental Health Services. (2012). SAMHSA's working definition of recovery updated. Retrieved from http://blog.samhsa.gov/2012/03/23/defintion-of-recovery-updated/#.VctivlViko

Suleman, A., & Whiteford, G. E. (2013). Understanding occupational transitions in forced migration: The importance of life skills in early refugee resettlement. *Journal of Occupational Science, 20*, 201-210.

Tansella, M. (1986). Community psychiatry without mental hospitals—the Italian experience: a review. *Journal of the Royal Society of Medicine, 79*(11): 664-669.

Thomas, Y., Gray, M., & McGinty, S. (2011). Occupational therapy at the "cultural interface": Lessons from research with Aboriginal and Torres Strait Islander Australians. *Australian Occupational Therapy Journal, 58*, 11-16.

Tickle-Degden, L. (2013). Nuts and bolts of conduction feasibility studies. *American Journal of Occupational Therapy,* Vol. 67, 171-176. doi: 10.5014/ajot.2013.006270.

Townsend, E. A., & Polatajko, H. J. (2007). Enabling occupation II: Advancing an occupational therapy vision for health, well-being & justice through occupation. Ottawa, ON: CAOT Publications.

Turner, A. (2007). Health through occupation: Beyond the evidence. *Journal of Occupational Science, 14*, 9-15.

Turner, T. (2004). The history of deinstitutionalization and reinstitutionalization. *Psychiatry 3*(9), 1-4.

Watson, R., & Swartz, L., (Eds.). (2004). *Transformation through occupation: Human occupation in context.* London: Whurr Publishers.

Waugh, E., & Mackenzie, L. (2011). Ageing well from an urban Indigenous Australian perspective. *Australian Occupational Therapy Journal, 58*, 25-33.

Whalley Hammell, K. R. (2013). Client-centred practice in occupational therapy: Critical reflections. *Scandinavian Journal of Occupational Therapy 20*(3), 174-181. doi:10.3109/11038128.2012.752032.

Whitehead, C. (2007). The doctor dilemma in interprofessional education and care: How and why will physicians collaborate? *Medical Education, 41*, 1010-1016.

Wilcock, A. A. (2002). *Occupation for health: A journey from prescription to self-health.* (Vol. 2). London: British Association and College of Occupational Therapists.

Wilding, C., May, E., & Muir-Cochrane, E. (2005). Experience of spirituality, mental illness and occupation: A life-sustaining phenomenon. *Australian Journal of Occupational Therapy, 52*, 2-9.

Wilkinson, R. G., & Marmot, M. G. (2003). *Social determinants of health: the solid facts.* World Health Organization. Retrieved from www.euro.who.int/data/assets/pdf_files/0005/98438/e81384.pdf

Williams, A., Fossey, E., & Harvey, C. (2010). Sustaining employment in a social firm: Use of the Work Environment Impact Scale v2.0 to explore views of employees with psychiatric disabilities. *The British Journal of Occupational Therapy, 73*(11), 531-539.

Willoughby, C., Polatajko, H., Currado, C., Harris, K., & King, G. (2000). Measuring the self-esteem of adolescents with mental health problems: Theory meets practice. *Canadian Journal of Occupational Therapy, 67*, 230-238.

Wisenthal, A., & Krupa, T. (2013). Cognitive work hardening: A return-to-work intervention for people with depression. *Work, 45*, 423-430.

World Federation of Occupational Therapists. (2006). Position statement on Human Rights, 2006. Retrieved from www.wfot.org/ResourceCenter.aspx

World Health Organization. (1986). Ottawa charter for health promotion. Retrieved from www.who.int/healthpromotion/conferences/previous/ottawa/en/.

World Health Organization. (2005). Mental health policies and programmes in the workplace. Mental Health Policy and Service Guidance Package. Retrieved from www.who.int/mental_health/policy/workplace_policy_programmes.pdf.

World Health Organization. (2010). *Framework for action on interprofessional education and collaborative practice.* Geneva: Department of Human Resources for Health. Retrieved from www.who.int/hrh/resources/framework_action/en.

World Health Organization. (2013). *International Classification of Diseases.* Retrieved from www.who.int/classifications/icd/en/

Yerxa, E. J. (1967). 1966 Eleanor Clarke Slagle lecture. Authentic occupational therapy. *American Journal of Occupational Therapy. 21*(1), 1-9.

Yerxa, E. J. (1990). An introduction to occupational science, a foundation for occupational therapy in the 21st century. *Occupational Therapy in Health Care, 6*, 1-17.

Yerxa, E. J. (1998a). Health and the human spirit for occupation. *American Journal of Occupational Therapy, 52*, 6, 412.

Yerxa, E. J. (1998b). Occupation: The keystone of a curriculum for a self-defined profession. *American Journal of Occupational Therapy, 52*(5), 365.

Zemke, R., & Clark, F. (1996). *Occupational science: The evolving discipline.* Philadelphia: F.A. Davis.

section II

Transdisciplinary Models and Frameworks

In Section II, we examine transdisciplinary models and their relationship to psychosocial occupational therapy concepts and practices. These models cross defined knowledge, research, and practice disciplines to integrate efforts to meet common goals. We examine both how these models influence occupational therapy practice and how occupational therapy theory and practice inform the development and application of the models. Although occupational therapists who use and develop these models do so using an occupational lens, the defining principles and beliefs upon which the models rest are shared across disciplinary boundaries, allowing some degree of cohesion, vision, and opportunity for debate around concepts that can be commonly understood. Transdisciplinary models aim to provide coordinated and integrated approaches and services that can address complex needs, based on a set of shared values and beliefs.

The first of these models, the Recovery Model, is examined in Chapter 3. It is currently the guiding vision for mental health service delivery internationally, and the most widely applied approach to mental health systems and service delivery in today's mental health policy and practice context. Occupational therapists have been leaders in the field of recovery, in part because of the alignment of the core values and principles across these two arenas. Both occupational therapy and recovery approaches are deeply committed to optimizing people's potential, hope and optimism about the future, maintaining and enhancing social connections; forming of identity beyond "patient"; empowerment; and finding a sense of meaning and purpose in life. The chapter illustrates the dynamic and transformational nature of recovery and delineates how occupational engagement influences this process. Although the model is transdisciplinary, the chapter presents contrasting views of recovery and attends to the tensions between scientific and humanitarian conceptualizations. It prepares occupational therapy practitioners to use their knowledge of occupation to develop recovery-oriented interventions and to evaluate and adapt these services across contexts and populations.

Chapter 4 describes two transdisciplinary models of disability, the World Health Organization's International Classification of Functioning, Disability and Health (ICF), and the Social Model of Disability. These selected frameworks have received international recognition, and as such they have the potential to advance integrated views of function and well-being while at the same time inviting an ever-changing and evolving view of these concepts. While each model is universally accepted, they are very different from one another. The ICF is a taxonomy, or framework, for describing and measuring health and disability at individual and population levels, without addressing cause and effect. The Social Model, on the other hand, is a political model, in that it argues that political, social and community contexts create and sustain disability. Each model is useful for occupational therapy in different ways. The former enables a view of the consequences of health conditions as extending beyond the disorder and highlights that functional, activity, and participation-related consequences can have a profound impact, whereas the latter helps us understand and act on barriers to participation. The chapter considers how the psychological, emotional, and social factors central to occupation are addressed within each of these models and discusses how the models can be applied to psychosocial occupational therapy practice.

Each of these three transdisciplinary models—the Recovery Model, the ICF, and the Social Model of Disability—enable occupational therapists to develop enabling occupational therapy practices in the psychosocial arena, based on a view of the individual relative to the larger context in which occupational function and disruption are experienced.

Recovery Frameworks

Deborah Pitts, PhD, OTR/L, BCMH, CPRP and
Erin McIntyre, OTD

Recovery is a process, a way of life, an attitude, and a way of approaching the day's challenges. It is not a perfectly linear process. At times our course is erratic and we falter, slide back, regroup and start again. The need is to meet the challenge of the disability and to reestablish a new and valued sense of integrity and purpose within and beyond the limits of the disability; the aspiration is to live, work, and love in a community in which one makes a significant contribution. (Patricia Deegan as cited in Ralph, Kidder, & Phillips, 2000, p. 6)

OBJECTIVES

The objectives of this chapter are as follows:
- » Define core elements of the recovery process.
- » Contrast competing frameworks of recovery: clinical and personal.
- » Consider the influence of occupational engagement on recovery.
- » Identify implications for the recovery perspective on mental health services.
- » Identify and describe specific recovery-oriented interventions.
- » Identify and describe specific measures of recovery and recovery-oriented services.

Krupa, T., Kirsh, B., Pitts, D., & Fossey, E. *Bruce & Borg's Psychosocial Frames of Reference: Theories, Models, and Approaches for Occupation-Based Practice, Fourth Edition* (pp 37-56).

BACKGROUND

Recovery for persons labeled with psychiatric disabilities has been clearly documented (Deegan, 1988; Harding, Brooks, Ashikaga, Strauss, & Breier, 1987a, 1987b), and engagement in occupation is argued as both a means to and evidence of recovery (Davidson & Strauss, 1997; Davidson et al., 2005; Laliberte-Rudman, 2002; Young, & Ensing, 1999). The importance of the recovery concept has grown considerably over the past two decades: recovery has been adopted as an organizing framework for publicly funded mental health services internationally (Substance Abuse and Mental Health Services Administration [SAMHSA], 2010a). Evidence-based interventions (EBIs) have been developed to support recovery (Bond et al., 2004; Drake et al., 2001; Eklund, 2001) and most often include strategies for sustained and successful participation in meaningful activities and social roles (i.e., occupations; SAMHSA, 2008a, 2008b). International, national, and local initiatives are promoting the implementation of recovery-oriented services (Davidson, Tondora, Lawless, O'Connell, & Rowe, 2009), in some instances mandating the use of evidence-based interventions in publicly funded mental health practice settings (Department of Health and Human Services, 2003, 2005; Goldman et al., 2001; Isett et al., 2007). This chapter will provide a review of the emergence of the recovery perspective, an understanding of what is meant by recovery, the influence that occupational engagement can have in people's recovery experiences, an overview of recovery-oriented services, and implications for occupational therapists as they practice in such services.

Since the early 1990s, there has been an intentional and thoughtful effort within the international mental health consumer, practitioner, and research community to define and describe what mental health recovery is and how it happens (Anthony, 1993; Bellack, 2006; Corrigan, Giffort, Rashid, Leary, & Okeke, 1999; Davidson, 2003; Davidson et al., 2005; Deegan, 1988, 1996; Jacobson & Greenley, 2001; Liberman & Kopelowicz, 2005; Resnick, Rosenheck, & Lehman, 2004; Young & Ensing, 1999). Much of this effort has focused on the recovery experience of persons labeled with what have been called "serious and persistent" and/ or "enduring" psychiatric disorders (e.g., schizophrenia) served largely by publicly funded mental health services.

Definition of Recovery

Pat Deegan's definition of recovery was selected as the opening quote for this chapter given her important role as someone with lived experience who has contributed significantly to our understandings of recovery. She emphasizes the dynamic and transformational nature of recovery. One of the most oft-cited definitions of recovery was offered by Anthony, a leading scholar in the field of psychiatric rehabilitation (1993) in his *Recovery from Mental Illness: The*

Guiding Vision of the Mental Health Service System in the 1990s, which presented the following:

> Recovery is described as a deeply personal unique process of changing one's attitudes, values, feelings, goals, skills, and/or roles. It is a way of living a satisfying, hopeful, and contributing life even with limitations caused by illness. Recovery involves the development of new meaning and purpose in one's life as one grows beyond the catastrophic effects of mental illness. (p. 11)

Although they are spoken from different "voices," both Deegan's and Anthony's definitions highlight that recovery affirms that people who experience mental illness can live lives filled with meaningful social connections and occupational participation.

Whereas there is no fully agreed on definition of recovery, there is an emerging consensus regarding the dimensions and key elements of the experience of mental health recovery. Leamy, Bird, Le Boutillier, Williams, and Slade (2011) conducted a systematic review and narrative synthesis and identified five recovery *processes*, including connectedness, hope and optimism about the future, identity, meaning in life, and empowerment (p. 448).

Connectedness represents the importance of the social support that emerges in meaningful relationships with others, both peers and non-peers, and being part of the community of mental health recovery (Leamy et al., 2011). This recovery process is grounded in the very human need for social connections. It challenges common assumptions that individuals labeled with mental disorders are "asocial." Esso Leete, whose first person account is one of the earliest and often cited, noted that "a supportive, accepting, and loving relationship with others…has been the key in my recovery" (as cited in Davidson, 2003, p. 161). Davidson and Strauss (1997, p. 28) argue that having someone who believes in the person in recovery offers that person a sense of hope regarding the possibility of an "active sense of self," and as a result serves as a catalyst for the person's recovery experience. An understanding of this recovery process has informed research efforts to better understand the relational nature of service provision (Longhofer, Kubek, & Floersch, 2010), and the inclusion of peer providers within mental health service delivery (Swarbrick & Schmidt, 2010), particularly in the public mental health delivery system.

Hope and optimism about the future is represented by an individual's "belief in the possibility of recovery," "motivation to change," "positive thinking and valuing success," and "having dreams and aspirations" (Leamy et al., 2011, p. 448). Hope is understood to be a key source for initiating and sustaining engagement in the hard work of recovery. Deegan (1996) has so powerfully framed the loss of hope that the experience of living with mental illness can bring as being "hard of heart" (p. 4). In her recovery story, Deegan (1988) also articulates the important role that hope played in getting her active again:

Hope is the turning point that must quickly be followed by the willingness to act...I began in little ways with small triumphs and simple acts of courage...I rode in the car, I shopped on Wednesdays, and I talked to a friend for a few minutes...I took responsibility for my medications, took a part-time job, and had my own money...I went to school to become a psychologist so I could work with people experiencing difficulties. One day at a time, with multiple setbacks, we rebuild our lives. We rebuild our lives on the three cornerstones of recovery—hope, willingness to act, and responsible action. (pp. 11-19)

Identity is represented by the individual's efforts at "*rebuilding/redefining [a] positive sense of identity*" and "*overcoming stigma*" (Leamy et al., 2011, p. 448). The experience of mental illness, both the actual lived experience and the experience of being labeled, has a significant impact on an individual's sense of self (Davidson & Strauss, 1997). In addition, certain mental disorders first emerge during adolescence and/or young adulthood: a key period for identity development. First-person accounts highlight the experience of the illness as becoming central and all consuming: "*your label is a reality that never leaves you; it gradually shapes an identity that is hard to shed*" (Leete, 1989, p. 199). Developing an identity beyond that of "mental patient" therefore becomes a critical aspect of recovery (Argentzell, Håkansson, & Eklund, 2010; Borg & Davidson, 2007).

Meaning in life is represented by an individual's efforts to incorporate and/or make sense of the "meaning of the mental illness experience" and to build or rebuild a "meaningful life" with "social roles/goals." It also takes account of a role for "spirituality" as a source of recovery (Leamy et al., 2011, p. 448). Profound human experiences, like experiencing and being labeled with mental illness, call for sense making. It has been argued that having some way of understanding one's experience may be more important than accepting one particular perspective or explanation about what has happened (Estroff, 1989). Disengagement from work, school, and other social roles, as well as daily life routines revolving around managing one's illness, are a common experience. While this withdrawal has been found to be adaptive (Corin & Lauzon, 1991; Deegan, 1996), re-engagement in valued social roles and goals is seen as another critical aspect of recovery (Leufstadis, Erlandsson, Bjorkman, & Eklund, 2008; Sutton, Hocking, & Smythe, 2012).

Empowerment is represented by the individual taking "personal responsibility," "control over [their] life," and "focusing upon strengths" (Leamy et al., 2011, p. 448). First-person accounts have documented the lost sense of control that happens given the nature of mental illness itself, the responses of others around them and the mental health system in their efforts to protect the individual from harm (Deegan, 1988; Leete, 1989; Stainsby, 1992). As in other experiences of disability, self-determination has been identified as critical to the recovery process (Cook & Jonikas, 2002). This is seen as a particularly important given the assumptions that insight and awareness are impacted in the context of mental illness (Amador, 2000; Davidson, 2003) and the presence of involuntary commitment laws often tied to assertive community treatment approaches (Allen & Smith, 2001). This aspect of recovery encompasses the responsibility and engagement in management of one's illness, including biomedical and other management strategies. Shared decision making has emerged as a core value and explicit method for promoting such empowerment (Drake & Deegan, 2008; Drake, Deegan, & Rapp, 2010).

KEY COMPONENTS/CONCEPTS

Stages of Recovery

An alternative to the notion of recovery processes identified above is the perspective that recovery is experienced in phases and/or stages. This perspective continues to acknowledge the non-linear and dynamic nature of recovery. One of the earliest stage models was developed by Davidson and Strauss (1997) informed by their longitudinal research focused on recovery. They proposed that recovery involved the development of a "new functional sense of self" and identified the following four dimensions or phases of recovery:

1. *Discovering a more active self* refers to the individual's awareness that he or she is more than the illness. This awareness seems to emerge at a time in the experience of the illness when the individual perceives him- or herself to have the capacity for more. This awareness may be quite profound or be just an inkling of an idea. A critical influence on this perception appears to be the active presence of others in the person's support network who believe in him or her and his or her ability to re-engage in occupation. This is highlighted in the following quote by Deegan:

    As for myself, I cannot remember a specific moment when I turned that corner from surviving to becoming an active participant in my own recovery process...One thing I can recall is that the people around me did not give up on me. They kept inviting me to do things. I remember one day, for no particular reason, saying yes to helping with food shopping. All I would do was push the cart. But it was a beginning. And truly, it was through small steps like these that I slowly began to discover that I could take a stand toward what was distressing me. (1996)

2. *Taking stock of the self* refers to a review of one's strengths and limitations for engaging in daily life. It is

TABLE 3-1					
COMPARISON BETWEEN STAGES OF RECOVERY IN FIVE STUDIES					
ANDRESEN ET AL. (2003)	**DAVIDSON AND STRAUSS (1992)**	**BAXTER AND DIEHL (1998)**	**YOUNG AND ENSING (1999)**	**PETTIE AND TRIOLO (1999)**	**SPANIOL ET AL. (2000)**
Stage 1: Moratorium		Crisis recuperation			Overwhelmed by the disability
Stage 2: Awareness	Awareness of a more active self		Initiating recovery	Meaning of illness	
Stage 3: Preparation	Taking stock of self; putting self into action	Decision Rebuilding independence		What now?	Struggling with the disability
Stage 4: Rebuilding	Appealing to the self	Awakening Building healthy interdependence	Regaining and moving forward	Reconstructing identity	Living with the disability
Stage 5: Growth			Improving quality of life		Living beyond the disability

From Andresen, R., Oades, L., & Caputi, R. "The experience of recovery from schizophrenia: Towards an empirically validated stage model," *Australian & New Zealand Journal of Psychiatry, 37*(5), p. 591. Copyright © 2003 by Sage Publications Inc. Reprinted with permission.

proposed that before individuals can get active again, they must evaluate what they bring to the process and what additional skills and support they will need. Sensibilities about the readiness to engage again may be tenuous or over the mark. In this phase, the person continues to be vulnerable and having others believe in him or her remains critical. Stigma and pessimistic or critical views from members of the person's support network can undermine the continued efforts at occupational engagement.

3. *Putting the self into action* refers to the person actually engaging or re-engaging in occupation. Again, they note the person's ongoing vulnerability and the importance of being able to successfully engage as important to sustain his or her efforts at recovery. It is emphasized that the level of engagement at times may seem modest and incremental, but is important to the recovery process because, as presented below, they are actions initiated by the individual.

> It is being active, and I take pride and I'm independent to a certain extent like in my jazz music, like I'll turn on my jazz radio, and I'll love it…it's my interest. I turn the radio on myself…I'm responsible, I enjoy the music, I make notes and draw while I'm hearing it then I turn it off, then I have some evidence, I've got something done, I've been productive, I have the drawings to look at. Maybe they're damn fine drawings…It was for me and by me. (Davidson & Strauss, 1997, p. 32)

4. *Appealing to the self* refers to the person's ability to use his or her new sense of self as functional to buffer him- or herself against the ongoing effects of the illness. This dimension is particularly important to occupational therapy for it proposes a role for occupation as a protective influence for the person in recovery.

> So then I drink the coffee, it's not all that awful, I'm in a contest of will with the world, with nature, whatever, and I say to myself: "Well, damn it, you just calm down and drink your coffee." And I say to myself: "You'll just have to wait 5 minutes." So I wait. And then the roommate's still bugging me out and then I have the control, the self-esteem, the confidence, and it's manageable. (Davidson & Strauss, 1997, p. 34)

Australian researchers Andresen, Oades, and Caputi (2003; Table 3-1) compared their research findings that proposed a five-stage model of recovery with that of Davidson and Strauss, as well as four other studies that proposed a phased or staged model of recovery.

Ridgway and colleagues, as part of the Recovery Paradigm Project (1999), also proposed a stage or phased approach. The work of this project is notable, both because it was an early effort by mental health consumers to represent their experience of recovery, and because it made evident the notion that persons in recovery could have a life beyond the mental health delivery system of care. This perspective on recovery highlights the transitions and/or movement from a life focused on illness and disability to

	TABLE 3-2	
RECOVERY PARADIGM PROJECTS' RECOVERY THEMES		
MAJOR THEMES	**THE JOURNEY FROM…**	**TO…**
Reclaiming positive sense of self in spite of the challenge of psychiatric disability	Resignation	Hopefulness and realistic optimism
	Alienation	Meaning and purpose
	Mental patient	Identity beyond disorder including battling external and internalized stigma and reclaiming self-respect
Actively self-managing one's life and mental health disorder	Passive adjustments	Active consumerism
	Stress-vulnerability	Self-management and hardiness
	Self-neglect	Positive lifestyle, self-care and wellness
Reclaiming a life beyond the system	Life spent in program environments	Life space in community
	Withdrawal and inertia	Active participation in meaningful activities
	Social isolation	Relationships and sense of community

From "Deepening the mental health recovery paradigm, defining implications for practice: A report of the Recovery Paradigm Project," by P. Ridgway. 1999. Copyright © 1999 by Lawrence, KA: University of Kansas School of Social Welfare. Reprinted with permission.

one focused on action and participation. Table 3-2 identifies the major themes identified by the participants of this Recovery Paradigm Project, along with the sub-themes represented by *journeys*.

Contrasting Views on Recovery

As efforts to define and describe recovery have evolved, contrasting views of recovery have been identified. These contrasting views are mostly typically represented as dichotomous, informed by fundamentally different views regarding the recovery experience. Bellack (2006) identifies these contrasting views as either scientific or consumer conceptualizations of recovery. He emphasizes that when "comparing consumer-oriented and scientific definitions of recovery, it is important to recognize that they have evolved from very different perspectives, different historical contexts, and with different goals" (p. 434).

Scientific (Bellack, 2006) or *clinical* (Slade, 2009) definitions of recovery have been developed for research purposes, emphasizing outcomes of recovery and include efforts to develop standard, operational definitions. For example, Liberman, Kopelowicz, Ventura, and Gutkind (2002) have identified the following as key criteria to be considered in recovery: sustained levels of symptom remission as rated on a symptom rating scale, engagement in at least 20 hours of productive activity weekly, living on one's own without assistance, and participation in social activities at least once a week. These definitions of recovery tend not to address the subjective experience of recovery, which may be very meaningful to mental health consumers. They may, however, address what is referred to as family burden. Furthermore, these definitions have been developed via a consensus process, but have yet to be supported via research (Bellack, 2009; Slade, 2009).

In contrast, *consumer-oriented* (Bellack, 2006) or *personal* (Slade, 2009) definitions of recovery have been heavily influenced by the mental health consumer movement, which is often considered to be a civil rights movement (Chamberlin, 1997a), a movement that sought to change perceptions about mental illness and mental health policies. These definitions have attended to both internal experiences of recovery (i.e., a sense of self) and external factors that may act as resources or barriers to recovery (i.e., financial resources, stigma, and discrimination). These definitions frame recovery as a process that happens over time in a non-linear way, and as a result are seen as nonspecific and are of limited value as research criteria. The perspective offered in this chapter clearly is informed by this consumer or personal perspective on recovery. Gordon (2013) draws on her experience as a mental health consumer and recovery researcher to argue that the process-outcome debate regarding recovery is problematic, and that "it is essential to the progress of recovery-based services that the mental health field avoid the trap of dualistic, either-or approach to recovery" (p. 270).

Dickerson (2006) expressed deep concern that the recovery perspective did not address the experience of all persons living with, and challenged by, mental illness, nor the very real socioeconomic barriers of poverty experienced by those living on government-supported disability payments in particular. Lal (2010), a Canadian occupational therapy researcher, also challenged the recovery perspective regarding the degree that it addresses the needs of seniors, minorities, children and youth, recent immigrants, and refugees.

KEY DEVELOPERS/THEORISTS

While contributions to the development of the recovery perspective have been widespread and include many individuals with lived experience, three key contributors to the development of our contemporary understandings are identified here—Patricia Deegan, Larry Davidson, and William A. Anthony. Each of these individuals has contributed philosophical and practice guidance that has informed the development of recovery-oriented services internationally.

Patricia Deegan, PhD is an internationally recognized mental health consumer advocate who began her mental illness and recovery journey at the age of 17 when she was labeled with schizophrenia. In her first-person accounts, Deegan tells the compelling story about being told to ready herself for a life of disability (Deegan, 1988). In spite of this dire prediction, one that many people have reported in their first encounter with the mental health system, Deegan went on to complete her PhD in clinical psychology and has made substantial contributions to recovery-oriented practice. Early on, her key contribution was in telling her story in a way that was profoundly accessible to mental health practitioners. Over the years, she has re-told and re-shaped her recovery journey story, including identifying as a trauma survivor and includes her experience with occupational therapy:

> Later in my recovery, I became willing to do psychotherapy in order to work through a history of child abuse. This was long and difficult work and I am glad I embarked on it after I had established myself in a meaningful career and had a strong network of friends. I needed to be firmly planted in the present as an adult, in order to look back at the trauma in my childhood. In the course of doing the trauma work, I sought out the help of an occupational therapist who specialized in sensory defensiveness in adults. She helped me learn a myriad of coping strategies including use of a

sand blanket, joint compression, tactile brushing, and the use of a sensory diet to help me modulate sensory input and affective arousal. These strategies have proved tremendously helpful and are a part of my everyday recovery "toolkit." (Deegan, 2001)

Deegan's key scholarship and contribution to recovery-oriented practice has been her commitment to strengthening mental health providers' readiness to make the necessary human connections to support recovery. This begins with her *The Lived Experience of Rehabilitation* (Deegan, 1988), continues with her *Recovery: A Journey of the Heart* (Deegan, 1996), her development of the National Empowerment Center's Hearing Voices that are Distressing Workshop (www.power2u.org), her collaborative development of the Intentional Care approach (www.advocatesinc.org/Resources-IntentionalCare/#), and extends to her recent work on shared decision making between mental health consumers and providers (Deegan & Drake, 2006; Deegan, Rapp, Holter, & Riefer, 2008).

Larry Davidson, PhD, is a phenomenological psychologist and prolific writer and collaborator. His long-time collaboration with Yale University colleague John Strauss, MD, provided some of the earliest articulations of what recovery meant for persons labeled with schizophrenia (Davidson & Strauss, 1997). He has continued to collaborate internationally with other schizophrenia and recovery researchers (including occupational therapists), such as David Roe (Israel), Marit Borg (Scandinavia), and Terry Krupa and Ellie Fossey (Canada and Australia). A key focus of his research has been to make the lived experience of mental illness more evident. Drawing on his phenomenological roots, he showed how necessary and critical an understanding of the subjective experience of illness and recovery is to designing meaningful and truly supportive recovery-oriented services (Davidson, 2003). Davidson is a strong advocate for occupational therapy in the mental health field, acknowledging that:

> When I started my training to become a clinical psychologist who wanted to specialize in working with individuals with serious psychiatric disabilities, it was often the occupational therapist on the team that I went to when I was having difficulties helping a client…It was the role of the occupational therapist to conduct functional assessments and to pay attention to how the person got along on an everyday basis. What did he do? How did she spend her time? What accommodations might this person need to function more effectively? These were the questions that seemed to matter most to the person, and certainly mattered to me. (Davidson as cited in Krupa et al., 2010)

In addition, to his continued research collaborations, Davidson has sought to influence systems of care.

Much of this work has taken shape in his collaboration with the Connecticut Department of Mental Health and Addiction Services and culminated in the publication of *A Practical Guide to Recovery-Oriented Practice: Tools for Transforming Mental Health Care* written in collaboration with Janis Tondora, Martha Staeheli Lawless, Maria J. O'Connell, and Michael Rowe. More recently, he has taken the lead in SAMHSA's Recovery to Practice Initiative (www.samhsa.gov/recoverytopractice/), which has sought to change mental health practice by enlisting key professional organizations, including the American Psychiatric Association, American Psychiatric Nurses Association, American Psychological Association, Council on Social Work Education, and the National Association of Peer Specialists.

William A. Anthony, PhD, is a psychiatric rehabilitation researcher and advocate who began his mental health practice in rehabilitation counseling. He is best known for serving as the Director of Boston University's Center for Psychiatric Rehabilitation (http://cpr.bu.edu/), which over the years became the preeminent source for psychiatric rehabilitation interventions and professional development resources. He was instrumental in shaping the interdisciplinary profession of psychiatric rehabilitation and advocating for its inclusion in the evolving U.S. mental health service system. He served as the editor of the *Psychiatric Rehabilitation Journal*, helping to develop its role as primary professional publication for staying current on recovery-oriented services.

IMPORTANT EVOLUTIONARY POINTS

Ridgeway (2001) and others (Bellack, 2006; Jacobson & Greenley, 2001) argue that the recent (1990s to present) turn to recovery as a viable outcome for persons labeled with mental illness emerges from several converging events. First, the broad dissemination of first-person accounts of recovery during the 1980s (see for example, Deegan, 1988; Houghton, 1982; Leete, 1989) provided clear and poignant descriptions of the lived experience of recovery, positioned people with mental illnesses as authorities in their recovery journeys, and identified how service systems helped and hindered recovery. Second, qualitative studies documented the experience of recovery (Davidson & Strauss, 1997; Young & Ensing, 1999). These qualitative studies in particular furthered our understanding of the process of recovery, including introducing a perspective that recovery happens in phases or stages. Finally, the empirical evidence beginning with the foundational work of Harding and her colleagues (1987a, 1987b) showed that recovery was possible. Harding's work in particular demonstrated that, even with persistent and serious mental illness, positive functional changes and quality of life were possible. When taken together, these sources for recovery have provided both the

humanitarian, as well as the "science" upon which the current perspectives on recovery are developing.

Another way to make sense of the evolution of the contemporary recovery perspective is to situate it within the shifts and changes in psychiatric practice itself (Davidson, Rakfeldt, & Strauss, 2010; Rutman, 1987), as well as broader sociopolitical movements (Chamberlin, 1997a, 1997b). Histories of psychiatry, as well as occupational therapy, provide an early perspective on recovery in response to what is known as moral treatment. Moral treatment has been variously characterized as a combination of the reduction of the use of restraint, increased opportunities for occupational engagement, and increased access to interpersonal connections with caring mental health providers, including peers in recovery (Bockoven, 1963; Davidson et al., 2010). Davidson et al. (2010) highlight their sense of the "lessons learned" regarding recovery that emerged from moral treatment and resonates well with occupational therapy:

- Many people recover from serious mental illness, either with or without treatment.

- Even when acutely ill, many people with serious mental illness retain certain of their mental faculties intact, with domains of health and competence coexisting with domains of dysfunction and impairment.

- Some individuals recovering from serious mental illness may be particularly well suited to taking care of others suffering from these conditions because they will have more empathy and compassion for their struggles and will likely treat them with more dignity, respect, and kindness.

- When provided the opportunity, most people with serious mental illness remain capable of working without any particular accommodations or supports.

- Engaging in work that the person finds interesting and/or enjoyable appears to promote recovery, perhaps more than any other single factor (p. 59).

Although moral treatment was abandoned by psychiatry in the later part of the 19th century, it informed the Progressive Era mental hygiene movement of the early 20th century within which the profession of occupational therapy took shape in the United States (Kielhofner & Burke, 1977). Adolf Meyer's psychobiological perspective— "common sense" psychiatry—provided a key framing for understanding the experience of mental illness and recovery during this time (Meyer, 1957). Meyer argued for what he called problems with living rather than fixed diagnostic categories, and emphasized that a person's history or biography was critical in making sense of his or her current distress (Lidz, 1966). Influenced by his pragmatist philosophy, Meyer believed that embodied action led to habits of the mind and emphasized our use of time including the importance of a "balance of work, rest, play and sleep" (Meyer, 1922). Davidson et al. (2010) argue for another

Progressive Era phenomenon, the settlement house as represented by Jane Addams Hull House as helping to shape the contemporary recovery movement. Hull House is, of course, important for occupational therapy given Eleanor Clarke Slagle, a key player in early occupational therapy in the United States, worked and took her occupations course there. Again, Davidson and his colleagues (2010) identify the following "lessons learned" regarding recovery from this period:

- People do not always have to be removed from their current life circumstances to receive assistance in addressing and overcoming difficulties.

- People can be assisted in managing their own difficulties and lives, rather than to have those difficulties, and their lives as a whole, taken over by others (p. 97).

- Mental illnesses, like life itself, are most likely multifaceted and multidimensional phenomena that involve biological, psychological, and sociocultural components.

- Having first-person experiences of mental illness, whether in one's own life or in the life of a friend or loved one, can be used advantageously in shedding light on the nature of mental illness, especially on the fact that it is an aspect of human experience and does not reduce the person afflicted to subhuman or alien existence.

- People can make progress by identifying and building on their personal assets and strengths (p. 143).

In many countries, deinstitutionalization has represented a key structural shift in the history of mental health service delivery that gave space for the emergence of contemporary community-based approaches (Rutman, 1987). In addition, the larger sociopolitical movements of the 1960s and 1970s, including the mental health consumer and/or psychiatric survivor's movement, also represent important macro influences on our understanding of mental illness and recovery. Here, Davidson (2010) and colleagues' "lessons learned" regarding recovery emphasize cautions:

- Institutions do more harm than good, adding to the burden of disease a sense of demoralization, hopelessness, and helplessness.

- Rather than promoting recovery, adopting the identity of a "mental patient" poses an additional barrier or obstacle to recovery.

- If agency plays a key role in recovery, then the restoration of person's sovereignty and civil rights needs to precede, rather than follow, recovery (p. 177).

OCCUPATIONAL ENGAGEMENT AND RECOVERY

Evidence of the influence of occupation on recovery is clearly articulated in first person accounts. For example Joan Houghton (1982) emphasized that "to maintain a sense of well-being, I have had to change my lifestyle and my priorities. My illness has taught me (the hard way) the importance of meaningful work, good patterns of rest and sleep, exercise, diet, and self-discipline" (p. 549). Similarly, Esso Leete (1989) captures the rich role that occupations play in recovery:

> To maintain my mental health...I have...had to plan for the use of my time. When one has a chaotic inner existence, the structure of a predictable daily schedule makes life easier. Now, obviously structured activity can be anything, but for me it is work—a paying job, the ultimate goal. It gives me something to look forward to every day and a skill to learn and to improve. It is my motivation for getting up each morning. In addition, my hours are passed therapeutically as well as productively. As I work, I become increasingly self-confident and my self-image is bolstered. I feel important and grown up, which replaces my sense of vulnerability, weakness, and incompetence. Being a member of the work force decreases stigma and contributes to acceptance by my community, which in turn makes life easier. (p. 197)

Research on recovery and the occupational experiences of persons with mental illness's related disabilities has come primarily from international occupational therapy researchers in Canada, UK, Australia, and Scandinavia (Chaffey & Fossey, 2004; Eklund, Hansson, & Ahlqvist, 2004; Kennedy-Jones, Cooper, & Fossey, 2005; Kirsh & Cockburn, 2007; Krupa, 2004; Krupa, Radloff-Gabriel, Whippey, & Kirsh, 2002; Laliberte-Rudman, Yu, Scott, & Pajouhandeh, 2000; Lloyd, Bassett, & King., 2002; Mee, Sumsion, & Craik, 2004; Rebeiro, 1999), as well as other recovery researchers (Carless & Douglas, 2008). A brief summary of some of the research findings, drawn from qualitative studies exploring the experience of occupational engagement and recovery, offers evidence that intentional engagement in occupation within supportive environments supports the recovery process:

- Occupation provides a sense of achievement that builds self-efficacy (Carless & Douglas, 2008; Krupa, 2004;

TABLE 3-3		
COMPARISON OF RECOVERY ASSUMPTIONS AND OCCUPATIONAL THERAPY ASSUMPTIONS		
Assumptions	Recovery (Anthony, 2000)	Occupational therapy (Polatajko, 1992)
Self-determination	Can occur without professional intervention	Individuals have the right to autonomy
Social support	Common denominator is the presence of people who believe in and stand by the person in need of recovery	Individuals are social beings
Process, not cause-effect	Vision of recovery is not a function of one's theory about the causes of mental illness	Value of human life is on meaning
Focus on strengths	Can occur even though symptoms reoccur	Individuals have abilities and competencies
Uniqueness	Unique process	Each individual is a unique whole
Client-centered	Demands that a person has choices	Each individual has the right to autonomy
Iatrogenesis	Consequences of the illness are sometimes more difficult for recovery than illness itself	Individuals shape and are shaped by their environment.

From Reberio-Gruhl, K. L. "The recovery paradigm: Should occupational therapists be interested?", *Canadian Journal of Occupational Therapy*, 72 (2), pp. 98. Copyright © 2005 by Sage Publications Inc. Reprinted with permission.

Leufstadis et al., 2008; Mee & Sumsion, 2001; Mee et al., 2004; Roe & Chopra, 2003), and personal mastery (Argentzell et al., 2010). Work in particular, has been linked to recovery (Krupa, 2004).

- Occupation facilitates formation of identity beyond that of "mental patient," (i.e., the sense of "being normal"; Andresen et al., 2003; Argentzell et al., 2010; Carless & Douglas, 2008; Krupa, 2004; Lloyd, Wong, & Petchkovsky, 2007; Mee et al., 2004; Ridgway, 2001).

- Occupations provide opportunity for maintaining and enhancing social connections, reduce the strain of social isolation, and buffer the impact of public stigma (Argentzell et al., 2010; Carless & Douglas, 2008; Leufstadis et al., 2008; Lloyd et al., 2007; Sutton et al., 2012).

- Participation in occupation provides temporal support in the form of structure and organization to one's day, helps to "keep busy" (Argentzell et al., 2010; Carless & Douglas, 2008; Leufstadis et al., 2008; Mee et al., 2004; Sutton et al., 2012).

- Occupation can provide a sense of control, self-direction, and empowerment (Carless & Douglas, 2008; Deegan, 2005; Krupa, 2004; Lloyd et al., 2007; Young & Ensing, 1999).

- Occupation fosters hope, provides sense of meaning/purpose, especially spiritual occupations (Argentzell et al., 2010; Leufstadis et al., 2008; Lloyd et al., 2007; Mee

& Sumsion, 2001; Sutton et al., 2012), and possibilities for future participation and sense of hope (Carless & Douglas, 2008; Deegan, 2005).

- Participation in occupation facilitates symptom management or acts as a coping strategy (Argentzell et al., 2010; Carless & Douglas, 2008; Krupa, 2004; Leufstadis et al., 2008; Lloyd et al., 2007; Young & Ensing, 1999).

Providing a framework for understanding occupational therapy in relation to recovery, Rebeiro-Gruhl (2005) examined both the Recovery Model as explicated in psychosocial rehabilitation (Anthony, 2000) and occupational therapy (Polatajko, 1992) to compare the core assumptions underlying each. This comparison is summarized in Table 3-3.

EVALUATION PROCESSES FOR OUTCOMES

Efforts to measure recovery outcomes are fraught with the same tensions identified previously regarding what counts as recovery (e.g., symptom remission vs. participation-focused outcomes, including full citizenship, and for some full separation from the mental health system; Ralph, Kidder, & Phillips, 2000). Despite these tensions, there have been efforts to develop tools

---

BOX 3-1. MEASURES TO ASSESS RECOVERY OUTCOMES

The Stages of Recovery Instrument (STORI) (Andresen et al., 2006) is designed to capture the following stages of recovery from the consumer's perspective: *moratorium (a time of withdrawal characterized by a profound sense of loss and hopelessness); awareness (realization that all is not lost, and that a fulfilling life is possible); preparation (taking stock of strengths and weaknesses regarding recovery, and starting to work on developing recovery skills); rebuilding (actively working toward a positive identity, setting meaningful goals and taking control of one's life); and growth (living a full and meaningful life, characterized by self-management of the illness, resilience and a positive sense of self).* The STORI comprises 50 items, each of which is rated on a 6-point Likert scale. Sample questions include "I don't think people with mental illness can get better," "I feel my life has been ruined by this illness," "because others believe in me, I've *just started* to think maybe I can get better," "I am learning new things about myself as I work toward recovery."

The Recovery Assessment Scale (Corrigan et al., 2004) is designed to assess various aspects of recovery from the perspective of the consumer, with a particular emphasis on hope and self-determination. The original instrument comprises 41 items, and a shorter version containing 24 items is also available. In both versions, each item is rated on a 5-point Likert scale. It covers five domains: personal confidence and hope, willingness to ask for help, goal and success orientation, reliance on others, and no domination by symptoms. Sample questions include "I have a desire to succeed," "even when I don't care about myself, others do," and "I am the person most responsible for my own improvement."

---

that capture various dimensions and/or stages of recovery. Examples of outcomes measures that have been identified as being brief and easy to use, taking a consumer perspective, and having scientific strength include the Stages of Recovery Instrument (Andresen et al., 2006) and the Recovery Assessment Scale (Corrigan, Salzer, Ralph, Sangster, Keck, 2004). Brief descriptions of these are provided in Box 3-1.

PRACTICE DEVELOPMENTS

Efforts at incorporating practices informed by the recovery paradigm have been taken up at all levels of the mental health services (DHHS, 2003, 2005). There is now a rich set of materials available to ready mental health practitioners to establish practice competencies that will support persons labeled with mental illness related disabilities in their recovery journey. Over the last three decades, there has been a proliferation of journal publications and books on the experience of recovery (Davidson, 2003) as well as workbooks for self-managed and professionally guided recovery-oriented interventions (Davidson et al., 2009). These practice developments are framed here at various levels—system, program, and provider.

Recovery-Oriented Mental Health Delivery Systems

At the national, regional, and local level, mental health system authorities have adopted recovery as a guiding approach for mental health services. Values to guide the development and implementation of recovery-oriented services have been identified (Anthony, 1993). For example, the U.S.-based National Empowerment Center (www.power2u.org), a consumer-run technical assistance organization, advocates that "a recovery-based mental health system would embrace the values of self-determination, empowering relationships based on trust, understanding and respect, meaningful roles in society, and elimination of stigma and discrimination" (Fisher & Chamberlin, n.d., p. 1). The SAMHSA adopted a National Consensus Statement on Mental Health Recovery (Box 3-2), which defines components of recovery and outlined principles to guide service delivery.

Recovery-Oriented Programs and Services

In addition to public policy initiatives to promote recovery (DHHS, 2003, 2005), identifying specific characteristics of programs that can facilitate recovery have also been identified (Ridgway, 1999). Best practices that are most likely to provide the contextual supports needed by persons labeled with a mental health–related disability to develop the internal resources and behavioral repertoire to achieve their recovery goals are being developed and tested (Davidson et al., 2005; Davidson et al., 2009; Slade, 2009). However, the fit between recovery and evidence-based practices has been questioned (Anthony, Rogers, & Farkas, 2003), and how available evidence-based interventions resonate with the recovery perspective continues to be explored (Bond et al., 2004; Farkas, Gagne, Anthony, & Chamberlin, 2005). For example, one of the most widely disseminated evidence-based practices is *assertive community treatment* (ACT; SAMHSA, 2008a). This community mental health

BOX 3-2. NATIONAL CONSENSUS STATEMENT ON MENTAL HEALTH RECOVERY

Self-Direction: Consumers lead, control, exercise choice over, and determine their own path of recovery by optimizing autonomy, independence, and control of resources to achieve a self-determined life. By definition, the recovery process must be self-directed by the individual, who defines his or her own life goals and designs a unique path toward those goals.

Individualized and Person-Centered: There are multiple pathways to recovery based on an individual's unique strengths and resiliencies as well as his or her needs, preferences, experiences (including past trauma), and cultural background in all of its diverse representations. Individuals also identify recovery as being an ongoing journey and an end result as well as an overall paradigm for achieving wellness and optimal mental health.

Empowerment: Consumers have the authority to choose from a range of options and to participate in all decisions—including the allocation of resources—that will affect their lives, and are educated and supported in so doing. They have the ability to join with other consumers to collectively and effectively speak for themselves about their needs, wants, desires, and aspirations. Through empowerment, an individual gains control of his or her own destiny and influences the organizational and societal structures in his or her life.

Holistic: Recovery encompasses an individual's whole life, including mind, body, spirit, and community. Recovery embraces all aspects of life, including housing, employment, education, mental health, and health care treatment and services, complementary and naturalistic services, addictions treatment, spirituality, creativity, social networks, community participation, and family supports as determined by the person. Families, providers, organizations, systems, communities, and society play crucial roles in creating and maintaining meaningful opportunities for consumer access to these supports.

Nonlinear: Recovery is not a step-by-step process but one based on continual growth, occasional setbacks, and learning from experience. Recovery begins with an initial stage of awareness in which a person recognizes that positive change is possible. This awareness enables the consumer to move on to fully engage in the work of recovery.

Strengths-Based: Recovery focuses on valuing and building on the multiple capacities, resiliencies, talents, coping abilities, and inherent worth of individuals. By building on these strengths, consumers leave stymied life roles behind and engage in new life roles (e.g., partner, caregiver, friend, student, employee). The process of recovery moves forward through interaction with others in supportive, trust-based relationships.

Peer Support: Mutual support—including the sharing of experiential knowledge and skills and social learning—plays an invaluable role in recovery. Consumers encourage and engage other consumers in recovery and provide each other with a sense of belonging, supportive relationships, valued roles, and community.

Respect: Community, systems, and societal acceptance and appreciation of consumers—including protecting their rights and eliminating discrimination and stigma—are crucial in achieving recovery. Self-acceptance and regaining belief in one's self are particularly vital. Respect ensures the inclusion and full participation of consumers in all aspects of their lives.

Responsibility: Consumers have a personal responsibility for their own self-care and journeys of recovery. Taking steps towards their goals may require great courage. Consumers must strive to understand and give meaning to their experiences and identify coping strategies and healing processes to promote their own wellness.

Hope: Recovery provides the essential and motivating message of a better future—that people can and do overcome the barriers and obstacles that confront them. Hope is internalized; but can be fostered by peers, families, friends, providers, and others. Hope is the catalyst of the recovery process.

Reprinted with permission from Substance Abuse and Mental Health Services Administration (2006). http://store.samhsa.gov/shin/content//SMA05-4129/SMA05-4129.pdf

intervention uses a team-based, transdisciplinary approach to reduce hospitalization and promote community integration of people with mental illness who have been high users of intensive services. Despite the evidence and international adoption of this practice, the degree to which ACT is recovery oriented has been questioned (Drake & Deegan, 2008; Kidd et al., 2010; Salyers & Tsemberis, 2007), especially given the perception that it is too medical-model oriented

---

Box 3-3. Qualities of Recovery Facilitating Environments

- Challenging environments that promote participation, learning, and striving
- Hopeful environments that promote positive expectations that inspire and encourage
- Resource-rich environments that meet basic needs, provide choices, opportunities, and needed supports
- Caring environments that are respectful and compassionate
- Environments that provide opportunities for meaningful participation and significant contribution
- Environments that help people feel powerful
- Environments that connect people to one another in meaningful ways

---

(Gomory, 2005). In response to these challenges, there have been efforts to document ways in which ACT teams can practice a recovery-oriented approach (Cuddeback et al., 2013; Salyers et al., 2013). Occupational therapists have also explored this question in light of their philosophy and practice values (Krupa et al., 2002).

With a focus on developing programs and services that are enabling of recovery, attention has been paid to the qualities of environments and contexts that are likely to promote recovery. Box 3-3 summarizes specific qualities that have been associated with recovery-enabling environments.

Supported life approaches, given their emphasis on full community integration, personal choice, and the provision of supports in the natural environment, are seen as having good alignment with the recovery orientation. These evidence-based approaches target different life domains and include supported employment (SAMHSA, 2009), supported housing (SAMHSA, 2010b), and supported education (SAMHSA, 2012). Since being identified, these evidence-based practices have been promoted in professional publications and toolkits have been developed and are available via the web (www.samhsa.gov). In addition, government mental health authorities have initiated strategic efforts to bring these evidence-based practices to their service providers (see for example, NASMHPD, 2004).

Intervention manuals that target illness management and recovery have also been developed, disseminated, and tested. Examples include the Wellness Recovery Action Plan (WRAP; Copeland, 2001), SAMHSA's Illness Management and Recovery Intervention (SAMHSA, 2008b), and the Center for Psychiatric Rehabilitation's Recovery Workbook (Spaniol, Koehler, & Hutchinson, 2009).

- *Wellness Recovery Action Plan* (WRAP; Copeland, 2001) represents one of the earliest of these approaches and was developed by Mary Ellen Copeland. Copeland has leveraged her recovery experience, and the recovery experience of other mental health consumers, to design an approach to dealing with difficult feelings and maintaining wellness in the face of mental ill-

ness. She and her colleagues at The Copeland Center (http://copelandcenter.com/) have developed a range of recovery resources that target the needs of different populations. An important aspect of the WRAP approach is its self-management approach, which aligns well with the growth of peer-support as a key aspect of recovery-oriented practices. A growing body of research evidence is demonstrating that WRAP has good potential to positively influence recovery by, for example, facilitating hope, providing self-management strategies, and facilitating recognition of early warning signs (Cook et al., 2010).

- *The Recovery Workbook: Practical Coping and Empowerment Strategies for People with Psychiatric Disabilities* (Spaniol, et al., 2009) was developed and is available from the Center for Psychiatric Rehabilitation (http://cpr.bu.edu/). It represents an evidence-based recovery curriculum that facilitates reflection and action toward recovery, increased knowledge and control, management of life's stresses, enhanced personal meaning, building personal support, and setting personal goals. The workbook can be used as part of a consumer-led workshop, course, or conducted seminar, or as a self-study course by individual consumers. Barbic, Krupa, and Armstrong (2009) conducted a multicenter, prospective, single-blind, randomized controlled trial of implementation of the Recovery Workbook training with persons receiving assertive community treatment. They found positive change in perceived level of hope, empowerment, and recovery for the intervention group.

- *SAMHSA's Illness Management and Recovery (IMR; SAMHSA, 2008b)* was developed from a comprehensive review of the research on teaching illness management strategies. It is available from SAMHSA (http://store.samhsa.gov/product/Illness-Management-and-Recovery-Evidence-Based-Practices-EBP-KIT/SMA09-4463). The IMR intervention is informed by a core set of recovery-oriented values and includes various modules that can be delivered either in a group or individual format. Sample module topics include Coping with Problems and Persistent Symptoms, and Building Social Support. Research has documented its effectiveness (Mueser et al., 2004; Mueser et al., 2006).

Although addressing illness management is important in the support of recovery, occupational therapy researchers have been engaged in the development of interventions to target participation outcomes. Indeed Davidson, in his forward to Krupa and colleagues' (2010) *Action Over Inertia* manualized intervention, argues that this is an important role for occupational therapy research and intervention development.

> It is occupational science and therapy as a field that offers the most experience and expertise in issues of everyday life that the rest of psychiatry is just now beginning to grapple with. (p. vi)

Action Over Inertia: Addressing the Activity-Health Needs of Individuals with Serious Mental Illness (Edgelow & Krupa, 2011; Krupa et al., 2010) is available from the Canadian Occupational Therapy Association (www.caot.ca/index.asp). This workbook is informed by occupational therapy's belief and profound commitment to facilitating engagement in occupation to support health and well-being. The intervention approach highlights the importance of explicitly linking occupational engagement to recovery in mental health service delivery. In addition, it draws on research that empirically and qualitatively documents the link between participation and health for persons with serious mental illness. Finally, it draws on research evidence regarding ways to address the common volitional disruptions experienced by persons with serious mental illness. The workbook is intended as a guide for occupational therapists and other mental health practitioners. Key elements of the intervention are identifying and understanding an individual's current activity patterns and activity preferences; activity "experiments" to jump start engagement in activity; education regarding the link between activity, health, and mental illness; and planning and supporting longer term activity engagement efforts. A pilot study that used a randomized controlled design demonstrated efficacy and clinical utility (Edgelow & Krupa, 2011).

Efforts to measure the degree to which mental health services have fully adopted and implemented a recovery-orientation have been developed to meet the needs of policy makers and accreditation organizations (Campbell-Orde, Chamberlin, Carpenter, & Leff, 2005; Ralph et al., 2000). Examples of such instruments include the Recovery Oriented Systems Indicators Measure (Campbell-Orde et al., 2005) and the Recovery Self-Assessment (Davidson et al., 2009; O'Connell, Tondora, Croog, Evans, & Davidson, 2005). Brief descriptions of these instruments are offered in Box 3-4.

Recovery-Oriented Providers and Practitioners

Patricia Deegan has offered some of the most meaningful guidance for the front-line practitioner in supporting persons labeled with psychiatric disorders as they engage in their recovery efforts. In particular, *Recovery as a Journey of the Heart* (Deegan, 1996) draws on her existential-phenomenological perspective to ready recovery-oriented practitioners for their work:

> I would say that when those of us with psychiatric disabilities come to believe that all of our efforts are futile; when we experience that we have no control over our environment; when nothing we do seems to matter or to make the situation better; when we follow the treatment teams' instructions and achieve their treatment goals for us and still no placement opens up in the community for us; when we try one medication after another after another and none of them seem to be of any help; when we find that staff do not listen to us and that they make all of the major decisions for us; when staff decide where we will live, with whom we will live; under what rules we will live, how we will spend our money, when we will have to leave the group home, and at what time we will be allowed back into it, etc. etc. etc., then a deep sense of hopelessness, of despair begins to settle over the human heart. And in an effort to avoid the biologically disastrous effects of profound helplessness, people with psychiatric disabilities do what other people do. We grow hard of heart and attempt to stop caring. (p. 94)

She goes on to offer the following guidance about how to enter into recovery-oriented relationships with persons who are hard of heart:

- Understand the existential significance of the hard-of-heart behavior and the very real risk that we are asking people to take when inviting them to care about something again.

- Suspend any perceptions of the person as fragile, or as what used to be known as a "chronic mental patient" and see them as a survivor with all that entails.

- Understand that practitioners do not have the power to change or motivate a person with a mental health-related disability who is hard of heart, but they do have power to change their environment (p. 95).

Deegan's guidance supports the importance of hope identified earlier in this chapter as important to the experience of recovery, and understood as often emerging out of relationships with important others (Davidson,

---

BOX 3-4. MEASURES TO ASSESS IMPLEMENTATION OF RECOVERY-ORIENTATION

Recovery Oriented Systems Indicators Measure (Campbell-Orde et al., 2005) was developed by Steven J. Onken and Jeanne M. Dumont. It includes a 42-item consumer self-report that includes eight domains: person-centered decision-making and choice, invalidated personhood, self-care and wellness, basic life resources, meaningful activities and roles, peer advocacy, staff treatment knowledge, and access. In addition to the consumer self-report, there is an administrative profile with six domains: peer support, choice, staffing ratio, system culture and orientation, consumer inclusion in governance, and coercion.

Recovery Self-Assessment (Davidson et al., 2009; O'Connell et al., 2005) captures the perceptions of persons in recovery, practitioners, family members, significant others, advocates, and agency directors. It contains 36 items and is available in four different versions for multiple stakeholders. Analysis of the items can be understood across four factors: roles and responsibilities in recovery addressing risk taking, decision making, etc.; nonlinearity of the recovery process addressing the role of illness and symptom management; the roles of self-definition and peers addressing a person's activities in defining identity for self, etc.; and expectations regarding recovery. Sample questions from the Practitioner Version include "people in recovery can choose and change, if desired, the therapists, psychiatrist, or other service provider with whom they work," "Staff and agency participants are encouraged to take risks and try new things," etc.

2003). Russinova (1999) argued that a practitioner's "hope-inspiring competence" (p. 50) influences the effectiveness of recovery-oriented services. She identifies that recovery-oriented practitioners need to do the following:

- *Believe in the potential for recovery*, especially for those that are hard of heart. These beliefs are profoundly influenced and shaped by professional training and subsequent work experience.

- *Have the capacity to tolerate the uncertainty regarding future outcomes.* This is particularly critical given that the factors that determine recovery are not completely known. As a result, we have to work without knowing for certain the outcome or speed of recovery.

- *Have motivation for promoting better outcomes.* This requires containment of our own feelings of helplessness with the often slow improvement seen in recovery and "good memory" for small achievements.

- *Hope-inspiring resourcefulness*, for utilizing their interpersonal resources (Box 3-5), and for mobilizing a person's internal resources for recovery (Box 3-6).

Efforts to measure provider capacities and qualities continue to be developed (Box 3-7). For example, occupational therapist Shu-Ping Chen (2011), concerned that the practice of recovery in the inpatient setting had received relatively little attention, has developed a recovery competency framework for inpatient mental health providers, and pilot tested an associated recovery educational program to meet inpatient needs (Chen, Krupa, Lysaght, McCay, & Piat, 2014).

A key target of this research is what is generally referred to as the "therapeutic alliance." For example, Russinova, Rogers, Cook, Ellison, and Lyass (2013) have developed the Recovery Promoting Relationships Scale. Other research targets include the development of provider-self assessment tools to assess recovery knowledge and attitudes, for example the Recovery Knowledge Inventory (Bedregal, O'Connell, & Davidson, 2006; Davidson et al., 2009).

Peer Providers as Essential to Recovery Support

There is clear consensus that peer providers are an essential component of contemporary recovery-oriented practice. Both peer providers themselves and the mental health system have developed a better understanding of how best to use and support peer providers (Swarbrick & Schmidt, 2010). The support available from peer providers that practice within mental health programs differs from the peer support available in self-help groups like Recovery International (www.lowselfhelpsystems.org/) or Schizophrenia Anonymous. Peer providers within the mental health programs, as recognized job positions, have to contend with the same challenges that other mental health providers experience, (i.e., billing, documentation, ethical issues). In recent years, peer providers have been organizing. For example the International Association of Peer Supporters (http://inaops.org/) was founded in 2004, and advocates for peer specialist certification. In the United States, several states have developed such certifications, the

---

Box 3-5. Hope-Inspiring Strategies for Using Interpersonal Resources for Recovery

- Believe in person's potential and strength
- Value the person as a unique human being; accepting the person for who he or she is
- Listen non-judgmentally to the person's experiences
- Tolerate the uncertainty about future developments in the person's life
- Accept "de-compensation" and failure as part of the recovery process
- Trust the authenticity of the person's experiences
- Express a genuine concern for the person's well-being
- Use humor appropriately

From Russinova, Z. "Providers' hope-inspiring competence as a factor optimizing psychiatric rehabilitation outcomes," *Journal of Rehabilitation, 16*(4), 50-57. Copyright © 1999 by National Rehabilitation Association. Reprinted with permission.

Box 3-6. Hope-Inspiring Strategies for Mobilizing Internal Resources for Recovery

- Help person to set and reach concrete goals
- Help person to develop better coping skills
- Help person to recall previous achievements and positive experiences
- Use techniques for changing the person's negative perceptions of events and self
- Help person to accept failures and learn from them
- Help person to make sense of suffering related to his or her mental illness
- Help person to find meaning and purpose in life
- Support the person's spiritual beliefs

From Russinova, Z. "Providers' hope-inspiring competence as a factor optimizing psychiatric rehabilitation outcomes," *Journal of Rehabilitation, 16*(4), 50-57. Copyright © 1999 by National Rehabilitation Association. Reprinted with permission.

Box 3-7. Measures to Assess Provider Recovery Capacities and Qualities

The Recovery Promoting Relationships Scale (Russinova et al., 2013) assesses provider's competencies that enhance recovery (i.e., enhancing client's hopefulness, empowerment, and self-acceptance), as well as those that build and maintain a strong therapeutic or working alliance. This scale is completed by the person in recovery about a specific provider with whom he or she is working, and can be administered anytime in the relationship. Sample questions, answered on a 5-point Likert scale, include "my provider helps me recognize my strengths," "my provider helps me feel I can have a meaningful life," and "my provider really listens to what I have to say."

Recovery Knowledge Inventory (Bedregal et al., 2006) is a 20-item provider assessment that assesses a provider's understanding across four different recovery domains: (1) roles and responsibilities in recovery, (2) non-linearity of the recovery process, (3) the roles of self-definition and peers in recovery, and (4) expectations regarding recovery. Sample questions include "the concept of recovery is equally relevant to all phases of treatment," "It is often harmful to have too high expectations for clients," etc.

most well-known being the Georgia Certified Peer Specialist Project (www.gacps.org/). Guidance has been developed for supporting and supervising peer providers, especially facilitating role clarification, boundary management and scope of practice (Swarbrick & Schmidt, 2010).

CONCLUSION

This chapter has provided an overview of recovery as a guiding vision for mental health service delivery internationally. The chapter positions occupational therapy as being particularly relevant to the advancement of the recovery vision, given the close connection between recovery and engagement in personally and socially meaningful activities. Beyond the philosophy and ideals of recovery, a range of intervention approaches consistent with recovery has been developed and the evidence base for their effectiveness is growing. Many of these interventions are transdisciplinary and will involve occupational therapists working collaboratively with other practitioners, including peer-providers, in the delivery of these services. Within occupational therapy, recovery-oriented approaches and evidence are growing.

LEARNING ACTIVITIES/ DISCUSSION QUESTIONS

1. It can be challenging to deliver recovery-oriented occupational therapy services in particular health or social service environments. Choose one of the following environments and (1) investigate how recovery-enabling practice is challenged, and (2) suggest how recovery-oriented practice might be promoted.

   a. Inpatient mental health units

   b. Forensic mental health services

   c. Shelters and other services for people who are homeless.

2. There are several excellent high-profile films available that demonstrate recovery in the context of serious mental illness. *A Beautiful Mind* is perhaps one of the best known films. Watch the film and consider how an occupational therapist working with Dr. Nash might have used recovery-oriented practice to enable his engagement in meaningful occupations.

3. The vision and practice of recovery has some similarities to chronic disease management. What are their similarities? Differences?

REFERENCES

Allen, M., & Smith, V. F. (2001). Opening Pandora's box: The practical and legal dangers of involuntary outpatient commitment. *Psychiatric Services, 52*(3), 342-346. doi: 10.1176/appi.ps.52.3.342

Amador, X. F. (2000). *I am not sick, I don't need help!: Helping the seriously mentally ill accept treatment: a practical guide for: families and therapists.* Peconic, NY: Vida Press.

Andresen, R., Caputi, P., & Oades, L. (2006). Stages of recovery instrument: Development of a measure of recovery from serious mental illness. *Australian and New Zealand Journal of Psychiatry, 40*(11-12), 972-980. doi: 10.1080/j.1440-1614.2006.01921.x

Andresen, R., Oades, L., & Caputi, P. (2003). The experience of recovery from schizophrenia: towards an empirically validated stage model. *Australian and New Zealand Journal of Psychiatry, 37*(5), 586-594. doi: 10.1046/j.1440-1614.2003.01234.x

Anthony, W. (1993). Recovery from mental illness: The guiding vision of the mental health system in the 1990's. *Psychosocial Rehabilitation Journal 16*(4), 11-23.

Anthony, W. (2000). A recovery-oriented service system: setting some system level standards. *Psychiatric Rehabilitation Journal, 24,* 159-168.

Anthony, W., Rogers, E. S., & Farkas, M. (2003). Research on evidence-based practices: Future directions in an era of recovery [electronic version]. *Community Mental Health Journal, 39*(2), 101-113.

Argentzell, E., Håkansson, C., & Eklund, M. (2010). Experience of meaning in everyday occupations among unemployed people with severe mental illness. *Scandinavian Journal of Occupational Therapy, 19*(1), 49-58. doi: 10.3109/11038128.2010.540038

Barbic, M. S. S., Krupa, P. D. T., & Armstrong, P. D. I. (2009). A randomized controlled trial of the effectiveness of a modified recovery workbook program: Preliminary findings. *Psychiatric Services, 60*(4), 491-497. doi: 10.1176/appi.ps.60.4.491

Bedregal, L., O'Connell, M., & Davidson, L. (2006). The recovery knowledge inventory: Assessment of mental health knowledge and attitudes about recovery. *Psychiatric Rehabilitation Journal, 30*(2), 96-103.

Bellack, A. S. (2006). Scientific and consumer models of recovery in schizophrenia: Concordance, contrasts, and implications [electronic version]. *Schizophrenia Bulletin, 32,* 432-442.

Bockoven, J. S. (1963). *Moral treatment in American psychiatry.* New York: Springer Publishing.

Bond, G., Salyers, M., Rollins, A., Rapp, C., & Zipple, A. (2004). How evidence-based practices contribute to community integration. *Community Mental Health Journal, 40*(6), 569-588.

Borg, M., & Davidson, L. (2007). The nature of recovery as lived in everyday experience. *Journal of Mental Health, 17*(2), 129-140. doi: 10.1080/09638230701498382

Campbell-Orde, T., Chamberlin, J., Carpenter, J., & Leff, H. S. (2005). *Measuring the promise: A compendium of recovery measures* (vol. II). Cambridge, MA: The Evaluation Center @ HSRI.

Carless, D., & Douglas, K. (2008). Narrative, identity, and recovery from serious mental illness: A life history of a runner. *Qualitative Research in Psychology, 5*(4), 233-248.

Chaffey, L., & Fossey, E. (2004). Caring and daily life: Occupational experiences of women living with sons diagnosed with schizophrenia. *Australian Occupational Therapy Journal, 51*(4), 199-207. doi:10.1111/j.1440-1630.2004.00460.x

Chamberlin, J. (1997a). The ex-patient's movement: Where we've been and where we're going. In L. Spaniol, C. Gagene, & M. Koehler (Eds.), *Psychological and social aspects of psychiatric disability* (pp. 541-551). Boston, MA: Center for Psychiatric Rehabilitation.

Chamberlin, J. (1997b). Rehabilitating ourselves: The psychiatric survivor movement. In L. Spaniol, C. Gagene, & M. Koehler (Eds.), *Psychological and social aspects of psychiatric disability* (pp. 522-526). Boston, MA: Center for Psychiatric Rehabilitation.

Chen, S., Krupa, T., Lysaght, R., McCay, E., & Piat, M. (2011). The development of recovery competencies for in-patient mental health providers working with people with serious mental illness. *Administration and Policy in Mental Health, 40*, 96-116.

Chen, S., Krupa, T., Lysaght, R., McCay, E., & Piat, M. (2014). Development of a recovery education program for in-patient mental health providers. *Psychiatric Rehabilitation Journal, 37*, 329-332.

Cook, J. A., Copeland, M. E., Corey, L., Buffington, E., Jonikas, J. A., Curtis, L., Grey, D. D., & Nichols, W. H. (2010). Developing the evidence base for peer-led services: Changes among participants following Wellness Recovery Action Planning (WRAP) education in two statewide initiatives. *Psychiatric Rehabilitation Journal, 34*(2), 113-120.

Cook, J. A., & Jonikas, J. A. (2002). Self-determination among mental health consumers/survivors: Using lessons from the past to guide the future. *Journal of Disability Policy Studies, 13*(2), 88-96. doi: 10.1177/10442073020130020401

Copeland, M. E. (2001). Wellness recovery action plan: A system for monitoring, recruiting and eliminating uncomfortable or dangerous physical symptoms and emotional feelings. In C. Brown (Ed.), *Recovery and wellness: Models of hope and empowerment for people with mental illness* (pp. 127-150). New York: Haworth Press.

Corin, E., & Lauzon, G. (1991). Positive withdrawal and the quest for meaning: the reconstruction of experience among schizophrenics. *Psychiatry 55*(3), 279-281.

Corrigan, P. W., Giffort, D., Rashid, F., Leary, M., & Okeke, I. (1999). Recovery as a psychological construct. *Community Mental Health Journal, 35*(3), 231-239.

Corrigan, P. W., Salzer, M., Ralph, R. O., Sangster, Y., & Keck, L. (2004). Examining the factor structure of the recovery assessment scale. *Schizophrenia Bulletin, 30*(4), 1035-1041.

Cuddeback, G. S., Morrissey, J. P., Domino, M. E., Monroe-DeVita, M., Teague, G. B., & Moser, L. L. (2013). Fidelity to recovery-oriented ACT practices and consumer outcomes. *Psychiatric Services, 64*(4), 318-323. doi: 10.1176/appi.ps.201200097

Davidson, L. (2003). *Living outside mental illness: Qualitative studies of recovery in schizophrenia.* New York: New York University Press.

Davidson, L., Borg, M., Marin, I., Topor, A., Mezzina, R., & Sells, D. (2005). Processes of recovery in serious mental illness: Findings from a multinational study. *American Journal of Psychiatric Rehabilitation, 8*(3), 177-201.

Davidson, L., Harding, C., & Spaniol, L. (2005). *Recovery from severe mental illness: Research evidence and implications for practice* (vol. 1). Boston, MA: Center for Psychiatric Rehabilitation, Sargent College of Health and Rehabilitation Science, Boston University.

Davidson, L., Rakfeldt, J., & Strauss, J. (2010). *The roots of the recovery movement in psychiatry: Lessons learned.* Hoboken, NJ: Wiley-Blackwell.

Davidson, L., & Strauss, J. (1997). Sense of self in recovery from severe mental illness. In L. Spaniol, C. Gagne, & M. Koehler (Eds.), *Psychological and social aspects of psychiatric disability* (pp. 25-39). Boston: Center for Psychiatric Rehabilitation.

Davidson, L., Tondora, J., Lawless, M., O'Connell, M., & Rowe, M. (2009). *A practical guide to recovery-oriented practice: Tools for transforming mental health care.* New York: Oxford University Press.

Deegan, P. (1988). Recovery: The lived experience of rehabilitation. *Psychosocial Rehabilitation Journal, 11*, 11-19.

Deegan, P. (1996). Recovery as a journey of the heart. *Psychiatric Rehabilitation Journal, 19*(3), 91-97.

Deegan, P. (2001). Recovery as a self-directed process of healing and transformation. In C. Brown (Ed.), *Recovery and wellness: Models of hope and empowerment for people with mental illness* (pp. 5-22). New York: Haworth Press.

Deegan, P. (2005). The importance of personal medicine: A qualitative study of resilience in people with psychiatric disabilities. *Scandinavian Journal of Public Health, 33*, 29-35.

Deegan, P. D. P., & Drake, M. D. P. D. R. (2006). Shared decision making and medication management in the recovery process. *Psychiatric Services, 57*(11), 1636-1639. doi: 10.1176/appi.ps.57.11.1636

Deegan, P. D. P., Rapp, P. D. C., Holter, P. D. M., & Riefer, M. S. W. M. (2008). Best practices: A program to support shared decision making in an outpatient psychiatric medication clinic. *Psychiatric Services, 59*(6), 603-605. doi: 10.1176/appi.ps.59.6.603

Department of Health and Human Services. (2003). The President's New Freedom Commission on Mental Health achieving the promise: Transforming mental health care in America: Department of Health and Human Services.

Department of Health and Human Services. (2005). Transforming mental health care in America—The federal action agenda: First steps: Department of Health and Human Services.

Dickerson, F. B. (2006). Commentary: Disquieting aspects of the recovery paradigm. *Psychiatric Services, 57*(5), 647. doi: 10.1176/appi.ps.57.5.647

Drake, R., & Deegan, P. (2008). Are assertive community treatment and recovery compatible? Commentary on "ACT and recovery: Integrating evidence-based practice and recovery orientation on assertive community treatment Teams." *Community Mental Health Journal, 44*(1), 75-77.

Drake, R., Deegan, P., & Rapp, C. (2010). The promise of shared decision making in mental health. *Psychiatric Rehabilitation Journal, 34*(1), 7-13. doi: 10.2975/34.1.2010.7.13

Drake, R. E., Goldman, H. H., Leff, H. S., Lehman, A. F., Dixon, L., Mueser, K. T., & Torrey, W. C. (2001). Implementing evidence-based practices in routine mental health service settings. *Psychiatric Services, 52*(2), 179-182. doi: 10.1176/appi.ps.52.2.179

Edgelow, M., & Krupa, T. (2011). Randomized controlled pilot study of an occupational time-use intervention for people with serious mental illness. *The American Journal of Occupational Therapy, 65*(3), 267-276. doi: 10.5014/ajot.2011.001313

Eklund, M. (2001). Psychiatric patients occupational roles: Changes over time and associations with self-rated quality of life. *Scandinavian Journal of Occupational Therapy, 8*(3), 125-130.

Eklund, M., Hansson, L., & Ahlqvist, C. (2004). The importance of work as compared to other forms of daily occupations for wellbeing and functioning among persons with long-term mental illness. *Community Mental Health Journal, 40*(5), 465-477.

Estroff, S. E. (1989). Self, identity, and subjective experiences of schizophrenia. *Schizophrenia Bulletin, 15*(2), 189-196.

Farkas, M., Gagne, C., Anthony, W., & Chamberlin, J. (2005). Implementing recovery oriented evidence based programs: Identifying the critical dimensions. *Community Mental Health Journal, 41*(2), 141-158.

Fisher, D., & Chamberlin, J. (n.d.). *Consumer-directed transformation to a recovery-based mental health system.* Lawrence, MA: National Empowerment Center. Retrieved from www.power2u.org/downloads/SAMHSA.pdf.

Goldman, H. H., Ganju, V., Drake, R. E., Gorman, P., Hogan, M., Hyde, P. S., & Morgan, O. (2001). Policy implications for implementing evidence-based practices [electronic version]. *Psychiatric Services, 52*(12), 1591-1597. doi: 10.1176/appi.ps.52.12.1591

Gomory, T. (2005). Assertive community treatment (ACT): The case against the "best tested" evidence-based community treatment for mental illness. In S. Kirk (Ed.), *Mental disorders in the social environment: Critical perspectives* (pp. 165-189). New York: Columbia University Press.

Gordon, S. E. (2013). Recovery constructs and the continued debate that limits consumer recovery. *Psychiatric Services, 64*(3), 270-271. doi: 10.1176/appi.ps.001612012

Harding, C. M., Brooks, G. W., Ashikaga, T., Strauss, J. S., & Breier, A. (1987a). The Vermont longitudinal study of persons with severe mental illness, I: Methodology, study sample, and overall status 32 years later [electronic version]. *American Journal of Psychiatry, 144*(6), 718-726.

Harding, C. M., Brooks, G. W., Ashikaga, T., Strauss, J. S., & Breier, A. (1987b). The Vermont longitudinal study of persons with severe mental illness, II: Long-term outcome of subjects who retrospectively met DSM-III criteria for schizophrenia [electronic version]. *American Journal of Psychiatry, 144*(6), 727-735.

Houghton, J. F. (1982). Maintaing mental health in a turbulent world. *Schizophrenia Bulletin, 8*, 548-552.

Isett, K. R., Burnam, M. A., Coleman-Beattie, B., Hyde, P. S., Morrissey, J. P., Magnabosco, J.,…Goldman, H. H. (2007). The state policy context of implementation issues for evidence-based practices in mental health. *Psychiatric Services, 58*(7), 914-921. doi: 10.1176/appi.ps.58.7.914

Jacobson, N., & Greenley, D. (2001). What is recovery? A conceptual model and explication. *Psychiatric Services, 52*(4), 482-485. doi: 10.1176/appi.ps.52.4.482

Kennedy-Jones, M., Cooper, J., & Fossey, E. (2005). Developing a worker role: Stories of four people with mental illness. *Australian Occupational Therapy Journal, 52*(2), 116-126. doi:10.1111/j.1440-1630.2005.00475.x

Kidd, S. A., George, L., O'Connell, M., Sylvestre, J., Kirkpatrick, H., Browne, G. & Thabane, L. (2010). Fidelity and recovery orientation in assertive community treatment. *Community Mental Health Journal, 46*, 342-350.

Kielhofner, G., & Burke, J. (1977). Occupational therapy after 60 years: An account of changing identity and knowledge. *American Journal of Occupational Therapy, 31*(10), 675-689.

Kirsh, B., & Cockburn, L. (2007). Employment outcomes associated with ACT: A review of ACT literature. *American Journal of Psychiatric Rehabilitation, 10*(1), 31-51.

Krupa, T. (2004). Employment, recovery, and schizophrenia: Integrating health and disorder at work. *Psychiatric Rehabilitation Journal, 28*(1), 8-15. doi: (Document ID: 703215031).

Krupa, T., Edgelow, M., Chen, S., Mieras, C., Almas, A., Perry, A.,…Bransfield, M. (2010). *Action over inertia: Addressing the activity-health needs of individuals with serious mental illness.* Ottawa, ON: CAOT Publications.

Krupa, T., Radloff-Gabriel, D., Whippey, E., & Kirsh, B. (2002). Reflections on occupational therapy and assertive community treatment. *Canadian Journal of Occupational Therapy, 69*(3), 153-157.

Lal, S. (2010). Prescribing recovery as the new mantra for mental health: Does one prescription serve all? *Canadian Journal of Occupational Therapy, 77*(2), 82-89. doi: 10.2182/cjot.2010.77.2.4

Laliberte-Rudman, D. (2002). Linking occupation and identity: Lessons learned through qualitative exploration. *Journal of Occupational Science, 9*(1), 12-19.

Laliberte-Rudman, D., Yu, B., Scott, E., & Pajouhandeh, P. (2000). Exploration of the perspectives of persons with schizophrenia regarding quality of life. *American Journal of Occupational Therapy, 54*(2), 137-147.

Leamy, M., Bird, V., Le Boutillier, C., Williams, J., & Slade, M. (2011). Conceptual framework for personal recovery in mental health: systematic review and narrative synthesis. *British Journal of Psychiatry, 199*(6), 445-452. doi: 10.1192/bjp.bp.110.083733

Leete, E. (1989). How I perceive and manage my illness. *Schizophrenia Bulletin, 15,* 197-200.

Leufstadis, C., Erlandsson, L., Bjorkman, T., & Eklund, M. (2008). Meaningfulness in daily occupation among individuals with persistent mental illness. *Journal of Occupational Science, 15*(1), 27-35.

Liberman, R. P., & Kopelowicz, A. (2005). Recovery from schizophrenia: A concept in search of research. *Psychiatric Services, 56*(6), 735-742. doi: 10.1176/appi.ps.56.6.735

Liberman, R. P., Kopelowicz, A., Ventura, J., & Gutkind, D. (2002). Operational criteria and factors related to recovery from schizophrenia [electronic version]. *International Review of Psychiatry, 14*(4), 0954-0261.

Lidz, T. (1966). Adolf Meyer and the development of American psychiatry. *American Journal of Psychiatry, 123*(3), 320-332. doi: 10.1176/appi.ajp.123.3.320

Lloyd, C., Bassett, H., & King, R. (2002). Mental health: How well are occupational therapists equipped for a changed practice environment? *Australian Occupational Therapy Journal, 49*(3), 163-166. doi:10.1046/j.1440-1630.2002.00332.x

Lloyd, C., Wong, S. R., & Petchkovsky, L. (2007). Art and recovery in mental health: A qualitative investigation. *British Journal of Occupational Therapy, 70,* 207-214.

Longhofer, J., Kubek, P. M., & Floersch, J. (2010). *On being and having a case manager: A relational approach to recovery in mental health.* New York: Columbia University Press.

Mee, J., & Sumsion, T. (2001). Mental health clients confirm the motivating power of occupation. *British Journal of Occupational Therapy, 64,* 121-128.

Mee, J., Sumsion, T., & Craik, C. (2004). Mental health clients confirm the value of occupation in building competence and self-identity. *British Journal of Occupational Therapy, 67*(5), 225-233.

Meyer, A. (1922). The philosophy of occupation therapy. *Archives of Occupational Therapy, 1*(1), 1-10.

Meyer, A. (1957). *Psychobiology: A science of man.* Springfield, IL: Charles C. Thomas.

Mueser, K. T., Corrigan, P. W., Hilton, D. W., Tanzman, B., Schaub, A., Gingerich, S.,... Herz, M. I. (2004). Illness management and recovery: A review of the research. *Focus, 2*(1), 34-47.

Mueser, K. T., Meyer, P. S., Penn, D. L., Clancy, R., Clancy, D. M., & Salyers, M. P. (2006). The illness management and recovery program: Rationale, development, and preliminary findings. *Schizophrenia Bulletin, 32*(suppl_1), S32-43. doi: 10.1093/schbul/sbl022

National Association of State Mental Health Program Directors. (2004). Implementing Recovery-Based Care: Tangible Guidance for SMHAs.

O'Connell, M., Tondora, J., Croog, G., Evans, A., & Davidson, L. (2005). From rhetoric to routine: Assessing perceptions of recovery-oriented practices in a state mental health and addiction system *Psychiatric Rehabilitation Journal, 28*(4), 378-386.

Polatajko, H. (1992). Naming and framing occupational therapy: A lecture dedicated to the life of Nancy B. *Canadian Journal of Occupational Therapy, 59,* 189-200.

Ralph, R. O., Kidder, K., & Phillips, D. (2000). Can we measure recovery? A compendium of recovery and recovery-related instruments. Cambridge, MA: The Evaluation Center @ HSRI.

Rebeiro, K. L. (1999). The labyrinth of community mental health: In search of meaningful occupation. *Psychiatric Rehabilitation Journal 23*(2), 143-152.

Rebeiro Gruhl, K. L. (2005). The recovery paradigm: Should occupational therapists be interested? *Canadian Journal of Occupational Therapy, 72,* 96-102.

Resnick, S. G., Rosenheck, R. A., & Lehman, A. F. (2004). An exploratory analysis of correlates of recovery. *Psychiatric Services, 55*(5), 540-547. doi: 10.1176/appi.ps.55.5.540.

Ridgway, P. (1999). Deepening the mental health recovery paradigm, defining implications for practice: A report of the Recovery Paradigm Project. Lawrence, KS: University of Kansas School of Social Welfare.

Ridgway, P. (2001). ReStorying psychiatric disability: Learning from first-person recovery narratives. *Psychiatric Rehabilitation Journal, 24*(4), 335-343.

Roe, D., & Chopra, M. (2003). Beyond coping with mental illness: Toward personal growth. *American Journal of Orthopsychiatry, 73*(3), 334-344.

Russinova, Z. (1999). Providers' hope-inspiring competence as a factor optimizing psychiatric rehabilitation outcomes. *Journal of Rehabilitation, 16*(4), 50-57.

Russinova, Z., Rogers, S., Cook, K., Ellison, M. L., & Lyass, A. (2013). Conceptualization and measurement of mental health provider's recovery-promoting competence: The recovery promoting relationships scale (RPRS). *Psychiatric Rehabilitation Journal, 36*(1), 7-14.

Rutman, I. (1987). The psychosocial rehabilitation movement in the United States. In A. Meyerson & T. Fine (Eds.), *Psychiatric disability: Clinical, legal, and administrative decisions* (pp. 197-220). Washington, DC: American Psychiatric Association.

Salyers, M. P., Stull, L. G., Rollins, A. L., McGrew, J. H., Hicks, L. J., Thomas, D., & Strieter, D. (2013). Measuring the recovery orientation of assertive community treatment. *Journal of the American Psychiatric Nurses Association, 19*(3), 117-128. doi: 10.1177/1078390313489570.

Salyers, M. P., & Tsemberis, S. (2007). ACT and recovery: Integrating evidence-based practice and recovery orientation on assertive community treatment teams. *Community Mental Health Journal, 43*(6), 619-641.

Slade, M. (2009). *Personal recovery and mental illness: A guide for mental health professionals.* New York: Cambridge University Press.

Spaniol, L., Koehler, M., & Hutchinson, D. (2009). *The recovery workbook: Practical coping and empowerment strategies for people with psychiatric disabilities* (revised edition). Boston, MA: Center for Psychiatric Rehabilitation.

Stainsby, J. (1992). Schizophrenia: Some issues. *Schizophrenia Bulletin, 18*(3), 543-546.

Substance Abuse and Mental Health Services Administration. (2008a). *Assertive community treatment evidence-based practice toolkit.* Rockville, MD: DHHS.

Substance Abuse and Mental Health Services Administration. (2008b). *Illness management and recovery toolkit.* Rockville, MD: DHHS.

Substance Abuse and Mental Health Services Administration. (2009). *Supported employment: Evidence-based toolkit.* Rockville, MD: Center for Mental Health Services, SAMHSA, US DHHS.

Substance Abuse and Mental Health Services Administration. (2010a). *SAMHSA joins together with national behavioral health provider associations to promote mental health recovery.* Washington, DC: SAMHSA

Substance Abuse and Mental Health Services Administration. (2010b). *Permanent supportive housing evidence-based practices.* Rockville, MD: Center for Mental Health Services, SAMHSA , US DHHS.

Substance Abuse and Mental Health Services Administration. (2012). *Supported education evidence-based practices kit.* Rockville, MD: Center for Mental Health Services, SAMHSA, US DHHS.

Sutton, D. J., Hocking, C. S., & Smythe, L. A. (2012). A phenomenological study of occupational engagement in recovery from mental illness. *Canadian Journal of Occupational Therapy, 79*(3), 143-150.

Swarbrick, M., & Schmidt, L. (2010). *People in recovery as providers of psychiatric rehabilitation: Building on the wisdom of experience.* Linthicum, MD: United States Psychiatric Rehabilitation Association.

Young, S. L., & Ensing, D. S. (1999). Exploring recovery from the perspective of people with psychiatric disabilities. *Psychiatric Rehabilitation Journal, 22*(3), 219-232.

Suggested Readings

Davidson, L., Harding, C., & Spaniol, L. (Eds). (2006). *Recovery from severe mental illness: Research evidence and implications for practice, volume 2.* Boston: Boston University, Center for Psychiatric Rehabilitation.

Ralph, R. O., & Corrigan, P. W. (2005). *Recovery in mental illness: Broadening our understanding of wellness.* Washington, DC: American Psychological Association.

Ridgway, P., McDiarmid, D., Davidson, L., & Bayes, J. (2002). *Pathways to recovery: A strengths recovery self-help workbook.* Lawrence, KS: Kansas University School of Social Welfare.

Spaniol, L., Bellingham, R., Cohen, B., & Spaniol, S. (2003). *The recovery workbook II: Connectedness.* Boston: Boston University Center for Psychiatric Rehabilitation.

4

Transdisciplinary Models of Disability
Applications to Psychosocial Practice

Terry Krupa, PhD, OT Reg (Ont), FCAOT and
Ellie Fossey, PhD, MSc, DipCOT (UK)

Life has generally been good to me. I've tried to live a life of faith and hope that things will be better in the future. Even though I have a diagnosis of schizophrenia, I try to move forward and not wear my hidden disability on my sleeve but rather use coping skills I've learned to function in broader society. While in the past, I have suffered with auditory hallucinations and delusions, I seem to have these issues dealt with appropriately by using medication, talk therapy, reflection and positively reframing thoughts. Anxiety and depression have bothered me on and off for the past 20 years. They have impacted my ability to work consistently and at a normal pace—sometimes I just need more time. I recently completed an online course but needed double the standard time to prepare for the exams—but I did pass. I don't want to be continuously on the go—I need my down time. Setbacks seem to be cyclical in nature with many good times and some not so good times. Having great friends and a rich support network really helps. A positive attitude and projecting empathy for others as well as having a friendly disposition leads to success. My support system encourages my strong work ethic and I've tried to master entrepreneurship and risk taking and incorporate those learned skills in my life. There is always tomorrow and new challenges and opportunities to tackle. (M. MacPherson)

OBJECTIVES

The objectives of this chapter are as follows:

» Describe two international, transdisciplinary models of disability.

» Consider how each of these models can be applied to psychosocial occupational therapy practice.

» Provide examples of practices, practice tools, and other resources that have evolved from these models.

Krupa, T., Kirsh, B., Pitts, D., & Fossey, E. *Bruce & Borg's Psychosocial Frames of Reference: Theories, Models, and Approaches for Occupation-Based Practice, Fourth Edition* (pp 57-72).

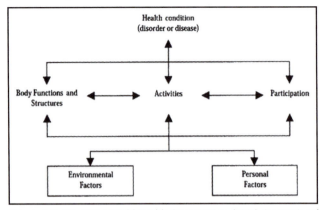

Figure 4-1. ICF. (From World Health Organization. (2001). *International Classification of Functioning, Disability and Health (ICF)*. Geneva, Switzerland: World Health Organization. Reprinted with permission.)

The chapter's opening quote highlights that people who experience mental health problems and/or mental illness can also experience significant disability. Historically the concept of disability has been linked to health conditions that affect the physical function of the body. Mental health problems or mental illness are not routinely associated with disability, even by those people with lived experience. Indeed, historically the broad field of disability has not integrated disruptions in mental health within their conceptualization of disability. Accordingly, advances in disability-related theory, knowledge and practice are not routinely applied to psychosocial practice, and relevant advances in psychosocial knowledge and practice have been poorly accessed by the broader field of disability.

Universal models of disability have the potential to advance integrated views of human health, function, and well-being internationally. This chapter will consider how the psychological, emotional, and social factors central to occupation are addressed within established and evolving models of disability. It will link key psychosocial occupational therapy concepts to these models and evaluate the consistency of these transdisciplinary models of disability with occupational therapy practice in the psychosocial domain. Finally, it will demonstrate how these models might be applied within psychosocial occupational therapy to both understand occupational function and disruption, and to develop enabling occupational therapy practices.

The chapter will focus specifically on two transdisciplinary models related to disability: the International Classification of Functioning (ICF) from the World Health Organization (WHO, 2001), and the Social Model of Disability (Bickenbach, Chatterji, Badley, & Üstün,, 1999; Oliver, 1996). These selected frameworks have received international recognition and they illustrate the rapidly evolving nature of the very large field of disability theory.

INTERNATIONAL CLASSIFICATION OF FUNCTIONING

Background

The ICF is a taxonomy, or a classification of health and health-related domains. It is the framework of the WHO for describing and measuring health and disability at both individual and population levels (Figure 4-1).

The domains are classified in the ICF from body, individual, and societal perspectives by means of two sections. The first section addresses functioning and disability by providing a categorization of body functions and structure, and a categorization of domains of activity and participation. Because human function and disability occur in a context, the second part of the ICF also includes personal and environmental contextual factors. The classification is available as an online, open-access publication (WHO, 2013a). The wide distribution of the ICF is consistent with the intent of the WHO to create a classification that will be used as an international standard for common language for epidemiological, clinical, service development, and research purposes.

ICF View of Health and Disorder

The ICF was developed with a view to defining how the consequences of health conditions extend beyond the disorder or illness, and highlights that functional, activity, and participation-related consequences can have an impact that is as profound, or even more profound, than the illness itself (Üstün, Chatterji, Bickenbach, Kostanjsek, & Schneider, 2003). The classification provides an organized and comprehensive description of human function and its restrictions as universal human experiences. The authors of the ICF highlight that the categories of the ICF are not meant to classify people, or to define standards of normality for function, but rather to describe the situation of people within a wide range of health-related domains. Based on this perspective, the ICF definition of disability is "difficulty in functioning at the body, person, or societal levels, in one or more life domains, as experienced by an individual with a health condition in interaction with contextual factors" (Leonardi, Bickenbach, Üstün, Kostanjsek, Chatterji, & MHADIE Consortium, 2006, p. 1220). As a universal model of disability, it should be as relevant and applicable to the functional consequences of health conditions that are psychosocial, or mental health-related in nature, as it is to other types of health conditions.

Theoretical Assumptions

The ICF is essentially a taxonomy, a very detailed classification system of the consequences of health and health-related conditions, and the contextual factors that influence these. It does not suggest the cause of these consequences, nor does it develop anything but a very cursory understanding of the relationship between these categories.

Even though the ICF classification is very detailed, the amount of detail is somewhat uneven across the classification. The domains and categories that appear to be most well developed are those that are perhaps most closely associated with traditional biomedical classifications, and those that are least developed have historically been less subject to exploration with respect to health and function. For example, body structures and functions are very detailed, while personal factors are described but not categorized in any organized way. This is probably an artifact of the historical prominence of biomedical models. With the ongoing development of the ICF model there has been a growing body of knowledge to develop and categorize personal factors (see for example Geyh et al., 2011).

The ICF describes situations that are relevant across the broad range of health and health-related conditions and in this way is meant to enable a comprehensive, or "full health experience," perspective on human function. The use of such a classification could ensure, for example, that service planning, practices, policies, and research related to people with mental health problems or mental illnesses goes beyond body level disruptions of symptoms and impairments to consider activities, participation, environmental, and personal components of function.

In practice, there can be an inaccurate assumption that certain types of activities and participation are irrelevant in the context of mental health conditions. A good example is the case of the mobility, which may be overlooked as an issue in psychosocial practice. The ICF mobility domain includes consideration of moving around using transportation, including driving and using public transportation (d470). These are both activities that can be experienced as problems by people with mental health conditions and significantly limit their participation in meaningful occupations. For example, people who experience high levels of anxiety (classified as a type of emotional function, b152), might have significant problems using public transit, particularly at times of overcrowding, or experience severe restrictions in their ability to drive, such as avoidance of highway driving. Similarly, people who live in poverty may not be able to afford such transit.

The ICF is based on the assumption that issues in function can emerge without the presence of disruptions at the level of body functions and structures. So people with mental health problems may experience significant limitations in activities and participation, even when no disruption in mental functions is present. This can be considered a particularly problematic issue for people with mental illness given the extent to which they are subject to societal stigma and discrimination that restricts their occupations and community participation even when they experience no impairments related to the illness. The ICF identifies societal attitudes (e460) as an environmental factor that can act as a barrier to activities and participation. So, for example, a young man who has experienced a first episode of psychosis might find himself prohibited from returning to his college studies because of stigma and discrimination (which are environmental factors), even though his mental illness is well controlled.

The ICF classification differentiates between *performance*, or what an individual actually does in the current context, and *capacity*, which indicates how the person is likely to function if the environment was adjusted. In addition, it makes note of function with or without assistive devices. Contemporary psychosocial practice has made significant advancements in the development of environmental adjustments, or accommodations and assistive devices, which can enable people with mental health issues to engage successfully in important community occupations. So, for example, a person who is coming back to work following a significant bout of depression might also be recovering from associated problems with higher level cognitive functions (b166), which could be accommodated by providing the individual with an organizing schedule to assist with arranging the time and space needed to carry out multiple tasks (d220).

Key Components

Figure 4-1 provides a pictorial diagram of the main components of the ICF. The components of the model are arranged hierarchically, so that within each major component there are a variety of domains divided further into categories. The key components are described briefly here and their application to psychosocial practice is illustrated by means of a practice vignette of Catherine presented in Box 4-1.

Part I of the ICF model presents the components associated with function and disability. Physiological functions of the body (including psychological and emotional functions) and anatomical parts of the body are located within the body structures and functions of the model. Impairment is the concept used to describe any significant deviation in generally accepted standards for body function or structure. Our vignette of Catherine describes that she has been diagnosed with major depression, a significant health condition that is known to be prevalent in society. Our current knowledge about depression suggests that it is a leading cause of disability internationally (Üstün, Ayuso, Chatterji, Mathers, & Murray, 2004). While Catherine's depression is her primary diagnosis, depression is a common secondary diagnosis for many health conditions

BOX 4-1. VIGNETTE: CATHERINE—ICF APPLICATION

Catherine is a 38-year-old woman who is currently on a disability leave from her job as a clerical assistant in a university department because of depression. She has a long history of living with depression and has been able to manage the illness well with medications and psychotherapy when needed. She had two previous short-term leaves from her job. This episode of the illness is a different experience for Catherine. It occurred in the context of separation from her husband that has been full of conflict. She is worried about her financial security and her future generally. The leave from work came at a bad time when the department was under considerable pressures related to the start of the school year. She is the mother of three children aged 6 to 10 and is finding it difficult to keep up with their needs, and she is unhappy with how she is managing typical household routines and the fact that she is asking the children to do more for themselves. Her energy level is very low; she has trouble getting out of bed in the morning, and she has eliminated social and community activities that had been a typical part of her occupational routine. Overall, her self-confidence has plummeted and she is finding herself unable to make even simple decisions. Although she has many friends, she is maintaining only superficial contact with them because she doesn't want to be a burden on them. Several of her friendships have been affected by the separation because they involved contacts with her and her husband as a couple. She says she finds it difficult to think of having friends and fun when she has children to care for and they should be her first priority. In fact, she finds that she derives little pleasure even from the activities she finds most meaningful. Catherine worries about losing custody of her children, feeling incompetent as a mother, and that she will be unable to manage financially if she does not soon return to work.

including heart disease (Elderon & Whooley, 2013), stroke (Hackett, Yapa, Parag, & Anderson, 2005), and Parkinson's disease (Zesiewicz & Hauser, 2002). Consequently, occupational therapists can expect to encounter depression and its sequelae in a variety of practice contexts. Because the classification of the ICF is not organized according to any specific health condition, it can enable therapists to recognize functional consequences of depression, even where it is not the primary diagnosis.

The vignette indicates that Catherine is experiencing several impairments related to her depression, and the ICF provides a framework for identifying and describing these. The impairments experienced by Catherine are, for the most part, identified under the category of mental functions in the ICF (b1). Specifically the vignette highlights that she experiences problems with energy and drive (b130). She describes fatigue that limits her performance and participation. In addition, she has difficulties with motivation. Although she continues to place a high value on her family and work activities, she is currently not experiencing them as particularly pleasurable. The vignette suggests Catherine may be experiencing problems with cognitive functions (b164) and in particular higher level cognitive functions associated with decision making. In addition there is some suggestion that her thought functions are affected, and in particular she is prone to highly negative thoughts about herself and her value to others. All of these impairments of body function are common in depression.

In the ICF, activities refer to the execution of tasks or actions, while participation refers to involvement typical in life situations. Activity limitations and participation restrictions are the concepts used in the ICF to describe problems experienced in these domains, and problems are evaluated within generally accepted standards within context, compared to individuals without health conditions. From an occupational therapy perspective, activities and participation are of particular concern because they have to do with the occupations that comprise daily life and contribute to personal and social health and well-being. They will be an important focus of occupational therapy services.

The ICF categories provide us with an organizational framework to identify and describe Catherine's functional issues, activity limitations, and participation restrictions, as well as areas of strength. The vignette indicates that Catherine is experiencing problems with carrying out daily routines (d230). She is particularly concerned about her domestic life activities (d6) and cites issues related to household tasks (d6630-d649) and assisting her children (d660). A major life area (d8) that is restricted is work and employment (d840-d859), and even though there is every reason to believe that she will return to her job, at the moment she is unable to fulfill the required duties. Similarly, her community, social, and civic lives (d9) have been significantly curtailed. Although it appears that she has had good interpersonal relations, in her current situation there has been a significant disruption in her social relationships (d750).

Part II of the model includes environmental factors (physical, social, and attitudinal) that are external to the individual but have an impact on all components of human function and disability. Using the ICF categories for environment factors draws our attention to several aspects of the vignette. Catherine's supports and relationships (e3) have been highly disrupted with the dissolution of her marriage, indicating that a relationship that might once have been an important source of support is now further compromising her ability to experience wellness and engage in important occupations (e310). We know little about the actual attitudes of others in her environment (e4), although Catherine herself seems to be concerned that others at work and in her social network judge her poorly. Other environmental concerns in this vignette include the laws and policies that will govern her access to finances within her changing family structure (e310) and the labour policies that will protect and support her return to work (e5902).

Part II of the ICF also includes personal factors that are individual factors, unrelated to the health condition or state, which nonetheless affect function and disability. Unfortunately, at this point in time these factors are not systematically defined and organized within the ICF. This is an important limitation of the model because these personal factors are highly relevant to understanding psychosocial health and well-being. These personal factors include age, education, lifestyle, habits, social background, education, life events, race/ethnicity, and sexual orientation. Our vignette of Catherine actually provides little personal information, although we can perhaps make the assumption that she has had some good experiences with coping with depression that will be an advantage to her today.

Key Developers

The ICF is only one of several comprehensive models of function, disability, and participation, although it is perhaps the mostly widely known and applied. Other general models of disability that have been used widely in the rehabilitation fields include those developed by Nagi (1979), Verbrugge and Jette (1994), and the model known as the Disability Creation process (sometimes referred to as the Quebec model; Fougeyrollas, Cloutier, Bergeron, Cote, & St. Michel, 1998).

Occupational therapy scholars have made significant contributions to the development and applications of the ICF internationally. The literature on the ICF has a large pool of papers that connect the model to occupational therapy theory and practice. This scholarship covers a wide range of topics from applications of the ICF to occupational therapy with particular health conditions (Kirchberger, Stamm, Cieza, & Stucki, 2007), using the ICF to understand challenges in service delivery (Shaw, Leyshon, & Liu, 2007), the application of the framework across the life span, and in particular the children and youth version of the ICF (Bendixon & Kreider, 2011), to examining the extent to which the ICF is understood and utilized by occupational therapists (Farrell, Anderson, Hewitt, Livingston, & Stewart, 2007).

In psychosocial occupational therapy practice, scholarly contributions related to the ICF have included demonstrations of the application of the ICF as a universal framework to promote cross-cultural understanding of the function, disability, and participation issues experienced in the context of mental health problems (Vrooman & Arthanat, 2008); the contribution of client self-assessment as a qualifier in understanding satisfaction in important activity and participation domains (Haglund & Faltman, 2012); the link between common assessments in psychosocial practice and the ICF categories (Haglund, 2008); illustration of the potential of the ICF to describe the experience of living with a mental health condition (Creek, 2008); and the relevance of activities and participation as developed within the ICF in mental health inpatient or institutional settings (Daremo & Haglund, 2008).

Important Evolutionary Points

The ICF can best be described as an ongoing work in progress and it has been, and continues to be, subject to critique and revision. Producing a comprehensive and universal framework focusing on human function has proven to be a difficult and complicated process. Earlier versions of the framework were highly influenced by biomedical interpretations of function flowing from disease states, and failed to consider function as highly contextualized. They were also developed from a normative interpretation that focused on disability rather than human function generally (see for example, Üstün et al., 2003). This is an important point; the current version of the ICF highlights that difficulties in function are part of the human condition, and not only the experience of people with significant health conditions. This is especially noteworthy in the mental health field because interpretations of mental disorders and their consequences are often seen to be alien to everyday human experience; these views fuel societal forces of stigma and discrimination. This creates a situation where people with problems of mental health and mental illness are subject to disrespect, devaluation, and paternalism even within the health services and professions, like occupational therapy, that are charged with promoting human health, well-being, and dignity (Krupa, 2008).

Revisions of the ICF have benefited from ongoing feedback from multiple stakeholder groups including professional disciplines such as occupational therapy and disability advocacy groups, and people with lived experience of disability. This may help to explain why the framework has been widely accepted internationally. This does not mean the framework is free from critique, and indeed ongoing debates stand to make important contributions to the future evolution of the framework. For example, the meanings associated with participation have been poorly represented in frameworks such as the ICF that have tended to focus on performance. This can have particular relevance for psychosocial practice where the meanings experienced through occupational participation are as relevant as performance. Catherine provides a good example. She finds meaning in her occupations, in particular she places a high value on the role of mother, but her perceptions that she could lose this meaningful occupation likely contributes to her psychological and emotional distress. This connection is not captured in the ICF classification system, but depends on collaborative interpretations between the occupational therapist and Catherine. Other critiques of the ICF question the legitimacy of a classification related to disability, arguing that any classification of human differences has the potential to be marginalizing, even if this is not the intent (Whalley-Hammell, 2004).

Expected Outcomes

The ICF is a comprehensive framework for understanding human functioning; it does not carry the immediate connections to outcomes that we associate with conceptual models that underlie change in occupational therapy practice. It is meant to have an international and system-wide influence, leading to improvements related to the lived experience of disability and the delivery of services and supports. These include the development of a shared language and agreement around core concepts for human function; assessments, goal setting practices, treatment and monitoring practices consistent with the framework; attention to the comprehensive outcomes associated with human function; the development of disability policy and law; and promotion of international research on human function (WHO, 2013b).

SOCIAL MODEL OF DISABILITY

Background

The social model focuses discussions about disability on the political, social, and community contexts within which disability is created and sustained. According to the social model, activity limitations and participation restrictions occur where human differences are ignored, poorly considered, or oppressed and marginalized in the design of our social worlds. The social model is, at its core, a political model that highlights that the barriers people with disability face in daily community life largely emerge within and from social structures that create and sustain a marginalized status. From an occupational therapy perspective, the social model provides the profession with a framework for understanding and acting upon a broad range of barriers to full functioning and participation in society. It has also served as a model for critiquing the profession as being complicit, even if unintentionally, in sustaining forces that oppress people with disability in daily life (Kielhofner, 2005). For example, occupational therapists who prioritize clinical explanations of occupational issues over social explanations can disempower people by continuing to see them as the source of a problem.

The social model is highly relevant in the area of psychosocial practice. People with mental illness have been shown to have high rates of exclusion from important community roles, opportunities, and resources. High proportions of people with mental illness exist among populations who are homeless, in receipt of government disability pensions, and those who have low life expectancy, indicating high levels of marginalization. This suggests that forces beyond the functional consequences of the health disorder itself are at play and meaningful progress is unlikely if the practice arena does not attend to how occupational experiences are socially restricted.

View of Health and Disorder

The social model is based on the assumption that disability is a social phenomenon, constructed within societal structures and processes. The model does not contest that people will experience impairments related to health conditions, or that they will experience limitations in activity and participation. However, unlike more individually focused models that place the source of the activity and participation limitations within the person, perhaps as something to be "fixed" or "compensated for," the social model argues that these are largely socially constructed limitations.

Key Components/Concepts

Because the social model is concerned with revealing the ways that society is organized and structured to create and sustain limitations in activity and participation, the key concepts of the model relate to these core barriers and discriminatory practices. To help organize our thinking about how societies are disabling, proponents of the social model have developed frameworks that identify key societal factors involved. In psychosocial practice, identifying these factors explicitly helps us to understand how people with problems of mental health or mental illness are subject to disabling environments that reduce their access to important occupational opportunities and resources. Examples are included in the following:

- *Attitudinal factors* are shared thoughts, beliefs, and opinions, that underlie actions and behaviors. In the psychosocial arena, there is a particular concern about widely held stigmatizing attitudes that underlie discrimination. For example, shared stigmatizing beliefs can feed into the idea that people with mental illness should be kept at the margins of important community activities roles and resources. They include, for example, assumptions that people with mental illness lack the competence to participate, they are dangerous and not to be trusted, they are somehow deserving of their problems, and their problems are unmanageable or untreatable (Corrigan, Markowitz, Watson, Rowan, & Jubiak, 2003). It has proven remarkably difficult to shake these shared stigmatizing beliefs. Powerful forces, such as media reports using language that dehumanizes people and incites fear in the public, are capable of contributing to these forces of social exclusion (Whitley & Berry, 2013). A particularly powerful impact of such stigma is that it can be received and integrated by people with mental health problems or mental illnesses in such a way that they come to believe it themselves, a phenomenon referred to as self-stigma (Watson, Corrigan, Larson, & Sells, 2007). Similarly, people who are in their social networks, like family, friends, and even health providers, can be subject to processes of devaluation and discrimination (associative stigma; Pryor, Reeder, & Monroe, 2012), weakening their capacity to serve as supports. In this way, people can be excluded from important participation, opportunities, and resources without the presence of very obvious discriminating practices.

- *Environmental factors* refer to elements of the design of societies and communities that influence accessibility to full social life. There is increasing awareness of how the built environment affects occupational participation in psychosocial practice. For example, the crowded, enclosed design of much public transit may compromise its accessibility to people who experience high levels of anxiety, and the construction of high-density, low-income neighborhoods lacking in socioeconomic diversity can provoke unpleasant emotions such as anxiety, feelings of suspiciousness, and ultimately restrict participation (see for example, Boydell, Gladstone, Crawford, & Trainor, 1999).

- *Institutional factors* are those social structures that formalize the way people access full social participation. These structures can be very explicit, as is the case with formal policies and procedures, but they can also be implicit, meaning that there can be a shared understanding of rules or norms that govern participation, even if they are not present in formal documents. Sometimes institutional factors that sustain forces that marginalize people in psychosocial practice can best be described as silence or a lack of explicit policy. For example, people with mental illness have been shown to have unequal access to important health and treatment resources compared to other health conditions (Desai, Stefanovics, & Rosenheck, 2005), yet governments have tended not to make explicit policy to improve equity, even where policy is based on principles of equity. Similarly, compared to physical health concerns, there has been limited attention to standards related to the psychological and emotional health and safety of

workplaces. Recent development of such standards in Canada (Mental Health Commission of Canada, 2013) has gained international attention, but to date the uptake of these standards remains voluntary rather than a requirement of workplaces in Canada.

These factors serve as a good guide for transdisciplinary dialogue and efforts to address the full community participation of people living with psychosocial health concerns. In reality, these restrictions are complex social processes that are likely grounded in the interaction of all of these factors. The vignette in Box 4-2 provides a good example of how one workplace, committed to ensuring the full participation of its workforce, developed formal policies and procedures. The example highlights how, within their interest in maintaining levels of productivity and order in the workplace, they assertively examined how their beliefs and assumptions might be discriminating against people with psychosocial health issues to create more inclusive policies and procedures.

Theoretical Assumptions

The theoretical foundation of the social model of disability does not deny that problems in health exist, or that they can have significant implications for the individual in his or her daily life. Rather they question the extent to which the discourse about human function, activities and participation is explained as an individual problem and not as a social response to human difference. In addition to drawing attention to disabling social conditions, such as discrimination, systemic disadvantage, poverty, etc., the social model challenges the way health-related practices can obscure these social influences. In this way, the social model serves as a foundation for an ongoing critique of health and social service systems. For example, in Chapter 3, the idea of recovery was highlighted as a guiding vision of mental health service delivery. Contemporary views of recovery describe the nature of the personal changes that occur as an individual to develop an identity that is less defined by illness and more defined by hope, personal responsibility, and meaningful activities and participation. Critiques of this view of recovery, informed by a social view of disability, point out that the transformative power of recovery as a path to empowerment, autonomy, and self-direction is threatened by professional views that "softened the more provocative aspects of the empowerment perspective" and more narrowly framed recovery as "a process of coming to accept mental health problems and adapting to live with them" (Masterson & Owen, 2006, p. 30).

Key Developers

The social model of disability originated in the 1970s with ongoing development by disability scholars and advocates such as Oliver (1996), Barnes and Mercer (2004), and

> # Box 4-2. Vignette: The Social Model in Practice: Inclusive Workplace Policies and Procedures
>
> The managers of a hotel were concerned about the number of occasions staff called in sick just before the start of their shifts, and even after their shifts started. This led to considerable problems in arranging coverage. In response, the workplace instituted a policy that stated all staff must call in at least 1 hour before the start of the shift to report an absence. The policy explicitly stated that failure to do so on two occasions would result in dismissal. The policy was perceived as fair given the impact of the behavior on workplace productivity and because employees were given the opportunity to be responsible for their actions. It was assumed that failure to comply would be evidence of irresponsibility, unreliability, and a lack of commitment to the workplace and the work team. In instituting the policy managers paid close attention to occasions when the policy was broken, and it seemed to them that people with mental health concerns were largely being affected. They considered if perhaps the policy was somehow faulty and disadvantaging certain people. They asked if something could be inhibiting people from calling in. They wondered if perhaps the power relations between the front-line supervisors and issues related to stigma might be systematically working against people with mental health concerns. They thought of ways these interpersonal relations might be taken into account and changed the policy to read: Staff, or their delegates, must call in when the worker will be absent from work for personal or health reasons. They hoped that this policy might decrease the impact of stigma or difficult relations with supervisors to lead to a desired behavior on the job—and a "win-win" situation for everyone.
>
> Adapted from Krupa, T., & Lysaght, R. (2011). *Case studies on information rich, inclusive workplaces: How employers, co-workers, unions, employer associations, occupational health professionals, and disability organizations can work together to create an environment that supports people with disabilities who have intermittent work capacity.* Human Resources and Skill Development Canada. [HRSDC Contract number: 7616-10-0017].

Marks (1997). In the mental health field, Beresford (2002) pointed out the relevance of the social model, but highlighted the extent to which social constructions of disability also emerge from the extent to which people with mental illness are devalued within society and subject to forms of control with legal and health systems. Applications of the philosophy and ideas of the social model to the psychosocial field have been proliferating, A few examples follow:

- High-profile movements by people with lived experience who have focused on the rights of people with mental illness as citizens in their communities, and on the importance of their active involvement in social change (see for example, Chamberlin, 1998; Pilgrim & Waldron, 1998) and greater ownership over the systems of treatment and care (Chamberlin, 1998; Nelson, Ochocka, & Janzen, 2006).

- Focused efforts to shift and resist negative attitudes about mental illness through a range of "pride activities" that counteract forces of shame that keep the voices and experiences of people with mental illnesses hidden from view, and subsequently poorly addressed. These activities include memoirs about mental illness, public presentations and narratives from people with lived experience, and even organized public events such as parades (Glaser, 2008).

- The application of a citizenship perspective in the design and delivery of health-related and social services to ensure that such services are governed by outcomes directed to protecting rights and enabling full community participation and access to valued resources (Hopper, 2007; Huxley & Thornicroft, 2003; Nelson, Lord, & Ochocka, 2001).

- Focused efforts to understand and address the attitudinal and structural foundations sustaining stigma and discrimination related to problems of mental health have proliferated over the past decade (Thompson et al., 2002; Thornicroft, 2006). To date, national anti-stigma initiatives have been launched in the United States, Canada, New Zealand, Australia, the United Kingdom, and Ireland.

Occupational therapists have made significant contributions to the advancement of the social model of disability. Jongbloed and Chricton (1990), for example, critiqued the way disability is viewed and ultimately approached in rehabilitation professions, such as occupational therapy. In the psychosocial practice arena, there are several examples of occupational therapy efforts to critique and develop the delivery of occupational therapy services from perspectives that are consistent with the social model. One of the most compelling examples has been the work of Townsend (1998) who identified the processes by which psychosocial practice in the profession can become organized to, albeit unintentionally, undermine the full participation of people with mental illness and ultimately contribute to the forces

TABLE 4-1	
ADDRESSING DISEMPOWERMENT IN THE ROUTINE DELIVERY OF PSYCHOSOCIAL OCCUPATIONAL THERAPY PRACTICE	
EMPOWERMENT-CONSTRAINING PRACTICE	**EMPOWERMENT-ENABLING PRACTICE**
• Objectifying participants: Casting individuals as objects of occupational therapy practice	• Inviting people to be active participants in envisioning and developing opportunities and potentials
• Individualizing action: Viewing addressing occupational issues on an individual level	• Enabling opportunities for individual and collective actions to develop opportunities and potentials
• Controlling collaboration: Hierarchy in decision making that minimizes the authority of the individual receiving services	• Encouraging collaborative decision making in relation to individual and service planning
• Simulating real life: Change is promoted through situations that imitate those in real-life	• Addressing individual and group occupational issues in real-life contexts and in real-time need
• Risking liability: Organizing and implementing services to manage risk	• Supporting risk-taking to enable change and growth
• Promoting marginal inclusiveness: Enabling limited and fringe forms of community participation	• Universal access and participation is championed
Reprinted with permission from Townsend, E. "Good Intentions Overruled: A Critique of Empowerment in the Routine Organization of Mental Health Services." Copyright © 1998 by University of Toronto Press.	

of disempowerment and exclusion. Table 4-1 provides a brief overview of these processes. For example, Townsend identified occupational therapists' use of simulated activities to enable positive change in occupation as a potentially disempowering process if it fails to translate to what people actually need, want, and are expected to do in their real community lives.

Evolutionary Points

The social model of disability has sparked considerable dialogue and debate since its emergence, and subsequently its theoretical foundations and applications have evolved. Contemporary considerations of the social model include the extent to which mental health issues intersect with other factors such as gender and race to lead to social inequities (Morrow & Weisser, 2012). Occupational therapists stand to make important contributions to the evolution of the social model. By carefully considering how particular populations are routinely disadvantaged in service delivery models, the profession can both demonstrate a genuine respect for the very real social barriers that people face, identify their needs, and contribute intervention approaches to promote their health and well-being. A good example is the work of

Helfrich, an American occupational therapist, and her colleagues who identified how the daily living skills of women in abusive domestic situations are systematically undermined within threatening and violent partner relations as a form of ongoing control. Using a participatory approach, they adapted and tested a life skills curriculum to meet their needs (Gorde, Helfrich, & Finlayson, 2004).

In many cases, these evolutions in practice are not necessarily explicitly tied to the social model, but nevertheless they are highly consistent with the social model. They frequently start as innovative ideas to create new service structures, but ultimately have a profound effect on the way disability in psychosocial practice is understood and addressed.

Expected Outcomes

Applications of the social model of disability are expected to lead to elimination of the many social and structural barriers to the activities and participation of people who experience mental health problems. Applied to service delivery systems, the expectation is that the social model will lead to a valuing of outcomes that are indicative of full social inclusion, full access to opportunities and resources, and other indicators of full citizenship. In this way, models of service delivery in psychosocial occupational therapy practice are increasingly being called upon to provide evidence that they are having a significant outcome on social inclusion and participation. This, in turn, presses for service delivery models that will include attention to social factors. For occupational therapists, this means moving beyond narrow definitions of service as "clinically" focused on individuals, to practice that is sensitive and responsive to these complex social processes.

PRACTICE DEVELOPMENTS

Although neither transdisciplinary model of disability is considered a practice model, they have served as a basis for, or inspired the development of, a range of knowledge or tools that can be applied directly to practice by occupational therapists and others in a transdisciplinary context. Only a brief sample of some of these practice developments is provided here.

The ICF has, perhaps, witnessed the most prolific development of practice tools. This is not surprising given that the developers of the ICF explicitly focused on its potential to positively influence service development and delivery. Practice tools emerging from the ICF framework include instruments that provide a comprehensive assessment of function using their universal language of health, activity, and participation to promote interdisciplinary work. The WHO Disability Assessment Schedule 2 for example is a 12- or 36-item measure designed to assess behavioral limits and restrictions on activities and participation of an individual independent of the health condition or diagnosis (WHO, 2013c).

Recognizing that in practice settings the application of the ICF to specific health conditions may be a complex process, the WHO has initiated a "core set" project, where rigorous and participatory processes are used to identify the most common categories relevant to specific health conditions, thereby providing some level of standardization in the application of the ICF. These core sets are available through the ICF Research Branch online website (www.icf-research-branch.org). In mental health, for example, the ICF has produced core sets for both depression and bipolar disorder. The brief core set for depression is presented here in Table 4-2. Referring back to the vignette of Catherine, many of these core categories are reflected: issues with optimism, energy level and motivation, solving problems and making decisions, managing daily routines and activities levels, and handling stress, as well as issues related to a range of important social relationships and maintaining employment. Other categories are not explicitly mentioned in the vignette, but may prompt consideration from the occupational therapist to consider, such as functions of attention and activities of self-care.

The recent development of a core set for multidisciplinary vocational rehabilitation crossed all health conditions to identify the most common categories relevant to describe and measure the function of people receiving vocational rehabilitation services (Table 4-3). Occupational therapists from around the world were well represented on the international expert panel that finalized the core sets for vocational rehabilitation (Finger et al., 2012), but the validity of the core set as a tool for occupational therapy practice has yet to be established. Of particular interest in this core set is the extent to which the core categories are psychological and emotional in nature, suggesting that psychosocial concerns are prevalent in addressing employment and work-related activities, across health conditions.

While key occupational therapy conceptual models have typically included environmental factors as central determinants of human occupation, the broad societal context of these environmental factors can compromise a therapist's sense of being able to truly "make a difference." The influence of the social model of disability has engendered practice contexts that enable occupational therapists to develop and implement practice consistent with its philosophical foundations. For example, empowerment has translated to a population level movement to organize people with disabilities against disabling, discriminating, and oppressive social structures. The influence of the social model has also been seen in the development of social policy that has legitimized and protected the rights of people with disability. In response, occupational therapists have become involved in acting as catalysts and advocates to facilitate these movements. Swarbrick and Pratt (2006), for example, describe the role that occupational therapists have played in the development of community-based services that are run by, and for, people with mental illness.

CONCLUSION

Each of the transdisciplinary models of disability has elements that will resonate with psychosocial occupational therapy theory and practice. The ICF, for example, offers a focus on function, activity, and participation that is highly consistent with the profession's focus on occupation. The ICF stands to raise the profile of activity limitations and participation restrictions that have long received limited attention in health fields that have largely been dominated by biomedical concerns. In psychosocial practice in particular the ICF provides a useful framework for connecting mental health and mental illness within the broader field of disability. For example, the model provides a means to link the symptoms and impairments common to mental illnesses with activity limitations and participation restrictions and to stress the similarities across physical and mental health conditions, rather than their differences. The ICF is, however, lacking in its development of the personal

TABLE 4-2

ICF CORE CATEGORIES FOR DEPRESSION

ICF CORE CATEGORY AND NUMBER	DEFINITION
Body function: Body functions are the physiological and psychological functions of body systems	
b1263 Psychic stability	Mental functions that produce a personal disposition that is even-tempered, calm, and composed, as contrasted to being irritable, worried, erratic, and moody
b1265 Optimism	Mental functions that produce a personal disposition that is cheerful, buoyant and hopeful, as contrasted to being downhearted, gloomy, and despairing
b1300 Energy level	Mental functions that produce vigor and stamina
b1301 Motivation	Mental functions that produce the incentive to act; the conscious or unconscious driving force for action
b1302 Appetite	Mental functions that produce a natural longing or desire, especially the natural and recurring desire for food and drink
b140 Attention functions	Specific mental functions of focusing an external stimulus or internal experience for the required period of time
b147 Psychomotor functions	Specific mental functions of control over both motor and psychological events at the body level
b1521 Regulation of emotion	Mental functions that control the experience and display of affect
b1522 Range of emotions	Mental functions that produce the spectrum of experience of arousal of affect or feelings such as love, hate, anxiousness, sorrow, joy, fear, and anger
Activities and participation: Activity is the execution of a task or action by an individual; participation is involvement in a life situation	
d163 Thinking	Formulating and manipulating ideas, concepts, and images, whether goal-oriented or not, either alone or with others, such as creating fiction, proving a theorem, playing with ideas, brainstorming, meditating, pondering, speculating, or reflecting
d175 Solving problems	Finding solutions to questions or situations by identifying and analyzing issue, developing options and solutions, evaluating potential effects of solutions, and executing a chosen solution
d177 Making decisions	Making a choice among options, implementing the choice and evaluating the effects of the choice, such as selecting and purchasing a specific item, or deciding to undertake and undertaking one task from among several tasks that need to be done
d2301 Managing daily routine	Carrying out simple or complex and coordinated actions in order to plan and manage the requirements of day-to-day procedures or duties
d2303 Managing one's own activity level	Carrying out actions and behaviors to arrange the requirements in energy and time day-to-day procedures or duties
d240 Handling stress and other psychological demands	Carrying out simple or complex and coordinated actions to manage and control the psychological demands required to carry out tasks demanding significant responsibilities and involving stress, distraction or crises such as driving a vehicle during heavy traffic or taking care of many children
d350 Conversation	Starting, sustaining, and ending an interchange of thoughts and ideas carried out by means of spoken, written, sign, or other forms of language, with one or more people one knows or who are strangers, in formal or casual settings

(continued)

TABLE 4-2 (continued)	
ICF CORE CATEGORIES FOR DEPRESSION	
ICF CORE CATEGORY AND NUMBER	**DEFINITION**
d510 Washing oneself	Washing and drying one's whole body or body parts, using water and appropriate cleaning and drying materials or methods, such as bathing, showering, washing hands and feet, face and hair, and drying with a towel
d570 Looking after one's health	Ensuring physical comfort, health, and physical and mental well-being, such as maintaining a balanced diet, and an appropriate level of physical activity, keeping warm or cool, avoiding harms to health, following safe sex practices, including using condoms, getting immunizations and regular physical examinations
d760 Family relationships	Creating and maintaining kinship relationships, such as with members of the nuclear, extended, foster, and adopted family and step-relationships, more distant relationships such as second cousins, or legal guardians
d770 Intimate relationships	Creating and maintaining a relationship based on emotional and physical attraction, potentially leading to long-term intimate relationships
d845 Acquiring, keeping, and terminating a job	Seeking, finding, and choosing employment, being hired and accepting employment, maintaining and advancing through a job, trade, occupation, or profession, and leaving a job in an appropriate manner
Environmental factors: Environmental factors make up the physical, social, and attitudinal environment in which people live and conduct their lives. The factors are focused on improving functioning, providing support, etc.	
e1101 Drugs	Any natural or human-made object or substance gathered, processed, or manufactured for medicinal purposes, such as allopathic and naturopathic medication
e310 Immediate family	Individuals related by birth, marriage, or other relationship recognized by the culture as immediate family
e320 Friends	Individuals who are close and ongoing participants in relationships characterized by trust and mutual support
e325 Acquaintances, peers, colleagues, neighbors, and community members	Individuals who are familiar to each other, in situations of work, school, recreation, or other aspects of life and who share demographic features such as age, gender, religious creed, or ethnicity or pursue common interests
e355 Health professionals	All service providers working within the context of the health system
e410 Individual attitudes of immediate family members; e415 extended family members; e420 friends; health professionals	General or specific opinions and beliefs of immediate/extended family members/friends/health professionals about the person or about other matters that influence individual behavior and actions
e580 Health services, systems and policies	Services, systems and policies for preventing and treating health problems, providing medical rehabilitation, and promoting a healthy lifestyle
Reprinted with permission from Cieza, A., Chatterji, S., Andersen, C., Cantista, P., Herceg, M., Melvin, J., Stucki, G., & de Bie, R. (2004). ICF Core Sets for depression. *Journal of Rehabilitation Medicine, 44 Sup*, 128-134.	

TABLE 4-3

ICF CORE SET FOR VOCATIONAL REHABILITATION: A GUIDE WITH DEFINITIONS

ICF CODE NUMBER AND CATEGORY	DEFINITION OF ICF CORE CATEGORY
Activity and participation: Activity is the execution of a task or action by an individual; participation is involvement in a life situation	
d155 Acquiring skills	Developing basic and complex competencies in integrated sets of actions or tasks so as to initiate and follow through with the acquisition of a skill, such as manipulating tools or playing games like chess
d240 Handling stress and other psychological demands	Carrying out simple or complex and coordinated actions to manage and control the psychological demands required to carry out tasks demanding significant responsibilities and involving stress, distraction, or crises, such as driving a vehicle during heavy traffic or taking care of many children
d720 Complex interpersonal interactions	Maintaining and managing interactions with other people, in a contextually and socially appropriate manner, such as by regulating emotions and impulses, controlling verbal and physical aggression, acting independently in social interactions, and acting in accordance with social rules and conventions
d845 Acquiring, keeping, and terminating a job	Seeking, finding, and choosing employment, being hired and accepting employment, maintaining and advancing through a job, trade, occupation or profession, and leaving a job in an appropriate manner. Includes seeking employment, preparing a resume or curriculum vitae, contacting employers and preparing interviews, maintaining a job, monitoring one's own work performance, giving notice, and terminating a job
d850 Remunerative employment	Engaging in all aspects of work, as an occupation, trade, profession or other form of employment , for payment, as an employee, full or part time, or self-employed, such as seeking employment and getting a job, doing the required tasks of the job, attending work on time as required, supervising other workers or being supervised, and performing required tasks alone or in groups
d855 Non-remunerative employment	Engaging in all aspects of work in which pay is not provided, full-time or part-time, including organized work activities, doing the required tasks of the job, attending work on time as required, supervising other workers or being supervised, and performing required tasks alone or in groups, such as volunteer work, charity work, working for a community or religious group without remuneration, working around the home without remuneration
Environmental factors: Environmental factors make up the physical, social, and attitudinal environment in which people live and conduct their lives	
e310 Immediate family	Individuals related by birth, marriage, or other relationship recognized by the culture as immediate family, such a spouses, partners, parents, siblings, children, foster parents, adoptive parents, and grandparents
e330 People in positions of authority	Individuals who have decision-making responsibilities for others and who have socially defined influence or power based on their social, economic, cultural, or religious roles in society, such as teachers, employers, supervisors, religious leaders, substitute decision-makers, guardians, or trustees
e580 Health services, systems, and policies	Services, systems, and policies for preventing and treating health problems, providing medical rehabilitation and promoting a healthy lifestyle

(continued)

TABLE 4-3 (continued)
ICF CORE SET FOR VOCATIONAL REHABILITATION: A GUIDE WITH DEFINITIONS

ICF CODE NUMBER AND CATEGORY	DEFINITION OF ICF CORE CATEGORY
e590 Labor and employment services	Services, systems, and policies related to finding suitable work for persons who are unemployed or looking for different work, or to support individuals already employed who are seeking promotion.
Body functions: Body functions are the physiological and psychological functions of body systems	
b130 Energy and drive functions	General mental functions of physiological and psychological mechanisms that cause the individual to move toward satisfying specific needs and general goals in a persistent manner. Includes function of energy level, motivation, appetite, craving, and impulse control.
b164 Higher-level cognitive functions	Specific mental functions especially dependent on the frontal lobes of the brain, including complex goal-directed behaviors such as decision-making, abstract thinking, planning and carrying out plans, mental flexibility, and deciding which behaviors are appropriate under what circumstances; often called executive functions.
b455 Exercise tolerance functions	Functions related to respiratory and cardiovascular capacity as required for enduring physical exertion. Includes functions of physical endurance, aerobic capacity, stamina, and fatiguability.
Reprinted with permission from Finger, M. E., Escorpizo, R., Glässel, A, Gmünder, H. P., Lückenkemper, M., Chan C., Fritz J, Studer, U., Ekholm, J., Kostanjsek, N., Stucki, G., & Cieza, A. (2012). ICF Core Set for vocational rehabilitation: results of an international consensus conference. *Disability and Rehabilitation, 34* (5): 429-438.

factors associated with human function, and this is a limitation for occupational therapists who look for and enable personal strengths and capacities to support occupational transformations. In addition, the ICF does not attend to the individual's actual *experience* of activities and participation, and is silent on matters of "meaning," "choice," and "patterns of activity," all considered central organizing forces for well-being in human function and participation for occupational therapists.

Consistent with the social model of disability, comprehensive occupational therapy conceptual modes include direct consideration of the social environmental context within which occupation occurs. A good example of this is the Person-Environment-Occupation Model detailed in another chapter in this text. Although the profession has not named society as the central source of disability, consideration of the social and environmental context is considered a necessary perspective from which to view problems in occupation by most of the foundational conceptual models used by occupational therapists. The evolution of the social model has led to the development of a knowledge base related to how society is disabling, and growing evidence of how to effectively reduce these barriers. This

has been particularly important in the psychosocial arena where people with problems of mental health and mental illness have experienced exceptionally high levels of discrimination and marginalization. However, operating solely, or even predominantly, from a social perspective may be impossible for occupational therapists who largely work in health systems that press for individually focused explanations for occupational problems.

LEARNING ACTIVITIES/ DISCUSSION QUESTIONS

1. The vignette of Catherine presented an example of how the ICF might be used to define the functioning, activities, and participation of a woman with a primary diagnosis of major depression. Apply the framework to an individual you know or have worked with in occupational therapy, who has experienced major depression along with another health condition such as diabetes mellitus, chronic back pain, or cardiac problems.

2. Imagine that you are the occupational therapist working with Catherine. How might the social model of disability inform your practice? Identify three specific things you might do, consistent with the social model, if you were working with Catherine.

3. The personal factors that enable or constrain function, activity, and participation have, to date, been relatively underdeveloped within the ICF. List the personal factors you think should be included in the ICF.

4. How do you think people with the lived experience of mental illness might view these two models—the ICF and the social model of disability? Find a first-person account by someone with lived experience and compare it to your thoughts on this.

REFERENCES

Barnes, C., & Mercer, G. (2004). *Implementing the social model of disability: Theory and research.* Leeds, UK: The Disability Press.

Bendixon, R. M., & Kreider, C. M. (2011). Review of occupational therapy research in the practice area of children and youth. *American Journal of Occupational Therapy, 65*(3), 351-359.

Beresford, P. (2002). Thinking about "mental health": Towards a social model. *Journal of Mental Health, 11*(6), 581-584.

Bickenbach, J. E., Chatterji, S., Badley, E. M., & Üstün, T. B. (1999). Models of disablement, universalism and the international classification of impairments, disabilities and handicaps. *Social Science & Medicine, 48,* 1173-1187.

Boydell, K. M., Gladstone, B. M., Crawford, E., & Trainor, J. (1999). Making do on the outside: Everyday life in the neighborhoods of people with psychiatric disabilities. *Psychiatric Rehabilitation Journal, 23*(1), 11-18.

Chamberlin, J. (1998). Citizenship rights and psychiatric disability. *Psychiatric Rehabilitation Journal, 21,* 405-408.

Cieza, A., Chatterji, S., Andersen, C., Cantista, P., Herceg, M., Melvin, J., Stucki, G., & de Bie, R. (2004). ICF core sets for depression. *Journal of Rehabilitation Medicine, 44 Sup,* 128-134.

Corrigan, P., Markowitz, F. E., Watson, A., Rowan, D., & Jubiak, M.A. (2003). An attribution model of public discrimination towards persons with mental illness. *Journal of Health and Social Behavior, 44*(2), 162-179.

Corrigan, P., & Watson, A. (2002). Understanding the impact of stigma on people with mental illness. *World Psychiatry, 1*(1), 16-20.

Creek, J. (2008). Living with depression: Function, activity and participation. *World Federation of Occupational Therapy Bulletin, 57,* May 12-16.

Daremo A., & Haglund, L. (2008). Activity and participation in psychiatric institutional care. *Scandinavian Journal of Occupational Therapy, 15*(3), 131-142.

Desai, R. A., Stefanovics, E. A., & Rosenheck, R. A. (2005). The role of psychiatric diagnosis in satisfaction with primary care: data from the department of Veterans Affairs. *Medical Care. 43,* 1208-1216.

Elderon, L., & Whooley, M. A. (2013). Depression and cardiovascular disease. *Progress in Cardiovascular Diseases, 55,* 511-523.

Farrell, J., Anderson, S., Hewitt, K., Livingston, M. H., & Stewart, D. (2007). A survey of occupational therapists in Canada about their knowledge and use of the ICF. *Canadian Journal of Occupational Therapy, 74,* 221-232.

Finger, M. E., Escoprizo, R., Glässel, A., Gmünder, H., Lückenkemper, H., Chan, C.,...Cieza, A. (2012). ICF core set for vocational rehabilitation: Results of an international consensus conference. *Disability & Rehabilitation, 34*(5), 429-438.

Fougeyrollas, P., Cloutier, R., Bergeron, H., Cote, J., & St. Michel, G. (1998). *The Quebec classification: Disability creation process.* Quebec: International Network on the Disability Creation Process.

Geyh, S., Peter, C., Muller, R., Bickenbach, J. E., Kostanjsek, N., Üstün,...Cieza, A. (2011). The personal factors of the International Classification of Functioning, Disability and Health in the literature—A systematic review and content analysis. *Disability and Rehabilitation, 33,* 1089-1102.

Glaser, G. (2008). "Mad pride fights a stigma." *New York Times.* Retrieved from www.nytimes.com/2008/05/11/fashion/11madpride.html?_r=0

Gorde, M., Helfrich, C. A., & Finlayson, M. (2004). Trauma symptoms and life skill needs of domestic violence victims. *Journal of Interpersonal Violence, 19*(6), 691-708.

Hackett, M. L., Yapa, C., Parag, V., & Anderson, C. S. (2005). Frequency of depression after stroke: A systematic review of observational studies. *Stroke, 36,* 1330-1340.

Haglund, L. (2008). The ICF vs. occupational therapy instruments similarities from a mental health perspective. *World Federation of Occupational Therapy Bulletin, 57,* May, 5-11.

Haglund, L. & Faltman, S. (2012). Activity and participation—Self-assessment according to the International Classification of Functioning: A study in mental health. *British Journal of Occupational Therapy, 75*(9), 412-418.

Hammel, J., Magas, S., Heinemann, A., Whiteneck, G., Bogner, J., & Rodriguez, E. (2008). What does participation mean? An insider perspective from people with disabilities. *Disability & Rehabilitation, 30*(19), 1445-1460.

Hopper, K. (2007). Rethinking social recovery in schizophrenia: what a capabilities approach might offer. *Social Science & Medicine, 65,* 868-879.

Huxley, P., & Thornicroft, G. (2003). Social inclusion, social quality and mental illness. *British Journal of Psychiatry, 182,* 289-290.

Jongbloed, L., & Chricton, A. (1990). A new definition of disability: Implications for rehabilitation practice and social policy. *Canadian Journal of Occupational Therapy, 57*(1), 32-38.

Kielhofner, G. (2005). Rethinking disability and what to do about it: Disability studies and its implications for occupational therapy. *American Journal of Occupational Therapy, 59,* 487-496.

Kirchberger, I., Stamm, T., Cieza, A., & Stucki, G. (2007). Does the comprehensive ICF core set for rheumatoid arthritis capture occupational therapy practice? A content-validity study. *Canadian Journal of Occupational Therapy, 74*(5), 267-280.

Krupa, T. (2008). Part of the solution…or part of the problem? Addressing the stigma of mental illness in our midst. *Canadian Journal of Occupational Therapy, 75*(4), 198-205.

Krupa, T., & Lysaght, R. (2011). *Case studies on information rich, inclusive workplaces: How employers, co-workers, unions, employer associations, occupational health professionals, and disability organizations can work together to create an environment that supports people with disabilities who have intermittent work capacity.* Human Resources and Skill Development Canada. [HRSDC Contract number: 7616-10-0017].

Leonardi, M., Bickenbach, J., Üstün, T. B., Kostanjsek, N., Chatterji, S., & MHADIE Consortium. (2006). The definition of disability: What's in a name? *Lancet, 368*, 1219-21.

Marks, D. (1997). Models of disability. *Disability and Rehabilitation, 19*(3), 85-91.

Masterson, S., & Owen, S. (2006). Mental health service user's social and individual empowerment: Using theories of power to elucidate far-reaching strategies. *Journal of Mental Health, 15*(1), 19-34.

Mental Health Commission of Canada. (2013). *Psychological health and safety in the workplace—Prevention, promotion, and guidance to staged implementation.* Calgary, AB: Mental Health Commission of Canada.

Morrow, M., & Weisser, J. (2012). Towards a social justice framework of mental health recovery. *Studies in Social Justice, 6*(1), 27-43.

Nelson, G. B., Lord, J., & Ochocka, J. (2001). *Shifting the paradigm in community mental health: Towards empowerment and community.* Toronto: University of Toronto Press.

Nelson, G. B., Ochocka, J., & Janzen, R. (2006). A longitudinal study of mental health consumer/survivor initiatives: Part 1-Literature review and overview of the study. *Journal of Community Psychology, 34*, 247-260.

Nagi, S. Z. (1979). The concept and measurement of disability. In E. D. Berkowitz (Ed), *Disability Policies and Government Programs.* New York: Praeger.

Oliver, M. (1996). *Understanding disability: From theory to practice.* Basingstoke: MacMillan.

Pilgrim, D., & Waldron, L. (1998). User involvement in mental health service development: How far can it go? *Journal of Mental Health, 7*(1), 95-104.

Pryor, J. B., Reeder, G. D., & Monroe, A. E. (2012). The infection of bad company: Stigma by association. *Journal of Personality and Social Psychology, 102*, 224-241.

Shaw, L., Leyshon, R., & Liu, M. (2007). Validating the potential of the International Classification of Functioning, Disability and Health to identify barriers to and facilitators of consumer participation. *Canadian Journal of Occupational Therapy, 74*(Special Edition), 255-266.

Swarbrick, P., & Pratt, C. (2006). Consumer-operated self-help services: roles and opportunities for occupational therapists and occupational therapy assistants. *OT Practice, 11*(5).

Thompson, A. H., Stuart, H., Bland, R. C., Arboleda-Florez, J., Warner, R., & Dicks, R. (2002). Attitudes about schizophrenia from the pilot site of the WPA worldwide campaign against the stigma of schizophrenia. *Social Psychiatry and Psychiatric Epidemiology, 37*, 475-482.

Thornicroft, G. (2006). *Shunned: Discrimination against people with mental illness.* Oxford: Oxford University Press.

Townsend, E. (1998). *Good intentions overruled: A critique of empowerment in the routine organization of mental health services.* Toronto: University of Toronto Press.

Üstün, T. B., Ayuso, J. L., Chatterji, S., Mathers, C., & Murray, C. J. (2004). Global burden of depression in the year 2000. *British Journal of Psychiatry, 184*, 386-392.

Üstün, T. B., Chatterji, S., Bickenbach, J. E., Kostanjsek, N., & Schneider, M. (2003). The International Classification of Functioning, Disability and Health: a new tool for understanding disability and health. *Disability & Rehabilitation, 25*, 565-571.

Verbrugge, L. M., & Jette, A. M. (1994). The disablement process. *Social Science & Medicine, 38*, 1-14.

Vrooman, K. E., & Arthanat, S. (2008). ICF and mental functions: applied to cross cultural case studies of schizophrenia. International Encyclopedia of Rehabilitation. Center for International Rehabilitation Research Information and Exchange (CIRRIE). Retrieved from http://cirrie.buffalo.edu/encyclopedia/en/article/308/.

Watson, A. C., Corrigan, P., Larson, J. E., & Sells, M. (2007). Self-stigma in people with mental illness. *Schizophrenia Bulletin, 33*, 1312, 1318.

Whalley-Hammell, K. (2004). Deviating from the norm: a sceptical interrogation of the classificatory practices of the ICF. *British Journal of Occupational Therapy, 67*, 408-411.

Whitley, R., & Berry, S. (2013). Analyzing media representation of mental illness: Lessons learnt from a national project. *Journal of Mental Health, 22*(3), 246-253.

World Health Organization. (2001). *International Classification of Functioning, Disability and Health (ICF).* Geneva, Switzerland: World Health Organization.

World Health Organization. (2013a). International Classification of Functioning, Disability and Health (ICF). Retrieved October 12, 2013, from www.who.int/classifications/icf/en/

World Health Organization. (2013b). ICF Application Areas. Geneva: World Health Organization. Retrieved from www.who.int/classifications/icf/appareas/en/index.html

World Health Organization. (2013c). WHO Disability Assessment Schedule 2.0 WHODAS 2.0. Retrieved on October 12, 2013 from www.who.int/classifications/icf/whodasii/en/

Zesiewicz, T. A., & Hauser, R. A. (2002). Depression in Parkinson's disease. *Current Psychiatry Reports, 4*(1), 69-73.

section III

Occupational Models and Frameworks

In this section, we present models and frameworks that are occupation focused; that is they are explicitly concerned with occupational performance and/or human experience of occupations. These models and frameworks have been selected because they have all, in some way, made significant contributions to the advancement of psychosocial practice. Because it was not possible to present the full array of occupation-focused models and frameworks, readers are encouraged to familiarize themselves with others that advance psychosocial practice; for example the Kawa Model presents a compelling framework that shifts the view of occupation from an individualistic one to collective and interdependent perspectives that may resonate cross culturally.

This section starts with chapters focused on meaning and motivation, two foundational constructs important to developing a full understanding of human occupation. Taken together, meaning and motivation help us to understand why humans engage in occupations, why they select or prefer particular occupations over others and why they will persevere with occupations even in the face of significant challenges. Meaning and motivation can also help us to understand why the people we serve as occupational therapists can become seriously disengaged from occupations. These chapters provide examples of how this occupational disengagement can present across a range of health and social circumstances and suggest intervention approaches to enable positive occupational experiences. Chapter 7 demonstrates how a generic model, the Person-Environment-Occupation Model, can be applied to understand and address the occupational issues experienced by people with mental illness. Chapter 8 presents the Canadian Model of Occupational Performance and Engagement with a focus on specific aspects of the model that have contributed to psychosocial practice. These include, for example, the development and applications of important constructs such as client-centred practice and empowerment, spirituality, enablement, and engagement. The Model of Human Occupation, presented in Chapter 9, has perhaps had the most profound impact on psychosocial practice. With its focus on the processes that interact to result in meaningful human occupation, the founders of this model distinguished and developed distinct aspects of this process—volition, habituation, and performance—in occupation, and created a range of intervention approaches and tools to support these processes. Finally, Chapter 10 focuses on temporal aspects of occupation, showcasing theory and practice in occupational therapy that attends to the personal and social implications of the daily rhythms of human occupation.

5

Occupation and Meaning

Ellie Fossey, PhD, MSc, DipCOT (UK); Terry Krupa, PhD, OT Reg (Ont), FCAOT; and Larry Davidson, PhD

Fiona: Now I'm doing something that I'm passionate about, and I'm happy.... I just feel so at home... I really enjoy it. I get a tremendous lot of feedback from seeing someone learn, and from having some acknowledgment that I've helped them in the process.... I spark off young people. They give me energy, and, um, I love teaching because of it.

Peter: I was feeling a sense of being under siege or feeling threatened; whereas now I feel a sense of, like, the outside world is not a threatening place. It's like an enjoyable place; it's almost like a playground where I'm finding all these [new] levels of fulfilment and enjoyment. (Quotes from Fiona and Peter, cited in Fossey, 2009, p. 263 & 312)

Life is never made unbearable by circumstances, but only by lack of meaning and purpose. (Viktor E. Frankl, Man's Search for Meaning)

OBJECTIVES

The objectives of this chapter are as follows:

» Describe ways in which meaning is understood in occupational therapy, distinguishing between meanings in occupation, meaning in life, meaning of life, and spirituality.

» Identify interdisciplinary perspectives of meaning.

» Identify sources of meaning in everyday occupations and discuss how meaning impacts activity choices, engagement, and sustained involvement.

» Discuss the evolution of occupational perspectives of meaning and key occupational therapy contributors.

» Discuss meaning and loss of, or lack of, meaning in relation to health and well-being.

» Describe how occupational therapists can support engagement in potentially meaningful occupations.

Krupa, T., Kirsh, B., Pitts, D., & Fossey, E. *Bruce & Borg's Psychosocial Frames of Reference: Theories, Models, and Approaches for Occupation-Based Practice, Fourth Edition* (pp 75-92). © 2016 SLACK Incorporated.

BACKGROUND

The term *meaning* in everyday language suggests something of significance, importance, and value. Meaning is understood to be a complex construct with multiple elements, including subjective experience, an inextricable link to context, and links to intention and purpose. Meaning is embedded in sociocultural knowledge that may be taken for granted, or not always explicit.

This chapter opens with quotations that illustrate some differing elements of meaning. Fiona and Peter both speak about their work in a project exploring everyday life from the perspective of adults with mental health issues in Australia (Fossey, 2009). Fiona describes the personal meaning of teaching for her, highlighting social aspects of its meaning—her interactions with the students and feeling "at home" in the place where she works. Peter's quote illustrates that meanings are not fixed but created, and transformed through engagement with the social world. Peter describes finding new "levels of enjoyment and fulfilment" through his job that were previously limited by his disengagement from the "outside world" during a prolonged period of unemployment and mental ill-health. Peter and Fiona convey a sense of valuing engagement in occupations that bring personal and social meaning to their everyday experience. The final quote, from the seminal work by Viktor Frankl, highlights that meaning is fundamental to well-being, and never more so than when humans are faced with circumstances of suffering.

In this chapter, the focus is on the notion of meaning as it relates to occupation. In occupational therapy, the concept of meaning is seen as inextricably linked to people's specific ways of participating in daily life. So when occupational therapists talk about *meaningful occupation*, they are referring to occupations that have personal and social significance, importance, and value. Even though the notion of meaningful occupation has long been prominent in occupational therapy discourse, the profession's dominant focus, even now, has been on objective functioning and performance issues. This has tended to overshadow the importance of clients' experiences of their everyday occupations in terms of their subjective or personal meaning (Doble & Santha, 2008; Hasselkus, 2002; Polatajko et al., 2007). Furthermore, Hasselkus (2006) has argued the very ordinariness, or everyday-ness, of what people do in their daily lives may have made it difficult for the profession to establish its credibility and gain respect within medical spheres, and more broadly, in society. So, despite the significance in human life of "the small experiences of everyday life and everyday occupation [that] have complexity, beauty, meaningfulness, and relevance to health and wellbeing that belies their aura of ordinariness and routine" (Hasselkus, 2006, p. 630), it has been difficult to give the idea of *meaning,* as it relates to occupation, shape and

definition as the central focus of an occupational therapy practice framework.

Current perspectives on occupation recognize that the notion of performance is in itself inadequate to understand the complexities of occupation. The need to reconceptualize occupation based on the subjective qualities of people's experiences of doing, rather than activity-based categorizations (such as self-care, leisure, and work), is being increasingly argued, along with the view that greater emphasis in occupational therapy practice must be placed on seeking to understand how people experience and find meaning in their doings (Doble & Santha, 2008; Hammell, 2009; Hasselkus, 2006; Jonsson, 2008). This central position of meaning as a foundation for occupation is reflected in the framework for psychosocial occupational therapy practice presented in Chapter 1. It is also evident in occupation-focused practice models, such as the Model of Human Occupation (Kielhofner, 2008b), in which processes of doing, experiencing, and meaning-making are seen as interconnected in how people experience and find meaning in occupation. In addition, concepts of spirituality and occupational engagement, as introduced into the Canadian Model of Occupational Performance and Engagement, also point to the meaning and experiential dimensions of engaging in occupations of daily life (Polatajko et al., 2007). This shift in focus toward the subjective experience and qualities of engagement in occupation holds promise for more fully developing a conceptual framework of meaning and occupation.

An appreciation of meaning as it relates to occupation is of particular relevance for occupational therapy in contemporary mental health practice, where the notion of recovery and supporting persons in their own recovery is a major focus. As detailed in Chapter 3, the process of recovery is typically seen to involve processes of meaning-making, self-discovery, growth, and transformation (Davidson, O'Connell, Tondora, Lawless, & Evans, 2005; Deegan, 2001; O'Hagan, 2001; Turner-Crowson & Wallcraft, 2002), whereas research suggests that the process of recovering occurs through everyday life interactions and activities (Borg & Davidson, 2008; Leufstadius, Erlandsson, Bjorkman, & Eklund, 2008; Sutton, Hocking, & Smythe, 2012). These ideas hold particular relevance to people experiencing prolonged illness, disability, or changed life circumstances (such as loss of employment, retirement, bereavement) that drastically alter or constrain their capacity to engage in and experience meaning in their daily activities. Positive adaptation in such altered conditions depends on being able to integrate these experiences in a way that allows for finding meaning (Borell, Asaba, Rosenberg, Schult, & Townsend, 2006; Jonsson, 2010; Psarra & Kleftaras, 2013), so it becomes important to explore how people go about rethinking their occupational engagement (Borell et al., 2006; Persson, Andersson, & Eklund, 2011). Occupational therapists who deepen their knowledge of the meaning and

TABLE 5-1
POSSIBLE MEANINGS OF PARTICIPATING IN EVERYDAY OCCUPATIONS
FOR PARTICIPATION TO BE MEANINGFUL, IT NEEDS TO OFFER THE PERSON OPPORTUNITIES
For becoming better at something and/or accomplishment
For connection with others and a sense of belonging
For expressing self, aptitudes, talents, and interests
For exercising agency and/or authority
For appreciating beauty and experiencing joy
For connecting to something larger than oneself
For rest, reflection, and quietude
For caring for and being good to oneself
For caring for/helping others out, and being cared for by others
For contributing in family, community, and society
For prospering socially and economically

experiential dimensions of occupation are in a good position to support people in regaining experiences of meaning, satisfaction, and well-being in daily life within contexts of ill-health, disability, or altered life circumstances.

THEORETICAL ASSUMPTIONS UNDERLYING MEANING AS IT RELATES TO OCCUPATION

There are a number of key ideas connecting meaning and occupation; these are briefly outlined below.

Occupational engagement is a widely used term in occupational therapy, but it is not often defined. As described in Enabling Occupation II, occupational engagement is to "involve oneself or become occupied, to participate" (Polatajko et al., 2007, p. 26) and is considered to encompass qualities such as the nature, intensity, extent of, and degree of establishment of a person's engagement in an occupation. Thus, the concept of occupational engagement focuses our attention on the experiential and meaning-related dimensions of occupation. In turn, this highlights that occupation cannot be fully understood without reference to the individuals engaged in it. In other words, the insider perspective of engaging in occupations is central to understanding the experience and meaning derived by the individual (Hammell, 2009; Jonsson, 2008).

People actively make meaning of what they do and experience. Indeed, the quest for and creation of meaning is viewed as central to being human, and to understanding the ways in which people think and act (Bruner, 1990;

Frankl, cited in Hasselkus, 2002). Meaning is also a relatively abstract notion, so that meanings are not always explicit. Therefore, the legitimacy and importance of meaning as a significant human phenomenon has been subject to question. Yet meaning is real in the sense that it is experienced and draws on real world knowledge from everyday experiences, even though it may not always be easily communicated (Hasselkus, 2002, p. 2).

Meanings Associated With Engagement in Everyday Occupations

The meanings ascribed to occupations are idiosyncratic and highly individual, but experiences and meanings are also strongly connected to social context and culture. This means we may identify a number of common or shared dimensions of meaning, even though the specific experience of meaning linked to engaging in particular occupations will be individual. For instance, in two qualitative studies exploring what participation means from an insider's perspective (Borell et al., 2006; Hammel et al., 2008), adults experiencing prolonged health conditions and disability described participation as "active and meaningful engagement," "taking initiative and making choices," "being a part of" something whether that be an activity, social scene, or group, and "doing something for others." They also emphasized experiential qualities of participation (e.g., fun, interacting, enriching, satisfying) and the expression of values related to choice and control, access and opportunity, connection and inclusion, and reciprocity and respect, rather than the specific activities in which they were involved (Hammel et al., 2008). Elaborating on this idea, Table 5-1 briefly lists a number of widely understood dimensions of meaning associated with engagement in everyday occupations.

Everyday occupations become sources of meaning in rich and complex ways (Hasselkus, 2002). Occupations may be identified with several different sources of meaning; for example, gardening may provide an income and means to contribute to the community if an individual works for the city park, and it may also offer quiet leisure and time to reflect, to accomplish something, or to enjoy or connect with nature when one gardens in his or her yard (e.g., Unruh & Hutchinson, 2011; Unruh, Smith, & Scammell, 2000). Similarly, people may ascribe multiple meanings to one occupation. For example, a student may view studying particular subject matter as a means of expressing talents or meeting a challenge, while the same student may view the course of study as part of a larger meaningful context, such as becoming equipped for a chosen career and contributing to society. Importantly, other contextual elements of occupation, such as the objects used, the other people involved, and places in which occupations take place, also contribute to the personal, social, and cultural sources of meaning ascribed to people's doings (Hasselkus, 2002). For instance, wearing favorite clothes to school, using the family's treasured tea set in hosting a tea ceremony, doing something with others with whom one has a sense of belonging, and being in a place associated with pleasurable, uplifting, or painful memories each imbue the occupation engaged in with particular meaning for the individual involved. In addition, the objects themselves may hold meaning as a way to express identity in an occupational sense, that is, who one is and what one does may be expressed through clothing, possessions, and so forth (Hocking, 2000; Kielhofner, 2008b).

Meaning and Subjective Experience

Meaning is considered a central driving or motivating force for choosing, engaging, and sustaining involvement in occupations. In other words, what people do in daily life, their experiences of engagement, and the meanings they ascribe to those experiences are important because they guide how subsequent participation in occupations is anticipated, chosen, experienced, and made sense of (Kielhofner, 2008a). Accordingly, positive experiences of engaging in occupations (e.g., pleasure, enjoyment, achievement, satisfaction, and so forth), along with their perceived personal and social value, contribute to the meaning ascribed to these occupations. In turn, these meanings promote the development of interests, appraisals of capability, and confidence that support a person's further pursuit and commitment to those occupations in the longer term.

Meanings ascribed to everyday occupations (such as those listed in Table 5-1) also have relevance for appreciating people's occupational choices, patterns of participation and evolving sense of identity over the lifespan, albeit that the meanings expressed through particular occupations or their relative importance may change during a person's lifetime. For instance, taking pleasure in music as a child may be expressed in learning to play an instrument or singing in a school choir; these same occupations could either become this person's career as an adult or remain pastimes expressed through playing, singing, or attending musical performances, allowing the person to retain a sense of liking music or being musical. Thus, meaning-making in occupations can also serve to connect an individual's past, present, and envisioned future, and to create and maintain a sense of identity and continuity in life over time (Christiansen, 1999; Kielhofner et al., 2008).

Meaning and subjective experience are intimately connected. When people engage in occupations to which they ascribe meaning in a positive sense, they experience and may express thoughts and feelings that are positive (as Fiona' and Peter's quotes illustrate). Unfortunately the ability to express the experience of meaning in occupation is often constrained by the limits of language. For instance, while terms such as pleasure, enjoyment, and satisfaction are frequently used, they do not reflect the full spectrum of positive subjective experiences. Thus, the word "satisfaction" might adequately summarize our feelings when we do well on an exam, but might not capture the sum of feelings associated with receiving the diploma or degree on graduation day.

Engagement in meaningful occupations also does not protect individuals from unpleasant experiences and feelings. For example, a student taking a test or attending graduation might experience anxiety in either of these circumstances, but at the same time view them as positive experiences.

Meaning in Everyday Life and Meaning of Life

The notions of meaning of occupation described in this chapter are more closely connected to the idea of "meaning in everyday life," than to the "meaning of life." King (2004) identified *experiencing everyday life* as one of three ways in which humans establish meaning in life, along with understanding self in the world and connecting to others. Meaning in life is conceptualized as an overarching framework associated with a variety of psychosocial elements that contribute to an individual's sense of purpose, fulfilment, order, integrity, and place in the world (Stockdale Winder, 1997). This is the kind of meaning in everyday life described in Peter's quote at the beginning of the chapter. The meaning of life, on the other hand, is typically more closely associated with the spiritual and religious realm (Unruh, Versnel, & Kerr, 2002), and concerned with responding to philosophical questions about the meaning of our existence, rather than with finding meaning in what one does in day-to-day life.

The View of Health/Disorder: Meaning in Occupation and Well-Being

Occupation has long been regarded as a vehicle for creating meaning and promoting well-being within occupational therapy literature (Hammell, 2004; Kielhofner, 1983, 2009; Meyer, 1922/1977). Furthermore, meaning is seen as having a key role in motivating and sustaining involvement in everyday occupations from which physical, psychological, and social benefits may be gained. In this way, meaningful occupational engagement is considered essential for enabling change and promoting development, transformation, and well-being (Hasselkus, 2002; Kielhofner, 1983, 2009; Wilcock, 2006). Evidence to support the importance placed by the occupational therapy profession on engagement in "meaningful" occupation is growing. For instance, first-person accounts and qualitative studies consistently suggest that meaningful engagement in occupations is a key element in recovery and in crafting a life beyond mental illness (Borg & Davidson, 2008; Davidson, 2003; Mezzina et al., 2006). Furthermore, in a Swedish study involving adults with persistent mental illness that explored the relationships among occupational performance, health, and well-being variables, Eklund and Leufstadius (2007) reported that the health-promoting elements of occupations were related to the ways in which occupations were perceived, rather than to doing them. Similarly, for experiences of aging, and persistent and degenerative health conditions, whether individuals continue to engage in particular occupations appears to depend on the meanings and value that individuals ascribe to their occupational experiences (see, for example, Keponen & Kielhofner, 2006; Öhman & Nygård, 2005; Persson, Erlandsson, Eklund, & Iwarsson, 2001; Wright-St. Clair, 2003, 2012).

Dimensions of Meaning as Psychosocial Determinants of Health

Each of the dimensions of meaning associated with participation in occupations (see Table 5-1) can be considered a psychosocial determinant of health, but the processes by which they each influence health and well-being will differ. Meanings of occupation that are associated with connections with others, for example, are linked to evidence that social connections can provide important sources of information, emotional and practical support to enable coping, modify stress, and encourage health-related living habits (Wilcock, 2006). On the other hand, meanings of occupation related to contributing to family, community, and society are believed to create access to important social supports and economic resources associated with survival and self-rated health. For some of these meanings of occupation,

the link to well-being is perhaps less obvious. For example, just viewing natural landscapes has been associated with positive affective changes and restoration, better attention, and decreased stress (Moll, Gewurtz, & Saltmarche, 2012).

Stress has long been recognized as a threat to health. Individuals experience stress in meeting the demands of daily life as they engage in occupations that they need to do, are expected to do, and want to do. The meanings ascribed to these occupations may be important mediators of the stress response and associated health outcomes. Current research has differentiated stress, labeling "good" stress as referring to situations wherein successfully responding to daily life demands has some associated benefit, whereas problematic or bad stress refers to experiences that are hard to handle and produce distress and lead to ongoing "wear and tear" on the body (McEwan & Gianoros, 2010). Meaning may be one of many psychosocial factors that enhances a sense of control, enables coping and resilience, and, in fact, may positively alter physiological stress responses that are known to affect health and longevity. For example, positive meanings associated with being a student might mediate the many demands and stresses that are inherent in the role, enabling individuals to apply effort and persevere in what they do.

On the other hand, daily life struggles related to ill health, disability, and altered life circumstances not only increase daily life demands and stresses, but also challenge or disrupt meaning. The consequence is that these meaning-related issues present challenges to health and well-being in and of themselves, regardless of the particular health condition or disabling circumstance.

Meaning, Loss of Meaning, and Meaninglessness

It is difficult to imagine well-being in occupational life in the absence of meaning. Indeed, to Viktor Frankl (1963), whose work drew on direct experience of internment in Nazi prison camps during World War II, where, even under such adverse conditions, it was both possible and necessary to make choices about meaning. Frankl highlighted that the search for meaning is part of the human condition, gives life its worth, and that meaning can be found in three ways: through doing deeds and creating work, through life experiences and encounters with people, and in suffering and adversity. Further, Frankl viewed life as made unbearable by a lack of meaning and purpose, rather than by circumstances per se. Also stemming from his work is the notion that meaninglessness reflects subjective states of boredom, apathy, and loss of direction in life's activities. So while Frankl's work focused on meaning in life, rather than occupation, his ideas are often cited in occupational therapy to emphasize the importance of restoring meaning and purpose through occupations as a worthwhile goal of therapy.

Baumeister's four human needs for meaning in life.

The importance of meaning-making for human beings is further developed by Baumeister (1991, cited in Christiansen, 1999). He proposed four human needs for meaning in life: first, that events have a purpose (related to goals and their fulfillment); second, that they are consistent with people's values (what is right and just); third, that people have a sense of control over events; and fourth, that their self-worth is affirmed. Furthermore, Antonovsky (1987) has argued that a sense of coherence in everyday life is essential for well-being and for overcoming adversity, and that one core element to this sense of coherence is finding everyday life situations meaningful, comprehensible, and manageable. Thus, meanings given to experiences can tell us not only about motives for action, but also about how people make sense of what is worthwhile and worth striving for. In turn, this shapes qualities of engagement such as effort, perseverance, and resilience in the face of difficulties or adversity. In other words, when events seem neither purposeful nor worthwhile to a person, then those events are likely to lose meaning, to seem pointless or not worth one's efforts. Hence, a sense of meaninglessness may occur "when the possibilities of a situation are not as expected and usual meanings have fallen apart" (Hasselkus, 2002, p. 3). Consequently, experiences of illness and disability may be profoundly meaning-altering experiences. For instance, Deegan (1988) provided a powerful personal account of how physical and mental disability can be such meaning-altering experiences as to leave individuals in states of profound inertia and anguish.

Some health conditions might primarily be regarded as "diseases of meaning" in the sense that they create unhappiness, alienation, and circumstances that threaten meaning (Christiansen, 1999), yet these meaning-related issues are by no means exclusive to the domain of health. Earlier it was acknowledged that multiple meanings can be ascribed to a single occupation. These meanings may or may not be congruent; in other words, there may be conflicting meanings associated with an occupation. For example, a form of employment that contributes to one's prosperity might also involve engagement in activities that are considered illegitimate socially, a situation that may lead to internal conflict, interpersonal conflict, victimization, and even threaten safety. Furthermore, the idea that occupations may be "demeaning" suggests that they can be experienced as undignified and belittling, and actually undermine the capacity to experience positive meanings in occupation. On the other hand, the impact of participating in a demeaning occupation may be offset by positive meanings associated with other activities—a person working at a low-level job to pay the bills may derive great meaning and pleasure from an artistic pastime. Thus, understanding the meaning associated with occupations is complicated and requires consideration of not only the totality of an individual's occupations, but also their social and cultural significance.

In occupational therapy literature, *occupational alienation* is a term used to describe and understand the undermining of meaning in occupation and resulting sense of meaning being absent in daily life occupations (Townsend & Wilcock, 2004). This idea of negative meaning experiences draws from an interdisciplinary perspective. For example, in sociology, *anomie* is a term coined by Durkheim to refer to instances in which there is a mismatch between social norms and rules and what people have opportunities to do that leads to experiences of alienation and purposelessness. When societies undergo significant changes in their social and economic structures and fortunes, anomie is believed to be more common because it becomes more difficult for individuals to achieve in daily life what is endorsed by personal and societal values. At a population level, these types of alienation result in increases in morbidity and mortality. For example, the social, economic, and political change occurring in response to the collapse of the Soviet Union in the early 1990s was associated with a range of negative health outcomes such as a decline in life expectancy (Kim & Pridemore, 2005).

A pattern of occupations devoid of meaning is associated with negative subjective experiences that are problematic for well-being. Occupational patterns lacking meaning have, for example, been connected to apathy and inertia. Antonovsky's (1987) aforementioned ideas may be helpful in understanding this. He proposed that meaning fosters the ability to develop a sense of coherence and to make sense out of chaos. Hence, when everyday occupations are meaningful, comprehensible, and manageable, this fosters a sense of coherence that positively affects health and well-being. Conversely, then, if everyday occupations become less comprehensible and manageable, or lose meaning due to changes in a person's capacities, subjective experiences of their world, or changed circumstances, this might be expected to have detrimental impacts on health and well-being. Disruptions in the pattern, extent, and quality of engagement in activities of everyday life can be profound for people experiencing ongoing health conditions. The quote from Peter, who appears in the introduction to this chapter, provides a further illustration (Box 5-1).

KEY DEVELOPERS/THEORISTS

No occupational therapy practice framework has yet been articulated to specifically focus on questions of *meaning* in occupation, or loss or lack thereof, and to give shape or guidelines to practice as it relates to addressing meaning issues. Nevertheless, meaningful occupation has long been considered central to occupational therapy practice. For instance, Meyer (1922/77), one of the founders of occupational therapy, emphasized the importance of creating opportunities for meaningful doing—as contrasted to activity prescription—as a means of healing. Later, the

---

BOX 5-1. PETER

Peter described a long period in his life after being diagnosed with schizophrenia when his occupations were very limited; he struggled to engage in any activity and to make sense of what was happening to him. At this time, in his words, "I was feeling a sense of being under siege, or feeling threatened, whereas now I feel a sense of, like, the outside world is not a threatening place." Having subsequently established a pattern of occupations including artistic, volunteering, and paid pursuits, in which he was finding pleasure, a sense of accomplishment, and connections with others, Peter sought to emphasize this contrast in his experience: "It's like an enjoyable place; it's almost like a playground where I'm finding all these levels of fulfilment and enjoyment" (Fossey, 2009, p. 312).

---

philosopher, Englehardt (1977, 1983) described occupational therapists as "custodians of meaning," believing that the purpose of occupational therapy was to create a context in which to engage clients in understanding and giving meaning to their lives. Yet, it is only with the resurgence of interest in occupation as the core of the profession that the creation and affirmation of meaning as it relates to occupation has become a focus for a greater depth of inquiry (Kielhofner, 1983). The move to a community focus involved the use of contexts in which experiences of meaning could more effectively be actualized and has, thus, further advanced the profession's focus on personal and social meanings of occupational engagement.

A number of occupational therapy scholars have written about meaning in occupation. Meaning in occupation has been linked to how people choose and orchestrate patterns of occupation and develop occupational identities over time (Christiansen, 1999; Kielhofner, 2008b; Laliberte-Rudman, 2002; Unruh, 2004). In addition, Hammel et al. (2008) have articulated dimensions of meaning experienced through occupation, arguing that these aspects of meaning may be seen as needs to be met in developing and sustaining well-being. Thus, drawing on earlier work by Wilcock (1998) and Rebeiro, Day, Semnuik, O'Brien, & Wilson (2001), Hammell (2004) proposed *doing, being, becoming,* and *belonging* as four dimensions of meaning that develop through occupational engagement. Occupation provides opportunities for *doing* that may be meaningful in an instrumental sense (e.g., to achieve, to develop skills); opportunities for *being* that can be meaningful in a reflective or contemplative sense; opportunities of *becoming* in the sense of the possibilities created for growth, self-discovery, transformation, and building an occupational identity; and opportunities for connecting with others and finding a sense of *belonging*.

example

Taking this further by drawing from recurrent themes in qualitative research focused on experiences of disability, Hammell (2009) proposed four experience-based categories of occupational engagement: restorative occupations; ways of fostering belonging, connecting, and contributing; engagement in doing; and ways of connecting the past and present to a hopeful future. Indeed, the growing body of qualitative research in the field is contributing to

understanding how people experience their occupational engagement. This is essential to the further development of the profession's knowledge base about meaning as it relates to occupation (Hammell, 2009; Jonsson, 2008).

More recently, occupational therapy scholars have also begun to suggest that the continuity of meanings in occupation may be challenged or disrupted in many other circumstances beyond those linked to health conditions or disability, such as situations of violence and conflict, migration, or colonization, and contexts that restrict freedoms and opportunities (Polatajko et al., 2007; Townsend & Whiteford, 2005). In such contexts, the inability to navigate or reconcile meaning in occupation can lead to disturbances of mental health (for example, depression), risky behaviors (such as substance misuse), and even pose a threat to pro-social behaviors. This more recent concern for population-level disturbances of meaning in occupation has contributed to emerging theory and practice related to occupational justice more fully developed in a subsequent chapter in this book.

Influential Interdisciplinary Perspectives of Meaning

Three interdisciplinary perspectives of meaning in particular have contributed to recent understandings of meaning and occupation in occupational therapy: phenomenological and narrative understandings of meaning, and studies of activity engagement informed by flow theory. Each offers a different way to both conceptualize and study the meanings ascribed to and derived from occupations.

Phenomenological Perspectives on Meaning

Phenomenology focuses on the ways that people experience their everyday lives and immediate social contexts, also referred to as their *life worlds*, meaning the world of daily activities, relationships, and pursuits that an individual encounters through direct experience (Jonsson & Josephsson, 2005). Although there are several approaches to

> # BOX 5-2. EXAMPLES OF PHENOMENOLOGICAL STUDIES RELATED TO MEANING AND OCCUPATION
>
> A Swedish study (Magnus, 2001) explored the occupation-related experiences of women with physical disabilities. With losses in occupation came losses in meaning that undermined their sense of identity. By using strategies to continue engagement in occupation that enabled their self-image as "whole" and "functioning" women, these women's occupational patterns evolved over time and integrated new meanings associated with positive self-identities.
>
> Hvalsoe and Josephsson (2003) explored the meaning in everyday occupations of unemployed men and women with long-standing mental ill-health in rural Denmark. Reported meaningful occupations included occupations that supported restoration; occupation that re-created everyday life with experiences of strengthened autonomy, identity, and connection with past values and interests; and occupations that reduced feelings of being an "outsider" and brought a sense of accomplishment and recognition by others.
>
> Lin et al. (2009) interviewed individuals living in a Canadian community who had mental health issues and had come in contact with the law. The study's findings suggested that meaningful occupational engagement included doing the right thing, connecting with others, and having opportunities for freedom and responsibility; whereas institutional and social restraints and lack of activities were challenges to meaningful engagement.
>
> A longitudinal study by Eriksson and Tham (2010) describes the recovery of everyday "doing" after life disruption as a result of stroke. They identified experiences of performing everyday occupations as characterized by encountering occupational gaps in formerly taken-for-granted activities; striving to narrow gaps in desired occupations; recognizing oneself in doing; and creating strategies to enable doing.
>
> In-depth interviews with persons experiencing mental health issues in Norway and New Zealand highlight that recovery is experienced through the effective pursuit of everyday life activities and relationships (Borg & Davidson, 2008; Sutton et al., 2012). Borg and Davidson (2008) identified four aspects of recovery as lived in everyday life: being normal—being an ordinary person carrying out ordinary activities; "just doing it"; finding ways to make life easier; and being good to yourself. Sutton et al.'s (2012) findings describe differing modes of occupational engagement with varying meanings, each with its place in supporting individuals in recovery (such as possibilities for grounding, becoming completely absorbed, for resting and quietude between more experiences of more intense engagement).

phenomenological research, broadly speaking, they all seek to describe individuals' experiences as they are lived, or what it is like for them in their own terms. The importance of phenomenological research for understanding everyday occupations is that it aims to reveal how taken-for-granted phenomena are lived and experienced (Hasselkus, 2006). Examples of phenomenological research from occupational therapy literature illustrate the interplay between self, doing, and the social world in the ways that people ascribe meaning to their everyday lives and experiences in a variety of social contexts including unemployment, ill health, or disability (Box 5-2).

As these examples show, phenomenological research is contributing to understanding phenomena of particular interest in occupational therapy; how people experience and find meaning in their occupations; and how disability, recovery, and well-being are experienced in the course of everyday life.

Narrative Understandings of Meaning and Identity

From early childhood through old age, stories and storytelling enable humans to make meaning of their actions and experiences (Bruner, 1990; Molineux & Rickard, 2003). People's stories of their experiences permit exploration of not only how events unfold in time and the meanings related to the occupations in which they engage, but also how people see themselves, or their agency in the situation (Molineux & Rickard, 2003). Thus, language used in storytelling, such as metaphors like "being stuck in the mud," "flying like the wind," "being out on a limb," "skating on thin ice," and "making mountains out of mole hills," reveal different meanings of engaging in occupations, or of struggles therein, and the sense of agency of the person involved. Because stories also connect events in time to create a meaningful whole, a narrative perspective on meaning also offers a way to appreciate how engagement in occupations contribute over time to a person's sense of identity and life story, which becomes the meaning framework guiding his or her personal choices and actions (Kielhofner et al., 2008; Molineux & Rickard, 2003).

For instance, drawing on narrative data from interviews with 32 Swedish adults in a 10-year longitudinal study of the transition from a working life to retirement, Jonsson (2008) identified that some occupations stood out from others over time in participants' stories for their engaging qualities. These "engaging occupations" occurred in many arenas, but had the following characteristics in common:

- Infused with positive meaning
- Experienced as highly meaningful
- Involved intense participation in duration and regularity
- Had evolved into a commitment or responsibility
- Consisted of a coherent set of activities
- Involved others who shared the same interest
- Created a sense of identity for the person

In contrast, killing-time occupations lack engagement and meaning beyond passing time, and neither they, nor occupations engaged in irregularly, were connected with descriptions of well-being (Jonsson, 2008). Negative experiences of killing-time occupations, or time that is empty with little sense of meaning, are also reported by people experiencing mental ill-health (e.g., Bejerholm & Eklund, 2004, 2006; Farnworth, Nitikin, & Fossey, 2003), but whether they, or people with other health conditions, would experience engaging occupations in similar ways to those identified by Jonsson remains to be established through further research.

Experience of Occupational Engagement Informed by Flow Theory

The concept of flow was introduced by Csikzentmihalyi to describe a peak experience where individuals become fully immersed in activity and experience a range of intrinsically pleasurable emotions. Csikzentmihalyi and colleagues used the Experience Sampling Method as a means to collect information about "in-the-moment" subjective experiences of what people do, which led to the articulation of flow theory (Jonsson & Josephsson, 2005). Briefly, the Experience Sampling Method involves using a device (e.g., phone, wristwatch) to prompt individuals at random intervals to fill out a questionnaire about what they are doing and their experience in that moment. Flow theory itself contends that experiences of engaging in activities depend on how an individual experiences the relationship between his or her skills (abilities to deal with the situation) and the challenges (opportunities for action) in doing that particular activity (Nakamura & Csikszentmihalyi, 2009). Accordingly, for example, differing levels of challenge in

relation to one's skills to meet those challenges in an activity may mean a person experiences anxiety (high challenge, low skill) or apathy (low challenge, low skill) and so forth. In conditions where an activity has clear goals, provides immediate feedback and the challenges for the person in doing the activity stretch his or her skills (but do not overtax them), flow may be experienced. A flow experience can occur with many different kinds of activity and is typically characterized as an experience of engagement that involves focused concentration in the present moment, a sense of control, and the merging of action and awareness so the person becomes fully absorbed and has a sense of losing track of time (Nakamura & Csikzentmihalyi, 2009). According to flow theory and research, such experiences of being fully absorbed in doing are meaningful as sources of enjoyment, pleasure, satisfaction and happiness, which in turn draw people to commit to, and persist with, activities that enable achievement and mastery of challenges, and are protective in relation to well-being (Nakamura & Csikszentmihalyi, 2009).

Flow theory does not directly inform a particular occupational therapy practice framework for explaining or enabling occupational engagement. However, Jonsson and Persson (2006) have used research based on flow theory to theorize how occupational balance might be understood in experiential terms. Others, too, have used this approach to investigate experiences of occupational engagement among people with HIV/AIDS (Kennedy & Vecitis, 2004) and activity experiences and mental health issues (Delespaul, 1995; McCormick, Funderburk, Lee, & Hale-Fought, 2005).

Flow theory is congruent, too, with occupational therapy's interest in creating just-right challenges. To operationalize this idea in practice, occupational therapists, like many other professions, have turned to the work of Russian psychologist, Lev Vygotsky, who advanced the practice of scaffolding within the zone of proximal development as a means to enable meaningful doing. At its core this refers to the idea of enabling the potential for future independent function by providing targeted support and collaboration (Davidson, Rakfeldt, & Strauss, 2010; Jonsson & Josephsson, 2005). The importance of creating just-right challenges highlights the close link between performance and experience of occupation.

Nakamura and Csikszentmihalyi (2009) also suggest three ways in which flow principles might be applied, each of which has relevance for occupational therapy:

1. To shape activity structures and environments to foster flow experiences, or to obstruct them less

2. To enable individuals to identify activities in which they may find enjoyment, and to learn how to invest in engaging in these activities

3. To orient therapy toward building on interests, strengths, and the skills and positive feelings that accompany flow experiences (p. 202)

In summary, the work of Csikszentmihalyi and colleagues suggests ways in which the process of engaging in an occupation can create subjective states that hold meaning and also influence well-being (Jonsson & Josephsson, 2005).

IMPORTANT EVOLUTIONARY POINTS

The notion of meaningful occupation has been considered important in occupational therapy since the profession's inception, when the healing potential of creating opportunities for meaningful doing within therapeutic settings was initially recognized. Historically, then, in occupational therapy the focus for understanding meaning was on identifying specific activities that could meaningfully engage clients. Occupational therapists sought primarily to use meaningful activity as a therapeutic medium, and to find ways to bring meaning-making into the goals and process of engaging clients in therapy. Pressures to align with narrow biomedical interpretations of health and to demonstrate efficiencies, costs, and tangible outcomes meant that the profession had to grapple with ways to maintain a focus on meaning. Recent decades have seen a re-emergence of a focus on occupation, development of occupation-related models of practice and research, and shifts in the focus on occupational therapy practice toward community and enabling people's occupational engagement with everyday life contexts. In this context, meaning needs to be understood as it relates not only to specific occupations, but also to the full pattern of occupations in which people engage in everyday life, their personal and social meanings, and links to well-being. In addition, the goals and process of therapy need to be oriented toward enabling people to meaningfully engage in self-chosen occupations within everyday life contexts.

PRACTICE APPROACHES— MEANING PERSPECTIVE OF OCCUPATION IN PRACTICE

Engagement in everyday occupations that hold personal and sociocultural meaning is known to support well-being. How to enable such engagement is at the core of occupational therapy practice with individuals, families, or groups of people who experience disruption or challenges in their everyday occupations. We know that the processes of recovering and experiencing health and well-being in the context of mental illness, other health conditions, and disability are supported by engagement in "meaningful" everyday life activities and relationships. Thus, important questions emerge: When a person's engagement in everyday activities

has been disrupted or challenged to the point where his or her participation in major domains of community life is profoundly curtailed or restricted, how are meaningful occupations to be identified? In addition, once such occupations have been identified, what can practitioners do to enable individuals to access and sustain involvement in them? More specifically, for practitioners who work within a person-centered approach, these questions can be framed: How do you facilitate an occupationally disengaged and potentially demoralized person to identify and set occupation-oriented goals for his or her own wellness plan? And, perhaps even more importantly, once such goals are identified, how do you assist the person in participating in the identified activities of interest? In other words, how do you assist the person in moving from here to there?

In response to these questions, a fruitful first step could be to explore possibilities for engagement in everyday activities in collaboration with the person. This might be termed a meaning-focused approach to occupation analysis. It goes beyond the profession's traditional idea of activity analysis that involves breaking a discrete activity into its constituent steps and analyzing its performance demands (physical, cognitive, neuro-behavioral, and so forth) as a basis for designing activity-focused interventions within therapeutic contexts (Creek & Bullock, 2008; Crepeau, 2003). Rather, a meaning-focused approach to occupation analysis focuses more closely on the experiential, social, and contextual dimensions that affect activity choices and engagement. It is oriented toward collaborating with persons experiencing ill-health or disability to enable self-determined engagement in everyday activities within community contexts of their choosing. This type of exploration creates possibilities to directly and systematically address the barriers to meaningful participation in everyday life and adds focus to everyday life activities and relationships to current person-centered, strengths-based, and wellness-oriented practices.

A clearly delineated meaning perspective from which to undertake such analyses for the purpose of enabling participation in everyday life situations has not yet been articulated. This would necessitate consideration of not only the personal meaning and significance of what is to be done, but also the experiential, emotional, interpersonal, and broader social contexts within which participation will be embedded. Furthermore, given its intent to facilitate individuals to identify and engage in self-chosen and personally meaningful activities, active collaboration with the person in the process of identifying possibilities for engagement and sources of meaning in occupations should be explicit and central to the process.

A meaning-focused perspective on occupational analysis might then be described as *the systematic consideration and promotion of an individual's possibilities for positive, self-directed engagement in personally meaningful everyday activities within real life contexts, incorporating social and contextual dimensions of his or her life experiences.* Of note, this places emphasis on the perspective that the everyday life activities to be enabled are naturally occurring, that is, part of the everyday world of experiences (as opposed to therapeutically controlled) in which meanings and communities are built (Hasselkus, 2006). This type of exploration involves viewing the activity as occurring within a specific context, and as it fits with the person who wishes to participate. Hence, this context, the person's point of view, and the personal and social significance of participation become central to the analytic lens. Given the importance of previous life experience and the idiosyncratic nature of the wellness journey, we are also describing a process that is not provider-driven, but rather one that is reflective, evaluative, exploratory, and, most importantly, collaborative. Indeed, the only way that a practitioner can know what personal meaning or significance a particular occupation holds for another person is by involving that person directly in the process of exploration itself.

EXAMPLES OF TOOLS

One way to approach developing this kind of collaborative understanding of meaning in everyday occupations is in an open-ended manner through talking with individuals about their everyday lives, for which the conversational structure and strategies provided in Table 5-2 may be a useful starting point.

A narrative (story-telling) approach to interviewing may also facilitate attending to individuals' unfolding stories. More specifically, narrative interviews enable us to appreciate how experiences are made sense of, and the ways in which people, actions, objects, places, and relationships become connected in meaning-making (Molineux & Rickard, 2003). An example of a narratively oriented, semi-structured interview developed in occupational therapy is the Occupational Performance History Interview-II (Kielhofner et al., 2004), described in more detail in Chapter 9 of this book. Using this interview may facilitate therapists' abilities to collaboratively develop an understanding of the unfolding meanings in a person's life story and actions, and as such the Occupational Performance History Interview-II may be valuable in recovery-focused mental health service provision (Ennals & Fossey, 2009), as well as in supporting people to make sense of experiences such as chronic pain, disability, and caregiving (Chaffey & Fossey, 2004; Keponen & Kielhofner, 2006).

In addition to interviewing, a number of structured tools have been developed in occupational therapy that focus on exploring meaningful occupational engagement, the value attached to occupations, and satisfaction with daily occupations with clients (Box 5-3). Such tools not only lend themselves to psychosocial practice as a brief and more structured means to collaborate with clients in identifying occupations that may hold meaning and value for them, but also to evaluate outcomes of occupational therapy.

EVALUATION PROCESSES FOR OUTCOMES

As noted previously, meaningful occupational engagement is thought to play central roles in motivating and sustaining involvement from which physical, mental, and social benefits may accrue, and in promoting development, transformation, and well-being (Hasselkus, 2002; Kielhofner, 1983, 2009; Wilcock, 2006). Hence, evidence of change or transformation in the meanings ascribed to occupational engagement is an important outcome in occupational therapy. Qualitatively different experiences of meaning in occupation over time are likely to be revealed in conversations between therapists and clients when a strong base of collaborative understanding has been established. However, several tools also exist that may be used to evaluate this type of change in a more structured manner to provide feedback to therapists and clients about progress being made. Examples include the EMAS (Goldberg, Britnell, & Goldberg, 2002), the OVal-9 (Persson & Erlandsson, 2010), the Profiles of Occupational Engagement (Bejerholm, Hansson, & Eklund, 2006), and Satisfaction with Daily Occupations (Eklund & Gunnarsson, 2007, 2008), each of which is described in Box 5-3.

EVIDENCE FOR THE APPROACH

As there is no occupational therapy practice framework that specifically addresses questions of meaning in occupation, or loss, or lack thereof, it is not possible to present evidence directly supporting a meaning-focused practice approach. Nevertheless, a growing body of qualitative research in occupational therapy (and other disciplines) from the perspectives of people experiencing a range of health conditions, disabilities, or altered life circumstances endorses the importance of meaningful engagement in everyday occupations for supporting recovery and well-being. So, this increasing focus on the subjective experience and qualities of occupational engagement holds promise for more fully developing a conceptual framework of the meaning and experiential dimensions of occupations in daily life.

An Application of Meaning Focused Practice—Kate

To illustrate some possibilities of a meaning-focused approach to exploring occupational engagement and its

TABLE 5-2
WAYS TO ELICIT CONVERSATION ABOUT HOW A PERSON EXPERIENCES EVERYDAY LIFE AND PARTICIPATION
A helpful conversational structure might be to begin with talking about the person's everyday activities in the present, then move to reflecting on his or her ways of participating in everyday activities from the past that were different, and then to what the person might like to add or change in the future if it were to become possible.
Consider it a conversation, not an interview, which may possibly occur across several encounters or over time, rather than as a "checklist" of topics to be covered or completed.
Some examples of possible opening questions that might be used as starting points in creating this type of conversation about the person's everyday life and activity participation include: • What are your days like at the moment? Or how do you spend your days at the moment? • What kinds of activities are you involved in? • Who do you spend time with? What kinds of activities do you do together? • What kinds of activities did you used to do? • What have you done that gave you a sense of enjoyment/achievement/ satisfaction? • What's been helpful in getting to do these things? • What is important to you in your life now? • What would you like to be doing in the future if it were to become possible? • What could be the issues to overcome? And what might help to make it happen? • What have we not covered that you think is important or would like me to know?
Helpful approaches to phrasing questions so as to elaborate your understanding of the person's everyday activities might include: • Practice phrasing questions using "what" and "how" to facilitate conversation (e.g., What is your work like? How do you get to your friend's place?). • Practice phrasing subsequent questions so that they explicitly build on what the other person's been saying (e.g., You just mentioned doing nothing much; what is doing nothing like? You spoke earlier of visiting your family sometimes; what kinds of things do you do when you visit them?).
Everyday activities can seem familiar to us, even a taken-for-granted part of life, and so this makes it easier for us to assume we know what someone else means when talking about his/her everyday activities. Being open to the possibility that your ideas may be different from the other person's ideas about everyday activities makes this less likely.
Adapted from Fossey, E. M. (2009). *Participating as resisting: Everyday life stories of people experiencing mental health issues.* Melbourne, Australia: The University of Melbourne.; Kielhofner, G., Mallinson, T., Crawford, C. Nowak, M., Rigby, P....Henry, A. (2004). *Occupational Performance History Interview II (OPHI-II) Version 2.1.* Chicago: MOHO Clearinghouse.; Davidson, L. (2003). *Living outside mental illness: Qualitative studies of recovery in schizophrenia* (Vol. 24). New York: New York University Press.; Bejerholm, U., Hansson, L., & Eklund, M. (2006). Profiles of Occupational Engagement in People with Schizophrenia (POES): The development of a new instrument based on time use diaries. *British Journal of Occupational Therapy, 69*(2), 58-68.

meaning, excerpts from a personal narrative are used (Vignette 5-1). Kate was interviewed as part of an Australian participatory research project exploring the everyday lives of people experiencing mental health issues (Fossey, 2009). This story highlights the experiential, social, and contextual dimensions of participation that affect activity choices and sustained engagement, to which occupational therapists must attend to enable others' self-determined engagement with everyday activities. First, the focus is on the experience of the activity, what the person might get out of the activity, its meanings, and his or her notions of how the activity is linked to experiences of health and well-being. These excerpts from Kate's story describe becoming part of something against the odds. Kate spoke of her long

BOX 5-3. EXAMPLES OF TOOLS DEVELOPED TO IDENTIFY OCCUPATIONS THAT MAY HOLD MEANING AND VALUE

Engagement in Meaningful Activities Survey (EMAS) (Goldberg et al., 2002)—This tool begins with an interview to identify activities that are meaningful to the person; then 12 statements about their meaningfulness are rated using a 5-point Likert scale from Never (1) to Always (5). The 12 EMAS items each begin with "The activities I do … " They include: The activities I do to take care of myself, to reflect the kind of person I am, to express my values, to express my creativity, to give me pleasure, to give me the right amount of challenge, to give me a sense of accomplishment, to contribute to feeling competent, to give me a feeling of control, to give me a sense of satisfaction, to help other people, and that are valued by other people. Positive relationships between engagement in meaningful occupations, measured with EMAS, life satisfaction and meaning in life, and also negative relationships with boredom and depression have been reported, with a recent study indicating that perceived meaning in occupations and occupational value may be important predictors of well-being (Eakman & Eklund, 2012).

Occupational Value (OVal-9) (Persson & Erlandson, 2010)—This is a 9-item self-reporting tool developed to evaluate the extent to which therapeutic intervention results in positive change in clients' experiences of everyday occupations. It is based on the Value, Meaning, and Occupation model (Persson et al., 2001), in which the experience of value in an occupation is seen as contributing to its meaningfulness, and as a propelling force for occupational engagement and well-being. Three potential sources in everyday occupations are described: the concrete or tangible value of occupational engagement (e.g., wages earned, products made, skills developed); the symbolic value of the occupation at a personal or a cultural level (e.g., a celebration, ceremony, a style of dancing); and their value as a self-rewarding experience (e.g., experience of being fully absorbed, inspired, relaxing).

The OVal-9 itself includes 9 items, each beginning "When I am engaged in this occupation I…" and covers some similar areas to EMAS above (e.g., feeling pleasure or satisfaction and expressing who I am), but also includes experiential dimensions, such as relaxing, releasing emotions, and becoming so engrossed that one forgets time, which reflect the influence of Csikzentmihalyi's work. Indeed, one suggested use of OVal-9 is with an experience sampling technique using a beeper device (like that used in Csikzentmihalyi's flow studies described above) as a means to explore how individuals' experience their repertoires of everyday occupations naturalistically (Persson & Erlandsson, 2010).

Profiles of Occupational Engagement (Bejerholm et al., 2006)—This structured tool was developed by drawing on qualitative research about the time use and occupational engagement of persons with schizophrenia (Bejerholm & Eklund, 2004, 2006). It involves use of a time diary to, first, gather information about the person's pattern of occupations, and second, to create a profile of the person's occupational engagement on nine dimensions such as the daily rhythm of activity, variety and range of occupations, place, social context, extent of meaningful occupations, and routines. See Chapter 10 for a more detailed description.

Satisfaction with Daily Occupations (Eklund & Gunnarsson, 2007, 2008)—This is a brief measure of whether or not a person engages in any of 9 main areas of occupation and the extent of the person's satisfaction in each. As such, it reveals relatively little detail about meaning in occupations. Nevertheless, it may be useful as a screening tool to prioritize working with clients for whom experiences of satisfaction in everyday occupations are lacking or to identify areas of occupation of most concern to clients.

experience of struggling to participate and battle with persisting mental health issues, and of finding that community choirs opened doors for her to new ways of pursuing longstanding interests, to contributing to something larger with others, and to achieving something that had once seemed impossible to her.

Kate's story highlights experiential and interpersonal aspects of participation and reveals meanings connected to her prior music-related experiences and social relationships that supported her experience of engaging in singing with a community choir. Stepping back to consider how Kate might have been supported to explore possibilities for participation in community activities, prior to her involvement with the choir, attention to each of these dimensions of participation could have been important to identify possibilities for participation that she might find meaningful.

One aspect would be to explore and reflect with Kate on her aspirations or dreams and activity-related experiences in relation to doing and being with others, the intent here not being to try to restore an "old" life but to learn

VIGNETTE 5-1. KATE

Kate* described how regular participation in community choirs became "major things for me." One choir met "just around the corner from me"; fortunate from Kate's perspective because she often felt unsafe in the neighborhood. She was introduced to another choir by a neighbor, who continued to accompany her to choir: "for the first time in my life I've actually had a male friend … I'm friends with his partner as well. And that's, like, huge … So that's been a very helpful relationship." Kate described how the choirs "have been really, really good for me." They connected her with a longstanding love of music and an image of herself as a singer, with opportunities to learn, and with "really, really nice people" and opportunities to build friendships, something that Kate described as difficult for many years prior:

"Always been interested in music … Dad played guitar, loved listening as a kid. I loved music as a kid; learned organ a little and loved playing; saw myself as a singer and used to hear orchestra as I was going off to sleep. Mum didn't think singing lessons were worthwhile, so I didn't have any as kid, and she didn't know about choirs. I've learned a lot more about music through community choirs, and my voice is developing." (Fossey, 2009, p. 243)

Performing at a community festival and at a major concert hall were experiences of singing with others and being part of "the community doing something good; it really did affect me," which inspired Kate to want to do something more in local communities. Contrasting these experiences with her daily battles—"it's a real struggle; it's a fight to get out"—Kate spoke of her sense of achievement and pleasure:

"Just recently through my other singing group, all singing groups from around [the area] joined together … They put on a performance once a year and they have a conductor and then, they have professional performers come on stage and sing … that just recently happened and actually I was performing. I was in the second row up on the Concert Hall. I just couldn't believe it. I just started crying on stage. It was like a really huge thing and I, like, had to have a lot of support, 'cause I had panic attacks. Like these were [at] the practices and I was round people I didn't know and I just clung to one of the ladies who's in our group. And, you know, I kept on biting her head off 'cause I was anxious. I'm not normally like that, except when I get anxious. … And then when it came to the day of the performance, I had no anxiety, and I thought, 'Oh, what the hell's wrong with me? I'm not even anxious!' This is not normal for me. It was so funny. I think I was just so tired and we'd practiced so much, like over-cramming for an exam, that I was like 'Ooohh!'… It was just an amazing experience! … When you know you sound good, I mean, it's not your own voice, it's many voices and you know many voices together sound fantastic. You're just, like, I can't believe I'm part of this! 'Cause a lot of the times in the choir, you know, you might have people that can't sing in tune, or whatever, and you know the quality's not very good but you're not there for that. You're there to enjoy yourself. But when you know you sound good… when it does sound good, you think, Oh! And when you hear people are genuinely clapping, that's a really good feeling!" (Fossey, 2009, p. 243)

*Pseudonym.

about her experiences, so as to appreciate her capabilities and what she might be drawn toward for the future. For example, reflecting with Kate about her experiences might have revealed her life-long affinity for music (i.e., listening, playing an instrument, singing), suggesting possible arenas in which to invite and explore options for participation. It might also have uncovered important interpersonal aspects that affect participation; for instance, that for Kate being around people could be anxiety provoking, making relationships difficult, but also that she had a friendship with a neighbor in a choir, with whom she might try out going to a community choir. In addition, in telling her story, Kate highlighted other contextual barriers that needed to be overcome, including neighborhood safety issues that limited her transport options—barriers that finding a community choir nearby and her neighbor's willingness

to assist with transport enabled her to overcome. Indeed, accessing this local community environment provided her with opportunities for accessing other locations, further from home, enabling Kate to rediscover a sense of herself as a contributing member of a larger community.

By focusing on the particular activity and context in which the person does or might participate (i.e., whether with the aim of enabling the person to initiate or sustain this activity), the exploration of participation barriers expanded beyond any performance issues, to identify all possible sources of meaning associated with well-being and fulfilment. It also more thoroughly considers contextual barriers to participation. Thus, both sources of barriers (be they social, material, personal and/or performance related) and potential sources of support, especially those within the person's natural environment, become particularly relevant, so that possibilities for enabling participation that is sustainable, meaningful, and satisfying can be discovered.

An important part of such an exploration is that it intentionally and deliberately attends to what people themselves (but sometimes also others who do activities with them) know about participating, and their own strategies and/or ways of going about participating. For instance, Kate's investigation of local community facilities and knowledge of her friend's choir membership were important resources in finding a way to pursue joining community choirs, and to gain the many subsequent benefits from this experience. Thus, when this is done, capabilities and natural supports can be acknowledged or recognized, supported, and a plan for what the person needs and wants her or his life to be like may begin to be built. Each of these aspects requires a contextualized and collaborative approach informed by an appreciation of the experiential qualities and potential sources of meaning associated with occupational engagement. Furthermore, this kind of practice involves making explicit that which is ordinary, taken-for-granted, or routine in everyday life. Like an ethnographer, the practitioner enters the process as if the participation situation is largely unknown, prepared to challenge prior knowledge and assumptions, to look with "fresh eyes" at the transactions between persons, their activities, and their environments. This extends to considering how the individual, through his or her involvement, will contribute to the participation context. It is from this perspective that exploring possibilities for enabling meaningful participation in everyday life challenges occupational therapy and mental health practices to focus not just on people experiencing mental ill-health and other disabling issues being located "in" the community, but on their becoming part "of" communities of their choosing (Davidson et al., 2010; Ware, Hopper, Tugenberg, Dickey, & Fisher, 2007).

CONCLUSION

Occupational therapists have available a range of tools for exploring the meaning dimensions of occupations in collaboration with clients, which may also be used to evaluate outcomes associated with meaning in occupational engagement. Furthermore, struggles in doing daily life in the context of ill-health, disability and altered life circumstances are known to increase daily life's demands and stresses, and there is increasing focus on factors such as meaning in stress research. While this interdisciplinary field is in its infancy, meaning and purpose in life should be integral components of intervention strategies intended to promote the capacity of individuals to adapt to daily living. This point should not be lost on occupational therapists working in health systems contexts with people who, in the

wake of significant health conditions and disability, find their occupations and their associated meanings significantly challenged, disrupted, or even lost.

LEARNING ACTIVITIES/ DISCUSSION QUESTIONS

1. Think about the activities you have engaged in over the past 2 weeks. Which of the meaning experiences listed in Table 5-1 have you experienced? Which have you not experienced? Consider how your meaning experiences influence your health and well-being.

2. Select one of the meaning experiences identified in this chapter and research what is known about its connection to health and well-being.

3. Form a discussion group to consider how the human experience of meaning evolves over the lifespan.

4. Select a first person account written by an individual whose activity and community participation was seriously affected by injury or a health condition. How did the person describe the effect on his/her meaning experiences? Did the person regain a sense of meaning through activity? How did this happen?

REFERENCES

Antonovsky, A. (1987). *Unraveling the mystery of health—how people manage stress and stay well*. San Francisco: Jossey-Bass Publishers.

Bejerholm, U., & Eklund, M. (2004). Time use and occupational performance among persons with schizophrenia. *Occupational Therapy in Mental Health, 20*(1), 27-47.

Bejerholm, U., & Eklund, M. (2006). Engagement in occupations among men and women with schizophrenia. *Occupational Therapy International, 13*(2), 100-121.

Bejerholm, U., Hansson, L., & Eklund, M. (2006). Profiles of occupational engagement in people with schizophrenia (POES): the development of a new instrument based on time-use diaries. *British Journal of Occupational Therapy, 69*(2), 58-68.

Borell, L., Asaba, E., Rosenberg, L., Schult, M.-L., & Townsend, E. (2006). Exploring experiences of "participation" among individuals living with chronic pain. *Scandinavian Journal of Occupational Therapy, 13*, 76-85.

Borg, M., & Davidson, L. (2008). The nature of recovery as lived in everyday experience. *Journal of Mental Health, 17*(2), 129-140.

Bruner, J. (1990). *Acts of meaning*. Cambridge, MA: Harvard University Press.

Chaffey, L., & Fossey, E. (2004). Caring and daily life: Occupational experiences of women living with sons diagnosed with schizophrenia. *Australian Occupational Therapy Journal, 51*, 199-207.

Christiansen, C. H. (1999). Defining lives: Occupation as identity: An essay on competence, coherence, and the creation of meaning. *American Journal of Occupational Therapy, 53*(6), 547-558.

Creek, J., & Bullock, A. (2008). Planning and implementation. In J. Creek & L. Lougher (Eds.), *Occupational therapy and mental health* (4th ed., pp. 109-130). Edinburgh: Churchill Livingstone.

Crepeau, E. B. (2003). Analyzing occupation and activity: A way of thinking about occupational performance. In E. B. Crepeau, E. S. Cohn & B. A. B. Schell (Eds.), *Willard & Spackman's occupational therapy* (10th ed., pp. 189-198). Philadelphia: Lippincott Williams & Wilkins.

Davidson, L. (2003). *Living outside mental illness: Qualitative studies of recovery in schizophrenia* (Vol. 24). New York: New York University Press.

Davidson, L., O'Connell, M. J., Tondora, J., Lawless, M., & Evans, A. C. (2005). Recovery in serious mental illness: A new wine or just a new bottle? *Professional Psychology: Research and Practice, 36*(5), 480-487.

Davidson, L., Rakfeldt, J., & Strauss, J. (2010). *The Roots of the Recovery Movement in Psychiatry: Lessons Learned.* Chichester: John Wiley & Sons Ltd.

Deegan, P. (2001). Recovery as a self-directed process of healing and transformation. In C. Brown (Ed.), *Recovery and wellness: Models of hope and empowerment for people with mental illness* (Vol. 17, pp. 5-21). New York: Haworth Press.

Deegan, P. E. (1988). Recovery: The lived experience of rehabilitation. *Psychosocial Rehabilitation Journal, 11*(4), 11-19.

Delespaul, P. A. E. G. (1995). *Assessing schizophrenia in daily life: The experience sampling method.* Maastricht: IPSER.

Doble, S. E., & Santha, J. C. (2008). Occupational well-being: Rethinking occupational therapy outcomes. *Canadian Journal of Occupational Therapy, 75*(3), 184-190.

Eakman, A. M., & Eklund, M. (2012). The relative impact of personality traits, meaningful occupation and occupational value on meaning in life and life satisfaction. *Journal of Occupational Science, 19*(2), 165-177.

Eklund, M., & Gunnarsson, A. B. (2007). Satisfaction with daily occupations: Construct validity and test-retest reliability of a screening tool for people with mental health disorders. *Australian Occupational Therapy Journal, 54*(1), 59-65.

Eklund, M., & Gunnarsson, A. B. (2008). Content validity, clinical utility, sensitivity to change and discriminant ability of the Swedish Satisfaction with Daily Occupations (SDO) instrument: A screening tool for people with mental disorders. *British Journal of Occupational Therapy, 71*(11), 487-495.

Eklund, M., & Leufstadius, C. (2007). Relationships between occupational factors and health and well-being in individuals with persistent mental illness living in the community. *Canadian Journal of Occupational Therapy, 74*(4), 303-313.

Englehardt, T. (1977). Defining occupational therapy: The meaning of therapy and the virtues of occupation. *American Journal of Occupational Therapy, 31*, 666-672.

Englehardt, T. (1983). Occupational therapists as technologists and custodians of meaning. In G. Kielhofner (Ed.), *Health through occupation: Theory and practice in occupational therapy* (pp. 139-144). Philadelphia: F. A. Davis.

Ennals, P., & Fossey, E. (2009). Using the OPHI-II to support people with mental illness in their recovery. *Occupational Therapy in Mental Health, 25*(2), 138-150.

Eriksson, G., & Tham, K. (2010). The meaning of occupational gaps in everyday life in the first year after stroke. *OTJR: Occupation, Participation & Health, 30*, 184-192.

Farnworth, L., Nitikin, L., & Fossey, E. (2003). Being in a secure forensic psychiatry unit: every day's the same, killing time or making the most of it. *British Journal of Occupational Therapy, 67*(10), 430-438.

Fossey, E. M. (2009). *Participating as resisting: Everyday life stories of people experiencing mental health issues.* The University of Melbourne, Melbourne.

Frankl, V. (1963). *Man's Search for Meaning.* Boston: Beacon Press.

Goldberg, B., Britnell, S., & Goldberg, J. (2002). The relationship between engagement in meaningful activities and quality of life in persons disabled by mental illness. *Occupational Therapy in Mental Health, 19*(2), 17-44.

Hammel, J., Magasi, S., Heinemann, A., Whiteneck, G., Bogner, J., & Rodriguez, E. (2008). What does participation mean? An insider perspective from people with disabilities. *Disability and Rehabilitation, 30*(19), 1445-1460.

Hammell, K. W. (2004). Dimensions of meaning in the occupations of daily life. *Canadian Journal of Occupational Therapy, 71*(5), 296-305.

Hammell, K. W. (2009). Self-care, productivity, and leisure, or dimensions of occupational experience? *Canadian Journal of Occupational Therapy, 76*(2), 107-114.

Hasselkus, B. (2002). *The meaning of everyday occupation.* Thorofare, New Jersey: SLACK Incorporated.

Hasselkus, B. R. (2006). 2006 Eleanor Clarke Slagle Lecture. The world of everyday occupation: Real lives, real people. *American Journal of Occupational Therapy, 60*(6), 627-640.

Hocking, C. (2000). Having and using objects in the Western world. *Journal of Occupational Science, 7*, 148-157.

Hvalsoe, B., & Josephsson, S. (2003). Characteristics of meaningful occupations from the perspective of mentally ill people. *Scandinavian Journal of Occupational Therapy, 10*, 61-71.

Jonsson, H. (2008). A new direction in the conceptualization and categorization of occupation. *Journal of Occupational Science, 15*(1), 3-8.

Jonsson, H. (2010). Occupational transitions: Work to retirement. In C. H. Christiansen & E. A. Townsend (Eds.), *Introduction to occupation: The art and science of living* (2nd ed., pp. 211-230). New Jersey: Prentice Hall.

Jonsson, H., & Josephsson, S. (2005). Occupation and meaning. In C. H. Christiansen, C. M. Baum & J. Bass-Haugen (Eds.), *Occupational therapy: Performance, participation, and well-being* (3rd ed., pp. 116-132). Thorofare, NJ: SLACK Incorporated.

Jonsson, H., & Persson, D. (2006). Towards an experiential model of occupational balance: An alternative perspective on flow theory analysis. *Journal of Occupational Science, 13*(1), 62-73.

Kennedy, B. L., & Vecitis, R. N. (2004). Contexts of the flow experience of women with HIV/AIDS. *OTJR: Occupation, Participation & Health, 24*(3), 83-91.

Keponen, R., & Kielhofner, G. (2006). Occupation and meaning in the lives of women with chronic pain. *Scandinavian Journal of Occupational Therapy, 13*, 211-220.

Kielhofner, G. (1983). *Health through occupation: Theory and practice in occupational therapy.* Philadelphia: F. A. Davis.

Kielhofner, G. (2008a). Volition. In G. Kielhofner (Ed.), *Model of Human Occupation: Theory and application* (4th ed., pp. 32-50). Baltimore, MD: Lippincott, Williams & Wilkins.

Kielhofner, G. (Ed.). (2008b). *Model of human occupation: Theory and application* (4th ed.). Baltimore, MD: Lippincott, Williams and Wilkins.

Kielhofner, G. (2009). *Conceptual foundations of occupational therapy* (4th ed.). Philadelphia: F. A. Davis.

Kielhofner, G., Borell, L., Holzmueller, R., Jonsson, H., Josephsson, S.,...Keponen, R. (2008). Crafting occupational life. In G. Kielhofner (Ed.), *Model of Human Occupation: Theory and application* (4th ed., pp. 110-125). Baltimore, MD: Lippincott, Williams and Wilkins.

Kielhofner, G., Mallinson, T., Crawford, C., Nowak, M., Rigby, M.,...Henry, A. (2004). *Occupational Performance History Interview II (OPHI-II) Version 2.1.* Chicago: MOHO Clearinghouse.

Kim, S., & Pridemore, W. A. (2005). Social change, institutional anomie, and serious property crime in transitional Russia. *British Journal of Criminology, 45*, 81-97.

King, G. A. (2004). The meaning of life experiences: Application of a meta-model to rehabilitation sciences and services. *American Journal of Orthopsychiatry, 74*, 72-88.

Laliberte-Rudman, D. (2002). Linking occupation and identity: Lessons learned through qualitative exploration. *Journal of Occupational Science, 9*(1), 12-19.

Leufstadius, C., Erlandsson, L., Bjorkman, T., & Eklund, M. (2008). Meaningfulness in daily occupations among individuals with persistent mental illness. *Journal of Occupational Science, 15*(1), 27-35.

Lin, N., Kirsh, B., Polatajko, H., & Seto, M. (2009). The nature and meaning of occupational engagement for forensic clients living in the community. *Journal of Occupational Science, 16*(2), 110-119.

Magnus, E. (2001). Everyday occupations and the process of redefinition: A study of how meaning in occupation influences redefintion of identity in women with a disability. *Scandinavian Journal of Occupational Therapy, 3*, 115-124.

McCormick, B. P., Funderburk, J. A., Lee, Y., & Hale-Fought, M. (2005). Activity characteristics and emotional experiences: Predicting boredom and anxiety in the daily life of community mental health clients. *Journal of Leisure Research, 37*(2), 236-253.

McEwan, B. S., & Gianaros, P. J. (2010). Central role of the brain in stress and adaptation: Links to socioeconomic status, health, and disease. *Annals of the New York Academy of Sciences, 1186*, 190-122.

Meyer, A. (1922/1977). The philosophy of occupational therapy. *American Journal of Occupational Therapy, 31*(10), 639-642.

Mezzina, R., Borg, M., Marin, I., Sells, D., Topor, A., & Davidson, L. (2006). From participation to citizenship: How to regain a role, a status, and a life in the process of recovery. *American Journal of Psychiatric Rehabilitation, 9*, 39-61.

Molineux, M., & Rickard, W. (2003). Storied approaches to understanding occupation. *Journal of Occupational Science, 10*(1), 52-60.

Moll, S., Gewurtz, R., & Saltmarche, E. (2012). Vitamin green: How viewing, being and "doing" in nature affects our health and wellbeing. *CrossCurrents, 16*(1).

Nakamura, J., & Csikszentmihalyi, M. (2009). Flow theory and research. In C. R. Snyder & S. J. Lopez (Eds.), *Handbook of positive psychology* (pp. 195-206). Oxford: Oxford University Press.

O'Hagan, M. (2001). *Recovery competencies for New Zealand mental health workers.* Wellington, New Zealand: Mental Health Commission.

Öhman, A., & Nygård, L. (2005). Meanings and motives for engagement in self-chosen daily life occupations among individuals with Alzheimer's disease. *OTJR: Occupation, Participation & Health, 25*(3), 89-97.

Persson, D., Andersson, I., & Eklund, M. (2011). Defying aches and reevaluating daily doing: Occupational perspectives on adjusting to chronic pain. *Scandinavian Journal of Occupational Therapy, 18*, 188-197.

Persson, D., & Erlandsson, L. K. (2010). Evaluating OVal-9, an instrument for detecting experiences of value in daily occupations. *Occupational Therapy in Mental Health, 26*(1), 32-50.

Persson, D., Erlandsson, L., Eklund, M., & Iwarsson, S. (2001). Value dimensions, meaning, and complexity in human occupation—A tentative structure for analysis. *Scandinavian Journal of Occupational Therapy, 8*, 7-18.

Polatajko, H. J., Backman, C., Baptiste, S., Davis, J., Eftekar, P.,...Harvey, A., (2007). Human occupation in context. In E. A. Townsend & H. J. Polatajko (Eds.), *Enabling occupation II: Advancing an occupational therapy vision for health, wellbeing and justice through occupation* (pp. 37-61). Ottawa: CAOT Publications ACE.

Psarra, E., & Kleftaras, G. (2013). Adaptation to physical disabilities: the role of meaning in life and depression. *European Journal of Counseling Psychology, 2*(1).

Rebeiro, K. L., Day, D. L., Semenuik, B., O'Brien, M. C., & Wilson, B. (2001). Northern initiative for social action: An occupation-based mental health program. *American Journal of Occupational Therapy, 55*(5), 493-500.

Stockdale Winder, F. (1997). *Meaning in Life: An exploration of the relevance of psychological theories to older women.* University of Saskatchewan, Saskatoon, Saskatchewan.

Sutton, D. J., Hocking, C. S., & Smythe, L. A. (2012). A phenomenological study of occupational engagement in recovery from mental illness. *Canadian Journal of Occupational Therapy, 79*(3), 142-150.

Townsend, E., & Whiteford, G. (2005). A participatory occupational justice framework: Population-based processes of practice. In F. Kronenberg, S. Simó Algado, & N. Pollard (Eds.), *Occupational therapy without borders: Learning from the spirit of survivors* (pp. 110-126). Edinburgh: Elsevier Churchill Livingstone.

Townsend, E., & Wilcock, A. A. (2004). Occupational justice. In C. H. Christiansen & E. Townsend (Eds.), *Introduction to occupation: The art and science of living* (pp. 243-273). Upper Saddle River, New Jersey: Prentice Hall.

Turner-Crowson, J., & Wallcraft, J. (2002). The recovery vision for mental health services and research: A British perspective. *Psychiatric Rehabilitation Journal, 25*(3), 245-254.

Unruh, A., & Hutchinson, S. (2011). Embedded spirituality: Gardening in daily life and stressful life experiences. *Scandinavian Journal of Caring Sciences, 25*(3), 567-574.

Unruh, A. M. (2004). Reflections on: "So...what do you do?" Occupation and the construction of identity. *Canadian Journal of Occupational Therapy, 71*(5), 290-295.

Unruh, A. M., Smith, N., & Scammell, C. (2000). The occupation of gardening in life-threatening illness: A qualitative pilot project. *Canadian Journal of Occupational Therapy, 67*(1), 70-77.

Unruh, A. M., Versnel, J., & Kerr, N. (2002). Spirituality unplugged: A review of commonalities and contentions, and a resolution. *Canadian Journal of Occupational Therapy, 69*(1), 5-19.

Ware, N. C., Hopper, K., Tugenberg, T., Dickey, B., & Fisher, D. (2007). Connectedness and citizenship: Redefining social integration. *Psychiatric Services, 58*(4), 469-474.

Wilcock, A. A. (1998). Reflections on doing, being, and becoming. *Canadian Journal of Occupational Therapy, 65*(5), 248-257.

Wilcock, A. A. (2006). *An occupational perspective of health* (2nd ed.). Thorofare, NJ: SLACK Incorporated.

Wright-St. Clair, V. (2003). Storymaking and storytelling: Making sense of living with multiple sclerosis. *Journal of Occupational Science, 10*(1), 46-51.

Wright-St. Clair, V. (2012). Being occupied with what matters in advanced age. *Journal of Occupational Science, 19*(1), 44-53.

The Drive and Motivation for Occupation

Terry Krupa, PhD, OT Reg (Ont), FCAOT

For 14 years the paralyzed man slouched in front of the television in the hell of his own despair and anguish. For months I sat and smoked cigarettes until it was time to collapse back into a drugged and dreamless sleep. But one day, something changed in us. A tiny, fragile spark of hope appeared and promised that there could be something more than all of this darkness. (Deegan, 1988)

OBJECTIVES

The objectives of this chapter are as follows:
- » Define motivation as it relates to occupational engagement.
- » Identify assumptions about healthy motivation in occupation.
- » Describe biological, psychological, and social theories of motivation.
- » Review assessment and practice principles of occupational therapy for enabling motivation for occupation.
- » Review assessment and practice principles of occupational therapy for enabling the ongoing investment in therapeutic processes of change.

Krupa, T., Kirsh, B., Pitts, D., & Fossey, E. *Bruce & Borg's Psychosocial Frames of Reference: Theories, Models, and Approaches for Occupation-Based Practice, Fourth Edition* (pp 93-106).
© 2016 SLACK Incorporated.

BACKGROUND

In Chapter 1, motivation was identified as a foundation for engagement in occupation. Motivation is the everyday concept we use to explain why humans do anything and helps explain how people do what they do. Motivation is considered a basic human drive that links human energy and effort to a purpose or goal direction and to particular behavior patterns (Wlodkowski, 1999). For example, we might use the term *motivation* to explain someone's activity patterns when they are characterized by a lack of persistence, or when specific activity patterns cannot be linked to individual preferences (Wlodkowski, 1985). We also use the concept of motivation to explain why people engage in behaviors and activities that we consider bad for health and well-being, such as substance misuse, gambling, and diet and physical activity patterns that are associated with morbidity and mortality. So, for example, we might comment that a person who has a dependence on illicit drugs has to find the motivation for change before her or she can kick the habit.

Motivation is a complicated and multi-dimensional construct. This chapter will focus on only two dimensions of motivation that are both common and challenging in occupational therapy practice. The primary focus of this chapter will be on motivation as it presents in individuals who demonstrate exceptional disengagement from occupations. The quote by Patricia Deegan that opens this chapter provides a stark view of apathy and disinterest as experienced by two people living with physical and mental disabilities. The quote is disturbing both in its characterization of despair and by how long this experience continued. It is also promising in that it suggests that change is a real possibility, never to be discounted.

A second focus of this chapter is motivation as it relates to the decisions people make to participate in and persist with therapeutic change. People refusing participation in therapeutic services known to support positive change, and/or non-adherence to these interventions, is an important issue in health care generally. Accordingly, there has been growing attention to developing strategies and approaches that promote the interest and active participation of people in therapeutic programs and services. Just as occupational therapists are challenged to find ways to support the motivation of individuals who are occupationally disengaged, so too they are challenged to find answers to the problem of motivation to participate in occupational therapy.

MOTIVATION AND OCCUPATIONAL DISENGAGEMENT

View of Health and Disorder

A central and longstanding assumption of occupational therapy is the belief that human beings are inherently occupational beings, driven to engage in occupations as a means to health, well-being, and survival (Townsend & Polatajko, 2007; Wilcock, 2006). The source of this drive is assumed to be the power of occupations to meet a range of important human needs. Some of these are very basic, such as needs related to food, safety, and security. Human well-being associated with these needs is fairly direct. For example, without accessing food and shelter, human life and welfare are seriously compromised. Other human needs that are met through occupation, such as belonging, achieving, and personal growth, and development are of a higher order in that they are considered integral to the long-term well-being and survival of humans, even though the link between specific occupations and activities today may not be obviously linked to well-being in the future. For example, working on a jigsaw puzzle or participating in a community fair may be immediately experienced as challenging and fun leisure activities, but may also be developing important skills, capacities, and resources that contribute to the ability to cope with challenge and adversity in the long term.

Developmentally, the drive for occupation is present from birth, expressed in its first rudimentary form as a baby's reflexive actions, such as sucking and crying, to stimulate the environment to meet needs. As infants develop, they demonstrate a growing diversity of behaviors, become progressively more goal oriented in their behaviors, and have the increasing capacity to connect their activities on any given day with benefits realized at a later time. Healthy children, by nature, are curious, exploratory, and persistent in their activities, and they display emotions that suggest they are engaged in these activities. Think, for example, of the screams of delight and persistence of a toddler who has just discovered that doors to cupboards can be opened and closed, or the focused attention of a child making the perfect mud pie.

Our assumptions about motivation throughout the life stages include the idea that there is considerable individual variation. We understand that there will be differences among people with respect to the diversity of their occupational involvements and the extent to which they outwardly display emotions associated with motivation. Yet we also know that human connection to occupation can be disrupted to the point where the capacity to experience health and well-being through occupation is seriously compromised. Disorder in this case might present as a very limited repertoire of goal-directed daily activities or a general pattern of apathy toward occupations. Disorder, as it applies to motivation, occurs when there is a pattern of indifference or avoidance toward activities associated with developmentally important activities and social roles or with activities that are valued by the individual. Disorders of motivation can extend to apathy toward activities we consider important to basic self-care and security, and present as self-neglect. Such conditions, which compromise self-actualization and well-being, are both puzzling and troubling, and occupational therapy can play an important role in ameliorating these situations in a manner that remains respectful of the individual.

Theoretical Perspectives on Motivation and Human Engagement in Occupation

Given the complexity and sophistication of human behavior and human occupation, no one theory provides a sound, all-encompassing explanation. Theoretical understandings of motivation can be loosely organized into three distinct but related categories: biological, psychological, and social.

Biological Theories

Biological theories are grounded in the assumption that motivation for occupation is fundamental to survival, and that from an evolutionary point of view, engagement in human occupations is instinctual—instincts for which humans are biologically "hard wired." These theories assume, for example, that motivation for occupation will contribute to natural processes of human selection, and that these in turn will contribute to the evolution of humans, and human societies that are continuously more adapted for well-being and survival (Wilcock, 2006). Drive theories associated with human behavior suggest that humans are moved by the urge to reduce bodily tensions, to maintain a state of equilibrium or homeostasis. So, for example, humans are assumed to engage in behaviors related to reducing the tensions associated with hunger, thirst, sex, and sleep. Body functions and structures that underlie processes associated with motivation for occupation have been identified. There are, for example, structural and physiological processes that govern hunger and eating as well as central nervous system structures and processes associated with the emotions experienced during human occupation. Disturbances of motivation can occur because of disorder at the level of these body functions and

structures. This means that it is possible that disturbances in motivation are a direct result of diseases, injuries, and other health-related conditions if they involve these body functions and structures. For example, central nervous system changes occurring in the context of schizophrenia, traumatic brain injury, and strokes have all been associated with motivational problems.

Psychological Theories

Psychological theories focus on the psychological and emotional processes underlying motivation for human behavior. Psychological theories, which focus on external incentives for behavior, suggest that valued incentives or perceived rewards received from the external environment contribute to human drive for activity and occupation. So for example, financial reward, material items, special treats and experiences, good grades, or scholarly awards can all serve as powerful motivators for human behavior. These ideas are more fully developed in the chapter in this book focusing on learning and occupation. Similarly, human activity can be motivated by the drive to avoid outcomes in the external environment that are perceived as harsh or punishing. Avoiding eviction, grade failures, or employment reprimands are all examples of human activity oriented to avoiding perceived negative consequences. Psychological theories that focus on the intrinsic sources of motivation explain that humans receive experiences of internal reward in the process of performing activity, separate from external outcomes (Ryan & Deci, 2000). These internal rewards can take many forms, but common terms used to describe this reward are *enjoyment*, *satisfaction*, *interest*, and *pride*.

Flow theory has contributed greatly to our understanding of the quality of the experience of activity engagement that is internally motivating (Csikszentmihalyi, 1991, 1993). Flow theory has been applied to occupational therapy (Rebeiro & Polgar, 1999; Reid, 2011). The premise of flow theory is that human activities are intrinsically rewarding when activities are goal directed, individuals become so engrossed in the activity that awareness merges with their actions, and activities present challenges that peak but do not overwhelm skills and capacities. In this way, humans experience a range of feelings while engaged in activity from feeling pleasure (e.g., fun, joy), to feeling good about oneself (e.g., feeling competent), feeling changed in positive ways (e.g., learning new skills), or perhaps feeling that important goals are being achieved (e.g., getting a desired job, securing a valued friendship group). It is these intrinsic motivators of human occupation that are most associated with the sustained commitment considered necessary for health and well-being through occupation.

In psychology and related disciplines, there has been much theoretical development of the psychological and emotional conditions that support or disturb motivation. For example, motivated human behavior is believed to be enabled by (1) the presence of goals or life tasks (often many simultaneously) that organize and give meaning to behaviors; (2) these goals or life tasks, and their associated behaviors, hold meaning and value for the individual; (3) the goals and/or life tasks offer opportunities for self-direction and agency; and (4) engagement in these goal-directed and meaningful behaviors engenders feelings of achievement and competence and self-worth (see for example, Wlodkowski, 1999). So it follows that significant disruptions in motivation can occur when goals and life tasks are disrupted, behaviors do not hold meaning for individuals, and when personal competence and self-esteem are compromised. These are situations that are frequently witnessed by occupational therapists in their day-to-day work. Many of these ideas are developed in more depth in Chapter 5.

Social Theories

Social theories explain the motivation for human activity in relation to broader social and cultural forces. While motivation is primarily considered an individual experience, foundational theories of motivation, such as that proposed by Maslow (1968), draw attention to how individual motivation must be understood in relation to the individual's position within the broader world. Maslow's famous model of human need positioned basic physiological needs, such as the need for food, water, and sex, as the foundation of the pyramid of needs. Following this are safety needs, which include security in relation to family, employment, property, etc. Love and belonging needs follow and highlight the importance of family, friendships, and intimacy to the human condition. Esteem and self-actualization needs, respectively, top the pyramid and include the importance of respect and recognition by others along with reaching personal potentials.

Social forces such as culture and social status help explain, for example, why individuals may commit themselves to particular human activities and activity patterns over others. While the idea that human motivation is aligned with goals, values, personal agency, etc., and is highly relevant in individualistic societies, people in collectivist societies or communities will be more oriented to aligning their goals, preferences, achievements, etc. with those favored by their social context (Iwama, 2006). This context includes families and communities, cultural values, and social norms.

Broader social structures, such as policies, legislation, and regulation can inhibit or facilitate human motivation. Laws specific to particular countries can enable or constrain human motivation for occupation for all citizens or for specific populations. For example, the World Development Report (World Bank, 2012) highlighted the need to improve the agency of women in developing countries in relation to a broad range of activities and opportunities fundamental to daily occupational and community life. The material

conditions of life are also believed to have a powerful influence on human motivation. A lack of finances can inhibit opportunities for occupations, but sustained experiences of abject poverty and financial dependence can both inhibit opportunity and crush intrinsic sources of drive for occupational engagement. Environments that are devoid of meaningful occupational opportunities, such as those common in long-term care or correctional institutions, can contribute to boredom, accompanied by disengagement and feelings of futility. Conditions of war and political unrest can create a situation where anxiety and fear override motivation. Environments that are psychologically and emotionally toxic, such as toxic workplaces, can influence motivation and ultimately undermine full participation. The final section of this textbook that focuses on social and ecological perspectives provides more detailed information about the social factors involved in motivation.

Although each of these theories related to human motivation for occupation is helpful, it is difficult to integrate them in a meaningful way to explain any discrete patterns of human activity. Frameworks that attempt to organize priorities of human need (such as that made famous by Maslow, 1968) are helpful, but still need to be applied in a judicious fashion. Maslow's hierarchy suggests that physiological needs (on the bottom of the pyramid) are the most basic and generally these needs must be met before activities associated with higher order needs can be engaged in and sustained. Yet, there are many everyday examples where needs considered a priority are delayed or ignored in favor of seemingly higher level priorities. You might, for example, be familiar with the experience of staying up late, fighting the urge to sleep, and the threat of early morning alarm clocks, to finish reading a good book or to find the last piece of the puzzle. In more serious life circumstances, narratives of the lives of prison camp survivors are often filled with stories of constructing opportunities for engaging in intellectual or creative activities, even in the face of extreme punishment and the loss of basic resources. Maslow's famous quote—"if you plan on being anything less than you are capable of being, you will probably be unhappy all the days of your life"—suggests that the pyramid of human need must be interpreted from a view of human fulfillment as a higher-order need that must ultimately be met, and the potential for doing so occurs even within problematic conditions of life.

The suggestion that the sources of reward can be categorized into those that are external or internal to the individual is far from simple. Incentives to act that are considered external to the individual have typically been considered to be less motivating than those that are intrinsic. In essence, the theory is that when human activity is pushed or pulled by outside reinforcers, it is unlikely to be sustained in the absence of those reinforcers and may even compromise intrinsic motivation for the activity. Yet, this does not always hold true in daily life occupations.

BOX 6-1. VIGNETTE: DION

Dion is 24 years old. He was working as a lab assistant until about 2 years ago when he experienced his first acute episode of psychosis. His current diagnosis is schizophrenia. A few months ago he began receiving a disability pension and this provides him with some financial security. Over the past 2 years, he has become quite isolated and very inactive. Outside of tending to his basic self-care and occasional contact with family who live several hours away, he has few work or leisure activities in his life. He rents a basement apartment in a house and so he has few home-related chores. His home is located in a poor district of town. He is troubled by feelings of ambivalence about following through with employment plans. He describes himself as having a "lack of purpose and direction," a disquieting feeling of "lack of enthusiasm," and an overall sense of "discomfort with himself." He is unsure if he will ever be able to manage any of the work and social activities he used to be involved with. He says these feelings predated his episode of psychosis, and he pinpoints Grade 10 as the beginning of changes in his drive and ambition. He had been oriented to attending university in preparation for a career. Although he states that a part of him desires to participate in the community, another part drives him to withdraw from social contacts and responsibilities. The information he has received about the illness has him worried that things "might not get much better."

For example, Ryan and Deci (2000) suggested that how an individual perceives and experiences the activities and its reinforcers is important to consider. So, in the case of paid work, for example, the financial reward is received, and this is an external incentive. Yet the incentive may actually be experienced as an internal reinforcer if the financial reward is experienced as a reflection of being socially valued and appreciated. Similarly, praise for an activity well done may be received from sources external to the individual, but complement internal, rewarding perceptions of achievement and belonging. In this way, praise, if it is consistent with the individual's own perception of his or her performance, may act more like an internal reinforcer than an external one.

Practice Developments

Therapeutic interventions designed to address issues related to profound problems in drive and motivation have received limited attention in the health care and rehabilitation literature. One therapeutic tool in occupational therapy—the therapeutic relationship—is at risk when clients experience disturbances in motivation in their daily lives. Motivational disturbances are complex and are likely the result of several, interacting underlying forces. With no one theoretical framework sufficing to explain significant motivation disruptions, therapists can mistakenly adopt simplistic or even non-empathetic or reproachful interpretations of motivational problems. In this way, motivational problems can become interpreted as willful resistance or non-compliance ("She's just being lazy," "He needs to pull up his boot straps," or "If she doesn't want to get better, I can't help"), and negatively affect the enabling qualities of the relationship.

In addition, significant motivational issues are not easily addressed within health systems and services that are time limited, have multiple policies and restrictions with respect to the organization of service delivery, or reward service interventions that are narrow in scope or highly technical (rather than humanistic) in nature. In this case, individuals with exceptional motivational problems can become perceived as a problem because they conflict with the organizational and administrative demands placed on the therapist.

Finally, if an individual is experiencing significant motivational problems in daily occupations, the qualities that characterize his or her motivation (e.g., apathy, limited expressions of satisfaction, reticence) are likely to extend into the therapeutic relationship itself and the therapist may experience the relationship as unpleasant, dull, and unrewarding, and perhaps even leading to feelings of incompetence. When a client's "unmotivated" behaviors prompt responses by the therapists that feed into maintaining these behaviors, a cycle of therapeutic disengagement becomes established. Developing a sound knowledge base about motivation as it affects occupation and skill in a broad range of related intervention approaches, along with ongoing reflection about the dynamics of the therapeutic relationship, is the best way to construct the therapeutic conditions that can enable positive change.

The two vignettes of Dion and Carl offer examples of disturbances in motivation in human occupation occurring within the context of health conditions (Boxes 6-1 and 6-2). They will serve as a springboard from which to learn about and apply theory and evidence-informed occupational therapy practices.

Assessment

Both of these vignettes present individuals with occupational patterns that suggest high levels of inactivity, a restricted range of activities, and disturbed emotional

Box 6-2. Vignette: Carl

It has been 4 months since Carl experienced a stroke. Carl had a long career as an editor. He retired last year and was looking forward to spending time with his wife, children, and grandchildren; working on his home and garden; and taking up some new hobbies. He was also looking forward to having time to read books of his own choice, and even trying his hand at writing some short stories. While his family members have been very worried about his post-stroke recovery, they have been particularly distressed with his general apathy. His daughter says, "It is just like Dad doesn't care about anything anymore." Carl is still highly dependent on his family to help him with his self-care, but they wonder if maybe he could be more involved in trying things out on his own, with their support. They note that even having his beloved grandchildren around can't seem to rouse him out of his indifference.

connections in activity. While Dion's brief vignette indicates that these patterns began several years ago, in his teenage years, Carl's vignette suggests an abrupt change. The vignettes show that feelings of distress can be associated with these disturbances in occupational engagement, both by the individual and by people in their families and social networks. In addition to the lived experience of drive and motivational disturbances, occupational therapists attend to observable behaviors that are assumed to indicate motivational issues. For example, the Volitional Questionnaire (de las Heras, Geist, Kielhofner, & Li, 2007), an assessment linked to the Model of Human Occupation, identifies a range of observable behaviors associated with motivated human activity, including showing curiosity, demonstrating pride, seeking out responsibilities, and staying engaged with activities until completion.

For the occupational therapist, the purpose of assessment will extend beyond merely naming the problem as one of profound occupational disengagement, to (1) developing an interpretation of contributing factors that need to be considered in intervention, and (2) identifying any particular strengths related to occupation that might be capitalized upon to enable motivation for occupation. Building an interpretation of contributing factors is based on the application of theories related to motivation. Using a comprehensive approach, we can build an interpretation about contributing factors that includes consideration of potential biological, psychological, and social contributing factors.

Biomedical considerations suggest that we attend to the possibility that body structures or functions associated with motivation might have been impacted in the context of disease, disorder, or injury. In Dion's situation, we could consider the possibility that his mental illness diagnosis can be associated with neural changes that can negatively affect the emotions, cognitive capacities (such as attention, planning, making decisions), and the energy levels responsible for motivated human occupation (Heckers, 2000). Although the current generation of anti-psychotic medications used to treat the symptoms of schizophrenia have been greatly improved compared to earlier medications, common side

effects of these treatments can still include feelings of fatigue and fogginess that can affect activity engagement. In the case of Carl, we know that apathy and indifference are not uncommon following stroke, with estimates of 20% to 25% (Jorge, Starkstein, & Robinson, 2010). This apathy can be associated with depression but can also present independently (van Dalen, van Charante, Nederkoorn, van Gool, & Richard, 2013). The brain pathology that might be associated with apathy in stroke is not altogether clear, but there is some evidence that right frontal lobe subcortical pathways can be involved (Brodaty et al., 2005).

Interpreting problems in drive and motivation as having some biological base is not without its problems in occupational therapy. First, the likelihood of receiving valid neurological testing to confirm that there is a clear biological basis for the motivational problems is slim. Second, biological explanations might leave the occupational therapist feeling disempowered, thinking that all the profession can do is wait to see if the underlying biomedical mechanisms for motivation and drive recover. The problem here, of course, is that the client becomes highly vulnerable to having his or her occupational needs ignored or poorly addressed. Note that the vignette of Dion suggests that he has received information about his illness that has left him feeling disempowered and somewhat hopeless with regard to his potential for occupational engagement. So, how can the occupational therapist frame biomedical interpretation of drive and motivation in a way that can support occupation-based practice? Acknowledging that there may be some biomedical basis for drive and motivation problems, in particular health conditions, can facilitate the development of a therapeutic relationship where the client feels listened to and understood. Psychological and emotional qualities we associate with motivation and drive are not *completely* absent in any health condition. Therefore, discovering, capitalizing on, and growing existing sources of motivation and drive are important. Finally, processes of improvement in serious and persistent health conditions are complex, and can be affected by a range of factors such as individual agency, social and cultural environment, opportunities, etc. In this context, enabling an individual's involvement in occupation might actually contribute to the recovery of the biomedical functions believed to underlie drive and motivation.

Psychological considerations for Dion and Carl include the assessment of psychological and emotional processes that may be influencing drive and motivation. In the case of Dion, we can assume that the loss of his main productivity role without any meaningful replacement has seriously compromised his goal-directed activities. The study suggests that in addition to an occupational profile that is reflective of a primary identity of "person with mental illness," Dion is experiencing compromised self-agency and self-efficacy. He speaks quite poignantly about the disruptions in emotional connections with activity that he has experienced. In addition, he presents as highly anxious, a distressing feeling that may also be constraining his occupational engagement. Compared to Dion, Carl is older with a rich history of occupational engagement. However, he has been transitioning to retirement and his occupational patterns in this new status had not been solidified when he experienced the stroke. Always highly self-sufficient and a provider for others, his high level of dependence on family may be affecting his self-esteem and contributing to feelings of shame and guilt that are associated with his presentation of apathy and indifference. The loss of particular abilities (e.g., physical or cognitive capacities) may be affecting his sense of self-efficacy.

Our vignettes suggest several social considerations for understanding drive and motivation for occupation. Dion's occupations have likely been affected by his poverty status. He lives in a poor socioeconomic district, which perhaps contributes to concerns about safety, and he may have few resources to support efforts to engage in occupations. Government disability pensions are well known to contribute to inactivity through policies that constrain participation (Krupa et al., 2012). He has a limited social network to support his activity involvement. The brief information we have about Carl suggests that, in comparison to Dion, he is well connected to a robust and supportive social network and a socioeconomic status that could provide materially for occupational engagement. However, we know little about the physical aspects of his home and community environment and the extent to which impairments associated with stroke might compromise important activities such as driving that have been central to his identity and activity patterns.

There is a range of standardized assessments available that provide some measurement of motivational problems related to specific health conditions. The Positive and Negative Syndrome Scale (Kay, Fiszbein, & Opler, 1987) and Scale for the Assessment of Negative Symptoms (Andreason, 1984) measure the observable signs of problems with motivation for people with schizophrenia including the blunting of affect, social withdrawal and passivity,

a lack of volition, and evidence of disrupted emotional connection to activities and people. The Apathy Evaluation Scale (Marin, Biedrzycki, & Firincioquallari, 1991) similarly measures dimensions, such as curiosity, the initiation of action, and emotions, associated with the motivational changes that occur in a broad range of health conditions with neurological and psychological implications such as cerebral vascular accidents, dementia, traumatic brain injury, Parkinson's disease, and mental illnesses such as depression and schizophrenia. The use of such standardized measurements can be important in developing a shared understanding of the nature of the functional changes associated with motivation, to serve as a baseline for sharing information interprofessionally, for understanding change over time, and for raising awareness of the significance and prevalence of motivational problems in a health care context. They are limited, however, in their ability to guide the development of person-centered intervention approaches.

Strengths-based and dynamic assessment processes are particularly useful for the occupational therapist working with individuals with significant patterns of occupational disengagement. Strengths-based assessments focus less on the pathology or disturbances experienced and observed and instead on revealing possibilities, identifying opportunities, and empowering individuals toward levels of self-agency we know are required to cause positive change (Blundo, 2001). How does the occupational therapist discover opportunities for enabling occupational engagement in the face of significant disruptions of drive and motivation? Our case vignettes offer a few examples. Dion, who once thought about furthering his studies, has had some good work experience, has some level of family connection, and has the self-awareness to be able to speak about the feelings he has associated with activities. Carl has a long-standing and broad range of interests and abilities and some plans for retirement. He has an involved family, apparently invested in supporting his occupational engagement, and the potential joy of grandchildren. These are all potential strengths that can serve as a springboard for intervention approaches that are both collaboratively determined and well supported. Table 6-1 identifies a range of strategies that an occupational therapist can use to reveal possibilities and opportunities for occupational engagement using a strengths perspective.

A dynamic assessment process provides the therapist and client with important information about the intervention approach that is likely to have the most impact (Missiuna, 1987). Whereas dynamic assessment processes in occupational therapy have traditionally been linked to the assessment of "performance" of occupations (Polatajko, Mandich, & Martini, 2000), in the case of occupational disengagement, there is equal attention to the "experience" of occupations, or the emotional connections that motivate and sustain engagement. In the case of drive and motivation, the therapist seeks to reveal intervention

TABLE 6-1
USING A STRENGTHS-BASED APPROACH TO ENABLE POSSIBILITIES AND OPPORTUNITIES FOR DEVELOPING MOTIVATION FOR OCCUPATION
Attending to evidence of interests, activities, meaning in the person's immediate environment, such as decorative objects, personal possessions, photos, books, etc.
Understanding past interests and activities
Prompting and listening to stories about life events and activities
Engaging in conversations about current events (world events, sports, community events, etc.)
Learning about cultural influences on activities
Observing interactions with immediate environment, including for example, people, animals, things

approaches that will enable responses consistent with motivated engagement in occupations. In our vignettes of Dion and Carl, for example, this might involve meeting outside of their homes within community environments that could spark interests, sharing humor and playfulness in an activity to elicit positive emotional responses, attending to the time of day/week that are best for activity involvement, and identifying the forms of feedback that have the most impact. Occupational therapists also have available to them a range of standardized tools to support these dynamic assessment processes. Leisure, interest, and role checklists (see for example, Leisure Scale [Beard & Ragheb, 1980], Occupational Self-Assessment [Baron, Kielhofner, Iyenger, Goldhammer, & Wolenski, 2006], Modified Interest checklist [Keilhofner & Neville, 1983], and Role Checklist [Oakley et al., 1986]) all engage individuals in evaluating their perceptions of possibilities and opportunities for occupational engagement. They should, however, be used with some caution with individuals who have significant issues with drive and motivation because they require considerable energy and have the potential to be deflating when the individual does not connect emotionally with the activity options presented.

Intervention Approaches

Collaborative, but systematic approaches that tie assessment to intervention processes to stimulate drive, motivation, and healthy activity patterns ensure client involvement in a manner that matches his or her capacities and emotional needs. Four approaches used by occupational therapists, and emerging from a variety of theoretical frameworks, are presented here. Although they are distinct approaches with their own knowledge base and body of evidence, they all have in common a focus on enabling sustained purposeful and goal-directed activity that promotes health and well-being. In addition, each of the approaches has assessment

processes that enable the ongoing evaluation of outcomes related to motivation and sustained activity engagement:

1. Systematic processes of goal setting and attainment have been developed for populations in health care where drive and motivation are prevalent issues. The standardized evaluation process, Goal Attainment Scaling (Kiersek & Sherman, 1968; Marson et al., 2009) has been used to engage service providers and their clients in collaboratively identifying explicit, manageable, and behavioral goals to provide some order and direction to activity and engagement that can be supported in the therapeutic relationship. The Goal Attainment Scaling provides a measure of goal achievement, for even small goals, and as such is sensitive to change.

Structured goal-oriented programs have been developed for a range of health-related conditions where motivational problems can be significant and identifying even small goals and supported sustained commitment will be challenged by a range of factors. For example, Nga and Tsang (2000) describe a theoretically grounded, four-stage goal program for individuals who are inpatients in mental health settings that includes (1) affirming personal worth, (2) imagining the future, (3) establishing a sense of control, and (4) setting goals for the future. Research of this program demonstrated its effectiveness in supporting goal setting and evidence of improved motivation for participation in rehabilitation to achieve these goals. Similarly, McPherson, Kayes, and Weatherall (2009) described "Identity-Oriented Goal Training" that had clients with acquired brain injury identify someone they admire and to use this individual as a metaphor for points of exploration on possible goal-directed behaviors. Qualitative evaluation of the process by these authors indicated that the approach was acceptable to both clients and health service providers. Goals were identified and were observed to be accompanied by improvements in motivation and affect. Challenges for service providers included the time required for the intervention and the change in approach from traditional forms of service delivery.

2. Action Over Inertia (Krupa et al., 2010) is an intervention approach designed to address the activity-health needs of individuals with serious mental illness who experience significant disengagement from activity patterns associated with health and well-being. The intervention includes The Activity Engagement Measure, which involves clients identifying particular experiences associated with activities that they would like to have in their lives. For example, the measure uses a 10-point scale as a basis for clients to consider whether they could benefit from more physical activity in their day, more social interactions, more meaningful activities, and access to a broader range of community environments. In this way, intervention approaches are directed to developing activity patterns that are likely to bring these experiences as an antidote to inertia in activities. The dimensions of experience are consistent with another validated measure of occupational engagement, the Profiles of Occupational Engagement in Schizophrenia (Bejerholm, Hansson, & Eklund, 2006). Pilot research on the Action Over Inertia intervention approach, using a randomized control trial design, demonstrated significant shifts in daily time use profiles, with community-dwelling adults with serious mental illness participating in the intervention showing less time in sleep and more time in activity compared to controls not receiving the intervention (Edgelow & Krupa, 2011).

3. An intervention approach known as Personal Projects, developed initially by Little and colleagues (2004), is based on the notion that humans experience well-being through their engagement in big or small projects that are personally salient and motivating. Theoretically, personal projects can be evaluated based on particular dimensions associated with well-being such as meaning, sense of community, efficacy, and others. Personal projects have been used by occupational therapists working in post-stroke rehabilitation, when individuals are at high risk for occupational disruption and apathy, to support and monitor the change in the quality of the experiences with activity engagement. Davis and colleagues (2013) described the process as involving clients in identifying goal-directed activities in daily life prior to the stroke and currently, and monitoring experiences with these projects that are associated with health and well-being such as control, identity, importance, and pleasure. These researchers were able to demonstrate that 12 months post-stroke,

study participants were able to reengage in activities that provided similar positive experiences to those pre-stroke. They recommend that personal projects may be a way to both monitor progress in relation to participation in meaningful activities and as a means to ensure that the activity-related support needs of clients are identified and addressed.

4. The Remotivation process is an intervention approach grounded theoretically in the Model of Human Occupation (de las Heras, Llerena, & Kielhofner, 2003). Using the Volitional Questionnaire (de las Heras et al., 2007), therapists observe and score behaviors that are indicative of values, interests, and personal causation. Interventions are matched to support activity engagement through phases of exploration, competence, and achievement. A qualitative study of occupational therapists applied this in a mental health context with individuals experiencing significant motivational problems related to depression. Therapists thought that the intervention enabled them to be more attuned to recognizing and addressing needs to support change in the therapeutic process (Pépin, Guérette, Lefebvre, & Jacques, 2008).

Practice Principles

The following section identifies a set of principles that underlie practice that is designed to positively influence the drive and motivation for occupational engagement:

- *Engage the individual in "doing"*: Reversing occupational patterns of inertia, indifference, and avoidance depends on the individual engaging in activity to experience the psychological, emotional, and social feedback likely to ignite motivation. Csikszentmihalyi (1990, 1993), in his seminal work on flow, for example, writes that activities have the potential to produce a range of positive experiences, from pleasure and joy, a sense of accomplishment, discovery, creativity, to a sense of harmony with others and personal control. It is these experiences that can lead to the drive for more complex and challenging activity engagement.

The key enabling skills of occupational therapy are focused on rousing individuals who are occupationally disengaged to action. Associated skills include inspiring, influencing, persuading, and encouraging. Exhorting is a particular enabling skill, perhaps first described in detail in Barris and colleagues' (1988) foundation text on psychosocial occupational therapy practice. Exhorting here refers to practices that engage individuals with significant motivational disruptions in activities that promote health and well-being, without crossing the boundaries to becoming judgmental and

TABLE 6-2	
POTENTIAL CHALLENGES TO ACTIVITY ENGAGEMENT	
CHALLENGES	**EXAMPLES**
Personal learning	Activities can require new knowledge or skills or even the need to practice old skills.
Material resources	Every activity will require access to material resources, such as transportation, equipment, clothing, etc.
Health management	Activities may require new health management strategies.
Emotional needs	Activities can stimulate feelings of worry, or negative thought patterns that counter positive emotions.
Managing social judgments	Activities may put people in touch with the misguided attitudes of others.
Activity modifications	Some elements of activities may need to be changed to support performance.
Social supports	Activities often require interactions with others or can be enhanced by support from others.

From Krupa, T. et al., *Action Over Inertia: Addressing the activity-health needs of individuals with serious mental illness*, Ottawa, Canada. Copyright © 2010 by CAOT. Reprinted with permission of CAOT Publications ACE.

coercive. At its core, exhorting is a relational skill that motivates others to action. Motivating activity engagement depends on creating conditions for motivation.

In this chapter, a range of such conditions have been identified and include connecting any activity to a purpose that holds personal and social meaning; ensuring that activities are compatible with cultural and personal values; ensuring that the activity challenges but does not overwhelm capacity; creating a sense of continuity, linking activities performed today to other promising opportunities in the future; and highlighting the positive experiences of engaging.

- *Conditions that have the potential to compromise activity engagement should be identified and addressed*: For individuals with significant motivational issues, even those activities that we perceive as small and inconsequential can hold considerable challenges, emerging from personal capacity issues, the nature of the activities, or the environmental context. Table 6-2 offers examples of typical challenges that can arise. Making potential challenges explicit provides the opportunity for the therapist to work collaboratively with an individual to address these concerns proactively.

- *Consider a wide range of occupational experiences associated with motivation*: The knowledge base of occupational therapy provides a rich understanding of the range of beneficial experiences associated with engagement in occupation. Where significant motiva-

tional issues exist with respect to occupational participation, the occupational therapist may need to generate many of these potential experiences to effect sustained motivation for occupation. For example, individuals with motivational issues may feel that their capacity to feel joy and pleasure is compromised, but still experience good feelings and well-being if an activity provides an opportunity to contribute in a way they find meaningful to their family or community.

- *Provide individuals served with information about motivation and activity engagement*: Evidence-based psychoeducation is based on the premise that people become empowered and energized when they have important knowledge to effect change in their lives (Baumi, Frobose, Kraemer, Rentrop, & Pitschel-Walz, 2006). The individuals served by occupational therapists and their families have the right to information relevant to their health and well-being, including information about understanding motivational issues affecting activity engagement. For example, understanding that motivational issues are a common concern in the daily lives of people with particular health conditions can help people to feel that they are not alone. It can also encourage their willingness to meet with others in similar circumstances who have experienced improvements in their activity engagement and to draw a sense of hope from these interactions.

- *Advocate to raise the priority of motivational issues and occupational engagement in program/service develop-*

ment: Motivational issues in the health care context are often given low priority, even when a significant portion of the population served experience these difficulties. People with significant motivational issues and occupational disengagement may themselves maintain a low profile and be unlikely to expect or demand services. In this regard, it is relatively easy for their needs to be poorly addressed. Creating a service context that enables the implementation of theory and evidence-informed approaches to address motivational issues depends on occupational therapists who can raise the profile and implement possibilities. The tools and intervention strategies offered in this text provide a foundation for developing program structures and demonstrating positive outcomes that can help to raise the profile of these issues.

ENABLING MOTIVATION FOR THERAPEUTIC CHANGE

View of Health and Disorder

In the health and social care context, it is not uncommon to hear concerns that some people receiving services are "unmotivated" to change behaviors that compromise their health and well-being. As mentioned at the beginning of the chapter, problems with motivation are often attributed to people who engage in potentially harmful activities such as drug, tobacco, and alcohol use or misuse, or who demonstrate a lack of physical activity and/or unhealthy dietary patterns. In service settings, the label "unmotivated" might also be applied to people who experience, or are at risk of experiencing, health-related impairments, or activity and participation limitations but who are uninterested or unwilling to engage in behaviors that could protect or improve their health and well-being. Occupational therapists will come into contact with a broad range of practice examples—from people apparently unwilling to wear protective gear like helmets while cycling, to not engaging in skin care routines to reduce the likelihood of pressure sores following spinal cord injuries, to limited adherence to recommended approaches to manage back pain. Not only do these "unmotivated" behaviors have negative health effects, they also can have a range of economic and social costs, including health care expenses, and the costs of lost productivity. Mastellos, Gunn, Felix, Car, and Majeed (2014) discuss the economic implications of obesity and lack of physical activity.

The fact that people will continue with these behaviors despite knowledge of the worst-case scenarios and public education about evidence-based treatments is a problem for service providers who are faced with addressing them within their practices. Explanations for these human behaviors have led to moralistic debates as to whether such behaviors are fundamentally individual or societal flaws or whether they are best explained as an individual's right to be self-determining and ultimately live by the consequences of those choices (Buchanan, 2008).

Theoretical Perspectives

Several theoretical models have been highly influential in the current understanding of why people engage in behaviors that are potentially harmful to health, or who do not capitalize on services and treatments that have the potential to lead to improvements in health and well-being. The Health Belief Model (Rosenstock, 1974) theorizes that human health behaviors will depend on the value individuals place on a particular health-related goal, and the extent to which they believe their behaviors will affect this goal. The model suggests that individuals will weigh their perceptions according to several dimensions: the potential severity of a health condition, the benefits of following a particular course of action, and the barriers. Particular cues can trigger changes in perception. If these cues affect the individual's sense of personal threat, behavioral change can occur. While evidence has provided support for the dimensions of health (Janz & Becker, 1984), the actual health-related perceptions of any individual will be affected by several factors. For example, adolescents are perhaps more likely to perceive themselves as invulnerable to severe health conditions (Rosenthal, Hall, & Moore, 1992) and given the health-related inequities in our health care systems, the perception of barriers to change can be expected to be influenced by race and ethnicity (Chen, Fox, Cantrell, Stockdale, & Kagawa-Singer, 2007).

The Theory of Planned Behavior (TPB; Ajzen & Madden, 1986) positions behaviors and behavioral intentions more within their social context. According to the TPB, behavioral intentions will be determined by the individual's attitude or evaluation of the particular behavior, and his or her perceptions of social norms or expectations related to the behavior. In addition, the extent to which individuals perceive that they can control the behavior will influence intentions and behaviors. In this way, the TPB considers personal volition as a potential barrier to behavioral change.

The Transtheoretical Model of Change contributes to our understanding of health related behaviors by suggesting that individual behavior changes depend on a state of "readiness" that can be defined according to specific stages and processes (Prochaska & DiClemente, 1982). This model is important in that it highlights that health-related behavior changes need to be understood as an interaction between individual variables, intervention approaches, and their relative timing.

Taken together, these theoretical perspectives have made significant contributions to the way we understand and act to influence health-related behaviors in health and social services. They suggest the importance of considering (1) the individual's own perception of the behaviors, and the meanings attributed to these; (2) the social-environmental context within which the behaviors exist and are sustained; (3) the external and internal barriers to behavioral change as perceived by the individual; and (4) readiness for change as a non-linear process.

Practice Developments

Assessment practices in the area of health-related behavior change suggest the importance of understanding how health-related intentions and behaviors are embedded in the day-to-day life of the individual. In this way, the occupational therapist comes to understand how these health-related behaviors are perceived and lived by the individual and how they emerge within, influence, and are influenced by the broader context for occupation. From this perspective, substance use is no longer understood solely as "unhealthy" behavior, but rather as a type of occupation that has meaning and purpose, associated tasks, and environmental contexts. For example, substance use and related behaviors might be perceived by an individual as a necessary action to support other pro-social activities, or perhaps the individual's primary social network might be largely organized around substance use. Likewise, lack of involvement in a program of return to work following a back injury might best be understood as having a particular meaning for the individual, shaped by beliefs, expectations of others ,and various environmental conditions.

The Stages of Change Model proposed by the Transtheoretical Model of Change (Prochaska & DiClemente, 1982) suggests the importance of occupational therapists assessing readiness for change. In this approach, the occupational therapist focuses on the ambivalence to change that underlies the particular stage of change and works to facilitate the individual's ability to resolve this ambivalence. Miller and Rollnick (1991) identify six stages of change and associated motivational tasks of the therapist. Stage 1, precontemplation, is a stage where the individual is not considering change seriously. The therapist's task is to promote doubt, by engaging the individual in considering the possible risks and problems associated with the behavior. Stage 2, contemplation, sees the individual considering change, although not yet committed. The therapist tries to both strengthen the individual's understanding of risks and problems associated with the behavior and to instill confidence that he or she has the ability to change behaviors. Stage 3 is determination, a stage that sees the individual invested in making a change; accordingly, the therapist acts to help the individual to make plans and set a course for action. Stage 4 is action, in which the individual moves to carry out plans, accompanied by the support of the therapist. Stage 5 is maintenance, where an individual who has been successful in changing his or her behaviors is faced

with keeping on course and avoiding relapse. The therapist in this stage can help the client to develop and implement strategies to avoid relapse. Finally, stage 6 refers to the very real potential for relapse and suggests that the therapist has an important role in helping the individual to frame its occurrence as a point for renewed commitment rather than resignation and despair.

A range of therapeutic strategies to enhance motivation for change are now available to occupational therapists. Although largely developed within the field of substance use, they have been applied more broadly in circumstances where particular behaviors have the potential to influence health and well-being. Stoffel and Moyers (2004) developed an evidence-based and occupationally oriented review of intervention approaches to facilitate behavior change in the context of substance use. Motivational strategies included the use of decision balance exercises to weigh the pros and cons of behaviors and skilled non-confrontational and empathic communication strategies, such as motivational interviewing (Miller & Rollnick, 1991) to positively influence intentions for change.

As each of the theoretical perspectives presented earlier suggest, intervention approaches will need to consider and address an individual's perceived barriers to change (both internal and external) to influence and sustain behavioral change. Occupational therapists may be in a particularly good position to identify and address barriers and concerns that emerge within the context of day-to-day occupations. So, for example, the individual considering changing substance use behaviors might benefit from occupational therapy assistance in understanding how engagement in particular occupations compels substance use, developing leisure activities and social networks that are free from alcohol or substance use, and learning the skills to refuse substances when they are offered. Similarly, an individual whose motivation for participation in a return-to-work program related to a back injury is tentative, might benefit from advocacy training and reasonable accommodations to support access to good working conditions upon a return to the workplace.

CONCLUSION

In this chapter, the factors underlying the motivation that underlies occupational engagement and activity patterns associated with health and well-being are presented as complex and interrelated. Subsequently, intervention approaches used by occupational therapists must be comprehensive while being informed by theory and evidence. Given that drive and motivational issues can be long-standing and sustained by a range of contextual conditions, approaches need to promote continuity over time. In short, the intervention approaches we use need to demonstrate the same level of persistence, dependability, and follow-through that we assume are qualities of motivated people. Addressing motivational issues is challenging, but given the impact of these issues on individual health and well-being and societal costs, occupational therapists who take up the challenge are in a good position to make an important difference.

Learning Activities/ Discussion Questions

1. What particular central nervous system structures and functions are linked to human motivation? Which of these have been associated with the following health-related conditions: traumatic-brain injury, schizophrenia, and stroke?

2. Read the journal article written by Deegan (1988) that is the source of the opening quote for the chapter. How did Deegan overcome the inertia that characterized her life following her first formal episodes of schizophrenia?

3. Think about a time when it was difficult for you to either change a behavior that was problematic, or when you didn't follow through with the recommendations of health professionals. Reflect on the factors that might have contributed to this. Consider what supports might have been helpful to you to improve your motivation.

4. Many people with significant disabilities are financially supported by government disability pensions. While these pensions are believed to provide much needed financial stability, they have also been criticized as robbing people of motivation to engage in important community activities. Find resources and/or discuss with others how this unintended and negative consequence might occur.

References

Andreasen, N. C. (1984). *Scale for the assessment of negative symptoms (SANS)*. Iowa City, University of Iowa.

Ajzen, I., & Madden, T. (1986). Prediction of goal-direction behavior: Attitudes, intentions and perceived behavioral control. *Journal of Experimental Social Psychology, 22*, 453-474.

Baron, K., Kielhofner, G., Iyenger, A., Goldhammer, V., & Wolenski, J. (2006). *A user's manual for the occupational self assessment (OSA) Version 2.2* Chicago: Model of Human Occupation Clearinghouse.

Barris, R., Kielhofner, G., Watts, J. H. (1988). *Occupational therapy in psychosocial practice*. Thorofare NJ: SLACK Incorporated.

Baumi, J., Frobose, T., Kraemer, S., Rentrop, M., & Pitschel-Walz, G. (2006). Psychoeducation: A basic psychotherapeutic intervention for patients with schizophrenia and their families. *Schizophrenia Bulletin, 32*(Suppl1), S1-S9.

Beard, J. G., & Ragheb, M.G. (1980). Measuring leisure satisfaction. *Journal of Leisure Research, 12*, 20-33.

Bejerholm, U., Hansson, L., & Eklund, M. (2006). Profiles of occupational engagement in people with schizophrenia, POES: Development of a new instrument based on time use diaries. *British Journal of Occupational Therapy, 69*, 58-68.

Blundo, R. (2001). Learning strengths-based practice: Challenging our personal and professional frames. *Families in Society: Journal of Contemporary Human Services, 82*(3), 296-304.

Brodaty, H., Sachdev, P. S., Withall, A., Altendorf, A., Valenzuela, M. J., & Loretntz, L. (2005). Frequency and clinical, neuropsychological and neuroimaging correlates of apathy following stroke—the Sydney Stroke Study. *Psychological Medicine, 12*, 1707-1716.

Buchanan, D. (2008). Autonomy, Paternalism and Justice: Ethical priorities in public health. *American Journal of Public Health, 98*, 15-21.

Chen, J. Y., Fox, S. A., Cantrell, C. H., Stockdale, S. E., & Kagawa-Singer, M. (2007). Health disparities and prevention: Racial/ethnic barriers to flu vaccinations. *Journal of Community Health, 32*, 7-20.

Csikszentmihalyi, M. (1990). *Flow: The psychology of optimal experience*. New York: Harper and Row.

Csikszentmihalyi, M. (1993). *The evolving self: A psychology for the third millennium*. New York: HarperCollins.

Davis, C. G., Egan, M., Duboulz, C.-J., Kubina, L-A., & Kessler, D. (2013). Adaptation following stroke: A personal projects analysis. *Rehabilitation Psychology, 58*(3), 287-298.

Deegan, P. (1988). Recovery: The lived experience of rehabilitation. *Psychosocial Rehabilitation Journal, 11*(4), 11-19.

de las Heras, C. G., Geist, R., Kielhofner, G., & Li, Y. (2007). *The volitional questionnaire (VQ) version 4.1* Chicago: Model of Human Occupation Clearinghouse.

de las Heras, C. G., Llerena, L., & Kielhofner, G. (2003). *A user's manual for remotivation process: Progressive intervention for individuals with severe volitional challenges*. Chicago, Illinois: The Model of Human Occupation Clearinghouse, Department of Occupational Therapy, College of Applied Health Sciences, University of Illinois at Chicago.

Edgelow, M., & Krupa, T. (2011). A randomized controlled pilot study of an occupational time use intervention for people with serious mental illness. *American Journal of Occupational Therapy, 65*(3), 267-276.

Heckers, S. (2000). Neural models of schizophrenia. *Dialogues in clinical neuroscience, 2*, 267-279.

Iwama, M. (2006). *The Kawa model: Culturally relevant occupational therapy*. Chicago: Churchill Livingston Elsevier.

Janz, N. K., & Becker, M. H. (1984). The health belief model: A decade later. *Health Education Quarterly, 11*, 1-47.

Jorge, R. E., Starkstein, S. E., and Robinson, R. G. (2010). Apathy following stroke. *Canadian Journal of Psychiatry, 55*(6), 350-354.

Kay, S. R., Fiszbein, A., Opler, L. A. (1987). The positive and negative syndrome scale (PANSS) for schizophrenia. *Schizophrenia Bulletin, 13*(2), 261–76

Kielhofner, G., & Neville, A. (1983). The modified interest checklist. Chicago: University of Illinois.

Kiresuk, T. J., & Sherman, R. E. (1968). Goal attainment scaling: A general method for evaluating comprehensive community mental health programs. *Community Mental Health Journal, 4*, 443-453.

Krupa, T., Edgelow, D., Radloff-Gabriel, D.,...Mieras, C. (2010). *Action over inertia: Addressing the activity-health needs of individuals with serious mental illness.* Ottawa: CAOT publications.

Krupa, T., Oyewumi, K., Archie, S., Lawson, S., Nandlal, J., & Conrad, G. (2012). Early intervention services for psychosis and time until application for disability income support: A survival analysis. *Community Mental Health Journal, 48*, 535-546.

Little, B. R., & Chambers, N. C. (2004). Personal project pursuit: On human doings and well-beings. In W. M. Cox, & E. Klinger (Eds.). *Handbook of motivational counseling: Concepts, approaches, and assessment.* (pp. 65-82). New York: John Wiley & Sons Ltd.

Marin, R. S., Biedrzycki, R. C., & Firincioquallari, S. (1991). Reliability and validity of the apathy evaluation scale. *Psychiatry Research, 38*(2),143-62.

Marson, S. M., Wei, G., & Wasserman, D. (2009). A reliability analysis of goal attainment scaling (GAS) weights. *American Journal of Evaluation, 30*, 203-216.

Maslow, A. H. (1968). *Toward a psychology of being.* New York: D. Van Nostrand Company.

Mastellos, N., Gunn, L., Felix, L. Car, J. Majeed, A. (2014). Transtheoretical model stages of change for dietary and physical exercise modification in weight loss management for overweight and obese adults. *Cochrane Database of Systematic Reviews, 2*.

McPherson, K. M., Kayes, N., & Weatherall, M. I. (2009). A pilot study of self-regulation informed goal setting in people with traumatic brain injury. *Clinical Rehabilitation, 23*, 296-309.

Miller, W. R., & Rollnick, S. (1991). Motivational interviewing: Preparing people to change addictive behavior. New York: Guilford Press.

Missiuna, C. (1987). Dynamic Assessment: A model for broadening assessment in occupational therapy. *Canadian Journal of Occupational Therapy, 54*(1), 17-21.

Nga, B. F., & Tsang, H. W. (2000). Evaluation of a goal attainment program using the goal attainment scale for psychiatric in-patients in vocational rehabilitation. *Work, 14*, 209-216.

Oakley, F., Kielhofner, G., Barris, T., & Klinger-Reichler, R. (1986). The Role Checklist: Development and Empirical Assessment of Reliability. *Occupational Journal of Research, 6*, 157-170.

Pépin, G., Guérette, F., Lefebvre, B., & Jacques, P. (2008). Canadian occupational therapists' experiences while implementing the model of human occupation remotivation process. *Occupational Therapy in Health Care, 22*, 115-124.

Polatajko, H. J., Mandich, A., & Martini, R. (2000). Dynamic performance analysis: A framework for understanding occupational performance. *American Journal of Occupational Therapy, 54*, 65-72.

Prochaska, J. O., & DiClemente, C. C. (1982). Transtheoretical therapy: Toward a more integrative model of change. *Psychotherapy: Theory, Research & Practice, 19*(3), 267-88.

Rebeiro, K., & Polgar, J. (1999). Enabling occupational performance: Optimal experiences in therapy. *Canadian Journal of Occupational Therapy, 66*, 14-22.

Reid, D. (2011). Mindfulness and flow in occupational engagement: Presence in doing. *Canadian Journal of Occupational Therapy, 78*, 50-56.

Rosenstock, I. M. (1974). Historical origins of the health belief model, *Health Education Monographs* 2, 328.

Rosenthal, D. A., Hall, C., & Moore, S. M. (1992). AIDS, adolescents, and sexual risk taking: A test of the health belief model. *Australasian Psychologist*, 166-171.

Ryan, R. M., & Deci, E. L. (2000). Intrinsic and extrinsic motivations: Classic definitions and new directions. *Contemporary Educational Psychology, 25*, 54-67.

Stoffel, V., & Moyers, P. (2004). An evidence-based and occupational perspective of interventions for persons with substance-use disorders. *American Journal of Occupational Therapy, 58*, 570-586.

Townsend, E. A., & Polatajko, H. J. (2007). *Enabling occupation II: Advancing an occupational therapy vision for health, well-being & justice through occupation.* Ottawa: Canadian Association of Occupational Therapists.

Wilcock, A. (2006). *An occupational perspective on health* (2nd ed.). Thorofare, NJ: SLACK Incorporated.

van Dalen, J. W., van Charante, E. P., Nederkoorn, P. J., van Gool, W. A., & Richard, E. (2013). Poststroke apathy. *Stroke, 44*, 851-860.

Wlodkowski, R. (1985). How to plan motivational strategies for adult instruction. *Performance Improvement, 24*, 1-6.

Wlodkowski, R. (1999). *Enhancing adult motivation to learn.* San Francisco: Jossey-Bass.

World Bank. (2012). *World development and report: Gender equality and development.* Retrieved from http://econ.worldbank.org.

Person-Environment-Occupation Model Applied to Mental Health

Patricia Rigby, PhD, OT Reg (Ont) and
Bonnie Kirsh, PhD, OT Reg (Ont)

I had successfully reapplied to university prior to the suicide attempt. My hands had healed by September, but I was a long way from being comfortable with the events. I remember stepping into a class of strangers the first day back at school. Carefully camouflaged in a long-sleeved shirt that hot September day, I felt the panic building as our first class let out for a break and I was no longer protected by the formality of the classroom. I had traversed the spectrum from psychiatric day hospital to university professional school in a few short months. From a demeaning lack of challenge to an intimidating sense of overload, there was no sign of a "best fit." (Hatchard & Missiuna, 2003, p. 10)

OBJECTIVES

The objectives of this chapter are as follows:

» To describe the elements of the Person-Environment-Occupation (PEO) model.

» To describe and explain PEO congruence or fit.

» To explore the theoretical underpinnings of the PEO model and examine the evidence to support the theoretical constructs of the PEO model.

» To examine how the PEO model is applied to psychosocial occupational therapy practice.

» To examine the evidence for using the PEO model in psychosocial occupational therapy practice.

Krupa, T., Kirsh, B., Pitts, D., & Fossey, E. *Bruce & Borg's*
Psychosocial Frames of Reference: Theories, Models, and Approaches for
Occupation-Based Practice, Fourth Edition (pp 107-121).
© 2016 SLACK Incorporated.

The Person-Environment-Occupation (PEO) model facilitates occupational therapists' understanding of the dynamic nature of occupational performance (Law et al., 1996; Strong et al., 1999). This model describes occupational performance—the doing or engagement in occupation—as the outcome of a transactional (interwoven) relationship experienced by persons with their occupations in the environments in which they live, work, and play. Optimal occupational performance occurs when there is a good "fit" or congruence in the PEO relationship. When applying the PEO model, the occupational therapist broadly examines the person, environment, and occupation factors that may be influencing occupational performance and the goodness of PEO fit. This analysis guides the therapist and the client to consider strategies for improving the PEO fit and enabling an optimal occupational experience.

The opening quote for this chapter emphasizes the importance of the notion of PEO fit in relation to the mental health recovery process and occupational performance in daily life. For the author of the quote, there was a lack of fit between the challenges presented by the demands of the social occupations in the university setting, and the author's ability and readiness to tackle them. The author goes on to say that returning to school offered her hope to move on with her life, but she was not yet stable enough to re-enter the school environment.

The core concepts and assumptions of the PEO model resonate for many occupational therapists working in mental health settings (e.g., Bejerholm & Eklund, 2006; Lexen, Hofgren, & Bejerholm, 2013; Peloquin & Ciro, 2013). They think this model is well suited to guide occupational therapy practice in mental health and to explain and advocate for the role of occupational therapy in mental health services. For example, Brown and Stoffel (2011) chose the PEO model to frame and organize their book, *Occupational Therapy in Mental Health: A Vision for Participation*. They emphasize the role of occupational therapy during the mental health recovery process and describe how therapists can apply the PEO model to support and enable clients on their journey toward recovery. Several authors (e.g., Brown, 2009; Merryman & Riegel, 2007; Stoffel, 2013) not only make a strong case for inclusion of occupational therapy in mental health services, they also describe how the PEO model is congruent with and can inform recovery models and funding programs in mental health. As they point out, the PEO model guides occupational therapy assessment and interventions toward enabling clients to achieve PEO fit, successfully engage in chosen occupations, and participate more fully in daily life.

This chapter introduces the key components, concepts, and assumptions of the PEO model and its theoretical foundations. It goes on to describe how the PEO model has been and could be used to guide psychosocial occupational therapy practice and research. It concludes with a review of evidence examining the relevance and usefulness of the PEO model for occupational therapy practice and research in mental health settings.

BACKGROUND

The PEO model was developed in the early 1990s by a group of Canadian occupational therapy researchers and clinicians to help frame and guide occupational therapy practice. Since the PEO model was first published (Law et al., 1996; Strong et al., 1999), it has been cited in over 600 publications internationally. It is widely used in research and clinical practice in occupational therapy and more broadly in rehabilitation. The PEO model and key theoretical assumptions of this model are integrated into the Canadian guidelines for client-centered practice (Canadian Association of Occupational Therapists [CAOT], 1997, 2002) and Enabling Occupation II (Townsend & Polatajko, 2007, 2013). This model is compatible with the International Classification of Functioning, Disability and Health (ICF; World Health Organization, 2001), which also acknowledges the interactions of person, environment, activity, and participation as they influence health and well-being. These relationships will be discussed further within the section on theoretical foundations and assumptions.

KEY COMPONENTS, CONCEPTS, AND ASSUMPTIONS

In occupational therapy practice, the principal goals for intervention are focused on enabling clients to engage in and perform occupations that have meaning and purpose in their lives (Townsend & Polatajko, 2013). The PEO model was created to focus on occupational performance and the factors influencing occupational performance and to enable and support client and family-centered practice (Law et al., 1996; Strong et al., 1999). This model supports the development of a partnership between the therapist and client (as well as the client's family when relevant). The client identifies and prioritizes his or her occupational goals and together, the therapist and client look at strengths and problems in occupational performance by assessing the environmental conditions and resources, analyzing occupational elements (e.g., challenges and demands of the occupation) and the client's personal capabilities and motivations that relate to performing the occupation (Strong et al., 1999). Once this information has been synthesized and analyzed, the therapist and client (and family, as applicable) can identify and implement intervention strategies. Using the PEO model expands the scope of possible interventions to enable occupational performance.

A simple Venn diagram (Figure 7-1) depicts the PEO model as three interdependent elements of person, environment, and occupation, and occupational performance is the outcome of the PEO relationship. In the diagram, the overlap of the three circles represents the goodness of fit or congruence among the three elements. Increasing the overlap of the circles to improve PEO fit will improve the quality of a person's experience doing or engaging in an occupation, and their level of satisfaction with their occupational performance. When there is poor congruence in the PEO relationship, occupational performance is diminished (Figure 7-2). The PEO relationship is dynamic because the three elements are continually changing and influencing each other. Thus, occupational performance and the degree of PEO fit are influenced by the passage of time and can change throughout the course of a day and over a lifetime.

The temporal aspect of the PEO model is relevant for occupational therapists working with clients during their mental health recovery journey. This journey may be prolonged and more challenging if the goodness of PEO fit becomes less optimal. Figure 7-3 shows how PEO fit can vary across the span of 18 months using the example of a young woman named Amita who is recovering from a severe depression and wants to return to work.

Prior to her hospitalization, Amita successfully worked as a sales assistant at a large department store. She now feels very anxious in busy public places and when communicating with people she doesn't know well. Her occupational therapist accompanied her on a visit to her former employer to discuss options for return to work for this company. The employer valued Amita's work and was eager to re-employ her but was at a loss as to how to do so without exposing her to the busy sales floor. He was worried that the stress might cause her to become ill again and that he would have to replace her, which was costly to his business. After some discussion involving the employer, Anita, and the occupational therapist, it was decided that Amita would return on a gradual schedule, first working two hours in the morning when the store was not yet busy, then moving on to work half-days and finally to full days. It was thought that a staged approach would effectively address the fit between Amita, the work, and the environment. Amita was pleased with these arrangements and adapted well to the first stage of working two hours in the morning; it was quieter at this time and the task demands (speed and quantity of work) were lower as well. However, as her hours increased, and as the store became busier with more to do in less time, Amita again experienced anxiety, which interfered with her work performance. She found herself making many mistakes and becoming abrupt with the customers. In this case, the change in PEO fit affected Amita's occupational performance. Realizing this relationship, Amita, her occupational therapist, and the employer reconvened to discuss solutions. Amita's occupational therapist suggested that she try working in a quieter section of the store, in a department with fewer sales and less walk-through traffic.

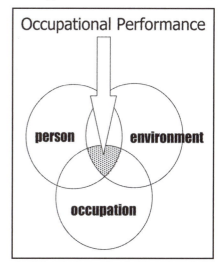

Figure 7-1. The Person-environment-occupation (PEO) model. (From Law, M. et al., "The Person-Environment-Occupation Model: A transactive approach to occupational performance," *Canadian Journal of Occupational Therapy, 63*(1), 9-23. Copyright © 1996 by SAGE Publications Inc. Reprinted with permission.)

Indeed, this environment provided the work conditions for Amita to successfully carry out her job duties and resume her role as a productive employee.

The PEO model is considered generic because it can be applied by occupational therapists across various settings with different populations and clients across the lifespan. It is purposefully flexible and the elements are broadly defined to allow adaptation and expansion for specific practice situations. As noted earlier, in many publications the PEO model has been applied broadly to frame evaluation and interventions or services in hospitals, the workplace, and in community and school-based settings; and to guide the development of research studies, new assessment tools, and occupational therapy curriculum in various academic programs around the world. The PEO model can be easily explained to and understood by clients, their families, and those outside the occupational therapy profession (Law et al., 1996; Strong et al., 1999), particularly when the Venn diagram is used (see Figures 7-1 to 7-3). This model can help others to understand the focus for, and unique contributions of, occupational therapy in mental health practice settings.

In the following discussion, each of the three components of the model is defined and described within the context of occupational experience.

Person

In the PEO model, a person is viewed as a composite of mind, body, and spiritual qualities, including values; beliefs and spirituality; and physical, cognitive, and sensory skills and abilities (Law et al., 1996). Persons assume a variety of

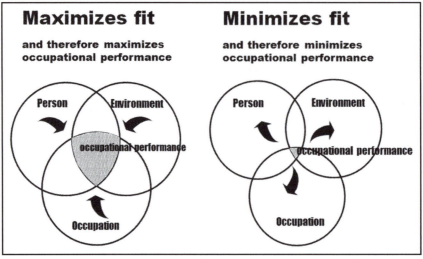

Figure 7-2. Changes in occupational performance as a consequence of variations in person-environment-occupation fit. (From Law, M., Cooper, B. Strong, S., Stewart, D., Rigby, P., & Letts, L. "The Person-Environment-Occupation Model: A transactive approach to occupational performance," *Canadian Journal of Occupational Therapy, 63*(1), 9-23. Copyright © 1996 by SAGE Publications Inc. Reprinted with permission.)

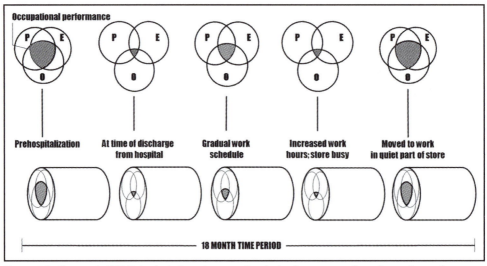

Figure 7-3. Changes in PEO fit for Amita's work occupation during her recovery from depression and return to work. (From Law, M., Cooper, B., Strong, S., Stewart, D., Rigby, P., & Letts, L."The Person-Environment-Occupation Model: A transactive approach to occupational performance," *Canadian Journal of Occupational Therapy, 63*(1), 9-23. Copyright © by 1996 SAGE Publications Inc. Reprinted with permission.)

roles simultaneously in daily life and these roles vary in their importance, duration, and significance. Personal experiences with personal skills and abilities, motivation, and self-concept influence occupational performance. Occupational therapists consider their clients' roles, responsibilities, and the various individual factors that can facilitate or hinder engagement in occupations that have meaning and importance to their clients. While this description appears to focus on the individual person, in the PEO model "person" can refer to individuals, groups, organizations, or communities, and can include anyone who experiences barriers to occupational performance or engagement.

Environment

Environment is also broadly defined to include cultural, physical, social, and institutional/organizational elements (Law et al., 1996). These elements can be viewed from the perspective of an individual, or groups of various sizes including a household or community group. The environment shapes human experience and behavior, and provides cues to people about what to do and what is expected of them. For example, a school auditorium can be used for gym class, dances, community meetings, and school exams; it is the physical setup of the auditorium that invites the particular behavior suited to it. In other words, people relate to environmental cues and behave accordingly. Elements of the environment can be viewed as barriers, resources, or supports to occupational performance; and it is important to understand clients' perceptions of, and the meaning they attach to, environments in which they live, work, and play (O'Brien, Dyck, Caron, & Mortenson, 2002). The occupational therapist might view specific elements of the environment as barriers or negative influences to a client's behavior, whereas the client may view those elements in a very different way; he or she may think they are important and have special personal meaning to him or her. For example, a client who is addicted to alcohol might value his local pub, and view those who work and frequent that pub as family even though others may see this environment as a risk to his well-being. Thus, it is important that the therapist acknowledges and respects her client's views and the meaning that the client attaches to places and spaces he frequents, and factors this into intervention planning (O'Brien, et al., 2002).

There is a growing body of research that demonstrates that the environment can be more amenable to change than the person, and that environmental interventions can have a very positive impact on occupational performance outcomes (e.g., Gillespie et al., 2009; Law, Di Rezze, & Bradley, 2010; Stark, 2004; Velligan, Mueller, Wang, Dicocco, & Diamond, 2006). Furthermore, O'Brien et al. (2002, p. 238) argue that the environment (e.g., barriers and negative social attitudes) may create disability as much, if not more, than the individual's impairments do. Thus, environment should be a focus for occupational therapy interventions.

Whereas some interventions with environments can be straightforward, such as accessing technical aids, other strategies are more complex and may require that the therapist assume advisory or advocacy roles to make changes to environments. Consider, for example, an occupational therapist who is consulting to employers or institutions to help them create psychologically healthy workplace and community settings or an occupational therapist who is advocating with government officials for changes to policies and services to better support people living with mental illnesses.

Occupation

The term *occupation* refers to everyday life activities that are goal directed, have meaning for the individual, and are culturally relevant (Law et al., 1996). In the PEO model, occupations are described as groups of self-directed functional tasks and activities in which a person engages to meet his or her needs for self-maintenance, expression, and fulfilment. Activities and tasks are nested within occupations; activities are the basic units of tasks and tasks are sets of purposeful, related activities. To illustrate this, consider the example of getting dressed for work, which is an occupation. This occupation includes the tasks of putting on a shirt, putting on pants, and putting on shoes. The activities for putting on a shirt include selecting the shirt in the closet, taking the shirt off the hanger, pulling the shirt over one's arms and over one's body, and buttoning the shirt.

People engage in various occupations for specific purposes to fulfil their roles and responsibilities in daily life (Strong et al., 1999). They can vary in importance, level of complexity, and demand characteristics. For example, preparing a gourmet meal for family and friends is more complex and likely more anxiety provoking than preparing a simple, familiar one. Occupations can provide structure and bring a rhythm to daily life (Bejerholm, 2007; Rebeiro, 1998). Evidence exists to support the relationship between occupation, health, and well-being (Gahnstrom-Strandqvist, Liukko, & Tham, 2003; Law, Steinwnder, & LeClair, 1998; Legault & Rebeiro, 2001). Furthermore, researchers have found that the strength of the effect of occupation on health depends on the relationship between the person, environment, occupation, and a balance of occupations in daily life (Law et al., 1998, p. 90). Engagement in occupations shapes our sense of self and identity (Krupa, McLean, Eastbrook, Bonham, & Baksh, 2003; Polatajko et al., 2013), and occupations that are meaningful to a person and congruent with one's values and identity have a positive influence on well-being (Anaby, Jarus, Backman, & Zumbo, 2010; Eklund & Leufstadius, 2007).

OCCUPATIONAL PERFORMANCE

As noted earlier, occupational performance is the outcome of the transaction of the person engaged in an occupation within an environmental setting (Law et al., 1996). Engaging in occupations provides the means to mental, physical, and spiritual health, and gives people a sense of meaning and purpose in life (Meyer, 1922/1977; Yerxa et al., 1990). It is considered a complex, dynamic process with both spatial and temporal qualities. It can be measured objectively through observation and subjectively through self-report. The occupational therapist can examine occupational performance by analyzing the degree of fit or congruence in the PEO relationship (see Figures 7-1 and 7-2) and the experience of occupational performance. The better the fit, the more optimal the person's occupational performance. When there is less congruence or poor PEO fit, occupational performance is less optimal.

THEORETICAL FOUNDATIONS

The theoretical underpinnings of the PEO model are found in the fields of human ecology, environmental psychology, psychology, and occupational therapy. Human ecology and environmental psychology involve multidisciplinary and interdisciplinary research from fields such

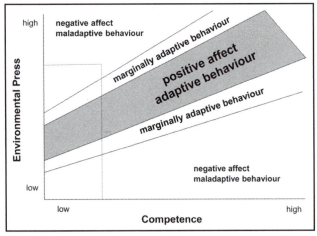

Figure 7-4. Lawton & Nahemow's (1973) ecological model of aging. The intersection of the two dashed lines demonstrates too much environmental press in relation to a person's competence; thus, poor person-environment fit. (Reprinted with permission from Lawton, M. P., & Nahemow, L. (1973). Ecology and the aging process. In C. Eisdorfer & M. P. Lawton (Eds.), *The psychology of adult development and aging* (pp. 619-674). Washington, DC: American Psychological Association.)

as psychology, sociology, anthropology, human geography, and architecture. This research enhances our understanding about the relationship between people; their natural, social, and built environments; and occupation. Law and colleagues (1996) drew upon the work of many prominent theorists and researchers including Bronfenbrenner (1977), Csikszentmihalyi (1990), and Lawton and Nahemow (1973) when developing the PEO model. Bronfenbrenner's (1977) ecological systems model describes the interrelationships between persons and the various levels of environment, including home, school, workplace, and the social and cultural structures of society. It also emphasizes the social nature of people as they interact within these various levels of the environment to develop and bring meaning to their lives. Lawton and Nahemow's (1973) ecological theory of aging describes the interactive relationship between an individual and the environment as it affects the degree of adaptation that the individual is able to achieve, particularly during the aging process. This theory of adaptation is similar to the views of Csikszentmihalyi (1990) in the field of psychology, who describes the relationship between the challenges of an activity and an individual's skills in his theory of flow. The work of these theorists offers relevant ideas for occupational therapists to consider both person and environment issues in practice, but also allows sufficient flexibility to include the concept of occupational performance as a critical outcome (Law et al., 1996).

The notion of person-environment fit as described by Lawton (1986) in the ecological model of aging, and Csikszentmihalyi's views about matching challenges of activities with the skills of a person in his model of flow (1990) helped shape the conceptualization of PEO fit (Rigby & Letts, 2003). Lawton (1986) argues that human behavior

and function result from the interaction between the competencies of the person and the demands or "press" of the environment, and the adaptation of the person to the environment (Figure 7-4). Adaptive behavior and positive affect are the outcomes of good person-environment fit. When a person's competencies are too low in relation to the demands of the environment, the person can experience maladaptive behavior, such as failure of performance, anxiety, and stress. This can be illustrated in the example of a frail elderly woman who was recently widowed and now lives alone. She rarely leaves her home because she finds it too stressful to go out without her husband's help and support; the physical and social demands of the environment are more than she can cope with. Thus she has become physically weakened, socially isolated and withdrawn, and is clinically depressed. There is a poor fit between her perception of her competencies and the social and physical demands of the environment beyond her home, as shown in Figure 7-4.

Similarly, in the model of flow, there is a good fit when a person's perceived skills match the challenges of a chosen activity (Csikszentmihalyi, 1990). Flow is experienced when one is fully absorbed and immersed in performing an activity, and feeling satisfaction with the experience. Like Lawton's model, when the challenges are too great and do not match the person's perceived skill level, the quality of the experience of doing the activity is less positive and the person experiences anxiety and distress. Thus, in the example above, the frail woman avoids social experiences in her community because she perceives that her social skills do not match the challenges of socializing, largely because she had deferred to and relied upon her husband in social situations.

While the authors of the PEO model found the ideas presented by Lawton, Nahemow, and Czikszentmihalyi very useful for conceptualizing PEO congruence or fit, they tailored their model to address the outcome of occupational performance, as described earlier in this chapter.

The PEO model is congruent with current global models of health, such as the revised International Classification of Functioning, Disability and Health (WHO, 2001), which also acknowledges the interactions of person and environment in the process of health and well-being. Thus, the PEO model is a synthesis of multidisciplinary approaches to person-environment relations and the unique perspective of occupational therapy.

THE PEO MODEL AND OCCUPATIONAL THERAPY PRACTICE IN MENTAL HEALTH SETTINGS

The PEO model is well suited to guide occupational therapists working with clients through the mental health recovery process because it supports a client-centered approach and facilitates understanding occupational performance and engagement issues from the perspective of a client's lived experience. A strong therapeutic alliance and effective therapist-client partnership can develop from a shared understanding of a client's issues and priorities (Strong & Rebeiro Gruhl, 2011). The PEO model also supports reflective, evidence-based practice by offering a comprehensive and systematic approach to the analysis of the complexities of human behavior while considering the influential relationships of the person with their occupations within the contexts of their daily lives at a micro or personal level, and more broadly at family, community, and societal levels. This approach expands potential options for interventions to include not only those directed at the client, but also those directed at the occupation and/or environment at the level of the individual client, and also at the level of institutions, organizations, and government.

The literature provides numerous examples of how the PEO model has been successfully applied to the mental health recovery process, and evidence to support using the PEO model to frame psychosocial occupational therapy practice; many of these are shared in this chapter. Several authors describe the unique and important role for occupational therapy in mental health settings by emphasizing that occupational therapy assessment and interventions address the person-environment-occupation factors that influence occupational performance and engagement (Brown, 2009; Krupa, Fossey, Anthony, Brown, & Pitts, 2009; Stoffel, 2013), and that improving occupational performance has a positive impact on quality of life and well-being (Bejerholm & Eklund, 2007; Krupa et al., 2009).

The PEO Model and the Recovery Process

The recovery process (discussed in detail in Chapter 3) involves transitioning from experiencing symptoms of mental illness through a reconstruction of one's life, toward a state of good health and well-being (Stoffel, 2013). Reconstruction entails reconstruction of identity, regaining hope, acceptance, a sense of agency, and coping (Bonney & Stickley, 2008). The recovery process is a journey that can last many months and years. It typically starts slowly, with the individual making gradual gains interspersed with setbacks and plateau periods along the way, as demonstrated in the personal story opening this chapter, shared by Hatchard and Missiuna (2003). Onken and colleagues (2007) propose using an ecological framework to examine the complex, transactional person-environment relationship influencing the mental health recovery process. The PEO model can take this ecological perspective a step further by viewing recovery as a multidimensional process that includes engaging in meaningful occupations, placing the client

at the center of the intervention, and designing context-based interventions to find the client's best fit for optimal occupational performance (Merryman & Riegel, 2007).

The PEO relationship is influential to an individual's recovery (Bejerholm, 2007; Lexen et al., 2013; Merryman & Riegel, 2007; Strong, 1998). If there is a misfit between the individual and their occupations and environments as a consequence of illness or its residual effects, occupational performance is hindered and disability can occur. Thus, when it comes to understanding disabilities, the person cannot be viewed as separate from the influences of his or her chosen occupations and the environments in which her or she lives (Bejerholm & Eklund, 2004; O'Brien et al., 2002; Strong et al., 1999). To achieve good PEO fit, individuals in recovery need access to carefully chosen environments that support their goals for recovery. By the same token, environments that are detrimental to health and well-being (e.g., those that are highly stigmatizing or discriminatory) must be altered or avoided. To engage in a process of recovery, individuals also need access to occupational roles and opportunities that hold meaning for them and support their goals (Anaby et al., 2010; Bejerholm & Eklund, 2007; Eklund & Leufstadius, 2007).

Brown (2009) provides a comprehensive case example to clearly illustrate how an occupational therapist can address the PEO elements influencing a client's occupational performance during the mental health recovery process, which readers may wish to access and review. In this example, Brown illustrates the therapist's approach to assessment and intervention options that address the person (e.g., skills acquisition and remediation of cognitive impairments), the occupation (e.g., adapting the process for completing the tasks and altering the way the task is completed), and the environment (e.g., organizing the tools and materials needed for the tasks and accessing social supports to help with task completion). She concludes the case example with strategies for achieving good PEO fit.

The PEO Model and Return to Work

Occupational therapists who assist clients in finding and keeping work may find the PEO model very useful to guide their assessments and interventions aimed at achieving a good match between a worker's personal preferences and capabilities, the job demands, and the workplace environment (Lexen et al., 2013; Rebeiro, 2001; Strong, 1998). In the workplace, job accommodations (changes to the workplace environment and/or in the way the job is done) are routinely applied to achieve a good PEO fit. Job accommodations can include flexible working hours (e.g., a later start and end to the day), a physical space that minimizes distractions, technical aids to compensate for organizational and cognitive deficits, or regular feedback meetings to ensure clear and consistent communication. Interventions directed at the worker may also be appropriate, including job training, assistance with social or daily living skills, and development of coping strategies to manage stress. The United States Department of Labor developed a website that provides searchable job accommodation recommendations to address specific work-related challenges (http://askjan.org/soar/index.htm). Strong and colleagues (1999) provide a useful case example that shows how the PEO model is applied to assessment, intervention, and follow-up with an individual named Spencer, who is recovering from schizophrenia.

Access to accommodation most often requires the client to disclose functional limitations and needs (although it does not require the disclosure of a particular illness or diagnosis). The decision regarding disclosure warrants careful consideration; each individual will need to decide whether to do so, how much to share, and whom to include. An assessment of the psychosocial work environment may provide some indication of the level of acceptance (or stigma) that the client may encounter as a result of such disclosure and may provide clues that occupational therapists can use to help clients prepare for workplace interactions.

Examples of Applying the PEO Model in Mental Health Settings

The following are a few published examples of how the PEO model has been applied in specific mental health settings. The first example is a self-development group intervention, which used the PEO model to provide structure and ensure that the sessions address the PEO relationship for individual participants and the group as a whole. It has been successfully run by occupational therapists in an intensive residential substance abuse recovery program (Peloquin & Ciro, 2013). This program targets recovery themes endorsed in the substance abuse and dependence literature, and uses arts and crafts media to engage the participants in occupation as a means to achieving therapeutic goals, and as metaphor and motivator for addressing the recovery themes (p. 84). Peloquin and Ciro conducted a retrospective study of 1488 post-intervention surveys completed by group participants and found that they were satisfied with the program and highly engaged in the self-development process.

Similarly, McWha, Pachana, and Alpass (2003) describe a hospital-based, occupational therapy activity group for older women who are experiencing depression. The therapists design and facilitate the group sessions to ensure a good fit in the PEO relationship for group participants. There are a variety of individual and group activities that can be graded and adapted to meet the interests and skill level of participants, and their readiness to participate. The therapists help to construct a supportive therapeutic environment that builds social relationships among the group members, where participants are expected to demonstrate respect, acceptance ,and interest in each other through group discussion and feedback. Study findings reveal that participants felt a sense of belonging in the group, and gained feelings of competency, enjoyment, and well-being; all of which contribute to their journey of recovery.

In another example, the PEO model was used to explain how pet ownership can provide a meaningful, socially valued occupation that supports community integration for persons with mental illness, and why pet ownership should be considered as a focus for recovery services (Zimolag & Krupa, 2009). Study findings show that pet owners demonstrated better social community integration than non-pet owners. Zimolag and Krupa describe PEO interventions to enable successful engagement in pet ownership, such as how this occupation can be graded from simple to more complex, the types of skills clients should develop, and how these can also be graded (e.g., cognitive, social, physical skills, and regulating one's affect), and the environmental conditions necessary to ensure the pet's comfort, safety, and health, which depend on the type of pet and whether ownership is shared (p. 34).

APPLYING THE PEO MODEL TO THE EVALUATION PROCESS

As noted earlier in this chapter, the PEO model can be used by occupational therapists to assess and analyze the PEO relationship with respect to whether there is a good PEO fit because this relationship influences occupational performance outcomes. By doing this, interventions can be chosen that attend to specific determinants of performance, such as modifying an occupation when a client feels overwhelmed by the demand characteristics of that occupation, and/or accessing environmental resources to support a client's engagement in the occupation. The occupational therapist can approach assessment in a few different ways. One way is to systematically examine the person, environment, and occupation elements separately using the PEO model application framework as described by Law and colleagues (1996) and illustrated in Figure 7-5. The occupational therapist would then pull the findings together to examine the PEO relationship and goodness of PEO fit. Another way is to examine the various layers of relationships across the person, environment, and occupational elements, such as focusing on the person-environment (PE), person-occupation (PO), and occupation-environment (OE) layers separately, and then pulling this knowledge together to reflect upon and evaluate the congruence of the PEO relationship, as described by Strong et al. (1999). Both approaches can be very useful when examining the demand characteristics of occupations and environments in relation to where clients are in the recovery process, their personal capacities, and their readiness to meet these demands. Occupational therapists can use both standardized and non-standardized assessments (e.g., observations and interview) to assess occupational performance, the PEO elements, and the PEO relationship. In the case example of Abdah, the community occupational therapist used the strategy described by Strong et al. (1999) to first examine the PO, OE, and PE relationships in her assessment of Abdah's occupational goal of maintaining a clean and tidy apartment (Figure 7-6). By examining the elements influencing PEO fit, the occupational therapist and Abdah can readily use this information to develop an intervention plan.

Two tools have been developed specifically using the PEO model as their theoretical underpinning. The first tool, the Profiles of Occupational Engagement in people with Schizophrenia (POES; Bejerholm & Eklund, 2006a; Bejerholm et al., 2006), is a 24-hour time-use diary that provides a profile of the rhythm of an individual's daily occupations and his or her occupational engagement. Respondents make notes for each hour in their diary about what they do, with whom, where, and how they perceived their performance of the occupations. The response categories correspond with occupational, environmental, and personal domains from the model, and together these shape an individual's occupational performance. The POES demonstrates good internal consistency and inter-rater reliability, and satisfactory content and construct validity (Bejerholm & Eklund, 2006a; Bejerholm et al., 2006). This tool enables the occupational therapist to assess occupational performance and engagement over time and examine life changes caused by factors influencing the PEO relationship. For example, the PEO relationship, and consequently occupational performance and engagement, would change when a person starts, stops, or changes taking antipsychotic medication, or loses a job, or begins to live alone for the first time. The POES can help occupational therapists "identify problems such as a lack of meaningful occupations, an imbalance between rest and activity, and few occupational and environmental opportunities, and thereby contribute to establishing relevant priorities and determining need areas that require further attention and assessments" (Bejerholm et al., 2006, p. 66).

The second tool, the Profiles of Occupational Engagement in People with Severe Mental Illness: Productive Occupations (POES-P) was adapted from the POES. It is a self-report diary for use in work or work-like settings with a focus on productive occupations (Tjornstrand et al., 2013). As with the POES, the PEO model provides the theoretical constructs for the POES-P time-use diary. The second part of this tool has a unique feature, in which the client rates their level of responsibility in eight dimensions of occupational engagement, such as his or her level of independence and initiative and the meaningfulness of the task. This tool can help the occupational therapist monitor a client's occupational performance and engagement within a program or new job, and also enables the occupational therapist, together with the client, to better

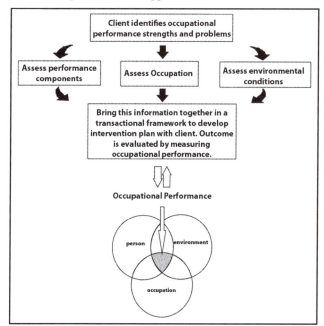

Figure 7-5. The application framework for the PEO model (From Law, M. et al., "The Person-Environment-Occupation Model: A transactive approach to occupational performance," *Canadian Journal of Occupational Therapy, 63*(1), 9-23. Copyright © 1996 by SAGE Publications Inc. Reprinted with permission.)

match occupations to the client's needs, skills, interests, and goals. The POES-P demonstrates good internal consistency, and adequate construct and convergent construct validity (Tjornstrand, Bejerholm, & Eklund, 2013).

EVIDENCE FOR THE APPROACH

There is growing evidence to support the relevance of the PEO model and its application to occupational therapy practice in mental health settings. As noted earlier, the PEO model has been used to explain and promote the value of occupational therapy in mental health, particularly during the recovery process; and to explain factors influencing the recovery process itself (e.g., Bejerholm, 2010; Brown, 2009; Merryman & Riegel, 2007; Stoffel, 2013). The PEO model has provided a useful framework for numerous studies. It has been used to (1) structure the study (e.g., Bejerholm & Eklund, 2004, 2007), (2) structure the development of assessment tools for research and occupational therapy practice in mental health (Bejerholm & Eklund, 2006a; Bejerholm et al., 2006; Hamera & Brown, 2000; Tjornstrand et al., 2013), (3) organize interview guides for qualitative studies and/or the approach to data analysis and interpretation (Bejerholm & Eklund, 2004; McWha et al., 2003; Strong, 1998), and (4) structure the interventions that are under investigation in studies (e.g., Egan, Kubina, Lidstone, Macdougall, & Raudoy, 2010; Lexen et al., 2013; Peloquin & Ciro, 2013). There is also evidence, as described later as

Case Study: Application of PEO Model to Occupational Therapy Assessment and Intervention

Abdah is a 40-year-old woman who was recently discharged from the inpatient schizophrenia unit at the city's psychiatric hospital. The hospital referred her to a community occupational therapist, who will be helping Abdah engage in occupations that are meaningful to her.

Since being back in her downtown apartment, Abdah has not really known what to do with her days and spends most of her time watching T.V. She left her apartment in a state of disarray when she was hospitalized and it is still in this state. She feels overwhelmed by the mess and by the busy streets and noise in her neighborhood, and she ends up staying inside and doing very little with her days.

When the community occupational therapist met with Abdah at her home, she noted that the apartment was untidy and disorganized. The sink was piled with dirty dishes, overflowing onto the countertops. Her bathroom was cluttered with toiletries, covering the sink, floor, and bathtub. Her personal belongings were all over the floor and on her furniture, and Abdah complained that she often struggles to find her belongings when she needs them.

Abdah reported that she gets anxious and depressed when she looks around and finds it hard to get going on the cleaning. She looks at her life regretfully, stating that she used to be on top of everything, and her apartment was clean even though she was busy all the time. Now, she sighs, even with nothing to do, she can't seem to manage it. Sometimes she gets a start on it, but then finds herself distracted by the T.V. She described herself as "useless" to the occupational therapist.

An examination of the PO interaction reveals that Abdah is having difficulty meeting the demands of the occupation. The chaos around her has overwhelmed her, and she seems to be immobilized by it. Although she has the skills to clean her apartment, she seems not to be able to put them into practice. As a result, she feels depressed and anxious, and her self-efficacy is suffering.

Looking at the OE interaction, Abdah spends her time in front of the TV and indeed is distracted by it when she gets started on occupations that could improve her situation. Even when she finds the energy to start cleaning, the TV that is usually playing in her small apartment draws her in, and the cleaning does not get done.

The PE interaction reveals that the environment is one that is not only overwhelming and anxiety provoking, but also unsafe and unhygienic. Reflecting on the notion that the cognitive deficits associated with schizophrenia may affect functional outcomes, the occupational therapist notes that people in similar situations have benefitted from a cognitive adaptation program that occupational therapists on her team are implementing and evaluating.

Intervention proceeds from here and focuses on improving occupational performance by removing constraints and developing supports to improve the quality of the PEO fit. The occupational therapist consults with team members to assess Abdah for the cognitive adaptation program and once deemed suitable, they apply some core principles that include person, occupation, and environment. Interventions include the following:

- Prompting and cueing in the environment to help Abdah complete tasks (e.g., using a voice alarm reminding her to clean her apartment)
- Helping Abdah develop schedules and checklists of activities that need to be done, including the T.V. shows that Abdah wants to watch built into the schedule as reward
- Arranging cleaning materials in a visible area in the kitchen/bathroom to prompt cleaning behavior
- Reuniting with family and friends so that Abdah can access support, include them in her life, and find even more reason to clean her apartment

The final phase would be evaluation and follow-up, where stages of improvement in the environment and in Abdah's activities and sense of well-being are monitored. Self-reports, journals, and formal scales could be used for these purposes. Ongoing follow-up and problem solving assistance would be provided to Abdah to improve the fit between the person, occupation, and environment.

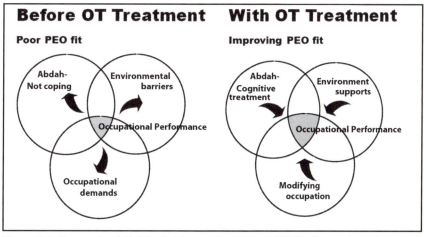

Figure 7-6. Case study of Abdah: Abdah experiences poor PEO fit after discharge home and improving PEO fit with occupational therapy intervention in the home setting.

well as earlier in this chapter, to support the central concepts and assumptions of the model, such as the influence of PEO fit on occupational performance; the influence of the elements of person, occupation, and environment on engagement in occupations; and the outcomes of quality of life and well-being.

Bejerholm (2007) used the PEO model to frame and guide the studies conducted for her doctoral thesis, in which she explored occupational perspectives on health and time use for people with schizophrenia (Bejerholm & Eklund, 2004, 2006a, 2006b, 2007; Bejerholm et al., 2006). She found that the PEO model illustrated the complex interplay of PEO factors influencing occupational performance and time use, and study results demonstrated a relationship between daily occupations and quality of life (Bejerholm & Eklund, 2004, 2006b). She also used the PEO model to structure the time use diary and the POES (described in the previous section of this chapter) developed for her thesis (Bejerholm & Eklund, 2006, 2006a). Bejerholm and Eklund (2007) found that persons with schizophrenia engage in occupations to a varying degree and higher levels of occupational engagement were associated with positive emotions, fewer psychiatric symptoms, and better ratings of quality of life.

The PEO model has also been used to examine return to work for persons with mental health issues (Lexen et al., 2013; Strong, 1998; Tjornstrand et al., 2013). Lexen et al. (2013) provide a good example of the utility of the PEO model to guide assessment and intervention in a return-to-work setting. They used a multiple case study method to explore elements of support and process within an Individual Placement and Support (IPS) program designed to help people with severe mental illness gain and keep employment. While previous IPS research has studied the match between a person with severe mental illness and the job, this study applied the PEO model to examine the match between the client's skills and preferences,

the work activities, and the work environment over time (Lexen et al., p. 436). One of the measures used in the study was the POES-P, described in the previous section of this chapter. Study findings demonstrate that an important predictor of success was when IPS services include an analysis of both the characteristics of the work environment and the job demands and responsibilities in relation to the client's interests, skills and abilities, and using this knowledge to achieve a good worker-job-environment match. Examples from the case studies are provided in this paper to illustrate how the PEO model was used to interpret the study findings. The study authors conclude that the PEO model was a very valuable theoretical framework to guide IPS programs.

OCCUPATION AND THE RECOVERY PROCESS

It is clear that occupation influences the recovery process. The link between occupation and quality of life and well-being for persons living with mental illnesses is well established (e.g., Eklund, Hansson, & Bejerholm, 2001; Eklund & Leufstadius, 2007; Rebeiro et al., 2001). Mental illness typically causes disruption to a person's daily occupations, and many experience an imbalance and/or deprivation in their occupational lives resulting from mental illness and life-changing experiences such as bereavement, job loss, migration, and poverty. Anaby and colleagues (2010) demonstrated that the following four characteristics of occupation influenced one's well-being: (1) the meaning of occupations to an individual (those congruent with one's values and identify), (2) the extent to which one's occupations are supported by others, (3) the efficacy of the occupation (the extent to which occupations are in progress toward a successful accomplishment), and (4) the structure of occupations (the level of organization and control). These characteristics influence and are influenced by PEO fit.

Occupational therapists not only recognize the therapeutic potential of occupation, but also of occupational balance in promoting recovery and well-being (Anaby et al., 2010; Polatajko et al., 2013; Wilcock, 2005). The notion of occupational balance has been the focus of many studies within and outside occupational therapy and occupational science, yet there is little consensus on its definition (Anaby et al., 2010). Christensen (1996) summarized the literature and proposed that occupational balance involves time use, the rhythm and patterns of daily occupations (e.g., rhythms between active and restful occupations, and patterns of sleep, self-care, work, and leisure activities), and the relationships among daily occupations (e.g., the impact of daily occupations on each other).

Occupational balance is also viewed as the balance between personal and environmental factors while engaging in occupations (Bejerholm, 2010; Christiansen & Matuska, 2006). In a study of occupational balance in people with schizophrenia, Bejerholm (2010) argues that "having occupational balance means a good correspondence between personal, environmental and occupational factors over a period of time" (p. 5). She found that the participants who engaged in occupations to a greater extent had better quality of life and sense of coherence and less negative symptoms than the group assessed as being under-occupied (p. 10). She goes on to recommend that occupational therapists assess both occupational balance and occupational engagement to help identify occupational problems such as imbalance between rest and activity, lack of meaningful occupations, and lack of occupational and environmental opportunities. This knowledge can be used to establish relevant priorities for intervention and to determine areas requiring further attention. Eklund and Leufstadius's study (2007) showed that the health-promoting ingredients in occupations seemed to be determined by the way occupations were perceived by an individual (and this in turn is influenced by society's perceptions of the occupation), rather than by the doing per se.

Research examining participation in day centers for people living with mental illness (Tjornstrand, Bejerholm, & Eklund, 2011, 2013a) demonstrated not only the value of day centers to the mental health recovery process, it also demonstrated the value of offering a variety of occupational opportunities with varying levels of occupational demand-related characteristics (e.g., level of responsibility, number of different tasks, degree of structure). A good PEO fit can be achieved for clients of the day center by matching occupations with the client's occupational interests and needs, and the environmental demands (e.g., physical, social, and organizational characteristics of the setting). This research helps to (1) validate a core assumption of the PEO model that optimal occupational performance and engagement

results from good PEO fit, and (2) show that occupational demands can be monitored and modified over time in day centers to match changes in a client's health, wellness, and readiness to take on greater occupational challenges.

The research reviewed in this section provides empirical evidence that occupational therapists should support their client to achieve good PEO fit and participate in satisfying and meaningful daily occupations because this can support their recovery and promote enhanced quality of life and well-being.

ENVIRONMENT AND THE RECOVERY PROCESS

Environments, which include physical, social, and political domains, determine PEO interactions and influence occupational performance and well-being. In the case of people living with mental illnesses, elements of the social and policy contexts in particular have been shown to influence recovery and occupational outcomes. Within the social environment, people living with mental illnesses experience high levels of stigma and discrimination and are often restricted from opportunities such as work, housing, education, and even social relationships. Evidence of stigma abounds; people with mental illnesses experience exceptionally high rates of unemployment compared to the general population (Smith & Twomey, 2002) and often report unsupportive relationships with coworkers and supervisors in the workplace (Stuart, 2004; Wahl, 1999). Advocacy groups have pointed out how "NIMBYism" (not in my backyard) denies them access to decent affordable housing (deWolff, 2008), and others report on the loss of friends and family due to fear or misinformation about mental illness (Standing Senate Committee on Social Affairs, Science and Technology, 2006). Stigma is one of the most profound barriers to the full social inclusion and community participation of persons with mental illness. It denies access to important community social roles and to equity and full participation in those roles. Stigma can also affect self-image when one starts to believe the negative views held by others, a phenomenon known as self-stigma.

In many jurisdictions, the policy context has been shown to present barriers to recovery as well. Many mental illnesses are episodic in nature and existing policies prevent people from engaging in meaningful occupations according to their changing status. For example, in Canada, the national disability plan restricts work for people with mental illnesses by equating eligibility with permanent disability. Specifically, eligibility for the Canada Pension Plan, Disability benefits involves acceptance of the designation of having a "severe and prolonged" disability, which indicates that regular gainful employment is not possible. This designation poses a dilemma for those who can work part-time or periodically according to the course of their illnesses because they must choose whether to work to their capacity without the security of benefits, or receive benefits and become marginalized from the workforce. A report by the Standing Senate Committee on Social Affairs, *Out of the Shadows at Last*, states: "To provide benefits only to someone while they are 100% disabled is discriminating, disempowering, and a disincentive to recovery" (Standing Senate Committee on Social Affairs, Science and Technology, 2006, p. 37). Other countries have made similar claims (Martin, Conley, & Noble, 1995), and mental health advocates across the globe are engaging in research and planning activities aimed at eliminating these environmental barriers to recovery.

CONCLUSION

This chapter has demonstrated that the PEO model is well suited to guide psychosocial occupational therapy practice, and provides a useful framework for research in mental health settings. It provides the occupational therapist with a systematic way to analyze and address the complex occupational performance issues experienced by persons experiencing mental illness, and to consider not only the person factors influencing a client's engagement in daily occupations, but also the occupational and environmental factors that can be supporting or hindering occupational performance during the recovery process.

LEARNING ACTIVITIES/ DISCUSSION QUESTIONS

1. Choose an occupational performance issue that you are currently experiencing. Using the PEO model, identify the person, environment, and occupation factors influencing your performance and describe the relationship of these factors to each other. Consider strategies involving the PEO relationship to improve your occupational performance.

2. Use the scholarly resources available to you to find an example (not described in the chapter) of how the PEO model has been applied to intervention in a mental health setting. Consider how the model influenced the intervention process.

REFERENCES

Anaby, D., Jarus, T., Backman, C., & Zumbo, B. (2010). The role of occupational characteristics and occupational imbalance in explaining well-being. *Applied Research in Quality of Life*, 5(2), 81-104.

Bejerholm, U. (2007). *Occupational perspectives on health in people with schizophrenia*. Lund, Sweden: Unpublished Doctoral dissertation, Lund University.

Bejerholm, U. (2010). Occupational balance in people with schizophrenia. *Occupational Therapy in Mental Health*, 26, 1-17.

Bejerholm, U., & Eklund, M. (2004). Time use and occupational performance among persons with schizophrenia. *Occupational Therapy in Mental Health*, 20, 27-47.

Bejerholm, U., & Eklund, M. (2006a). Construct validity of a newly developed instrument: Profile of Occupational Engagement in People with Schizophrenia, POES. *Nordic Journal of Psychiatry*, 60, 200-206.

Bejerholm U., & Eklund, M. (2006b). Engagement in occupations among men and women with schizophrenia. *Occupational Therapy International*, 13(2), 100-121.

Bejerholm, U., & Eklund, M. (2007). Occupational engagement in persons with schizophrenia: Relationships to self-related variables, psychopathology, and quality of life. *American Journal of Occupational Therapy*, 61(1), 21-32.

Bejerholm, U., Hansson, L., & Eklund, M. (2006). Profiles of occupational engagement in people with schizophrenia, POES: Development of a new instrument based on time-use diaries. *British Journal of Occupational Therapy*, 69, 1-11.

Bonney, S., & Stickley, T. (2008). Recovery and mental health: a review of the British literature. *Journal of Psychiatric and Mental Health Nursing*, 15, 140-153.

Bronfenbrenner, U. (1977). Toward an experimental ecology of human development. *American Psychologist*, 32, 513-531.

Bronfenbrenner, U. (2005). *Making human beings human: Bioecological perspectives on human development*. Thousand Oaks, CA: Sage.

Brown, C. (2009). Functional assessment and intervention in occupational therapy. *Psychiatric Rehabilitation Journal*, 32(3), 162-170.

Brown, C., & Stoffel, V. (2011). Occupational therapy in mental health: A vision for participation. Philadelphia, PA: F. A. Davis Co.

Canadian Association of Occupational Therapists. (1997). *Enabling occupation: An occupational therapy perspective*. Ottawa, ON: CAOT Publications ACE.

Christiansen, C. H. (1996). Three perspectives on balance in occupation. In R. Zemke, & F. Clark (Eds.), *Occupational science: The evolving discipline*, pp. 431-451. Philadelphia: F.A. Davis.

Christiansen, C. H., & Matuska, K. M. (2006). Lifestyle balance: A review of concepts and research. *Journal of Occupational Science, 13,* 49-61.

Csikszentmihalyi, M. (1990). *Flow: The psychology of optimal experience.* New York: Harper & Row.

De Wolff, A. (2008). We are neighbours. The impact of supportive housing on community, social, economic and attitude changes. Wellesley Institute. Retrieved from www.wellesleyinstitute.com/wp-content/uploads/2011/11/weareneighbours_0.pdf.

Egan, M. Y., Kubina, L-A., Lidstone, R. I., Macdougall, G. H., & Raudoy, A. E. (2010). A critical reflection on occupational therapy within one assertive community treatment team. *Canadian Journal of Occupational Therapy, 77*(2), 303-313.

Eklund, M. Hansson, L., & Bejerholm, U. (2001). Relationships between satisfaction with occupational factors and health-related variables in schizophrenia outpatients. *Social Psychiatry and Psychiatric Epidemiology, 36,* 79-85.

Eklund, M., & Leufstadius, C. (2007). Relationships between occupational factors and health and well-being in individuals with persistent mental illness living in the community. *Canadian Journal of Occupational Therapy, 74*(4), 70-79.

Gahnstrom-Strandqvist, K., Liukko, A., & Tham, K. (2003). The meaning of the working cooperative for persons with long-term mental illness: A phenomenological study. *American Journal of Occupational Therapy, 57*(3), 262-272.

Gillespie, L. D., Robertson, M. C., Gillespie, W. J., Lamb, S. E., Gates, S., Cumming, R. G., & Rowe, B. H. (2009). Interventions for preventing falls in older people living in the community. *Cochrane Database of Systematic Reviews,* (2), CD007146. doi:10.1002/14651858.CD007146.pub2.

Hamera, E., & Brown, C. E. (2000). Developing a context-based performance measure for persons with schizophrenia: The test of grocery shopping skills. *American Journal of Occupational Therapy, 54*(1), 20-25.

Hatchard, B., & Missiuna, C. (2003). An occupational therapist's journey through bipolar affective disorder. *Occupational Therapy in Mental Health, 19*(2), 1-17.

Kelly, M., Lamont, S., & Brunero, S. (2010). An occupational perspective of the recovery journey in mental health. *British Journal of Occupational Therapy, 73*(3), 129-135.

Krupa, T., Fossey, E., Anthony, W. A. Brown, C., & Pitts, D. B. (2009). Doing daily life: How occupational therapy can inform psychiatric rehabilitation practice. *Psychiatric Rehabilitation Journal, 32*(3), 155-161.

Krupa, T., McLean, H., Eastbrook, S., Bonham, A., & Baksh, L. (2003). Daily time use as a measure of community adjustment for persons served by assertive community adjustment for persons served by assertive community treatment teams. *American Journal of Occupational Therapy, 57*(5), 558-565.

Law, M., Cooper, B., Strong, S., Stewart, D., Rigby, P., & Letts, L. (1996). The person-environment-occupation model: A transactive approach to occupational performance. *Canadian Journal of Occupational Therapy, 63*(1), 9-23.

Law, M., Di Rezze, B., & Bradley, L. (2010). Environmental change to improve outcomes. In M. Law & M. A. McColl (Eds.), *Interventions, effects and outcomes in occupational therapy: Adults and older adults* (pp. 155-182). Thorofare, NJ: SLACK Incorporated.

Law, M., Steinwender, S., & LeClair, L. (1998). Occupation, health and well-being. *Canadian Journal of Occupational Therapy, 65,* 81-91.

Lawton, M. P. (1986). *Environment and aging* (2nd ed.). Albany NY: The Centre for the Study of Aging.

Lawton, M. P., & Nahemow, L. (1973). Ecology and the aging process. In C. Eisdorfer & M. P. Lawton (Eds.), *The psychology of adult development and aging* (pp. 619-674). Washington, DC: American Psychological Association.

Legault, E., & Rebeiro, K. L. (2001). Occupations as means to mental health: A single-case study. *American Journal of Occupational Therapy, 55,* 90-96.

Lexen, A., Hofgren, C., & Bejerholm, U. (2013). Support and process in individual placement and support: A multiple case study. *Work, 44*(4), 435- 448.

Martin, D., Conley, R., & Noble, J. (1995). The ADA and disability benefits policy. *Journal of Disability Policy Studies, 6*(2), 1-15.

McWha, J. L., Pachana, N. A., & Alpass, F. (2003). Exploring the therapeutic environment for older women with late-life depression: An examination of the benefits of an activity group for older people suffering from depression. *Australian Occupational Therapy Journal, 50,* 158-169.

Merryman, M. B., & Riegel, S. K. (2007). The recovery process and people with serious mental illness living in the community: An occupational therapy perspective. *Occupational Therapy in Mental Health, 23*(2), 51-73.

Meyer, A. (1922/1977). The philosophy of occupation therapy. *American Journal of Occupational Therapy, 31*(10), 639-642.

O'Brien, P., Dyck, I., Caron, S., & Mortenson, P. (2002). Environmental analysis: Insights from sociological and geographical perspectives. *Canadian Journal of Occupational Therapy, 64,* 229-238.

Onken, S. J., Craig, C. M., Ridgway, P., Ralph, R. O., & Cook, J. A. (2007). An analysis of the definitions and elements of recovery: a review of the literature. *Psychiatric Rehabilitation Journal, 31*(1), 9-22.

Peloquin, S. M., & Ciro, C. A. (2013). Self-development groups among women in recovery: Client perceptions of satisfaction and engagement. *American Journal of Occupational Therapy, 67*(1), 82-90.

Polatajko, H., Davis, J., Stewart, D., Cantin, N., Amoroso, B., Purdie, L., & Zimmerman, D. (2013). Specifying the domain of concern: Occupation as core. In E. Townsend & H. Polatajko (Eds.), *Enabling occupation II: Advancing an occupational therapy vision for health, well-being & justice through occupation* (2nd ed., pp 13-36). Ottawa, ON: CAOT Publications ACE.

Rebeiro, K. (1998). Occupation-as-means to mental health: A review of the literature, and a call for research. *Canadian Journal of Occupational Therapy, 65,* 12-19.

Rebeiro, K. (2001). Enabling occupation: The importance of an affirming environment. *Canadian Journal of Occupational Therapy, 68*(2), 80-89.

Rebeiro, K. L., Day, D. G., Semeniuk, B., O'Brien, M. C., & Wilson, B. (2001). Northern initiative for social action: an occupation-based mental health program. *American Journal of Occupational Therapy, 55,* 493-500.

Rigby, P., & Letts, L. (2003). Environment and occupational performance: Theoretical considerations. In L. Letts, P. Rigby, & D. Stewart (Eds.). *Using environments to enable occupational performance* (pp. 17-32). Thorofare NJ: SLACK Incorporated.

Smith, A., & Twomey, B. (2002). Labour market experience of people with disabilities. *Labour Market Trends*, August, pp. 415-527.

Standing Senate Committee on Social Affairs, Science and Technology. (2006). Out of the shadows at last: Transforming mental health, mental illness and addiction services in Canada. Retrieved from www.parl.gc.ca/content/sen/committee/391/soci/rep/rep02may06-e.htm.

Stark, S. (2004). Removing environmental barriers in the homes of older adults with disabilities improves occupational performance. *Occupational Therapy Journal of Research*, 24(1), 32-39.

Stoffel, V. C. (2013). Opportunities for occupational therapy behavioral health: A call to action. *American Journal of Occupational Therapy*, 67(2), 140-145.

Strong, S. (1998). Meaningful work in supportive environments: Experiences with the recovery process. *American Journal of Occupational Therapy*, 52, 31-38.

Strong, S., & Rebeiro Gruhl, K. (2011). Person-Environment-Occupation Model. In C. Brown, & V. Stoffel (Eds.), *Occupational therapy in mental health: A vision for participation* (pp. 31-55). Philadelphia, PA: F. A. Davis Co.

Strong, S., Rigby, P., Law, M., Cooper, B., Letts, L., & Stewart, D. (1999) Application of the person-environment-occupation model: A practical tool. *Canadian Journal of Occupational Therapy*, 66(3), 122-130.

Stuart, H. (2004). Stigma and work. *Healthcare Papers*, 5(2), 100-111.

Tjornstrand, C., Bejerholm, U., & Eklund, M. (2011). Participation in day centres for people with psychiatric disabilities: Characteristics of the occupations. *Scandinavian Journal of Occupational Therapy*, 18, 243-253.

Tjornstrand, C., Bejerholm, U., & Eklund, M. (2013a). Participation in day centres for people with psychiatric disabilities: A focus on occupational engagement. *British Journal of Occupational Therapy*, 76, 144-150.

Tjornstrand, C., Bejerholm, U., & Eklund, M. (2013b). Psychometric testing of a self-report measure of engagement in productive occupations *Canadian Journal of Occupational Therapy*, 80(2), 101-110.

Townsend, E., & Polatajko, H. (2007). *Enabling occupation II: Advancing an occupational therapy vision for health, well-being, & justice through occupation*. Ottawa, ON: CAOT Publications ACE.

Townsend, E., & Polatajko, H. (2013). *Enabling occupation II: Advancing an occupational therapy vision for health, well-being, & justice through occupation* (2nd ed.). Ottawa ON: CAOT Publications ACE.

Velligan, D. I., Mueller, J., Wang, M., Dicocco, M., & Diamond, P.M. (2006). Use of environmental supports among patients with schizophrenia. *Psychiatric Services*, 57(2), 219-224.

Wahl, O. (1999). Mental health consumers' experiences of stigma. *Schizophrenia Bulletin*, 25 (3), 467-478.

Wilcock, A.A. (2005). Occupational science: Bridging occupation and health. *Canadian Journal of Occupational Therapy*, 72, 5-12.

World Health Organization. (2001). *International classification of functioning, disability and health*. Geneva: WHO.

Yerxa, E. J., Clarke, F., Frank, G., Jackson, J., Parham, D., Pierce, D.,...Zemke, R. (1990). An introduction to occupational science: A foundation for occupational therapy in the 21st century. In J. A. Johnson & E. J. Yerxa (Eds.), *Occupational science: The foundation for new models of practice* pp. 1-18. New York: Haworth Press.

Zimolag, U., & Krupa, T. (2009). Pet ownership as a meaningful community occupation for people with serious mental illness. *American Journal of Occupational Therapy*, 63(2), 126-137.

Canadian Triple Model Framework for Enabling Occupation

Terry Krupa, PhD, OT Reg (Ont), FCAOT

A central principle in enabling occupation is to reduce the professional and managerial hierarchy which limits consumers' power. You work with people in need and other professionals, and you avoid labels which stigmatize people or portray them as passive and "patient," a label which is appropriate for someone being medically treated, but not someone actively engaged in occupation …. We need to make our collaboration clear, so that the expertise and complexity of this work are recognized. Explaining to others what is meant by enabling occupation helps. (George, an occupational therapist's narrative in Townsend, 1999)

Both theory and research demonstrate that an environment that provides opportunities for active engagement in life contributes to health, well-being, independence, and survival. We need to take another look at the trivialization of occupation. What could be less trivial than survival? (Yerxa, 1998, p. 417)

OBJECTIVES

This objectives of this chapter are as follows:

» Describe the Canadian Triple Model Framework for Enabling Occupation, with emphasis on its relevance to psychosocial occupational therapy practice.

» Define occupational engagement, which extends the focus of occupational therapy beyond occupational performance.

» Examine how the Triple Model Framework informs occupational therapy psychosocial practice.

» Examine applications of the Triple Model Framework in psychosocial practice.

Krupa, T., Kirsh, B., Pitts, D., & Fossey, E. *Bruce & Borg's Psychosocial Frames of Reference: Theories, Models, and Approaches for Occupation-Based Practice, Fourth Edition* (pp 123-133).
© 2016 SLACK Incorporated.

Background

The Canadian Triple Model Framework for Enabling Occupation (Townsend & Polatajko, 2007) was developed to guide occupational therapy in practice contexts characterized by sociocultural diversity, in recognition of the need to deliver occupational therapy services that are inclusive, equitable, and just. The framework consists of three distinct but related models (Figures 8-1 and 8-2; Tables 8-1 to 8-3). The first is the Canadian Model of Occupational Performance and Engagement (CMOP-E), a conceptual model, that defines how humans experience meaning through their occupations, and the transaction between person-level and environment-level elements that make this possible. The second is a practice model, the Canadian Process Practice Framework, which develops a generic, eight-step action pathway for delivering services that promote enablement of occupations in a client-centered manner. The third is a practice model, the Canadian Model of Client-Centered Enablement (CMCE), which identifies and develops a range of enablement skills that are integral to enabling occupations with sensitivity to collaboration, power, equity, and justice. Taken together, these models introduce several theoretical constructs that are highly relevant to psychosocial practice that will be discussed in more detail later in this chapter: engagement, spirituality, client-centered, and enablement. The final concept, justice, as it applies to occupation, is more fully discussed in the final section of this book.

Developed with input from over 60 Canadian occupational therapists, the Triple Model Framework was created with a view to advancing concepts, ideals, and assumptions about health, well-being, and justice through occupation, as well as illustrating their potential applications in diverse contexts.

The Triple Model Framework is a generic framework, and so it is not oriented to psychosocial practice per se. In this chapter, we show that there are at least three ways that this Triple Model Framework of enabling occupation advances practice in the psychosocial arena. First, within the framework there are particular ideals, concepts, and practice approaches that advance our understanding of the psychological, emotional, and social dimensions of human occupation. Second, as the opening quotes suggest, the framework was developed with a view to counteract the marginalization of occupation and occupational therapy practice within fields related to human health and well-being. It accomplishes this by both grounding the work explicitly in assumptions about health and occupation, and by distinguishing enablement of occupation from treatment services, as the core therapeutic process of the profession. Finally, the framework was developed to show the relevance of occupation to health in socially, culturally, and politically diverse practice contexts. This is accomplished largely by efforts to demonstrate the application of the three models to a range of practice scenarios, many outside of the traditional health field. For example, case illustrations of the framework in practice include examples of individuals who experience difficulties with occupational health in the context of immigration and political conflict.

Although the current Triple Model Framework was developed in 2007, it actually evolved over more than 30 years. From the very beginning, the framework's models were developed to guide practice in Canada. The historical progression of the framework is well recorded through formal documents, minutes of professional meetings, and associated occupational therapy scholarship. In 1983, the first guiding model, the Occupational Performance Model (Department of National Health & Welfare & Canadian Association of Occupational Therapists [CAOT], 1983), was developed and defined occupation as the core of the profession focused explicitly on the client-centered practice of occupational therapy. This concept was further developed in future guidelines (CAOT, 1991, 1993). In 1997, the guidelines were advanced to define "enabling occupation" as the central therapeutic process of the profession (CAOT, 1997). Since the publication of the original guidelines in 1983, several related resources and documents have been developed to advance their application. These include, for example, the Canadian Occupational Performance Measure (Law et al., 2005), guidelines for client-centered mental health practice (CAOT, 1993), and a document focused on outcome measurement (DNHW & CAOT, 1987). Since the publication of the most recent version of the enabling occupation framework, new efforts to address implementation challenges have emerged. For example, the Leadership in Enabling Occupation Model (Townsend, Polatajko, Craik, & von Zweck, 2011) has been developed to assist occupational therapists with moving the vision of health-promoting human occupation forward within contemporary health and social systems and structures.

View of Health and Disorder

The Canadian Triple Model Framework has been constructed from the premise that health and well-being are supported through participation in occupations that are meaningful, both personally and socially. Health and well-being, therefore, are equated with occupational well-being. Individuals can experience disease, illness, injury, disruptions in life and social circumstances, and other such threats, and still experience occupational health and well-being. This can happen in at least two ways. First, people can engage in occupations that provide conditions for improvement of their health conditions. For example, when a young man with schizophrenia participates in community activities that he finds meaningful, it provides a context for him to learn how to recognize and manage the symptoms of his illness, and provides him with

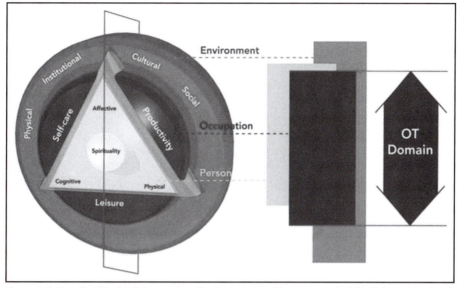

Figure 8-1. Canadian Model of Occupational Performance and Engagement (CMOP-E). (From Townsend, E., & Polatajko, H., "Enabling Occupation II: Advancing an occupational therapy vision for health, well-being and justice through occupation," Ottawa, Canada. Copyright © 2007 by CAOT Publications. Reprinted with permission.)

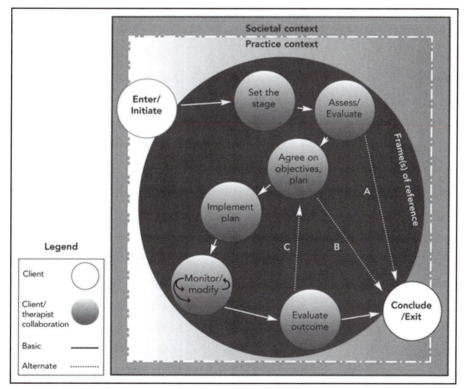

Figure 8-2. Canadian Practice Process Framework (CPPF). (From Townsend, E., & Polatajko, H., "Enabling Occupation II: Advancing an occupational therapy vision for health, well-being and justice through occupation," Ottawa, Canada. Copyright © 2007 by CAOT Publications. Reprinted with permission.)

relief from his symptoms. Likewise, a senior citizen who continues to participate actively in physical and mental activities that provide a challenge, may reduce the risks for cognitive and physical decline in aging. Second, in the course of experiencing significant life disruptions and transitions, losses, personal or social crises, engaging in meaningful occupations can bring well-being, stability, adaptation, life quality, and future possibilities. So for example, interventions focused on enabling the occupations of seniors can facilitate their ability to age successfully

	TABLE 8-1
	CANADIAN MODEL OF CLIENT-CENTERED ENABLEMENT: SKILLS OF ENABLING
KEY SKILLS	**RELATED ENABLEMENT SKILLS**
Adapt	Accommodate, adjust, "analyze and break down" occupations into doable components, configure and reconfigure, confirm, cope, observe, tailor
Advocate	Challenge, champion, develop (guidelines, policy, positions, regulations, reports), generate critical perspectives, politically strategize, prompt power sharing and empowerment, enlighten, lobby, make visible, mobilize, promote, raise consciousness
Coach	Encourage, guide, challenge, expand choices, hold accountable, see the big picture, listen, mentor, motivate, pose powerful questions, reflect, reframe, support
Collaborate	Communicate, cooperate, encourage, facilitate, form alliances, mediate, negotiate, partner, resolve competing interests, tap motivation
Consult	Advise, brainstorm options, confer, counsel, integrate, recommend, suggest, synthesize and summarize
Coordinate	Arrange, bring together, case coordinate/manage, develop and manage budgets, document, integrate, identify, interweave or weave together, allocate human, financial, space and material resources, lead, link, manage, network, orchestrate, organize, supervise, synthesize
Design/Build	Conceive, construct, create, develop, devise, fabricate, formulate, envision, evaluate, manufacture, plan, prescribe, propose, redesign, rebuild, strategize, visualize
Educate	Demonstrate, enlighten, instruct, inform, facilitate learning through doing, notify, present just-right-challenge, prompt learning of skills, prompt rote and repetitive learning, prompt transformative learning, simulate, teach, train, tutor
Engage	Build trust, challenge normal expectations, develop readiness and confidence, do with/in parallel, draw into performance in tests or use of technology, engage in "doing", identify occupational issues and potential, involve, occupy, optimize potential, socially mobilize, spark visions of possibility and hope, stimulate creative expression through occupation, prompt optimal participation, tap potential
Specialize	Facilitate body function, apply hands on techniques (e.g., asset-based practice, cognitive approaches, driver rehabilitation, ergonomics, group therapy, psychosocial rehabilitation, sensory integration)

Adapted from Townsend, E., & Polatajko, H., *Enabling Occupation II: Advancing an occupational therapy vision for health, well-being and justice through occupation*, Ottawa, Canada. Copyright © 2007 by CAOT Publications.

	TABLE 8-2
	CLIENT-CENTERED PRACTICE QUESTIONS
COMPONENT OF CLIENT-CENTERED PRACTICE	**EXAMPLES OF PRACTICE QUESTIONS**
Power	Do I use language that my clients will understand?
Listening and communicating	Do I truly listen to what my clients are trying to tell me, looking beyond their words to the meanings they are trying to convey?
Partnership	What do I bring to this partnership? What does my client bring to this partnership?
Choice	Am I providing opportunities for real choice when I work with this client?
Hope	How do I understand and express hope in working with this client?

Adapted from Sumsion, T., & Law, M., A review of evidence on the conceptual elements informing client-centred practice, *Canadian Journal of Occupational Therapy, 73*, 153-162. Copyright © 2006 by SAGE Publications.

TABLE 8-3	
STRATEGIES FOR MAXIMIZING CLIENT-CENTERED PRACTICE WHEN THE CLIENT EXPERIENCES COGNITIVE IMPAIRMENT OR ACUTE MENTAL INSTABILITY	
STRATEGY	**EXAMPLES**
Negotiated decision making (Moats, 2007)	Engaging family members or other significant social supports in the decision-making process, in a dynamic way that respects the individual's capacities Balance concerns about risk with the goal of autonomy through evaluation of occupation in the natural context with and without support
Graded decision making (Hobson, 1996)	Apply the principles of graded activity to the decision-making process, increasing the amount of structure used in the process to match client need
Advocacy (Hobson, 1996)	Where the competency of a client has been legally declared, continually evaluate the suitability of this declaration, and challenge it when appropriate. The goal is to ensure that the autonomy and dignity of clients is respected.
Framing the process (White, 2011)	Describe the goals and processes of occupational therapy in a way that is materially relevant to the client's lifestyle and life conditions
Keep aware of varying capacities for authentic collaboration (White, 2011)	Since the mental and affective capacities of individuals can vary, be prepared to adjust strategies to engage clients as needed.

in their homes and participate meaningfully in family and community activities. Likewise, they can facilitate the transition of adolescents and young adults with disability as they move from school to community work and living settings.

THEORETICAL ASSUMPTIONS

The Canadian Triple Model Framework is explicitly grounded in two central assumptions: that humans need occupation and that occupation has therapeutic value. These central assumptions are further grounded in the beliefs that occupations bring meaning to life, structure and organize daily routines and habits, and that they are highly personal and idiosyncratic (Townsend & Polotajko, 2007).

Beyond assumptions about occupation and health, the framework also makes explicit assumptions about the individuals that receive occupational therapy services. Specifically, it is assumed that (like all citizens) when it comes to their occupational lives, they have the need for autonomy and choice, and that they have knowledge and expertise that should be acknowledged and respected (Sumsion & Law, 2006). Furthermore, the framework

assumes that because meaningful occupations promote health and well-being, access to meaningful occupations represents a justice issue, and is thus subject to considerations of equity and fairness.

KEY THEORETICAL DEVELOPMENTS

The CMOP-E is the triple framework's conceptual model depicting person, occupation and environment components, and their relationships, that explain human occupation performance and engagement. Visually the model is depicted as a three-dimensional figure, reflecting a dynamic interaction between occupations (self-care, leisure, and productivity), personal level components (physical, affective, cognitive), and the essence of the person (spirituality), and environmental components (physical, institutional, cultural, and social; see Figure 8-1). The Canadian Practice Process Framework is the second part of the Canadian Triple Model Framework (Craik, Davis, & Polotajko, 2007); it is a generic process framework that defines eight action points for client-centered, goal-directed, and evidence-based occupational therapy practice (see Figure 8-2). Visually, the central role of the client in the collaborative relationship is highlighted in the model. The final part of the triple framework is the CMCE, which identifies enablement as the core competency of the profession and describes a range of core enablement skills (see Table 8-1). In addition, the CMCE is accompanied by descriptive categories outlining how occupational therapy practice can be enabling or disabling. For example, enablement is described as ineffective when it is characterized by alienation of the client through expert dominance, or by value clashes between the client and therapist.

As mentioned, each element of the Canadian Triple Model Framework reflects a generic model focused on occupation, but many of the beliefs and ideas central to the framework have contributed significantly to the development of psychosocial knowledge, theory, and practice in the profession. Specifically, many of these ideas and their applications have more firmly grounded occupational therapy knowledge and practice within the social, cultural, and political worlds where clients reside and participate. In the following section, these key ideas are described more fully.

Engagement

The triple framework, and specifically the CMOP-E, identifies occupational engagement as an integral element of human occupation and a legitimate focus of occupational therapy practice. This means that, beyond the profession's traditional focus on performance, human occupation also requires consideration of the human experience of occupation. Engagement is defined as the state of being actively involved or occupied. Rather than an "all or nothing" concept, people can have differing levels of engagement. Compare for example, the difference between being absorbed in an occupation to being passively involved. Identifying engagement as central to human occupation is important, because it is through engagement that we experience the full potential of possible health-promoting meanings associated with occupation.

Enabling

The Canadian framework calls upon occupational therapists to define their core competence as enabling occupation. Enabling as a focus of occupational therapy is distinguished from the more traditional idea that the profession provides treatment. While the concept of treatment suggests that service providers manage or care for people to address illness or health-related issues, the concept of enabling suggests that the therapeutic process is oriented to giving people the means to do or make some difference to their health and well-being. Consistent with psychosocial practice, enabling as an overall therapeutic approach has the potential to positively influence clients' autonomy, self-efficacy, coping, and problem solving.

The framework encourages therapists to intentionally construct their professional practice to create conditions that will enable engagement in and performance of meaningful occupation. The Canadian framework, particularly the CMCE, identifies and explicates the occupational therapy skills that are associated with enabling practice. The skill range is as follows:

- "Clinical" in nature, meant to therapeutically affect the function of the body in occupation (including, for example the many specific therapeutic intervention strategies and techniques developed throughout this book)
- Expand visions of possibilities in occupation
- Impart knowledge critical to engaging in meaningful occupations
- Develop authentic collaborations
- Change social and environmental conditions for occupation

Again, this broad range of enabling skills is constructed to increase the profession's sensitivity to the diversity of occupational needs and practice contexts that occupational therapists encounter.

Spirituality

Spirituality is perhaps one of the most challenging ideas for occupational therapy theory and practice captured within this Canadian Triple Model Framework. Spirituality as a central focus in human occupation emerged from the contention that the power of occupation to influence human and social health and well-being cannot adequately be understood within psychological, emotional, or social perspectives on function and participation. Instead, spirituality is viewed as the essence of the self, the sense of purpose and meaning, and the relationship of the self to larger society and the world. Humans express their spiritual nature through their occupations and their experience of these occupations (Baptiste, 2005; Egan & DeLaat, 1994; Kirsh, 1996). McColl (2000), in her Muriel Driver Lecture to Canadian occupational therapists, distinguished between "spirit" and "spirituality." Spirit is defined as a force that enlivens all living beings and is independent from individuals. Spirituality on the other hand, is a human condition that reflects sensitivity to this life force of spirit. McColl eloquently illustrates how these ideas move us beyond psychological notions of drive for occupation:

> However if we agreed that spirit is not within the person, but instead is an energy that passes between people and the world, then we might see it as transformative and inspirational, rather than simply motivational. I suggest that spirit acts through us, rather than in us. That is not to say that our free will is compromised by spirit, but that our potential is enhanced by it. (p. 220)

Translating spirituality into occupational therapy theory and practice has witnessed lively debates and discussions.

VIGNETTE 8-1. GINA

Gina is the mother of 30-year-old man with multiple chronic health conditions and limitations in function that affect his independence in self-care, and constrain his participation in community leisure and productivity. Until recently, her son lived at home, where Gina took care of all his daily living needs. Gina's daily life was taken up with caregiving for her son. Her vision of "mothering," coming from her own social-cultural beliefs and values, emerged from a view that mothers "take care" of their sons until they leave the house to start their own families. In practice, this vision left her exhausted, often at odds with other family members whose occupational lives were also constrained by this vision, and unable to consider other future possibilities.

Through her ongoing connections with influential people from her cultural community, discussions with her son's occupational therapist and other service providers, and the support of other family members, Gina agreed to have her son move into a supported community residence. She continued to visit her son regularly and defined a set of "mothering" activities that she would continue. This move provided her with the opportunity to take on new meaningful roles in her cultural community, including spearheading the development of approaches to regularly include people with disabilities (including her son) in their events and activities.

For example, discussions have emerged regarding the extent to which spirituality is distinct from religion, and about the extent to which spirituality demands a broad understanding of interprofessional practice that includes practitioners outside of the health service realm.

It seems that "seeing" and "working" with spirituality is not always obvious in the everyday practice of occupational therapists, but there have been circumstances and contexts that have helped with the advancement of applications of spirituality. For example, the idea that people who experience significant disability are vulnerable to spiritual crises that affect their capacity to have health through occupation is a common theme (Egan & DeLaat, 1994; McColl, 2000). Gina, in Vignette 8-1, illustrates this idea. Gina's situation suggests that her experience as a mother of a man with a significant health condition and disability engenders a spiritual crisis, where the meanings and purposes she derives through her occupations are challenged. The processes by which she reconstructs the beliefs and values that underlie these meanings and purposes can be understood as a type of spiritual transformation, where new meanings and purposes create other possibilities with the potential for considerable reward and well-being.

As a second example, it appears that the construct of spirituality holds considerable promise as a way to connect occupational therapy assumptions about occupational therapy with experiences of meaning and purpose in occupation cross-culturally. Hopkirk and Wilson (2014), for example, identified spirituality as an important connection between occupational therapy and Maori culture, illustrated by this quote from a study participant: "Spirit is unique—the life force—I can't describe it, but it drives all people the way we 'do.' It is the fire within—what you feed it will depend on what you do with it … It is a journey, spirit, activity, meanings all combine" (Interviewee A, p. 6).

Similarly, a study exploring brain injury from a First Nations perspective in Canada highlighted the significance of spirituality and spiritual guidance in conceptions of healing and wellness (Knightley et al., 2011). In this way, the concept of spirituality may present the profession with a worldview and language that resonates, and thus can be shared with many populations and cultures.

Client-Centered Practice and Empowerment

Throughout its evolution, the Canadian framework has championed the advancement of a therapist-client relationship that is authentically a collaborative and partnership approach, where clients are actively involved in negotiating goals and intervention approaches and exercising choice. Many of the people, groups, and communities that occupational therapists serve are either vulnerable, or experience disempowerment, in their daily lives. The impact of client-centered practice extends beyond the respect and power sharing of the client-therapist relationship. Indeed, the evidence-base that supports the development of a client-centered approach highlights its potential to increase personal agency and autonomy, self-confidence and self-efficacy, and ultimately improvements in function and expanded visions of future possibilities (Sumsion & Law, 2006). These are all person-level factors that are central to psychosocial health and well-being.

OCCUPATIONAL THERAPY PRACTICE

As mentioned earlier, the Canadian Triple Model Framework is a generic set of conceptual and practice models that are meant to inform and guide occupational therapy practice. Practice approaches and tools have emerged from these models, particularly in an effort to guide therapists in operationalizing the key constructs and assumptions. In this section, these practice applications are examined as they have been applied specifically in the mental health and psychosocial practice arena.

Practical Applications of Client-Centered Practice and Enabling Occupation in the Mental Health Arena

The profession has witnessed the development of skills and strategies specific to client-centered practice, with a view to ensuring that the ideals upon which this practice is based can be realized. For example, Table 8-2 provides a few examples of questions that therapists can pose to themselves to evaluate whether their practice is addressing the key dimensions of client-centered practice. Occupational therapists practicing in the psychosocial arena may often find that they are challenged in their efforts to deliver truly client-centered practice. One commonly cited reason for this is that, for a variety of reasons, their clients experience considerable limitations in their ability to exercise informed decision making, to be self-determining, and to envision possibilities. This may be because, in the context of mental illness, they experience cognitive impairments and/or periods of mental or emotional instability that can affect their insight into their occupational issues and needs, and this will influence the way they collaborate with therapists to envision and realize possibilities. In such situations, occupational therapists can find themselves struggling with the challenge of balancing choices and autonomy with risk to the client and perhaps even the community. Practice strategies have evolved to account for these challenges while maximizing the client-centered process. Table 8-3 provides a few examples of such practice strategies that are offered in the occupational therapy literature. For example, Hobson (1996) suggested that informed decision making related to occupation can be thought of as an activity that is amenable to grading. In this way, the occupational therapist can grade the amount of support provided in decision making, the structure of the process, the amount and nature of information provided, etc.

The Canadian Occupational Performance Measure (COPM) is an outcome measure that is aligned with the Canadian models of enablement. It was specifically designed to engage clients in a process of selecting meaningful occupational issues that they perceive as currently challenging, ranking the priority issues, and self-rating levels of performance and satisfaction. It offers the therapist and client a structured way to collaborate to set occupation-related goals and interventions. The measure has been widely researched and its utility with a wide range of clients and in a broad range of practice settings has been demonstrated (Carswell et al., 2004).

In mental health settings, approaches that promote the autonomy and self-determination of clients have taken center stage as the field has advanced a recovery orientation in service delivery. Kirsh and Cockburn (2009), in their review of the relevance of the COPM in mental health settings, highlight that (1) the movement to advance recovery is founded on the idea of helping people with mental illnesses to experience meaningful lives, and the COPM provides corresponding indicators for this vision; and (2) recovery practice is highly oriented to promoting choice, autonomy, and empowerment, all central principles of the COPM. The authors suggest that the tool does hold the potential to be a useful service or system-wide tool, to identify population-level information about occupational needs and issues and to evaluate the changes that occur over the course of service delivery. Occupational therapists are certainly well positioned to take a leadership role in the implementation of the COPM and to advance its potential as a measure within recovery for recovery-oriented service delivery.

Kirsh and Cockburn (2009) note that the COPM has been the outcome measure of choice among Canadian occupational therapists practicing in a range of mental health practice contexts. Outside of the Canadian context there is also growing evidence of its application. Warren (2002) described an interesting study focusing on the use of the COPM among a small group of mental health therapists in the United Kingdom who positively received the tool. Interestingly, their training in the use of the COPM also included information about client-centered practice as developed with the Canadian models; linking the tool explicitly to the philosophy and models of practice underlying it may be an important step in facilitating its uptake.

Vignette 8-2 provides an example of the application of the COPM. Catherine, a woman who is working with an occupational therapist to address concerns she has about daily life occupations, was first introduced in Chapter 4 of this book. Catherine is recovering from an acute episode of depression. As the vignette suggests, she has had a rich occupational life participating in a range of meaningful roles and activities. Her experience of depression, occurring in the context of the dissolution of her marriage, has left her unable to manage or fully enjoy activities and responsibilities she has largely managed effectively in the past. With her home management, family, employment, and social activities disrupted, the occupational therapist found Catherine to be highly distressed in the process of client-centered goal setting. The COPM provided the structure needed to identify the immediate and priority occupational issues from Catherine's perspective, and to design interventions and approaches that would not be overwhelming but bring

VIGNETTE 8-2. CATHERINE

Catherine is a 38-year-old woman who is currently on disability leave from her job as a clerical assistant in a university department because of depression. She has a long history of living with depression and has been able to effectively manage the illness with medications and psychotherapy when needed. She had two previous short-term leaves from her job. This episode of the illness is a different experience for Catherine. It occurred in the context of separation from her husband that has been full of conflict. She is worried about her financial security and her future generally.

The leave from work came at a bad time when the department was under considerable pressures related to the start of the school year. She was dealing with timetabling and room assignments for the next academic year and at the same time preparing letters for admission, responding to admission inquiries, and responding to the requests and needs of the student body. She works in a large office with three other clerical workers. The organization has no capacity for providing coverage for these workers. Catherine gets on well with the coworkers in her office, but she is certain that they are unhappy that she is taking time off.

She is the mother of three children, aged 6 to 10, and is finding it difficult to keep up with their needs. She is also unhappy with how she is managing typical household routines and the fact that she is asking the children to do more for themselves. Her energy level is very low, she has trouble getting out of bed in the morning, and she has eliminated social and community activities that had been a typical part of her occupational routine. Overall, her self-confidence has plummeted and she is finding herself unable to make even simple decisions. Although she has many friends, she is maintaining only superficial contact with them because she doesn't want to be a burden on them. She says she finds it difficult to think of having friends and fun when she has children to care for and they should be her first priority. In fact, she finds that she derives little pleasure even from the activities she finds most meaningful. Catherine speaks about losing the custody of her children, feeling incompetent as a mother and concern that she will be unable to manage financially if she does not soon return to work.

Catherine completed the Canadian Occupational Performance Measure. With her occupational therapist's support, she identified the following priority issues and then re-evaluated 4 weeks later:

PRIORITY OCCUPATIONAL PERFORMANCE ISSUE	SELF-RANKING OF PERFORMANCE TIME 1	SELF-RANKING OF PERFORMANCE TIME 2	SATISFACTION RANKING TIME 1	SATISFACTION RANKING TIME 2
Sharing breakfast with the children before they head for school	3	8	2	6
Organizing weekly "fun" family activities	1	7	1	8
Maintaining a tidy and organized home	3	5	2	5

rapid, positive changes in her occupational performance and experience. To address these focused, meaningful goals, the occupational therapist and Catherine agreed on a plan of action that included strategies to monitor her time use and effectively use her limited energy, cognitive behavioral strategies to counteract her tendency to perceive her efforts and experiences in a perfectionist and negative light, as well as social network approaches that constructed one or two family events that included friends and families

from her existing group of friends. As COPM goals were met, Catherine was able to move on to prioritizing work-related goals.

Research on the COPM has advanced our understanding of the challenges of implementing the COPM with particular populations. For example, a systematic review of research on the COPM by Parker and Sykes (2006) indicated that there can be difficulties with implementing the tool with individuals with limited insight, significant cognitive problems, and acute mental illness. The review also suggested that for individuals with prevalent symptoms of depression or psychosis, additional time may be required to complete the tool. This does not mean that the tool is unsuitable for this group of people. Indeed Warren's (2002) study found that clients with psychosis expressed satisfaction with the tool, pleased that it gave them the opportunity to see what they could continue to do well despite their illnesses. Future work on the COPM in this area could benefit from ongoing dialogue among therapists about the strategies they use to effectively collaborate with clients to implement the tool.

To date, the core construct of client-centered practice has been subject to the most direct application to practice. Other key constructs, such as spirituality and enablement, are comparatively new to the Canadian Triple Model Framework and their application to practice is understandably less developed. There are, however, emerging examples of practical applications of these ideas. Kirsh (1996), for example, has suggested the use of a narrative approach as a way to translate spirituality into practice, particularly given the ability of narratives to elicit experiences of meaning and purpose as they evolve over time.

CONCLUSION

This chapter describes the Canadian Triple Model Framework for enabling occupation, which includes three models designed originally to provide a shared vision and guidelines for Canadian practice. The models have gained the attention of occupational therapists internationally. This is a generic framework that develops particular values, ideals, assumptions, and practices that advance psychosocial practice in occupational therapy. In particular, the framework advances practice related to the experience and meaning of occupation, client choice and autonomy, and occupation as a justice issue. The COPM is a client-centered outcome measure with broad applications in practice. This chapter shows the application of the COPM to a practice situation in mental health practice and calls for ongoing efforts by occupational therapists to define the elements of practice that will enable even the most vulnerable clients to participate in the therapeutic relationship in an engaged and collaborative way.

LEARNING ACTIVITIES/ DISCUSSION QUESTIONS

1. The vignette of Gina in this chapter describes her experience of a crisis of spirituality and the transformative resolution of this crisis. Think about an individual you have seen in the course of your occupational therapy practice who has experienced a spiritual crisis. How did this person express this crisis occupationally? In ideal circumstances, what would an occupational therapist do to enable the resolution of this crisis?

2. In a group with other occupational therapists, discuss the following question: What pros and cons exist for the inclusion of spirituality as a core element of occupational therapy practice?

3. Consider the Canadian Practice Process Model. Describe how client-centered practice might be operationalized in each of the eight action steps.

4. Think of a person with a cognitive impairment and a mental illness who you have seen in occupational therapy practice. Identify the specific approaches you might use to successfully engage this individual in completing the Canadian Occupational Performance Measure.

REFERENCES

Baptiste, S. (2005). Spirituality in occupational therapy. In A. Meier, T. St. James O'Connor, & P., Van Katwyk (Eds.), *Spirituality and health: Multidisciplinary explorations.* Waterloo, ON: Wilfrid Laurier Press.

Canadian Association of Occupational Therapists. (1991). *Occupational therapy guidelines for client-centred practice.* Toronto: CAOT publications.

Canadian Association of Occupational Therapists. (1993). *Occupational therapy guidelines for client-centred practice.* Toronto: CAOT publications.

Canadian Association of Occupational Therapists. (1997/2002). *Enabling occupation: An occupational therapy perspective.* Ottawa, ON: CAOT Publications ACE

Canadian Association of Occupational Therapists. (2002). *Enabling occupation: An occupational therapy perspective.* Ottawa, ON: CAOT publications.

Carswell, A., McColl, M. A., Baptiste, S., Law, M., Polatajko, H. & Pollock, N. (2004). The Canadian Occupational Performance Measure: A research and clinical literature review. *Canadian Journal of Occupational Therapy, 71,* 210-222.

Craik, J., Davis, J., & Polatajko, H. (2007). Introducing the Canadian Practice Process Framework (CPPF): Amplifying the context. In E. Townsend & H. Polatjko (Eds.), *Enabling occupation II: Advancing an occupational therapy vision for health, well-being & justice through occupation.* Ottawa, ON: Canadian Occupational Therapy Association.

Department of National Health and Welfare & Canadian Association of Occupational Therapists. (1983). *Guidelines for client-centred practice of occupational therapy.* Ottawa, ON: DNHW & CAOT.

Department of National Health and Welfare & Canadian Association of Occupational Therapists. (1987). *Towards outcomes measures in occupational therapy.* Ottawa, ON: DNHW & CAOT.

Egan, M., & DeLaat, M. D. (1994). Considering spirituality in occupational therapy practice. *Canadian Journal of Occupational Therapy, 61*(2), 95-101.

Hobson, S. (1996). Being client-centred when the client is cognitively impaired. *Canadian Journal of Occupational Therapy, 63,* 133-137.

Hopkirk, J., & Wilson, L. H. (2014). A Call to Wellness—Whitiwhitia i te ora: Exploring Māori and Occupational Therapy Perspectives on Health. *Occupational Therapy International.* doi: 10.1002/oti.1373

Kirsh, B. (1996). A narrative approach to addressing spirituality in occupational therapy: Exploring personal meaning and purpose. *Canadian Journal of Occupational Therapy, 63,* 55-61.

Kirsh, B., & Cockburn, L. (2009). The Canadian Occupational Performance Measure: A tool for recovery-based practice. *Psychiatric Rehabilitation Journal, 32,* 171-176.

Knightley, M. L., King, G. E., Jang, S. H., White, R. J., Colantonio, A., Minore, J. B.,...Longboat-White, C. H. (2011). Brain injury from a First Nation's perspective: Teachings from elders and traditional healers. *Canadian Journal of Occupational Therapy, 78,* 237-45.

Law, M., Baptiste, S., Carswell, A., McColl, J. A., Polatajko, H., & Pollock, N. (2005). *Canadian Occupational Performance Measure.* Ottawa: CAOT publications.

McColl, M. A. (2000). Spirit, occupation and disability. *Canadian Journal of Occupational Therapy, 67,* 217-228.

Moats, G. (2007). Discharge decision-making, occupation and client-centred practice. *Canadian Journal of Occupational Therapy, 74,* 91-101.

Parker, D. M., & Sykes, C. H. (2006). A systematic review of the Canadian occupational performance measure: A clinical practice perspective. *British Journal of Occupational Therapy, 69,* 150-160.

Sumsion, T., & Law, M. (2006). A review of the evidence on the conceptual elements informing client-centred practice. *Canadian Journal of Occupational Therapy, 73,* 153-162.

Townsend, E. (1999). Enabling occupation in the 21st century: Making good intentions a reality. *Australian Journal of Occupational Therapy, 46,* 147-159.

Townsend, E. A., & Polatajko, H. J. (2007). *Enabling occupation II: Advancing an occupational therapy vision for health, well-being & justice through occupation.* Ottawa, ON: Canadian Occupational Therapy Association.

Townsend, E. A., Polatajko, H. J., Craik, J. M., & von Zweck, C. M. (2011). Introducing the Leadership in Enabling Occupation (LEO) model. *Canadian Journal of Occupational Therapy, 78*(4), 255-259.

Warren, A. (2002). An evaluation of the Canadian model of occupational performance and the Canadian occupational performance measure in mental health practice. *British Journal of Occupational Therapy, 65,* 515-521.

White, A. (2011). How occupational therapists engage clients with cognitive impairments in assessment. (Unpublished master's thesis). University of Auckland, Auckland, New Zealand.

Yerxa, E. (1998). Health and the human spirit for occupation. *American Journal of Occupational Therapy, 52,* 419-422.

9

The Model of Human Occupation
A Framework for Occupation-Focused Practice

Ellie Fossey, PhD, MSc, DipCOT (UK)

An occupational therapist's perspective: "What influenced my thinking in practice? How did I structure the way I worked with service users?... *I needed a defined assessment process that would give a broader understanding of occupational performance, something that highlighted more about the person than just identifying what they were engaged in doing. I realised* doing *was an important part of occupational therapy, but I wanted to know more about why service users were* doing *chosen occupations, how they were* doing *those occupations and what influenced their abilities to do* occupations.... *I consider the MOHO's assessments as my* toolbox *and choose the appropriate assessment based on what information I need to know, and the best way in which to gather this information.*" (Cook, 2012, p. 142; p. 143).

Following interviews informed by the Model of Human Occupation (MOHO), clients of a mental health service spoke of it being "good" or a "relief" to talk about their lives, including the very difficult or distressing aspects, their joys, hopes and dreams, "not just illness"; and it created an openness and different sense of connection with the occupational therapists in these interviews than was usual in their experience of mental health care. As Gwen expressed: I remember being quite happy after the interview, the more I learnt the stronger I felt. That maybe I can achieve more stuff than I really thought and be more focused on what I wanted to do in the future.... Maybe their role had changed. Questions were asked and maybe they [occupational therapists] changed the way they presented themselves.... It is hard to explain; not a friend, but more like a companion just having a chat, than being your worker, or a person superior. Even though OTs [occupational therapists] get paid and all that, it was a bit different. It seemed to me more like the walls had come down. (Ennals & Fossey, 2007, p. 17 and 18)

OBJECTIVES

The objectives of this chapter are as follows:

» Outline the theoretical origins and development of the Model of Human Occupation (MOHO) as an explanatory framework for understanding how people choose, organize, and perform occupations within their particular contexts, and over the course of their everyday lives.

» Describe personal and environmental factors that are addressed by MOHO and how they interact to shape a person's occupational life.

» Provide examples of practical tools and practices informed by MOHO.

BACKGROUND

This chapter focuses on the Model of Human Occupation (MOHO; Kielhofner, 2008a), an occupation-focused, theory-driven, and extensively researched approach to occupational therapy practice that is widely used in areas of practice where psychosocial issues are addressed. It opens with a quote from Sarah Cook, an occupational therapist, reflecting on why she was drawn to MOHO (Kielhofner, 2008) to structure her thinking and ways of working with service users in practice; this is followed by quotes from adults attending a community mental health clinic who participated in a study of the Occupational Performance History Interview from clients' and therapists' perspectives (Ennals & Fossey, 2007). These quotes draw our attention to the following features of MOHO as a framework for occupation-focused practice:

- Occupational therapists need frameworks to structure and guide their thinking and ways of working in practice that address *doing* and the complex range of factors that affect clients' doing in their particular situations—MOHO offers such a framework.

- Widely used by occupational therapists, MOHO provides a useful structure to guide occupation-focused practice with clients and a clear professional identity (Kielhofner, Forsyth, Kramer, Melton, & Dobson, 2009; Lee, Taylor, Kielhofner, & Fisher, 2008) that is deepened through its ongoing use in a reflexive way.

- MOHO places emphasis on the subjective and contextually embedded nature of participation in occupations, so that it supports therapists to attend to, and engage with, clients' lived experiences and everyday worlds, and to collaborate with them to enable change.

- Talking about their everyday lives is valued by clients; it offers possibilities for reflection and the development of new perspectives on their lives.

- MOHO provides an extensive range of tools that can be used to understand clients' occupational lives and

environments, and to inform how change may be facilitated.

Developed over 30 years through the scholarship of Dr. Gary Kielhofner in collaboration with many practitioners and researchers internationally, MOHO seeks to explain how people choose, organize, and orchestrate their everyday occupations to develop and sustain patterns of participation over their lives. It provides a framework for understanding threats to, or problems with, participation in occupations that people experience whether due to life transitions, changing capacities with ageing, ill-health, developmental delay, and environmental restrictions. It also provides evidence and practical tools to support client-centered and occupation-focused practice (Forsyth & Kielhofner, 2011).

VIEW OF OCCUPATION, AND HEALTH/DISORDER

MOHO was developed at a time when the predominant focus of much occupational therapy theory and practice was understanding and alleviating impairments, but also a time of re-emergent interest in occupation (Kielhofner et al., 2009). Hence, MOHO was developed with the intention to focus theory and practice on occupation. Within this framework, occupation broadly refers to a wide range of doing, including work, play, and activities of daily living, that occur within temporal, physical, social, and cultural contexts that shape and inform much of human life (Kielhofner, 2008b).

MOHO is informed by an occupational perspective of health. Put succinctly, participation in everyday occupations is understood as a fundamental human need, an important determinant of mental, physical, and social well-being, and an agent for restoring and maintaining health (Kielhofner, 2009; Polatajko et al., 2007; Wilcock, 2006). Consequently, MOHO is broadly applicable to people who face challenges to participate in everyday occupations, irrespective of diagnosis or health status. Indeed, it neither seeks to explain specific impairments of body structure or function, nor does it focus on the functional consequences of particular diagnoses or health conditions. Rather, MOHO provides a framework to understand and address the disruptions and challenges in choosing, organizing, and orchestrating the everyday occupations that people experience at times of life transitions, due to ill-health and disability or environmental restrictions. Therefore, MOHO is as applicable to addressing difficulties in everyday occupation that are psychosocial in nature, and that are faced by people experiencing mental illness, as it is to a range of other circumstances in which participation in everyday occupations is either challenging or restricted.

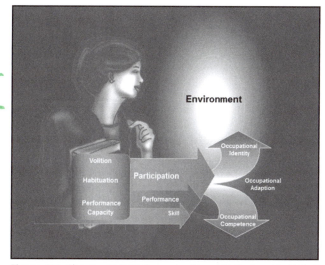

Figure 9-1. The Key MOHO Concepts. (From Kielhofner, G. (Ed.), *A model of human occupation: Theory and application (4th ed.)*, Baltimore, MD. Copyright © 2008 by Lippincott, Williams & Wilkins. Reprinted with permission.)

THE MODEL OF HUMAN OCCUPATION: THEORETICAL ASSUMPTIONS

The person, environment, and occupation are the focus of many theoretical frameworks that address occupation in occupational therapy literature (Baum & Christiansen, 2005; Brown, 2014; Townsend & Polatajko, 2007), albeit that they differ in how they view the interface among these three. MOHO was the first of these frameworks to draw on a systems theory perspective to conceptualize the interplay among personal factors, environmental factors, and what people do in daily life (i.e., their occupation) in a dynamic way that allows for appreciating and explaining the factors that contribute to how individuals' particular experiences in occupations unfold over time, and how change can occur. Thus, MOHO asserts the following:

- Persons and their environments are inextricably linked in a constantly unfolding dynamic that contributes to how persons choose, organize, and perform occupation within given contexts.

- What a person does in daily life (his or her occupation) results from the interplay of the person's inner characteristics (volition, habituation, performance capacity) and the environmental conditions.

- A person's inner capacities, motives, abilities, and routine ways of doing things are shaped, maintained, and changed through engaging in occupations.

- A person's inner characteristics (volition, habituation, performance capacity) and the environmental conditions are all involved in contributing to how changes unfold through occupational engagement (Kielhofner, 2009).

Given that MOHO has developed over more than 30 years, it is important to be aware when reading literature about MOHO that some concepts have been refined

or revised with the emergence of new thinking and evidence on its application in practice. The most current and informative reference is the fourth edition of *A Model of Human of Occupation, Theory and Application* (Kielhofner, 2008). For those wishing to learn more about how MOHO has changed over time, some of the major changes are noted later in this chapter. First, the current key concepts are described here.

Key Concepts

The key concepts in MOHO explain how the inner processes by which people are motivated toward, and choose to engage in, particular occupations (*volition*) organize their actions into patterns and routines (*habituation*) and use and experience their capacities' (*performance capacity*) interplay with characteristics of the environment to contribute to what we each do in daily life. In addition, individuals' cumulative experiences of participation in occupations and development of skilled performance of those occupations over time create a sense of who they are (*occupational identity*) and of being able to sustain participation in occupations consistent with this identity (*occupational competence*; Kielhofner, 2008a, 2009). Furthermore, when individuals experience disrupted participation or difficulties in performing occupations, MOHO provides a way to explain how volition, habituation, performance capacity, and environmental conditions contribute to this situation and impacts their sense of occupational identity and competence.

These key concepts are depicted in Figure 9-1. Each concept, and the ways in which they interact to affect a person's occupational life, is briefly described. Examples of their potential relevance understanding and addressing the difficulties in everyday occupations of a psychosocial nature are included.

Key Person-Related Concepts in MOHO

MOHO identifies three person-related concepts—*volition*, *habituation*, and *performance capacity*—that interact with each other and the environment, to explain how a person's particular occupations are chosen, organized, and performed in daily life.

Volition: Motivating and Choosing Occupations to Engage In

Volition describes how people are motivated toward, and choose, what particular occupations they do. It serves to guide immediate day-to-day choices about participation in activities (such as which toys to play with, meal to prepare, or restaurant to dine at), as well as the longer term commitments that people make to particular occupations (such as extended involvement as a young person in a specific sport or hobby, or as an adult in a particular career; Kielhofner, 2008c).

Volition consists of a person's thoughts and feelings about three issues: how capable and effective the person feels (*personal causation*); what the person considers important or meaningful (*values*); and what the person finds enjoyable and satisfying to do (*interests*). Together, these volitional thoughts and feelings occur through the following cycle:

- *Anticipating possibilities for doing* (e.g., looking forward to an upcoming outing, feeling excited about performing in a sports competition, worrying or feeling anxious about a classroom test or job interview)

- *Choosing what to do* (e.g., making plans for the outing, attending sports training sessions, practice doing the test or interview)

- *Experience while doing* (e.g., enjoying the outing, feeling tired and frustrated during training, feeling confident in a practice test or interview)

- *Interpreting the experience* (e.g., reflecting that outings are enjoyable when well planned, reflecting on poor training performance and committing to work harder before the competition, recalling that having practiced well means feeling better prepared for test or job interview; Kielhofner, 2009)

This means new or altered volitional thoughts and feelings emerge as individuals discover and develop their capacities, skills, and patterns of doing through engagement in occupations, but also that opportunities and resources in the environment play a critical role in creating possibilities for volitional development and change. For example, opportunities for engaging with differing objects and spaces in play support a child's awareness of his or her capacities and interests to develop. In comparison, in the transition to retirement, the kinds of environments in which a person engages in doing change and may contribute to a loss of feelings of capability or usefulness previously gained in the workplace. So, volitional thoughts and feelings have a pervasive influence throughout life on how people view the opportunities and challenges in their environments, what particular occupations people choose to do, and their experiences and views of their occupations (Kielhofner, 2009). Consequently, difficulties in choosing, committing to, and sustaining participation in occupations can arise when people experience changed life circumstances, illness, or disability if, for example, this leads to the following:

- The person's thoughts and feelings about his or her capabilities being undermined.

- The person's loss of sense of pleasure, achievement, or satisfaction accrued from performance.

- The person's participation in valued occupations becoming disrupted.

- The person lacking positive experiences of everyday occupations on which to base occupational choices, or having limited opportunity to exercise valued choices (Kielhofner 2008c).

It follows then that identifying or re-discovering occupations that bring experiences of pleasure, satisfaction, and success, and involvement in occupations that reconnect people with a sense of being able and valued are important in addressing volitional challenges. Indeed, these features are present in the lived experiences of recovering described by people experiencing mental illness, as well as the narratives of people managing ongoing health conditions, such as chronic pain, and occupational transitions, such as retirement (e.g., Davidson, 2003; Jonsson, Josephsson, & Kielhofner, 2001; Kielhofner et al., 2008; Persson, Andersson, & Eklund, 2011).

Habituation: Habits and Roles to Anchor and Organize Daily Life

Everyday life typically involves orchestrating a range of occupations, be they related to taking care of oneself or others, learning, earning an income, play, leisure or community involvement, and so on. The ways in which people organize their participation into patterns and routines is explained in MOHO by the concept of habituation. The importance of these routine aspects of daily life is that, once established, they allow us to efficiently carry out many actions in familiar situations, and to integrate multiple occupations (Kielhofner, 2008d). How people establish and maintain these patterns of action is shaped by *habits* and *roles*.

Habits represent a learned way of doing that becomes established through repeated performance in particular

---

BOX 9-1. DISTINGUISHING OBJECTIVE AND SUBJECTIVE UNDERSTANDINGS OF PERFORMANCE CAPACITY—AN ILLUSTRATION

In the following quotes from her narrative, Lisa described how she experienced the changes occurring in her memory. She spoke of feeling "somewhat of a chaos inside", and evoked images of "sticky mess" in her head and of "all small things become huge houses" to convey how she experienced her memory difficulties and struggles to manage daily life (Kielhofner, Borell, Holzmueller et al. 2008, p. 119). Understanding Lisa's cognitive function from an objective viewpoint would be important to appreciate the extent of change in her cognitive capacities (for which another model may be used). Using MOHO to attend to Lisa's lived experience of performance offers clues to one of the ways in which therapy might aim to support Lisa in managing her life: through identifying and implementing strategies that experientially reduce Lisa's sense of chaos and being overwhelmed in everyday tasks, for which not only Lisa's environment, but also her volition, habits and roles would need taking into account.

---

contexts. They include habitual ways of performing routine activities, of using time, and of behaving in specific familiar situations.

Roles represent social and cultural ideas about identity and associated expectations of what people should do and how they should behave (e.g., student, worker, retiree, parent). They are learned and internalized through interactions with others, and in turn serve as maps of how to behave in particular social contexts.

Being linked to time and place means that habits, routines, and roles bring temporal rhythm to daily life and are elicited by specific physical and social contexts (Clark, 2000; Kielhofner, 2008d). Thus, a loss or lack of valued social roles, as too frequently experienced by people with mental illness (Eklund, Leufstadius,& Bejerholm, 2009), can contribute to difficulties in structuring time use and maintaining patterns of routine activities. Furthermore, when a person's habitual ways of doing are disrupted by the onset of illness or impairments, actions become more effortful and much of the familiarity, relative ease, and efficiency in everyday life may be lost, so that daily life may no longer be taken for granted (Davidson, 2007; Kielhofner, 2008d). Changed environmental circumstances, like a person moving home, migrating to another country, or changing jobs, may likewise challenge the person's established patterns and routines , which may in turn contribute to daily life being experienced as less familiar, more demanding, and difficult to manage, at least until habits and roles can be reconstructed (Kielhofner, 2008d).

Performance Capacity: Use and Experience of Underlying Capacities in Performance

Performance capacity is concerned with how mental and physical abilities are used and experienced in performance. MOHO acknowledges that capacity for performance is affected by underlying sensory, musculoskeletal, neurological, cardiopulmonary, and other bodily systems since these capacities are called upon and exercised when people are engaged in doing occupations. MOHO also draws a distinction between objective and subjective understandings of performance (Kielhofner, 2009; Kielhofner et al., 2008).

Detailed explanations of how specific performance capacities and underlying body structures and functions contribute to performance from an objective viewpoint are beyond the scope of MOHO. Indeed, Kielhofner (2009) explicitly recommends occupational therapists use MOHO in combination with other frameworks that address specific capacities (i.e., biomechanical, motor control, cognitive) where necessary to guide their reasoning and use of assessments, activity analyses, and interventions in practice. In comparison, MOHO highlights the importance of attending to the lived experience of performance, particularly when people experience limitations in performance. That is, attending to how people's bodies feel to them and how people experience themselves in the world in a lived sense can enhance understanding of how altered experiences affect performance (Kielhofner, 2009). Thus, experiences such as sensory loss, memory difficulties, auditory hallucinations, chronic pain, or fatigue each may alter how person's lived experiences affect his or her world and performance. Box 9-1 provides an example.

KEY CONCEPTS IN MOHO CONCERNING ENVIRONMENT

MOHO emphasizes that what people do in daily life results from the dynamic interplay of person-related characteristics (volition, habituation, and performance capacity) with the particular features of their environments (Kielhofner, 2008c). The environment is conceptualized as those physical, social, cultural, economic, and political features of a person's context that influence choices and motivation, organization, and performance of occupation. For instance, economic and political conditions shape individuals' resources (including the spaces and objects available for use) and opportunities for doing; cultural and social groups (e.g., family, friends, neighbors, club/team members, coworkers) influence beliefs about what is important, what should be done, how it should be done, and the kinds of objects used in occupations.

The impact of features in a particular environment may be either to create opportunity, support, and direct a person's engagement in occupation or to constrain it. Thus, some features may create opportunities and resources that support individuals in choosing, doing, interacting with others, and sustaining motivation, whereas other features can limit or direct what people do in ways that either enable or constrain action and motivation (e.g., based on their physical features, social norms, rules, regulations, and laws). Nevertheless, the actual effect on a specific person depends on the interaction of his or her volition, habituation, and performance capacity with the particular environment (Kielhofner, 2008e). For example, individuals experiencing persistent mental ill-health, as well as people experiencing disability, all too often face economic, attitudinal, and systemic barriers to employment that constrain their options and resources for engaging in valued occupations (Fossey & Harvey, 2010; Gewurtz & Kirsh, 2009). Yet, even within these economic and political conditions, some individuals will sustain employment in workplaces where there are jobs suited to their interests and skills, and employers and coworkers provide an inclusive environment.

KEY CONCEPTS RELATED TO DOING AND CRAFTING AN OCCUPATIONAL LIFE

Dimensions of Doing: Occupational Participation, Performance, and Skill

MOHO identifies three interconnected levels at which it is possible to describe doing: skills, performance, and participation. Skills are conceptualized as the discrete goal-directed actions used in performing a specific task (occupational performance). For instance, performing a task, like making a phone call, involves a series of discrete actions, such as lifting, gripping, and manipulating a mobile phone in one's hand, initiating and sequencing the necessary steps to call the number, and speaking when the call is answered. In turn, performing a task, like making a phone call, may be one of a cluster of related activities or tasks undertaken in participating in an occupation, such as doing one's job, pursuing a hobby or sport, or caring

for a friend or family member (occupational participation; Kielhofner 2009).

Difficulties in performing skills can limit the effectiveness of a person's occupational performance, such as his or her efficiency, safety, or independence, but also affect the person's experience of participation. From a MOHO perspective, limited experience or confidence in using specific skills, impaired capacities, and environmental barriers may each contribute to these difficulties, so that appreciating how these personal and environmental factors interrelate is necessary to understand a person's difficulties in doing (Kielhofner, 2008f).

Crafting an Occupational Life: Occupational Identity, Competence, and Adaptation

Broadly speaking, MOHO conceptualizes occupations as having a dynamic and ongoing influence on our sense of who we are and what we are capable of as we develop and respond to life changes during our lives (Kielhofner, 2008f). In other words, our cumulative experiences of participating in occupations over time contribute to creating an occupational identity based in how we view ourselves, what we are capable of, and what we envision for ourselves in narrative terms (within a life story). Occupational identity then reflects the subjective meanings that occupations bring to one's life (Braveman, 2012; Kielhofner, 2008g; Kielhofner et al., 2008). In turn, the degree to which we are able to put that sense of identity into action through sustained participation contributes to a sense of occupational competence. For example, experiences of participating in work and fulfilling the responsibilities involved will support the development of a positive occupational identity as a worker; sustained participation in work at a standard that is personally satisfying and meets workplace expectations will contribute to a sense of occupational competence. Evidence for these two elements of occupational adaptation was developed through studies of the occupational performance history interview (Kielhofner, Mallinson, Forsyth 2001; see Table 9-1 for more details). Similar processes of realizing an occupational identity through everyday acts of doing, and through recrafting a positive sense of identity and competence through participating in meaningful and satisfying occupations are recognized as elements of experiencing recovery and well-being following mental illness (Davidson, 2003).

A particular characteristic of MOHO is that it provides a dynamic framework for appreciating and explaining the factors contributing to individuals' occupational lives, and how their particular experiences of disruptions or problems in occupations have unfolded over time, whether resulting from life transitions, changed capacities, or environmental circumstances. As this practitioner perspective illustrates:

	TABLE 9-1
	SOME EXAMPLES OF MOHO ASSESSMENTS RELEVANT TO PSYCHOSOCIAL PRACTICE
Model of Human Occupation Screening Tool (MOHOST) (Parkinson et al., 2006) Short Child Occupational Profile (Bowyer et al., 2008)	MOHOST is designed for adults and Short Child Occupational Profile for use with children with wide-ranging health conditions. Information gathered provides an overview of how factors in the areas of volition, habituation, performance and environment impact participation in occupation Designed to combine varied information sources (e.g., talking or engaging in occupations with the person, talking with family members and practitioners, chart review) and to integrate this information in a format readily understood by those in other professions and team colleagues Useful to screen referrals, explore needs and desired changes to participation in occupations, and identify participation-related outcomes (Cook, 2012)
Occupational Self-Assessment (OSA) (Baron et al., 2006) Child Occupational Self-Assessment (COSA) (Keller et al., 2005)	OSA is designed for adults and COSA for use with children with wide-ranging health conditions. Occupational competence in 21 everyday activities, the importance of these activities, and their priorities for change are self-rated. Like the Canadian Occupational Performance Measure, OSA and COSA encourage working in partnership and identification of participation-focused goals and plans (Kirsh & Cockburn, 2009), but they offer a potentially more structured approach to client-centered assessment. The legitimacy of clients' viewpoints may sometimes be questioned in psychosocial practice; clients nevertheless have a perspective of what is happening and what they think needs to change that is important to understand.
Role Checklist (Oakley et al., 1986)	Suitable for use with adolescents and adults A brief checklist gathering information about the perceived value and past, present, and anticipated future role participation in 10 roles Used to identify patterns in role involvement, such as role loss or over-commitment, and to assess role change outcomes (Kielhofner et al., 2008)
Occupational Performance History Interview II (Kielhofner et al., 2004)	A detailed semi-structured interview that explores the person's occupational history, focusing on occupational choices and experiences, daily living routines and environments, and changes brought about by health conditions and/or other life circumstances It yields a narrative life history and scales reflecting occupational identity, occupational competence and environmental impact on participation Helpful for building partnerships with clients and attending closely to their lived experiences; may also support clients and careers in making sense of these experiences and their impact on everyday life (Apte et al., 2005; Chaffey & Fossey, 2004; Ennals & Fossey, 2007; Kielhofner et al., 2008)
Occupational Circumstances Assessment Interview & Rating Scale (OCAIRS) (Forsyth et al., 2005)	Semi-structured interview gathers information about volition, habits and roles, environmental impact on participation, and readiness for change. Specific interview formats for use in forensic, mental health, and physical rehabilitation settings are available, as are guidelines for using OCAIRS in combination with either MOHOST or WRI. Used to gather a profile of strengths and challenges, identify long- and short-term goals, and inform therapy and discharge planning (Kielhofner et al., 2008)

(continued)

TABLE 9-1 (continued)	
SOME EXAMPLES OF MOHO ASSESSMENTS RELEVANT TO PSYCHOSOCIAL PRACTICE	
Worker Role Interview (WRI) (Braveman et al., 2005) Work Environment Impact Scale (WEIS) (Moore-Corner et al., 1989)	Two semi-structured interviews with a focus on the occupation of work WRI explores the impact of volition, habituation and perceptions of the work environment on psychosocial readiness for work (Lee & Kielhofner, 2010) WEIS explores the impact of workplace characteristics on participation and enables clients to identify workplace adjustments to experience success in employment; it is therefore more suited to workers with difficulties in current or recent jobs (Lee & Kielhofner, 2010; Wastberg et al., 2012; Williams et al., 2010)
School Settings Interview (SSI) (Hemmingsson et al., 2005)	Semi-structured interview designed to assess the impact of the school environment, including classrooms, playground and other facilities, on the student, and the need for reasonable accommodations in the school setting Designed to provide an opportunity for students with disabilities to voice their experiences, preferences, and needs (Kielhofner et al., 2008)
Residential Environment Impact Survey (REIS) (Fisher et al., 2008)	The REIS was developed to assess the residential environment in 24 areas, but also to determine its impact on residents through observation or interview. A short form is also available for use to understand the quality of an individual's home environment in terms of its impact on his or her participation in occupations that he or she needs, wants, or is expected to do (Parkinson et al., 2011a, 2011b).
Volitional Questionnaire (VQ) (de las Heras et al., 2007) Pediatric Volitional Questionnaire (PVQ) (Basu et al., 2008)	VQ is designed for use with individuals with whom assessment of volition through verbal report is not feasible; PVQ is similar and intended for use with young children (Kielhofner et al., 2008). VQ and PVQ gather in-depth information through observation about volition and the impact of environments on an adult or child's volition while engaged in occupations. The use of observation recognizes that clients communicate their interests, preferences, and volitional feelings through actions, when they may not do so verbally. Individuals are rated on 14 items reflecting these aspects of volition in behavioral terms. The remotivation process (de las Heras et al., 2003), an intervention protocol for addressing volitional challenges, uses the VQ or PVQ to guide the intervention and assess change (Kielhofner et al., 2008).
Assessment of Motor and Process Skills (AMPS) (Fisher, 1997; Fisher & Bray Jones, 2010a, 2010b)	AMPS is used to observe and evaluate the quality of a person's performance in culturally relevant and familiar personal or domestic activities of daily living tasks. It focuses on observable actions, namely motor and process skills, necessary for task performance, allowing the occupational therapist to identify strengths and difficulties that have an impact on physical effort, efficiency, safety, and independence in ADL task performance. Wide applicability exists for use with people of differing ages and diagnostic conditions to inform therapy and measure outcomes; there is extensive supporting research (www.innovativeotsolutions.com/content/).

"The dynamic aspect of the model, the interrelation between its components and its constant interaction with the environment, gives me a 'movie' about my client instead of a still picture." (Genevieve Pepin, cited on the MOHO website: www.cade.uic.edu/moho/resources/perspects/index.aspx). In turn, this means MOHO provides a dynamic way to consider how change can occur.

THE PROCESS OF CHANGE AND THERAPY

MOHO asserts that development and change are driven by clients' occupational engagement (i.e., by what clients do, think, and feel when engaged in occupations

Box 9-2. Dimensions of Occupational Engagement.

Choose / decide—Engaging in occupations presents wide-ranging options to enact choices and decisions of varying complexity about not only what to do, but also what tools and materials to use (e.g., toys to play with, clothes to wear, foods to cook, equipment for home maintenance tasks), how something might be done (e.g., whether done alone, in company, with assistance of a carer, use of a particular technique) and so on. Often exercising such choices in occupational engagement is critical to clients regaining a sense of control or power in their lives.

Explore—Investigating new options for what to do or how, trying out or experimenting with new ways of doing, and weighing up experiences and possibilities for participation allow informed decisions about occupational engagement

Commit—Committing to a course of action (e.g., to accomplish a goal like return to study or work, to take on a project, to make a change in daily routines to achieve a healthier lifestyle) is necessary to achieve and sustain change, whether that be over weeks, months or longer term.

Identify—Locating new information (e.g., from feedback, learning, examining alternatives) that offers a different perspective, new knowledge, solutions and/or meanings to guide subsequent actions

Negotiate—Involves finding the middle ground between different expectations, plans, wishes (e.g., with family members about managing chores, with work supervisors about how jobs are done, within social groups). Negotiating successfully with others is critical to occupational engagement in many social contexts, including an important contributor to change when a collaborative context for therapy is fostered.

Plan—Thinking through and planning new courses of action, so as to maximise the likelihood of success when attempting to do something new or a new way of doing.

Practice—Repeatedly engaging in a particular occupation so as to build and consolidate skill, or to improve the ease and effectiveness with which it is performed.

Re-examine—Appraising one's occupational engagement (e.g., ways of doing, thinking and feeling), so as to recognise strengths and issues and consider alternative options necessary to bring about change.

Sustain—Persisting or persevering with occupational performance or participation over time despite the effort involved or presence of difficulties (e.g., pain, slow progress, setbacks), so as to attain the benefits of sustained occupational engagement (e.g., new learning, achievement, satisfaction, friendship).

---

under particular environmental conditions (Kielhofner & Forsyth, 2008a). Consequently, volition, habituation, performance capacity, and environmental conditions are all involved in contributing to how change processes unfold. For this reason, how these person- and environment-related factors are interacting needs to be attended to during the course of therapy (Kielhofner, 2009; Kielhofner & Forsyth, 2008a). Moreover, MOHO identifies nine dimensions of occupational engagement that are important contributors to change during therapy or as a result of therapy, as briefly described in Box 9-2. For therapists, these dimensions provide a useful structure for thinking about how clients can achieve change through occupational engagement, and how therapy may be planned to support this. More detailed descriptions with client scenarios in Kielhofner and Forsyth (2008a) illustrate their use in practice.

Origins and Key Developers

Gary Kielhofner is the primary theorist and scholar associated with the MOHO, notwithstanding that many occupational therapy scholars and practitioners have contributed to its ongoing development. MOHO was first outlined in a series of papers by Kielhofner and two colleagues over 30 years ago (Kielhofner, 1980a; 1980b; Kielhofner & Burke, 1980; Kielhofner, Burke, & Heard, 1980). The first reference text on MOHO was published 5 years later (Kielhofner, 1985). Three further editions followed in 1995, 2002, and 2008, including substantial revisions to integrate emerging ideas, theory, and evidence from research and practice, and to elaborate its practice applications. The scholarship and extensive research that have contributed to MOHO's development as a framework for occupation-focused, client-centered, and evidence-informed practice reflect the late Dr. Gary Kielhofner's major academic accomplishments and contributions to occupational therapy over his career, but also the collaborative efforts of many occupational therapy practitioners and scholars internationally who have made, and continue to make, substantial contributions.

The early development of MOHO was influenced by the work in the late 1960s and 1970s of Dr. Mary Reilly, with whom Kielhofner studied as a graduate student. Reilly (1962) emphasized the importance of occupation as central to human life, achievement, and adaptation, reaffirming many of the ideas about occupation upon which the profession was founded in the early 20th century (including those of Adolf Meyer, an American physician and psychiatrist considered one of the founders of occupational therapy in the United States). Meyer had sought to understand how mental illness develops and manifests within the context of everyday life, and emphasized the need to understand patients as persons with biographies, everyday lives and social worlds, as well as their biology (Davidson, Rakfeldt, & Strauss, 2010). Furthermore, he considered that occupation served as an organizing force for health and adaptation by bringing structure and meaning to the use of time, and the means to exercise one's physical and mental capacities (Kielhofner, 1977). This idea underpins Reilly's call for occupational therapists to focus on occupation as a means to elicit healthy behavior and to facilitate clients' exploration and mastery of daily living, work, and play environments through occupational behavior (Reilly, 1962), as well as MOHO's view that occupational engagement is the central means by which human development and change occur. Thus, MOHO may be considered a further articulation of Meyer and Reilly's work, building on their ideas about occupation and health, including the following:

- Humans maintain themselves in the world of reality through being actively engaged in occupations that bring meaning, purpose, and pleasure to the use of time.

- Occupation engages and exercises the mind and body in an integrated fashion.

- Balanced use of capacities is essential to health, so that health in occupational terms is reflected in the pattern and organization of one's use of time in daily life.

- Enforced idleness (or lack of occupation) results in demoralization, breakdown of habits, physical deterioration, and loss of abilities, but so, too, activity imposed by others without the person's choosing may be detrimental to mental health and well-being.

- Specific physical and social contexts may contribute to difficulties in everyday living, but are also adaptable to create possible solutions, or a better fit between the person and the demands of the environment.

- The healing and restorative potential of occupation comes from opportunities to discover interest, try out and engage in freely chosen occupations—not from specific prescriptions of what to do or how to act in life (Davidson et al., 2010; Kielhofner, 1977, 2009; Meyer, 1922/1977).

In addition, MOHO draws strongly from an interdisciplinary knowledge base, in particular from psychology and social sciences. Systems thinking, theories of person-environment interaction from gerontology and psychology, motivation theories, and a developmental perspective have been drawn together to articulate how individuals choose, organize, and orchestrate their occupations, and how their patterns of participation develop and are sustained across the lifespan.

IMPORTANT EVOLUTIONARY POINTS

While a number of occupation-focused practice frameworks have since developed in occupational therapy, Bruce and Borg (2002) argued that MOHO led the way in articulating a practice focused on ideas about occupation and its healing potential on which the profession was founded. Its ongoing development through applications in practice and research over 30 years means many of the original MOHO concepts remain but there are also significant differences between MOHO as originally conceptualized and the most recent version (Kielhofner, 2008a). Some notable differences are discussed below.

Kielhofner and colleagues (1980, 1985) originally drew on general systems theory to provide an organizing framework for describing the MOHO concepts, and explaining relationships among them in terms of intake, throughput, and output mechanisms. Thus, the environment was viewed as a source of information taken in by the person (intake) and acted upon in performing an occupation (output), with volition, habituation, and performance subsystems being the throughput for processing information necessary to choose, organize, and perform occupations. The volition, habituation, and the mind-brain-body subsystems were also originally conceptualized as hierarchically organized. This is strikingly different to the way in which the relationships among MOHO concepts have been presented more recently. Instead, acknowledging the influence of dynamical systems thinking, Kielhofner (2008f) described the MOHO concepts as interrelated and mutually influenced, so that what a person does, thinks, and feels arises out of the ongoing and dynamic interplay between volition, habituation, performance capacity, and environmental context. Furthermore, change in any element of volition, habituation, performance capacity, or the environment can alter this dynamic, leading to change in the thoughts, feelings, and doing that make up one's occupational engagement (Kielhofner, 2008g). In turn, this allows for dynamic explanations of disruption and possibilities for positive change.

The ways in which doing, performance, and performance capacity are conceptualized in MOHO have also changed, and illustrate the contributions of other scholars' research to the theoretical development of MOHO. Originally, MOHO did not make a clear distinction between underlying performance capacities (e.g., sensory, musculoskeletal, neurological, cognitive) and the skills enacted during performance (e.g., lifting, gripping, initiating) of an occupation. The work of Dr. Anne Fisher and colleagues to develop the AMPS (Doble, 1991; Fisher, 1997; Fisher & Bray Jones, 2010a, 2010b) contributed taxonomies of motor and process skills, but also conceptualized skilled action as distinct from performance capacity. That is, skills are enacted in the midst of doing, so that characteristics of the person (volition, habituation, and performance capacity) and the environment together contribute to the possibilities for skilled action and the effectiveness of the skill performance (e.g., effort involved, efficiency, safety; Fisher, 2013; Kielhofner, 2008f). In practice, this serves to guide our thinking to more clearly distinguish evaluations and intervention that directly address impaired performance capacities, such as muscle strength or range of movement, from those that focus on the quality of a person's occupational performance under specific environmental conditions.

Performance capacity has also been redefined. Thus, more recently, MOHO has distinguished two understandings of performance capacity: an objective perspective of capacity to perform and a lived experience perspective of performing. A phenomenological understanding of "lived body" and the research of Swedish occupational therapists to understand subjective experiences of disability (e.g., Tham, Borell, & Gustavsson, 2000) have informed this shift in how performance capacity is conceptualized in MOHO. In these ways, MOHO explicitly looks beyond objective performance capacities or impairments to consider other factors in explaining the process of performing (doing), including the lived body experience, the enactment of skills under specific environmental conditions, as well as the person's volitional thoughts and feelings, habits, and routines.

Other developments reflect the extent to which scholarship and research has focused on practice applications of MOHO. An extensive range of assessment tools have been developed to support its use; examples are presented in Table 9-1, and MOHO is being used by occupational therapists to develop and deliver occupation-focused services for diverse child, adult, and older adult populations in clinical and community practice settings around the world. More recently, Abelenda, Kielhofner, Suarez-Balcazar, and Kielhofner (2005) and Kielhofner, de la Heras, and Suarez-Balcazar (2011) have illustrated the potential use of MOHO as tool for understanding social injustices, to empower people whose occupational engagement is disrupted by poverty, political, and other societal forces that create social injustice and to address barriers to social justice in their environments. The fourth edition of MOHO (Kielhofner, 2008a) explicitly identifies social, economic, and political conditions as environmental factors that may enable or constrain what people do and how occupations shape and sustain their lives, so that it better lends itself to applications focused on addressing occupational issues framed in social, political, and human rights-based terms (Kielhofner et al., 2011).

USING MOHO IN PRACTICE

Using MOHO to guide practice involves thinking with theory in practice, and moving back and forth between theory and the client's situation to inform one's reasoning (Kielhofner, 2009). Kielhofner and Forsyth (2008c) describe a therapeutic reasoning process to guide therapists' use of MOHO concepts in thinking about client situations, planning, and implementing therapy. This therapeutic reasoning process is intended to be client-centered in reflecting a deep appreciation for clients' circumstances and through involving the client insofar as is possible (Kielhofner, 2009). It is outlined in the following six steps:

1. Generating questions to guide information gathering
2. Gathering information on, from and with the client
3. Creating an understanding of the client
4. Generating therapy goals and strategies
5. Implementing and monitoring therapy
6. Determining outcomes of therapy

Several examples presented elsewhere show how these six therapeutic reasoning steps may be used to guide occupational therapy assessment with children experiencing difficulties in school, occupational therapy services in a chronic pain program, and occupational therapy practice with clients experiencing mental health issues at a community program and a MOHO-based supported employment service (Forsyth et al., 2014; Kielhofner, 2009; O'Brien et al., 2010). Box 9-3 presents a brief summary of each of the six steps of therapeutic reasoning.

GATHERING INFORMATION ON, FROM, AND WITH THE CLIENT

MOHO offers a useful conceptual framework for assessment to understand and address how ongoing health conditions interact with engagement in everyday occupations. These conditions often include enduring and potentially debilitating symptoms, such as pain or fatigue, which can not only significantly disrupt a person's participation, but also the meaning and satisfaction derived from occupations. As Sarah Cook (2012) reflected in the chapter's opening quote, MOHO provides an extensive "toolbox" of assessments for use in psychosocial practice, examples of which are briefly presented in Table 9-1. The use of MOHO to guide assessment is then briefly illustrated, using the example of chronic pain to highlight how a therapist might select from these tools in practice (Box 9-4).

BOX 9-3. THE SIX STEPS OF THERAPEUTIC REASONING

THERAPEUTIC REASONING STEPS	
Generating questions to guide information gathering	When seeking to learn about clients and their situations, therapists generate explicit questions to guide their therapeutic reasoning. MOHO concepts orient therapists to particular kinds of issues (e.g., clients' roles, routines, volitional thoughts and feelings) about which to frame questions to guide information gathering.
	It may be useful to create a set of MOHO-based questions to guide therapeutic reasoning in working with a particular client population. Examples for therapists using MOHO to guide their information gathering in working with older adults or children and their families can be found in Kielhofner and Forsyth (2008b).
Gathering information on, from, and with the client	Therapists may gather information using a range of unstructured and structured methods, the choices being guided by the questions previously generated. Many MOHO-based interview, self-report, and observational tools have been developed for this purpose (see Table 9-1 for examples).
Creating an understanding of the client	Therapists use and organize the information gathered to create a theory-based understanding of the client's occupational life and circumstances. Using MOHO at this step allows the therapist to develop a dynamic explanation of the factors contributing to how his or her particular experiences of disruptions or challenges in occupations, as well as strengths, can be built upon.
Generating therapy goals and strategies	The therapist's theory-based understanding of the client's occupational life and circumstances may guide identifying goals for therapy, what kinds of client occupational engagement will enable change (see Box 9-2 for examples), and what therapeutic strategies are used by the therapist to support the client's occupational engagement (see Box 9-5 for examples). The therapist's ability to respect the client's perspective and to collaborate with the client in this process is also critical.
Implementing and monitoring therapy	Implementing the planned actions and how the therapy unfolds to respond to client feedback, and adjust actions as new information or unanticipated issues emerge
Determining outcomes of therapy	Collecting information through unstructured and structured means to determine the extent to which the client's desired improvements and therapy goals were achieved

More detailed information about these and other MOHO-related tools can be accessed from MOHO Clearinghouse website (www.cade.uic.edu/moho).

PRACTICE APPROACHES

MOHO is used by occupational therapists to guide the development and delivery of occupation-focused services in diverse practice settings internationally. Many examples of its use in assessment, planning, and implementation of occupational therapy with diverse populations and occupation-related challenges are available. For instance, the key textbook (Kielhofner, 2008a) presents practice applications with child, adult, and older adult populations provided in hospital, rehabilitation, home care, long-term residential, and community-based settings. MOHO is also widely used in forensic settings (Munõz, 2011). Further examples relevant to psychosocial practice include the following:

BOX 9-4. SELECTING MOHO ASSESSMENTS: EXAMPLES OF WORKING WITH PERSONS IN PAIN

As an occupation-focused framework to guide assessment of persons in pain, MOHO provides occupational therapists with a way of explaining how a person's pain interacts with his or her engagement in everyday occupations, to compliment the assessment of pain symptoms and severity (Taylor & Fan, 2013). It provides a range of information-gathering tools from which to select for different circumstances:

- The Model of Human Occupation Screening Tool (MOHOST; Parkinson et al., 2006) may be selected, allowing the therapist to use multiple information sources to identify the extent to which pain is interacting with the person's motivation for occupation, habitual pattern of participation, performance skills (motor, process, communication and interaction), and environmental supports and barriers in everyday life (Taylor & Fan, 2013). MOHOST offers a brief structured way to identify key occupational issues and strengths, which can be useful for prioritizing areas for subsequent assessment (e.g., occupational performance, particular environments), as well communicating with the client and team (Forsyth, Kielhofner, Bowyer et al., 2008). The use of MOHOST may or may not strongly reflect the client's perspective, depending on the information sources used.

- The Occupational Self Assessment (OSA; Baron et al., 2006) is also relatively brief; its use would contribute to understanding the client's view of those everyday occupations that are important and his or priorities for change, so as to direct what supports and interventions are provided. For the purpose of understanding of the client's perspective of how chronic pain has impacted his or her occupational life over time, the Occupational Performance History Interview-II (OPHI-II; Kielhofner et al. 2004) may alternatively be used to gather detailed knowledge about the meaning of occupations in the context of chronic pain (Keponen & Kielhofner, 2006).

- The NIH Activity Record (ACTRE; Furst et al., 1987) could be used to enable the client to record his or her time use and the influence of pain and fatigue on each activity undertaken during the day, so as to enhance understanding of his or her patterns of doing and to support self-management of chronic pain in everyday life (Kielhofner, Forsyth, Suman et al., 2008). (See Chapter 10 for further details on ACTRE.)

- For clients who indicate difficulties performing occupations, Assessment of Motor and Process Skills (AMPS; Fisher & Bray Jones, 2010a, 2010b) may be selected to observe their occupational performance and obtain detailed information about its quality, specific skills difficulties and areas of strength, which can in turn be used in decision-making about the directions for therapy (Kielhofner, Cahill, Forsyth et al., 2008).

MOHO provides tools to support the person in pain to identify occupations that hold meaning and value; and to develop strategies that allow sustained participation in these occupations with greater ease and efficiency. It also complements using the Intentional Relationships model and cognitive-behavioral therapy to support clients who experience chronic pain (Taylor & Fan, 2013).

BOX 9-5. THERAPEUTIC STRATEGIES IDENTIFIED BY MOHO

Validating	Identifying	Giving feedback
Advising	Negotiating	Structuring
Coaching	Encouraging	Physically supporting

Reprinted with permission from Boyt Schell, B.A., Scaffa, M., and Gillen, G. (Eds.), *Willard & Spackman's Occupational Therapy (12th ed.),* Philadelphia. Copyright © 2014 by Lippincott, Williams & Wilkins.

- Illustrations of occupation-focused practice involving children with disabilities, adults diagnosed with mental illness, and older adults following the onset of disability (Forsyth & Kielhofner, 2011; Forsyth et al., 2014; Kielhofner et al., 2009; O'Brien et al., 2010)

- The development of the remotivation process, an approach to understand the volitional challenges of clients with any diagnosis and to provide interventions designed to support motivation for occupational engagement (de Las Heras, Llerena, & Kielhofner, 2003; Kielhofner, 2009)

- Uses of MOHO to understand and address the specific disruptions and challenges in everyday occupations experienced by people with persistent pain or fatigue (Taylor & Fan, 2013; Taylor & Kielhofner, 2003) and to explore employment readiness, return to work, and job tenure issues (Ekbladh, Thorell, & Haglund, 2010; Lee & Kielhofner, 2010; Prior et al., 2013; Williams, Fossey, & Harvey, 2012)

- Applications of MOHO to guide the development of wellness programs for older adults (Yamada, Kawamata, Kobayashi, Kielhofner, & Taylor, 2010), inpatient services for people experiencing acute mental illness (Melton, Forsyth, & Metherall, 2008), and employment services (Kielhofner et al., 2004, 2008)

Expected Outcomes and Evaluation Processes

MOHO offers a dynamic explanatory framework within which to understand people's occupational lives. It allows occupational issues and the contributing personal and environmental factors that affect occupational participation and performance to be identified, not only in the present, but also longitudinally. Furthermore, it provides a framework within which to identify mechanisms for enabling change in occupational engagement in a client-centered, occupation-focused manner, and tools and strategies supported by evidence for working with clients therapeutically to enable change (Kielhofner, 2009). Broadly speaking, MOHO focuses on creating opportunities for participation, enabling skill development, collaborative problem-solving, and use of strategies to make environmental adjustments (whether physical and/ or social), with the intended outcome of enabling people's participation in occupations that support recovery, health, well-being, and adaptation (Kielhofner, 2009).

Determining the outcomes of therapy is important to document progress toward and attainment of goals, whether or not one's practice is informed by MOHO. Reviewing the extent to which goals or desired outcomes have been achieved with clients, and re-administering initially conducted assessments to determine changes in scores, are both means by which therapy outcomes can be evaluated (Kielhofner, 2009). A number of MOHO assessment tools are suitable for the latter purpose (see Table 9-1 for examples). For instance, MOHO assessments may be selected for re-administration to identify whether changes in perceived role involvement, perceived

competence in everyday occupations, changes in the impact of volition, habituation, performance, and environment on participation, or changes in the quality of a person's performance in culturally relevant and familiar personal or domestic activities of daily living have been achieved.

Evidence for the Approach

There is more extensive research evidence related to MOHO than other contemporary occupation-focused practice frameworks at this point (Lee, 2010):

- Research that expands or provides support for the MOHO concepts, the relationships among them, and their capacity to predict client change proposed by MOHO as an explanatory framework

- Evidence supporting MOHO assessments as psychometrically sound tools for use in practice

- Studies that examine the practice application of MOHO or its assessments

- Studies to demonstrate the effectiveness of occupational therapy services informed by MOHO (Forsyth & Kielhofner, 2011; Lee, 2010)

It is beyond the scope of this chapter to review this evidence base in detail. Reviews can be found elsewhere (e.g., Kramer, Bowyer, & Kielhofner, 2008; Lee & Kielhofner, 2010), and a substantial bibliography related to MOHO research, assessment tools, practice applications, and supporting evidence can be accessed from MOHOWeb (www.cade.uic.edu/moho).

Conclusion

MOHO is a well-developed occupation-focused model that is widely used in occupational therapy practice generally but also particularly in areas of practice where psychosocial issues are addressed. The model provides a way of understanding how people choose, organize, and orchestrate their occupations and how occupations are refined and sustained over a lifetime. From a psychosocial perspective, the model provides way of understanding how personal attributes such as identity and self-efficacy beliefs, and conditions in the social context are associated with occupational experience and performance. A broad range of assessment and practice tools have been developed with a view to enabling the integration of MOHO theory into practice.

Learning Activities/ Discussion Questions

1. Think of a person (child or adult) accessing occupational therapy services with whom you have contact as an occupational therapy student or occupational therapist and consider the following questions:

    a. What is the person's occupational identity? (Think about what occupations the person identifies with. What roles does the person hold and/or are important in his or her life? Have either the person's occupations or roles changed or been disrupted recently?)

    b. What is the person's occupational competence? (Think about what the person says about him- or herself and how he or she sees his or her abilities, skills, talents, and responsibilities. Are the person's views consistent with what he or she does and envisions doing?)

    c. What are the present positive qualities or strengths for the person's occupational life? (Consider the person's occupational engagement in a range of relevant occupations, the person's interests, values, personal causation, habits, roles, performance capacities, skills, and environmental conditions).

    d. What are the challenges or difficulties engaging in occupations that this person faces? (Consider a range of relevant occupations, volition, habituation, performance capacity, skills, and environment to identify factors contributing to present challenges or difficulties).

2. Write a summary statement describing this person's occupational life, his or her strengths and challenges related to engaging in occupations—either using MOHO language or everyday language to convey MOHO concepts.

3. How might this person achieve change through occupational engagement—using the dimensions in Box 9-2 to structure your thinking, identify three specific things you might do to support this person in her/his occupational engagement (doing, thinking, and feeling).

4. How you might use MOHO concepts and assessments to contribute to your understanding of a person's lived experience of illness or disability and its impact on his or her participation in occupations of daily life?

References

Abelenda, J., Kielhofner, G., Suarez-Balcazar, Y., & Kielhofner, K. (2005). The model of human occupation as a conceptual tool for understanding and addressing occupational apartheid. In F. Kronenberg, S. Simó Algado, & N. Pollard (Eds.) *Occupational therapy without borders. Learning from the spirit of survivors* (pp. 183-196). Edinburgh: Churchill Livingstone/Elsevier.

Apte, A., Kielhofner, G., Paul-Ward, A., & Braveman, B. (2005). Therapists' and clients' perceptions of the Occupational Performance History Interview. *Occupational Therapy in Health Care, 19,* 173-192.

Baron, K., Kielhofner, G., Iyenger, A., Goldhammer, V., & Wolenski, J. (2006). *A user's manual for the Occupational Self Assessment (OSA)* (version 2.2). Chicago: Model of Human Occupation Clearinghouse.

Basu, S., Kafkes, A., Schatz, R., Kiraly, A., & Kielhofner, G. (2008). *The Pediatric Volitional Questionnaire (PVQ)* (version 2.1). Chicago: Model of Human Occupation Clearinghouse.

Baum, C. M., & Christiansen, C. (2005). Person-environment-occupation-performance: An occupation-based framework for practice. In C. H. Christiansen, C. M. Baum, & J. Bass-Haugen (Eds.), *Occupational therapy: Performance, participation, and well-being* (3rd ed., pp. 242-267). Thorofare, NJ: SLACK Incorporated.

Bowyer, P. L., Kramer, J., Ploszaj, A., Ross, M., Schwartz, O., Kielhofner, G., & Kramer, K. (2008). *The Short Child Occupational Profile (SCOPE)* (version 2.2). Chicago: Model of Human Occupation Clearinghouse.

Braveman, B. (2012). Development of the worker role and worker identity. In B. Braveman, & J. J. Page (Eds). *Work: Promoting participation and productivity through occupational therapy,* pp. 28-51. Philadelphia, F. A. Davis.

Braveman, B., Robson, M., Velozo, C., Kielhofner, G., Fisher, G., Forsyth, K., & Kerschbaum, J. (2005). Worker Role Interview (WRI) (version 10.0). Chicago: Model of Human Occupation Clearinghouse.

Brown, C. E. (2014). Ecological models in occupational therapy. In B. A. B. Schell, et al. (Eds.), *Willard and Spackman's occupational therapy* (12th ed., pp. 494-504). Philadelphia: Lippincott, Williams & Wilkins.

Bruce, M. A., & Borg, B. (2002). *Psychosocial frames of reference: Core for occupation-based practice* (3rd ed.). Thorofare, NJ: SLACK Incorporated.

Chaffey, L., & Fossey, E. (2004) Caring and daily life: Occupational experiences of women living with sons diagnosed with schizophrenia. *Australian Occupational Therapy Journal, 51,* 199-207.

Clark, F. (2000). The concept of habit and routine: A preliminary theoretical discussion. *Occupational Therapy Journal of Research. 20*(Supp. 1), 123S-137S.

Cook, S. (2012). Personal reflections on understanding and using the Model of Human Occupation in practice. In G. Boniface, & A. Seymour (Eds). *Using occupational therapy theory in practice* (1st ed., pp. 141-151). Hoboken, NJ: Wiley-Blackwell.

Davidson, L. (2003). *Living outside mental illness: Qualitative studies of recovery in schizophrenia* (vol. 24). New York: New York University Press.

Davidson, L. (2007) Habits and other anchors of everyday life that people with psychiatric disabilities may not take for granted. *OTJR: Occupation, Participation and Health, 27,* Suppl, 60S-68S.

Davidson, L., Rakfeldt, J., & Strauss, J. (2010). *The roots of the recovery movement in psychiatry: Lessons learned.* Chichester: John Wiley & Sons Ltd.

de las Heras, C. G., Geist, R., Kielhofner, G., & Li, Y. (2007). *The Volitional Questionnaire (VQ)* (version 4.1). Chicago: Model of Human Occupation Clearinghouse.

de las Heras, C. G., Llerena, V., & Kielhofner, G. (2003). *A user's manual for remotivation process: Progressive intervention for individuals with severe motivational challenges.* Chicago: Model of Human Occupation Clearinghouse.

Doble, S. E. (1991). Test-retest and inter-rater reliability of a process skills assessment. *Occupational Therapy Journal of Research, 11,* 8-23.

Ekbladh, E., Thorell, L., & Haglund, L. (2010). Return to work: The predictive value of the Worker Role Interview (WRI) over two years. *Work, 35,* 163-172.

Eklund, M., Leufstadius, C., & Bejerholm, U. (2009). Time use among people with psychiatric disabilities: Implications for practice. *Psychiatric Rehabilitation Journal, 32*(3), 177-191.

Ennals, P., & Fossey E. (2007). The Occupational Performance History Interview (OPHI-II) in adult community mental health settings: Consumers' and occupational therapists' perspectives. *Australian Occupational Therapy Journal, 54*(1), 11-21.

Farnworth, L. (2004). Time use and disability. In M. Molineux (Ed.) *Occupation for occupational therapists* (pp. 46-65). Hoboken, NJ: Blackwell Publishing.

Fisher, A. G. (1997). Multifaceted measurement of daily life task performance: Conceptualizing a test of instrumental ADL and validating the addition of personal ADL tasks. *Physical Medicine and Rehabilitation: State of the Art Reviews, 11,* 289-303.

Fisher, A. G. (2013). Occupation-centred, occupation-based, occupation-focused: Same, same or different? *Scandinavian Journal of Occupational Therapy, 20,* 162-173.

Fisher, A. G., & Bray Jones, K. (2010a). *Assessment of Motor and Process Skills. Volume. 1: Development, standardization, and administration manual* (7th ed.) Fort Collins, CO: Three Star Press.

Fisher, A. G., & Bray Jones, K. (2010b). *Assessment of Motor and Process Skills. Volume. 2: User manual* (7th ed.) Fort Collins, CO: Three Star Press.

Fisher, G., Arriaga, P., Less, C., Lee, J., & Ashpole, E. (2008). *Residential Environment Impact Survey (REIS)* (version 2.0). Chicago: Model of Human Occupation Clearinghouse.

Forsyth, K., Deshpande, S., Kielhofner, G., Henriksson, C., Haglund, L., Olson, L.,...Kulkarni, S. (2005) *The Occupational Circumstances Assessment Interview and Rating Scale (OCAIRS)* (version 4.0). Chicago: Model of Human Occupation Clearinghouse.

Forsyth, K., & Kielhofner, G. (2011). The model of human occupation: embracing the complexity of occupation by integrating theory into practice and practice into theory. In E. A. S. Duncan (Ed.). *Foundations for practice in occupational therapy* (5th ed., Chapter 6, pp. 51-80). Edinburgh: Elsevier.

Forsyth, K., Kielhofner, G., Bowyer, P., Kramer, K., Ploszaj, A., Blondis, M.,...Parkinson, S. (2008). Assessments combining methods of information gathering. In G. Kielhofner (Ed.), *Model of human occupation: Theory and application* (4th ed., pp. 288-310). Baltimore, MD: Lippincott, Williams & Wilkins.

Forsyth, K., Taylor, R. R., Kramer, J. M., Prior, S., Richie, L., Whitehead, J.,...Melton, J. (2014). The model of human occupation. In B. A. B. Schell, et al. (Eds.), *Willard and Spackman's occupational therapy* (12th ed., pp. 505-526). Philadelphia: Lippincott, Williams & Wilkins.

Fossey, E., & Harvey C. A. (2010). Finding and sustaining mainstream employment: A qualitative meta-synthesis of mental health consumer views. *Canadian Journal of Occupational Therapy, 77*(5), 303-314.

Furst, G., Gerber, L., Smith, C., Fisher, S., & Shulman, B. (1987). A program for improving energy conservation behaviors in adults with rheumatoid arthritis. *American Journal of Occupational Therapy, 41,* 102-111.

Gewurtz, R., & Kirsh, B. (2009). Disruption, disbelief and resistance: A meta-synthesis of disability in the workplace. *Work, 34,* 33-44.

Hemmingsson, H., Egilson, S., Hoffman, O., & Kielhofner, G. (2005). *The School Setting Interview (SSI)* (version 3.0). Chicago: Model of Human Occupation Clearinghouse.

Jonsson, H., Josephsson, S., & Kielhofner, G. (2001). Narratives and experience in an occupational transition: A longitudinal study of the retirement process. *American Journal of Occupational Therapy, 55*(4), 424-432.

Keller, J., Kafkes, A., Basu, S., Federico, J., & Kielhofner, G. (2005) *A user's manual for the Child Occupational Self Assessment (COSA)* (version 2.1). Chicago: Model of Human Occupation Clearinghouse.

Keponen, R., & Kielhofner, G. (2006). Occupation and meaning in the lives of women with chronic pain. *Scandinavian Journal of Occupational Therapy, 13,* 211-220.

Kielhofner, G. (1977). Temporal adaptation: A conceptual framework for occupational therapy. *American Journal of Occupational Therapy, 31,* 235-247.

Kielhofner, G. (1980a). A model of human occupation, part two. Ontogenesis from the perspective of temporal adaptation. *American Journal of Occupational Therapy, 34,* 657-663.

Kielhofner, G. (1980b). A model of human occupation, part three. Benign and vicious cycles. *American Journal of Occupational Therapy, 34,* 731-737.

Kielhofner, G. (1985). (Ed.) *A model of human occupation: Theory and application.* Baltimore, MD: Williams & Wilkins.

Kielhofner, G. (2008a). (Ed.) *A model of human occupation: Theory and application* (4th ed.). Baltimore, MD: Lippincott, Williams & Wilkins.

Kielhofner, G. (2008b). The basic concepts of human occupation. In G. Kielhofner (Ed.), *Model of human occupation: Theory and application* (4th ed., pp. 11-23). Baltimore, MD: Lippincott, Williams & Wilkins.

Kielhofner, G. (2008c). Volition. In G. Kielhofner (Ed.), *Model of Human Occupation: Theory and application* (4th edition ed., pp. 32-50). Baltimore, MD: Lippincott, Williams & Wilkins.

Kielhofner, G. (2008d) Habituation: Patterns of daily occupation. In G. Kielhofner (Ed.), *Model of human occupation: Theory and application* (4th ed., pp. 51-67). Baltimore, MD: Lippincott, Williams & Wilkins.

Kielhofner, G. (2008e). The environment and human occupation. In G. Kielhofner (Ed.), *Model of human occupation: Theory and application* (4th ed., pp. 85-100). Baltimore, MD: Lippincott, Williams & Wilkins.

Kielhofner, G. (2008f). Dimensions of doing. In G. Kielhofner (Ed.), *Model of human occupation: Theory and application* (4th ed., pp. 101-109). Baltimore, MD: Lippincott, Williams & Wilkins.

Kielhofner, G. (2008g). The dynamics of human occupation. In G. Kielhofner (Ed.), *Model of human occupation: Theory and application* (4th ed., pp. 24-31). Baltimore, MD: Lippincott, Williams & Wilkins.

Kielhofner, G. (2009). *Conceptual foundations of occupational therapy.* (4th ed.). Philadelphia: F. A. Davis.

Kielhofner, G., Borell, L., Holzmueller, R., Jonsson, H., Josephsson, S., Keppnnen, R.,...Nygard, L. (2008). Crafting occupational life. In G. Kielhofner (Ed.), *Model of human occupation: Theory and application,* (pp. 110-125). Baltimore, MD: Lippincott, Williams & Wilkins.

Kielhofner, G., Braveman, B., Finlayson, M., Paul-Ward, A., Goldbaum, L., & Goldstein, K. (2004). Outcomes of a vocational program for persons with AIDS. *American Journal of Occupational Therapy, 58,* 64-72.

Kielhofner, G., Braveman, B., Fogg, L., & Levin, M. (2008). A controlled study of services to enhance productive participation among people with HIV/AIDS. *American Journal of Occupational Therapy, 62,* 36-45.

Kielhofner, G., & Burke, J. (1980). A model of human occupation, part one. Conceptual framework and content. *American Journal of Occupational Therapy, 34,* 572-581.

Kielhofner, G., Burke, J., & Heard, I. C. (1980). A model of human occupation, part four. Assessment and intervention. *American Journal of Occupational Therapy, 34,* 777-788.

Kielhofner, G., Cahill, S. M., Forsyth, K., de las Heras, C. G., Melton, J., Raber, C., & Prior, S. (2008). Observational assessments. In G. Kielhofner (Ed.), *Model of human occupation: Theory and application* (4th ed., pp. 217-236). Baltimore, MD: Lippincott, Williams & Wilkins.

Kielhofner, G., de la Heras, C., & Suarez-Balcazar, Y. (2011). Human occupation as a tool for understanding and promoting social justice. In F. Kronenberg, N. Pollard, & D. Sakellariou (Eds.), *Occupational therapies without borders. Volume. 2: Towards an ecology of occupation-based practices* (pp. 269-277). Edinburgh: Churchill Livingstone/Elsevier.

Kielhofner, G., & Forsyth, K. (2008a). Occupational engagement: How clients achieve change. In G. Kielhofner, *A model of human occupation: Theory and application* (4th ed., pp. 171-184). Baltimore, MD: Lippincott, Williams & Wilkins.

Kielhofner, G., & Forsyth, K. (2008b). Therapeutic reasoning: Planning, implementing, and evaluating the outcomes of therapy. In G. Kielhofner, *A model of human occupation: Theory and application* (4th ed., pp. 143-154). Baltimore, MD: Lippincott, Williams & Wilkins.

Kielhofner, G., & Forsyth, K. (2008c). Therapeutic strategies for enabling change. In G. Kielhofner, *A model of human occupation: Theory and application* (4th ed., pp. 185-203). Baltimore, MD: Lippincott, Williams & Wilkins.

Kielhofner, G., Forsyth, K., Clay, C., Ekbladh, E., Haglund, L., Hemmingsson, H.,...Olson, L. (2008). Talking with clients: Assessments that collect information through interviews. In G. Kielhofner, (Ed.), *Model of human occupation: Theory and application* (4th ed., pp. 262-287). Baltimore, MD: Lippincott, Williams & Wilkins.

Kielhofner, G., Forsyth, K., Kramer, J., Melton, J., & Dobson, E. (2009). The model of human occupation. In E. B. Crepeau, E. S. Cohn, & B. A. Boyt Schell (Eds.), *Willard & Spackman's occupational therapy* (11th ed., pp. 446-461). Philadelphia, PA: Lippincott, Williams, & Wilkins.

Kielhofner, G., Forsyth, K., Suman, M. Kramer, J., Nakamura-Thomas, H. Yamada, T.,...Henry, A. (2008). Self-reports: Eliciting client's perspectives. In G. Kielhofner (Ed.), *Model of human occupation: Theory and application* (4th ed., pp. 237-261). Baltimore, MD: Lippincott, Williams & Wilkins.

Kielhofner, G., Mallinson, T., Crawford, C., Nowak, M., Rigby, M., Henry, A., & Walens, D. (2004). *Occupational Performance History Interview II (OPHI-II) (version 2.1).* Chicago: MOHO Clearinghouse.

Kielhofner, G., Mallinson, T., Forsyth, K., & Lai, J-S. (2001). Psychometric properties of the second version of the Occupational Performance History Interview (OPHI-II). *American Journal of Occupational Therapy, 55*(3), 260-267.

Kielhofner, G., Tham, K., Baz, T. & Hutson, J. (2008). Performance capacity and lived body. In G. Kielhofner (Ed.), *Model of human occupation: Theory and application* (4th ed., pp. 68-84). Baltimore, MD: Lippincott, Williams & Wilkins.

Kirsh, B., & Cockburn, L. (2009). The Canadian Occupational Performance Measure: A tool for recovery-based practice. *Psychiatric Rehabilitation Journal, 32*(3), 171-176.

Kramer, J., Bowyer, P., & Kielhofner, G. (2008). Evidence for practice from the model of human occupation. In G. Kielhofner (Ed.), *Model of human occupation: Theory and application* (4th ed., pp. 466-505). Baltimore, MD: Lippincott, Williams & Wilkins.

Lee, J. (2010). Achieving best practice: A review of evidence linked to occupation-focused practice models. *Occupational Therapy in Health Care, 24,* 206-222.

Lee, J. (2012). Occupational therapy conceptual practice models and related knowledge to support work practice. In B. Braveman, & J. J. Page (Eds.), *Work: Promoting participation and productivity through occupational therapy* (pp. 78-97). Philadelphia, F. A. Davis.

Lee, J., & Kielhofner, G. (2010). Vocational intervention based on the model of human occupation: A review of evidence. *Scandinavian Journal of Occupational Therapy, 17*, 177-190.

Lee, S. W., Taylor, R., Kielhofner, G., & Fisher, G. (2008). Theory use in practice: A national survey of therapists who use the model of human occupation. *American Journal of Occupational Therapy, 62*(1), 106-117.

Melton, J., Forsyth, K., & Metherall, A. (2008). Program redesign based on the model of human occupation: Inpatient services for people experiencing acute mental illness in the UK. *Occupational Therapy in Health Care, 22*(2-3), 37-50.

Meyer, A. (1922/1977). The philosophy of occupational therapy. *American Journal of Occupational Therapy, 31*(10), 639-642.

Moore-Corner, R., Kielhofner, G., & Olsen, L. (1998). *A user's guide to Work Environment Impact Scale (WEIS) (version 2.0)*. Chicago: Model of Human Occupation Clearinghouse.

Munõz, J. P. (2011). Mental health practice in forensic settings. In C. Brown, & V. C. Stoffel (Eds.). *Occupational therapy in mental health: A vision for participation* (pp. 526-545). Philadelphia: F. A. Davis.

Oakley, F., Kielhofner, G., Barris, R., & Reichler, R. K. (1986). The role checklist: Development and empirical assessment of reliability. *Occupational Therapy Journal of Research, 6*, 157-170.

O'Brien, J., Asselin, E., Fortier, K., Janzegers, R., Lagueux, B., & Silcox, C. (2010). Using therapeutic reasoning to apply the model of human occupation in pediatric occupational therapy practice. *Journal of Occupational Therapy, Schools, & Early Intervention, 3*(4), 348-365.

Parkinson, S., Fisher, G., & Fisher, J. (2011a) *Residential Environment Impact Survey—Short Form (REIS-SF) UK (version 2.2)*. Chicago: Model of Human Occupation Clearinghouse.

Parkinson, S., Fisher, G., & Fisher, J. (2011b). Development of an occupation-focused home assessment for use in mental health services. *Mental Health Occupational Therapy, 16*(1): 8-11.

Parkinson, S., Kielhofner, G., & Forsyth, K. (2006). *The Model of Human Occupation Screening Tool (MOHOST) (version 2.0)*. Chicago: Model of Human Occupation Clearinghouse.

Persson, D., Andersson, I., & Eklund, M. (2011). Defying aches and re-evaluating daily doing: Occupational perspectives on adjusting to chronic pain. *Scandinavian Journal of Occupational Therapy, 18*, 188-197.

Polatajko, H. J., Backman, C., Baptiste, S., Davis, J., Eftekar, P., & Harvey, A. (2007). Human occupation in context. In E. A. Townsend, & H. J. Polatajko (Eds.), *Enabling occupation II: Advancing an occupational therapy vision for health, wellbeing and justice through occupation* (pp. 37-61). Ottawa, ON: CAOT Publications ACE.

Prior, S., Maciver, D., Forsyth, K., Walsh, M., Meiklejohn, A., & Irvine, L. (2013). Readiness for employment: Perceptions of mental health service users. *Community Mental Health Journal*, DOI 10.1007/s10597-012-9576-0.

Reilly, M. (1962). Occupational therapy can be one of the great ideas of 20th century medicine. *American Journal of Occupational Therapy, 16*, 1-9.

Smith, N., Kielhofner, G., & Watts, J. (1986). The relationship between volition, activity pattern and life satisfaction in the elderly. *The American Journal of Occupational Therapy, 40*, 278-283.

Taylor, R. R., & Fan, C. W. (2013). Managing pain in occupational therapy: Integrating the model of human occupation and the intentional relationship model. In E. Cara and A. MacRae (Eds.), *Psychosocial approaches to occupational therapy* (3rd ed., pp. 573-642). Independence, KY: Cengage Learning.

Taylor, R. R., & Kielhofner, G. W. (2003). An occupational therapy approach to persons with chronic fatigue syndrome: Part two, assessment and intervention. *Occupational Therapy in Health Care, 17*(2), 63-87.

Taylor, R. R., Kielhofner, G., Abelenda, J., Colantuono, K., Fong, T., Heredia, R.,…Vacquez, E. (2003). An approach to persons with chronic fatigue syndrome based on the model of human occupation: Part one, impact on occupational performance and participation. *Occupational Therapy in Health Care, 17*(2), 47-61.

Tham, K., Borell, L., & Gustavsson, A. (2000). The discovery of disability: A phenomenological study of unilateral neglect. *American Journal of Occupational Therapy, 54*, 398-406.

Townsend, E. A., & Polatajko, H. J. (Eds.). (2007). *Enabling occupation II: Advancing an occupational therapy vision for health, wellbeing and justice through occupation* (pp. 37-61). Ottawa, ON: CAOT Publications ACE.

Wastberg, B. A., Haglund, L., & Eklund, M. (2012). The Work Environment Impact Scale—Self-Rating (WEIS-SR) evaluated in primary health care in Sweden. *Work: Journal of Prevention, Assessment & Rehabilitation, 42*(3), 447-457.

Wilcock, A. A. (2006). *An occupational perspective of health* (2nd ed.). Thorofare, NJ: SLACK Incorporated.

Williams, A., Fossey, E., & Harvey, C. (2010). Sustaining employment in a social firm: Use of the Work Environment Impact Scale v2.0 to explore views of employees with psychiatric disabilities. *British Journal of Occupational Therapy, 73*(11), 531-539.

Williams, A. E., Fossey, E., & Harvey, C. (2012). Social firms: Sustainable employment for people with mental illness. *Work: Journal of Prevention, Assessment, & Rehabilitation, 43*(1), 53-56.

Yamada, T., Kawamata, H., Kobayashi, N., Kielhofner, G., & Taylor, R. R. (2010). Programs to promote wellness for older people. *British Journal of Occupational Therapy, 73*(11), 540-548.

Patterns of Participation
Time Use and Occupational Balance

Ellie Fossey, PhD, MSc, DipCOT (UK) and
Terry Krupa, PhD, OT Reg (Ont), FCAOT

A person "maintains and balances [him/herself] in the world of reality and actuality by being in active life and active use.... There are many rhythms which we must be attuned to: the larger rhythms of night and day, of sleep and waking hours and finally the big four—work and play and rest and sleep, which our organism must be able to balance even under difficulty. The only way to attain balance in all this is actual doing.... Man learns to organize time and he does it in terms of doing things. (Meyer, 1922/1977, pp. 641-642)

Elvis: When you've got nothing to do ... and when you've got too much to do—they're not good for you. Nothing to do is not good, and too much to do is also not good. Basically, I don't want to be involved in those two ideas. Nothing to do's not me. I've always got something to do. I've got a whole place to clean if I want to clean it. And something to do, but not too much to do, is me as well. I look after me house, I cook for myself, I go for a walk if I can. I love [the lake] once in a while, feed the ducks once in a while, go to the city as much as possible. I'm sick. I've done less things and more things sometimes, but I try to make my days as beautiful as I can ... because without doing the things that keep you happy, satisfied and content in your day, you end up a wreck. (Quote from Elvis, cited in Fossey, 2009, p. 263 & 312)

OBJECTIVES

The objectives of this chapter are as follows:

» Describe ways in which time use and occupational balance are understood in occupational therapy.

» Identify interdisciplinary perspectives of time use and balance in everyday life.

» Discuss the evolution of temporal perspectives of occupation and key occupational therapy contributors.

(continued)

Krupa, T., Kirsh, B., Pitts, D., & Fossey, E. *Bruce & Borg's*
Psychosocial Frames of Reference: Theories, Models, and Approaches for
Occupation-Based Practice, Fourth Edition (pp 153-173).
© 2016 SLACK Incorporated.

» Distinguish between occupational balance, occupational imbalance, and related notions of lifestyle balance and work-life balance.

» Describe practice tools and methods for exploring time use and occupational balance issues.

» Describe occupational therapy practices that draw on an understanding of the temporal dimension of occupation and occupational balance to address engagement in meaningful and satisfying patterns of occupation.

BACKGROUND

Occupation has a number of differing characteristics that encompass what people do, when, where, how, and why they do it (Polatajko et al., 2007). The opening quotation of this chapter is from by a speech by Dr. Adolph Meyer, an important figure in American psychiatry, whose ideas about the importance of occupation for restoring and maintaining health significantly shaped the assumptions on which occupational therapy in the United States was founded (Kielhofner, 1977). The second quote is from an interview in which Elvis (pseudonym) was speaking about his activity participation as part of a research project about what everyday life is like from the viewpoint of adults with persisting mental health issues in Australia (Fossey, 2009). These quotes highlight essential themes to be explored in this chapter: a person's use of time is a valuable means by which to understand what he or she does in daily life; how the rhythms and patterns of participation everyday occupations are organized; and the idea that cultivating a balance in what one does is necessary for health and well-being.

Time and human action are inseparably linked in daily life (Kielhofner, 1977). Indeed, occupation may be defined as the actions of seizing, taking possession of, and occupying time, as well as space and place, in one's life (Oxford English Dictionary, cited in Fisher 1994). Interest in the temporal dimension of occupation was prominent in early psychosocial occupational therapy at the beginning of the 20th century, influenced by Meyer's (1922/1977) ideas quoted at the start of the chapter. Concepts relevant to the temporal dimension of occupation have since been integrated into several occupational therapy practice frameworks. For instance, the Model of Human Occupation (Kielhofner, 2008) addresses the ways in which people organize their participation into patterns and routines within daily life; and the Ecology of Human Performance framework considers the temporal context within which occupations are performed (Brown, 2014). Further, the Dynamic Occupation in Time framework (Larson, 2004; Larson & von Eye, 2010) highlights the interplay between occupation and subjective experience of time, for example, noting that engaging in occupation time may can be experienced as either longer or shorter compared to real time. While occupational therapy's view of elements of occupation, described in Chapter 1, suggests that human occupations offer opportunities to engage in a range of activities grounded in important human motives and meanings, it does not address how these are connected to time use and temporal patterns. To date, there is no fully developed psychosocial occupational therapy practice framework that specifically addresses the temporal patterning of occupations and occupational balance.

This chapter provides an overview of time use and occupational balance concepts relevant to understanding patterns of participation in daily life and how they may be affected by ill-health and disability, and considers their applications in occupational therapy practice. First, it describes people's time use patterns as an important perspective within which to explore what people do, with whom and where, as well as the temporal organization of daily life. Second, concepts of occupational balance and occupational imbalance as ways to understand patterns of participation and their potential effects on health and well-being are considered. Third, the chapter will demonstrate how an understanding of the temporal dimension of occupation and occupational balance may be applied in psychosocial occupational therapy to enable engagement in meaningful, satisfying, and health-promoting patterns of occupation.

TIME USE AND DAILY LIFE

Time is a universal dimension of experience: our actions both occur in time and mark time passing, so that its temporal nature is an important dimension of occupation (Kielhofner, 1977). Human experiences of time and ideas about time use are also embedded within historical, social, and cultural contexts (Christiansen, 2005). For instance, the invention of time-keeping technologies (e.g., clocks, watches) means that the 24-hour clock has become a dominant organizing feature of daily life in many societies to schedule occupations such as schooling, working, and shopping. In comparison, time use in other social contexts (e.g., at home, within families) may be organized in a less structured manner. Likewise, there are variations across societies and cultures, as well as between urban and rural communities, with respect to how activities are governed by the calendar, seasons, or the 24 hour clock, and how activities are connected to marking of the passage of time (e.g., ceremonies for significant events, spring and harvest festivities to mark changing seasons).

Broadly speaking, time-use studies investigate what people do and how they allocate their time to their differing activities. How people spend their time is of interest in many fields. For example, economists, planners, and policymakers use information about people's time use to quantify time spent in paid and unpaid work, shopping, travel, and entertainment, in order to identify needs for particular goods, facilities, and services. In comparison, understanding how time-use patterns relate to health and well-being is at the core of occupational therapists' interest in time use and patterns of participation in everyday life.

VIEW OF HEALTH AND DISORDER— TIME-USE PATTERNS

Relationships among activity participation, health, and well-being are complex, and there is no prescription for how to allocate time between activities for optimal health (Backman, 2004, 2010). Time use is considered to be linked to health and well-being principally because of what time use reveals about lifestyle, activity levels, and activity patterns.

- Time use allocation to particular activities permits the exploration of relationships between lifestyle and health. Lifestyle characteristics, such as activity levels, the extent of participation in particular types of activity (e.g., social activity, leisure, physical exercise) are related to longevity, health status, risks for various chronic health conditions, and measures of well-being (Christiansen, 2005).

- Higher levels of activity, in particular in socially valued, productive roles and activities that support social connections, appear to be associated with higher levels of satisfaction and community engagement (Eklund et al., 2009).

- Passive activity that involves limited challenge or skills (e.g., watching T.V.) may be useful as a form of resting, but is associated with lower levels of satisfaction, health, and well-being (Wilcock, 2006). For example, unemployed people report spending large amounts of time in non-directed activity (e.g., watching T.V., doing nothing in particular), have significant challenges establishing satisfying and productive occupational

patterns, and poor mental health and general health (Scanlan, Bundy, & Matthews, 2011).

- Limited occupation, that is, having little to do with one's time, is not considered good for one's health and can be difficult or distressing, creating a sense of killing time as illustrated by this quote—"And then I'll go and take a cup of coffee. So I'll walk around in town for a while. Then I'll take the metro home again. That will make the day pass. You can travel around a bit. You've got to find something to make time pass" (Participant cited in Jonsson, 2010, p. 220). Thus, prolonged low levels of activity are associated with loss of hope, meaning, connection to activity and its benefits, loss of capabilities, social isolation, a sense of alienation, and wasting one's life away (Krupa, McLean, Eastbrook, Bonham, & Baksh, 2003; Legault & Rebeiro, 2001; Wilcock, 2006). This experience has been described in studies of homelessness, where "passing time" contributes to a sense of lack of meaning (Illman et al., 2013).

- How people allocate time to activities, places, and interactions reflects the impact of illness, disability and socioeconomic restrictions on their activity participation and daily lives. In turn, patterns of time use may reflect poorer health or experiences of disability because they show the impacts on a person's activities of difficulties such as pain, fatigue, sleep, or mood problems. In this sense, time use patterns may indicate the extent of adjustment to daily living demands, disability, and participation restrictions (Harvey, Fossey, Jackson, & Shimitras, 2006; Harvey & Pentland, 2010; Krupa et al., 2003).

KEY CONCEPTS

A number of concepts relevant to understanding how people use their time underpin how the temporal dimension of occupational engagement is understood in occupational therapy.

Time Use

Time use typically refers to the allocation of time to different activities and is represented in terms of clock time, that is, as time has been divided and organized since societies first had chronometers by which to measure time (Farnworth & Fossey, 2003). Time use, then, is a way to represent what people do in daily life in terms of the amount and variation in their activities over a particular time period (e.g., a day, week), to describe the frequency, duration, sequence, and repetition of these activities, whether measured at an individual or population level (Harvey & Pentland, 2010).

The typical method used as a basis to study people's activities in this way is a *time budget* or *time diary* (Christiansen, 2005; Harvey & Pentland, 2010). Time use diaries are typically designed to record what a person does within blocks of time over the course of one or more days, and to allow the calculation of the person's total time spent in different categories of occupations over that period. They may be relatively simple structured forms on which to record time spent in particular categories of activity (e.g., work, domestic activity, social activity, leisure, sleep). Alternatively, a more open-ended approach might be used so that activities are described by the person completing the time diary form. As well as recording actual activities, time diaries are often designed to gather some contextual information, such as where with whom activities are being done. The amount of time allocated to differing activities can then be calculated from a completed time diary, for example, by using a set of categories to classify reported activity in order that time allocated to particular activities can be summed. One example is to use the four activity categories described by Aas (cited in Harvey & Pentland, 2010): *necessary* (to meet physiological and self-care requirements), *contracted* (work/study in exchange for pay or a qualification), *committed* (obligated but unpaid, such as housework, caring), and *discretionary/free-time* activities. While this type of approach is common in time use research (see, for example, Harvey et al., 2006; Krupa et al. 2003; Scanlan et al., 2011), coding time use in this way may differ from how people view their own time use so that some kinds of participation may be under- or over-represented (Harvey & Pentland, 2010). When time diaries are used in health contexts to explore individuals' patterns of occupations, their views about their time use are essential to its interpretation.

Occupational Pattern

People generally engage in a number of everyday occupations (some with daily regularity, some routinely but less often, others more flexibly), which become woven into a pattern of activity in time over the day, week, or longer. For example, the occupational pattern of a child attending school likely includes a routine of getting up, traveling to school and attending classes at regular times, but also includes other times during the day and on weekends that may be more flexibly used to play, hang out with friends, rest, and so forth. Occupational patterns often include the following features:

- *Enfolded activity*—this term describes doing that simultaneously involves more than one occupation. For example, when a parent simultaneously engages a young child in play while preparing a meal; or when an adult simultaneously listens to music and prepares for a meeting whilst traveling to work by bus. Thus, enfolded activity is frequently part of a person's occupational pattern (Polatajko et al., 2007).

- *Routines*—this terms refers to relatively fixed, temporally anchored patterns of occupations executed in customary sequences over the day, or longer periods, which create a sense of structure and order in daily life (Kielhofner, 2008).

Another concept related to the temporal dimension is how individuals subjectively experience the passage of time (*temporality*) during occupational engagement (e.g., experiences of time dragging, flying by, or standing still), and how individuals connect and give meaning to times past, present, and future (Clark, 1997; Larson, 2004). Therefore, temporality cannot be readily understood from information collected by means of time diaries alone, but rather involves understanding how people describe their time use patterns; this is because temporality is considered important as an indicator of the emotional experience of participation. For instance, activities in which time passes quickly may be viewed as pleasant, whereas a sense of time being scarce or rushed means participation is more likely to be experienced as stressful (Larson & von Eye, 2010). Furthermore, experiences of participation that involve similar levels of activity may be qualitatively different in their potential for engagement, such as sitting doing "nothing" in active contemplation compared with passing time with little or nothing to do.

Temporal Adaptation

This term was used by Kielhofner (1977) to describe the "integration of an entire spectrum of activities into one's life, the organization of which supports health on an ongoing basis" (p. 235). As this suggests, the interrelatedness between activities in one's daily life is an important consideration in health and well-being. This is explored further in the section of this chapter about occupational balance.

THEORETICAL ASSUMPTIONS

The amount of time allocated to particular activities cannot be assumed to indicate better health or quality of life (Harvey & Pentland, 2010). For example, physical activity and employment are each known to have positive health benefits, yet people sometimes participate in physical activity or in work in ways that compromise their well-being, perhaps by restricting their involvement in other activities important for their social relationships or experiencing enjoyment. That said, overall levels of activity do make a difference to reported levels of satisfaction and engagement. It is not merely what people do in their daily time use that affects their health and well-being, but the temporal organization and pattern to people's rounds of daily occupations that is important. This is because many activities have the potential to contribute to well-being, depending on characteristics such as their meaningfulness, including whether self-chosen or directed, engaging, enhancing social connections, or personal development.

People who experience significant disruptions to their patterns of participation in everyday occupations or conditions that restrict their opportunities for active engagement in everyday life (e.g., unemployment) are at risk of occupational imbalance and detrimental impacts on their health and well-being. Time-use studies involving adults experiencing disability in general find that their time use reflects both less varied occupations and less frequent participation compared with the general population (Christiansen, 1996; Farnworth, 2003; Pentland & McColl, 1999; Pagán, 2013). Typically, this means their time use patterns are characterized by less diversity of occupations, less time in paid work, fewer activities outside the home, and more time in household and personal care activities. Hence, it has been suggested disability appears to "steal" time in the sense that some everyday activities may be more time-consuming for disabled persons to accomplish and that additional activities may become a necessity, such as those related to medical care and self-management of health conditions (Pagán, 2013). An alternative explanation is that their altered time use pattern reflects the more restricted options available to adults who are under-employed or lacking paid work, and the disabling impacts of the substantial employment barriers faced by this population. This is borne out by Scanlan et al.'s (2011) time use study involving unemployed youth who likewise reported more time around home, watching TV or doing nothing, and sleeping compared to young people in employment. Similar findings are consistently reported across time use studies undertaken in Canada, England, Japan, Sweden, and the United States involving people with persistent mental health issues; in which the prevailing patterns of participation are dominated by sleep, quiet leisure activities (such as listening to music or radio, watching T.V.), and time at home; and restricted social interactions, productive, and community-based activities (Eklund et al., 2009; Harvey et al., 2006; Krupa et al., 2003). Notably, the majority of participants in these studies were also unemployed.

Many factors may have a bearing on time use patterns, including unemployment, poverty, and limited access to resources, factors in the social and cultural context, as well as personal preferences, age, prior experience and abilities, health and self-management strategies for minimizing stress and maintaining well-being (Christiansen, 2005; Harvey & Pentland, 2010; Minato & Zemke, 2004; Yanos, West, & Smith, 2010). Thus, disrupted and restricted patterns of participation reflect many barriers to occupational engagement and balance, some personal or related to health

conditions themselves but many external and often more restricting than the internal ones (Edgelow & Krupa, 2011). Thus, having experienced illness or disability does not mean people use their time in particular ways, nor does it mean that every person experiencing illness or disability will have an impoverished lifestyle (Eklund et al., 2009). Nevertheless, time use research does suggest the time use patterns, occupational balance, and engagement issues of people who are unemployed, who experience mental health issues, or other ongoing health conditions and disability warrant attention in psychosocial occupational therapy practice.

In the mental health field, there are also differing and contradictory views regarding the role of activity in promoting health. For example, stress paradigms have suggested that activities of daily life can be demanding and activity participation potentially stressful or overwhelming for people with persistent mental illness; that people with psychological and emotional challenges may have a low tolerance for active engagement; and accordingly, that their activity levels may require active monitoring to avoid exacerbating symptoms of distress and to maximize the beneficial effects of activity. In contrast, activity participation within community contexts is considered recovery-promoting since it enables the person to discover strengths, capabilities and an identity beyond mental illness, and to develop strategies and supports that maintain well-being (Borg & Davidson, 2008; Mezzina et al., 2006). Activity involvement is also the focus for addressing barriers to social and economic participation irrespective of ill-health. Further research to understand how people choose and manage both their activity participation and stresses in daily life in the context of mental health issues is important to disentangle these apparently contradictory views and to guide clients in making choices about how to use their time or develop occupational patterns to promote and maintain well-being.

OCCUPATIONAL BALANCE

Occupational balance is a fundamental concept underlying the way in which occupational therapists understand the relationship among occupations, health, and well-being. Meyer (1922/1977), in articulating his vision of occupational therapy at the beginning of the 20th century, not only spoke of the importance of considering how people use and organize their time, he also linked balanced use of time to maintaining well-being. He highlighted the negative health consequences of a lack of occupations that bring meaning and organization to daily life. The idea that a balance in what one does is good for one's health has been a longstanding theme across many disciplines. For instance, the notion of balance is evident in ancient Greek and eastern philosophies; it is also evoked in sociological discussions about the relationships between work and non-work domains of life (Matuska & Christiansen, 2008; Thompson & Bunderson, 2001; Wilcock, 2006). Furthermore, the idea that a balance in what one does is better for one's health has become popularized, at least within the privileged world (Backman, 2010; Matuska & Christiansen, 2008). Here we explore how occupational balance and lifestyle balance are understood from an occupational perspective.

VIEW OF HEALTH AND DISORDER—OCCUPATIONAL BALANCE AND IMBALANCE

From an occupational perspective, people engage in a repertoire of occupations related to their roles, interests, talents, resources, and opportunities; these occupations may be more or less elaborate, require varying degrees of organization, be undertaken with differing frequency, and change over the life course (Backman, 2010). This means both the nature of the occupations in a person's repertoire and how these occupations are orchestrated as part of daily life can be potential sources of well-being, or conversely of stress and ill-health. In relation to health and well-being, the concept of balance is used to describe these occupational patterns. In essence, *occupational balance* is viewed as beneficial for health and well-being and characterizes those occupational patterns that contribute to health and positive experiences related to well-being, such as satisfaction, meaning, and fulfilment. Conversely, *occupational imbalance* characterizes occupational patterns seen as undermining or detrimental to health and well-being.

KEY CONCEPTS AND THEORETICAL ASSUMPTIONS

Occupational balance is an evolving and not fully understood concept (Backman, 2010). Early ideas about occupational balance emphasized that a balance between work, rest, play, and sleep was necessary for health well-being (Meyer 1922/1977). Often this idea of a balance across major categories of activity has been linked to time use (Backman, 2004; Christiansen, 1996). In other words, occupational balance is assumed to mean that some appropriate distribution of time (hours) can and should be achieved between various domains of activity and commitments (work, domestic, family, recreation, community, and so on) for health and well-being. However, as seen in earlier discussion of time use patterns, how much time is spent in particular activities is only one aspect of people's patterns of participation in everyday occupations that contributes to

their health and well-being. Hence, occupational balance is increasingly viewed not so much in terms of time use but as concerned with how people experience their occupational patterns, and with the characteristics or qualities of occupational patterns that address needs or support health and well-being.

Occupational balance is therefore conceptualized in several different ways. Based on a concept analysis of how *occupational balance* is understood in occupational science and occupational therapy literatures, Wagman, Håkansson,, and Björklund, (2012) proposed occupational balance is an occupational pattern involving the right amount of occupation and the right variation between occupations as defined from an individual's own perspective. In addition, what constitutes the subjectively defined "right" amount and "right" variation in occupations relates to the following three aspects of occupational balance:

1. A balance of participation in different occupational areas (sometimes described as work/productive occupations, play/leisure, rest, sleep, and so forth)

2. A balance of occupations with different characteristics (such as use of different capacities, challenge, and other experiences)

3. Time spent in varied occupations, although not necessarily equal amounts of time

The above view of occupational balance suggests some of its characteristics, but it does not elaborate how different occupational areas or occupations with different characteristics may interact to affect individual's perception of occupational balance or occupational imbalance.

Occupational balance is further characterized as a pattern of occupations that includes varied, obligatory, and discretionary occupations, which are personally meaningful and satisfying, as when individuals perceive their patterns of occupations as harmonious, fulfilling, and aligned with their values and priorities (Backman, 2010; Matuska & Christiansen, 2008). To illustrate, for women recovering from stress-related disorders who participated in focus group research in Sweden, achieving balance and well-being in everyday life involved engaging in a repertoire of personally meaningful occupations that was harmonious, manageable, and respected their values, needs, and resources (Håkansson, Dahlin-Ivanoff, & Sonn, 2006). Many fluctuating factors also influence an individual's perceptions of occupational balance (e.g., changing circumstances and demands, personal values and priorities, cultural beliefs, socioeconomic conditions). Therefore, occupational balance is relative, (i.e., it is experienced in varying degrees; Backman, 2010).

In comparison, *occupational imbalance* has been described as the disproportionate involvement in particular occupations at the expense of other occupations, or involvement in a limited range of occupations (Backman, 2010; Wilcock, 2006). Thus, occupational imbalance tends to be viewed as a temporal concept concerned with how time is allocated to categories of activity (e.g., work, leisure, rest), and may imply either being under-occupied or being over-occupied (Backman, 2010; Bejerholm, 2010). Yet, as much as occupational balance also relates to how people experience their occupational patterns and the qualities of different occupations, occupational imbalance also needs to be viewed more broadly (Backman, 2010). Occupational imbalance then is the experience of occupational patterns that limit a person's expression of interests and values, use of capacities, and/or access to the physical, mental, and social benefits of varied occupations (Wilcock, 2006). Thus, occupational imbalance characterized by the absence of occupations with these qualities or by disproportionate participation in work/productive activities, leisure/play, and rest are considered risk factors for compromising well-being. Health may be compromised by occupational imbalance in a number of ways, for instance, health can decline when capacities are strained or under-used, and high and low levels of time pressure are associated with poorer mental health, while other consequences of an imbalance in occupations are thought to include stress, lack of energy, fatigue, burnout, and boredom (Christiansen & Matuska, 2006; Farnworth, 2003; Wilcock, 2006).

Two further perspectives of occupational balance and occupational imbalance may usefully inform psychosocial practice: a *chronobiological perspective* concerned with the synchrony between internal biological rhythms, activity patterns, and well-being; and the concept of *lifestyle balance* (Christiansen, 1996; Matuska & Christiansen, 2008). A *chronobiological perspective* highlights the potential importance of links between biological rhythms and activity patterns for well-being (Christiansen, 1996, 2005). Humans are subject to many daily physiological rhythms, such as the sleep-wake cycle and changing levels of arousal during the day (or activity/rest cycle), which may also be attuned to external influences such as light, temperature change, and regular social rhythms such as mealtimes and bedtimes. While little exploration of the impact of biological rhythms on occupational patterns has been undertaken in occupational therapy, disruptions to these cycles are known to affect activity patterns and well-being. A relatively familiar example is jet lag, whereby biological rhythms of a circadian nature (i.e., follow a 24-hour cycle) are disrupted by long distance travel across time zones, resulting in temporary disturbances to sleeping and eating patterns. Disturbances of time use patterns are also considered characteristic of some health conditions, for example, mood disorders and bipolar disorders are associated with altered sleep/wake or activity/rest cycles, and the establishment of regularity in daily routines may be part of

a relapse prevention strategy (Frank, Gonzalez, & Fagiolini, 2006). Similarly, occupational patterns that are out of sync with broader social patterns can alter sleep-wake cycles and compromise well-being. For example, people can find their sleep-wake cycle reversed in the absence of structured and obligatory occupational demands during the day, as may occur when their participation in productive activities is limited. In turn, their opportunities for social connections and community activities become compromised.

Related to occupational balance, the concept of *lifestyle balance* is described in terms of how repertoires or patterns of everyday occupations meet essential needs (Håkansson & Matuska, 2010; Matuska & Christiansen, 2008). The concept of lifestyle balance is situated within a literature about lifestyle factors that may promote health, reduce stress, and prevent illness (Backman, 2010; Matuska & Christiansen, 2008), and draws on related interdisciplinary research about physiological and psychological needs important for well-being (Christiansen & Matuska, 2006). Thus, Matuska and Christiansen defined a balanced lifestyle as "a satisfying pattern of [activities which are] healthful, meaningful and sustainable to an individual within the context of his or her current life circumstances" (p. 11). Furthermore, they propose five needs-based dimensions of occupational patterns as essential, including the concept that a person's repertoire of occupations enables him or her to do the following:

- Meet basic instrumental needs for sustained biological health and safety

- Have rewarding and self-affirming relationships with others

- Feel engaged, challenged, and competent

- Create meaning and a positive personal identity

- Organize time and energy in ways to enable personal goals and renewal

To experience lifestyle balance, then, involves being able to engage in occupational patterns that meet the above essential needs, whereas those who are not able to so, due to personal and environmental challenges and barriers, are less likely to experience lifestyle balance and may perceive poorer well-being. Phenomenological findings from Håkansson and Matuska's (2010) study of perceived lifestyle balance among women recovering from stress-related disorders lend support to these needs-based dimensions. They also have much in common with experiential qualities of occupational engagement that appear to support well-being identified in other qualitative research. For instance, pursuit of occupations that were engaging in terms of their intensity, positive meaning, commitment, connection to a community, and coherence as a whole supported older adults to develop fulfilling patterns of occupations in transitions to retirement (Jonsson, 2008, 2010).

KEY DEVELOPERS/THEORISTS

There is as yet no fully developed occupational therapy practice framework that specifically addresses the temporal patterning of occupations and occupational balance to provide guidelines for psychosocial practice as it relates to promoting healthy time use patterns, occupational balance, and well-being, or as it relates to addressing issues of loss or disruption of time use patterns, occupational imbalance, and disengagement. Nevertheless, these concepts have been influential since the occupational therapy profession's inception in the early 20th century through the work of occupational therapists like Eleanor Clarke Slagle, as well as psychiatrists of that time such as Dr. Adolf Meyer in the United States. Meyer linked ideas about time use patterns and a balance of occupations and health, viewing health as reflected in the organization of everyday use of time, for which a balance of occupations that require being, thinking, and doing is required. Conversely, he saw lack of occupation as detrimental for health, viewing enforced idleness (or lack of occupation) as contributing to demoralization, breakdown of habits, physical deterioration, and loss of abilities (Kielhofner, 1977; Wilcock, 2006). Furthermore, early occupational programs were based on the proposition that people's use of time and daily routines have health-sustaining and health-promoting potential, an idea that remains at the core of occupational therapy (Kielhofner, 1977).

Later, Kielhofner (1977) reintroduced the temporal dimension of occupation in daily life into occupational therapy discourse. He argued that the temporal dimension of occupation is concerned not only with the ways in which people organize their time use, but also that the human awareness and experience of time (temporality) allows us to make meaningful connections between past and present experiences and to project plans for action into the future. He considered individuals' use of time to be a function of their particular interests and goals, and to be strongly embedded within cultural values and norms about time (e.g., values about what constitutes "productive" use of time and "wasting" time varies among differing sociocultural groups and societies). Furthermore, he viewed the development of skills around organizing time to be an ongoing necessity as roles and occupations change, and a critical factor in adjusting to health conditions or following the onset of disability. For Kielhofner then, the conditions for psychosocial health are created by an interrelated balance of self-maintenance, work, and play that is individually satisfying and appropriate for the person's roles within society, and not just so much work, play and rest in terms of time allocation. Many time use studies have subsequently been undertaken by occupational therapy researchers, providing evidence that time use patterns became disrupted in diverse circumstances, for example, living with mental illness (Eklund et al., 2009), long-term pain (Liedberg, Hesselstrand, & Henriksson, 2004), unemployment (Scanlan et al., 2011), and living in an emergency shelter (McNulty, Crowe, Kroening, VanLeit, & Good, 2009).

A number of occupational therapy scholars have also written about occupational balance. Christiansen (1996) proposed three interdisciplinary perspectives from which balanced participation in occupations may be understood: the first is rooted in how time is allocated to different activities, whereas the second draws on biological knowledge concerned with synchrony between biological rhythms and activity patterns as previously described. The third perspective suggests the balance among a person's repertoire of goal-directed occupations (personal projects) as another way to view occupational balance. This perspective draws from a personal projects approach in psychology to view occupational balance as the extent to which occupations committed to in an ongoing way are complimentary or in conflict with each other. For example, the student who is committed to successfully completing study assignments, maintaining a healthy exercise regime, and keeping in regular contact with friends may at times experience these "projects" as in harmony or even supporting each other. On the other hand, these projects could also compete for the student's time, energy, and other resources, meaning that they are experienced as conflicting or discordant. In a study analyzing the personal projects of 120 adults (college students, employed, and retired persons), Christiansen et al. (1998) identified that meaning, structure, efficacy, social relations, and stressfulness were characteristics of participants' personal projects that influenced their subjective well-being, suggesting occupational balance might relate not only the extent to which one's personal projects compliment or conflict with each other, but also the extent to which those goal-directed occupations (personal projects) have qualities that support or undermine well-being.

The qualities of occupations and occupational engagement that contribute to occupational balance have been the subject of research by a number of other occupational therapy scholars. Examples include explorations of occupational balance from an experiential viewpoint (Jonsson & Persson, 2006) and research involving adults in transition to retirement (Jonsson, 2008, 2010) or health conditions such as stress-related disorders (Håkansson et al., 2006; Håkansson & Matuska, 2010), persistent mental illnesses (Bejerholm, 2010; Eklund, Erlandsson, & Leufstadius, 2010), rheumatoid arthritis (Forhan & Backman, 2010; Stamm et al., 2009), and multiple sclerosis (Matuska & Erickson, 2008). Taken together, this research indicates repertoires of occupations that include certain characteristics are more likely to contribute to a sense of occupational balance and well-being. These include: varying degrees of complexity, novelty, and time structure and regularity involved; varying depths of emotional, cognitive, and social involvement; scope to use one's capacities; social value; personal meaning; and connections with others.

Interdisciplinary interest, particularly within the social sciences, has also contributed to our understanding of people's use of time and balance in daily life. Time use studies in the social sciences have contributed substantial general population level data and knowledge to our understanding of human time use internationally, allowing for cross-cultural comparisons and consideration of time use differences related to age, gender, lifestyle, disability, and so forth (Harvey & Pentland, 2010). In addition, time allocation has often been central to sociological discussions about the relationships between work and other aspects of life, including: the extent of perceived balance between work and non-work domains of life; and whether there is sufficient time to meet work and home life commitments (Polatajko et al., 2007). The metaphor of balance is evoked with use of the term *work-life balance* in these discussions and, as within occupational therapy, is critiqued for neglecting the subjective meanings derived from work and non-work time (Thompson & Bunderson, 2001). However, whereas the concept of work-life balance focuses particularly on the occupation of paid work, occupational balance "considers life's occupations in the broadest sense" with potential applicability to people irrespective of age, roles, or employment status (Backman, 2010, p. 236). Nevertheless, to what extent occupational balance and imbalance hold relevance across sex, culture, ability, and privilege are open questions (Whiteford, 2009).

IMPORTANT EVOLUTIONARY POINTS

Interest in the temporal dimension of occupation was prominent in the vision and practice of early psychosocial occupational therapy. These ideas about the temporal organization of daily life have been examined in greater depth within occupational therapy and occupational science literatures over the past 30 years (Backman, 2010; Christiansen, 1996; Christiansen & Matuska, 2006; Kielhofner, 1977). Studies of the time use and activity patterns of people with a range of health conditions, as well as international time use research in the social sciences, have contributed much to what is known about time use in the context of disability, and within general populations (Farnworth, 2004; Harvey & Pentland, 2010). The focus on daily time-use in terms of time allocation or distribution among broad categories of activity (e.g., self-care, productivity, leisure, rest/sleep) in occupational therapy has been criticized (Jonsson, 2008) because of growing recognition that many of the ways in

which people occupy themselves are not readily defined in these terms (Hammel et al., 2008). In addition, these activity categories potentially undervalue occupations that people find important but define differently (e.g., caring for others, doing with others, reflecting, cultural practices) (Hammell, 2009). Furthermore, while time use patterns that reflect doing too little or doing too much are considered detrimental for health, emerging understandings of occupational balance and occupational imbalance highlight a range of other characteristics in patterns and qualities of people's occupational engagement as important for health and well-being. For these reasons, it is recommended to explore individuals' time use and experiences of occupational engagement in their own terms.

Widely used since occupational therapy's beginnings, occupational balance and imbalance are evolving concepts understood in the following ways:

- Occupational balance was initially thought of as a temporal concept related to how time is allocated among categories of occupations (Backman, 2004; Christiansen, 1996).

- More recently, occupational balance has been conceptualized as a balance among occupations that offer a mix of characteristics considered important for health and well-being, such as variety, challenge, meaningfulness, social connection, and so on (Stamm et al., 2009; Wagman et al., 2012), or as a relative phenomenon defined by individuals for themselves; that is, the extent to which individuals perceive their own patterns of occupations as harmonious, fulfilling, and congruent with their values and priorities (Backman, 2010; Håkansson et al., 2006).

- Conversely, occupational imbalance has been understood as the result of an over-abundance or dearth of occupations; it also characterizes patterns of occupations lacking in challenge, stimulation, and other qualities that support the use of capacities and bring health and well-being benefits (Backman, 2010; Bejerholm, 2010; Wilcock, 2006). Hence, Backman argues occupational balance and occupational imbalance are experienced in varying degrees, and should be thought of on a continuum affected by life circumstances, occupational choices, and resources.

- Drawing from interdisciplinary research about physiological and psychological needs important for well-being, the related concept of lifestyle balance is described in terms of how repertoires or patterns of everyday occupations meet essential needs (Håkansson & Matuska, 2010; Matuska & Christiansen, 2008). In other words, experiencing lifestyle balance involves being able to engage in occupational patterns that meet essential needs, whereas those who are unable to so, due to personal and environmental challenges and barriers, are less likely to experience life balance and may perceive a poorer sense of well-being.

From a psychosocial practice perspective, these ways of conceptualizing occupational balance and imbalance are not yet articulated as a specific practice framework. Nevertheless, they indicate important dimensions of occupational patterns to which occupational therapists may usefully attend in practice, including the variety, regularity, challenge, and other physical, mental, and social health and well-being benefits of participation reflected in a person's pattern of occupations. Further research is required to strengthen the evidence supporting these perspectives of occupational balance, and to examine the applicability of occupational balance and occupational imbalance for conceptualizing the relationships between occupational patterns, health, and well-being in both well populations and among those who experience prolonged health conditions, disability, or disadvantage in daily life.

EXPECTED OUTCOMES

Time use, or how people allocate their time, is not an outcome in itself. However, ill-health and experiences of disability can disrupt people's participation in everyday occupations in ways that are reflected in altered time use, for example, through restricting access to some occupations (e.g., paid work) or because a longer time may be taken to perform certain tasks. Thus, alterations in time use patterns can be an indicator of health status and quality of life (Harvey & Pentland, 2010). Psychosocial occupational therapy often aims to bring about change in either the extent or the pattern of a person's participation in everyday occupations, and so time use is a highly relevant outcome for evaluating occupational therapy interventions. Time use diaries provide a way to measure both the extent and pattern of what people do in daily life, without under- or over-emphasizing particular occupations as outcomes (Farnworth, 2004; Krupa et al., 2003). Time use diaries also provide an accessible way for occupational therapists to explore patterns of daily occupations in terms that readily make sense to clients themselves—doing too much, doing too little, not doing as much of what they wish to, and so forth (Farnworth, 2004).

Occupational therapists consider occupational engagement in a varied pattern of meaningful and satisfying occupations essential for health and well-being, so that changes in experiences of occupational engagement and participation are important to evaluate. Evaluation of the extent to which clients' perceptions of occupational balance or imbalance are changed is an important way in which to evaluate the outcomes of occupational therapy designed to improve experiences of occupational engagement and

participation, if explored and interpreted in a culturally and contextually sensitive way (Haertl, 2010).

Time use patterns and occupational balance are interconnected ways in which to think about the temporal nature of people's occupations. Time use provides a window on what people actually do in daily life, and the frequency, duration, sequence, and repetition in their repertoire of occupations. Thus, daily time use indicates the extent and variation in a person's activities, both of which contribute to health, well-being, and quality of life. The concept of occupational balance is complementary, and extends our understanding of the elements of occupational engagement that we should consider in enabling clients to regain or build patterns of participation in everyday occupations that promote health and well-being. Thus, occupational balance as a concept is concerned in part with how much time is spent in differing occupations and the variety in the individuals' repertoire of occupations, but also with the extent to which these occupations have characteristics that provide varied health benefits (physical, social, emotional, intellectual, etc.), and how individuals experience their repertoire of occupations (in terms of their harmony, conflict, etc.). An understanding of these concepts is important, then, to address occupational engagement issues in psychosocial practice.

PRACTICE DEVELOPMENTS

Time use offers a perspective through which to explore and appreciate what people do in daily life, their patterns of participation, and the extent of their engagement in occupations that support health and well-being. Neither the temporal dimension of occupation nor occupational balance can be considered practice models. Nevertheless, the application of these concepts within occupational therapy is longstanding since seeking to understand how people use their time offers a valuable approach to explore clients' involvement in everyday activities with them, and to identify disrupted activity patterns and disengagement from occupations that influence well-being (Edgelow & Krupa, 2011; Pentland & McColl, 1999; Box 10-1).

A range of practice tools and guides have been developed that occupational therapists can use in psychosocial practice to investigate time use and occupational balance with clients, and to support them in addressing identified difficulties, challenges, and aspirations.

EXAMPLES OF PRACTICE TOOLS AND GUIDES

Information may be gathered in a range of ways to explore time use patterns with clients in psychosocial

---

Box 10-1

Psychosocial practice informed by an understanding of individuals' time use patterns and occupational balance can serve to address issues and challenges related to occupational engagement that include the following:

- Very limited occupation or disengagement from occupations in one's daily life
- Patterns of participation that lack variety, challenge, satisfaction, fulfilment
- Patterns of participation that are missing in occupations with benefits in one or more areas of physical, social, emotional, or intellectual health and well-being
- Time use patterns affected by disrupted sleep/wake cycles or fluctuating experiences of a phenomena such as stiffness, pain, fatigue, low mood
- Difficulties organizing one's time use efficiently, or in a satisfying way

---

occupational therapy practice, including through interviews, observations, and structured methods. A common structured method is to use tools based on a time budget approach, generally referred to as time use diaries (Figure 10-1). Time use diaries are typically designed to record what a person does within blocks of time over the course of one or more days, and to allow the calculation of the person's total time spent in different categories of occupations over that period. They can be relatively simple structured forms on which to record time spent in particular categories of activity, such as work, domestic activity, social activity, leisure, or sleep. Alternatively, a time use diary may be more open-ended to allow the person completing it to describe the activities that he or she undertakes.

For time use research, a set of activity categories is often used to classify reported time use for the purpose of quantifying the amount of time allocation to differing activities (see, for example, Krupa et al., 2003; Minato & Zemke, 2004). When using time diaries in psychosocial occupational therapy practice, the purpose for asking a client to complete a time use diary is likely to learn about and review client's time use patterns together as a basis for identifying issues that he or she would like to address or areas in which he or she wishes for support to make change. In this context, a time use diary serves as a basis for exploring the person's own view of his or her time use, strengths, difficulties, and sense of occupational balance/imbalance (Eklund et al., 2009) and will often be best completed within face-to-face interactions with clients. This also allows for greater depth of exploration of the meaning and experiential aspects of occupation that are not only important elements of occupational balance conceptually, but also relate to perceptions of well-being (Eklund & Leufstadius, 2007; Eklund et al., 2009).

Two examples of tools developed by occupational therapists for gathering time use information are described next.

The Occupational Questionnaire

Originally developed by occupational therapists to use with adolescents or adults, the occupational questionnaire (OQ; Smith, Kielhofner, & Watts, 1986) records an individual's daily time use in half-hourly blocks through the day, providing information about the pattern of the person's activities categorized as work, leisure, daily living task, or rest (Eklund et al., 2009). The OQ also records self-ratings for enjoyment, importance, and competence in doing each activity. The NIH Activity Record (ACTRE; Furst, Gerber, Smith, Fisher, & Shulman, 1987) is similarly designed to the OQ, but was developed for use with individuals with physical impairments and disability and includes additional questions about pain, fatigue, difficulty of performance, and rest taken during activity performance. These questions mean the ACTRE provides valuable information about the impact of health issues and disability in everyday life (Kielhofner et al., 2008); it also provides a structure that could be readily modified to obtain information about other dimensions of experience, such as perceived stress, mood, and satisfaction, that are relevant to psychosocial practice (Farnworth, 2004). The OQ and ACTRE may be self-reported or completed in an interview, the latter being advantageous for ease of completion and to adequately contextualize a person's time use as a basis for informing interventions (Farnworth, 2003). Their use has been reported to understand the daily routines and activity participation of college students; community-dwelling adolescents; adults diagnosed with mental illness, spinal cord injuries, arthritis, chronic fatigue syndrome, cardiopulmonary disease, or post-stroke; as well as older adults in community settings and nursing homes (Kielhofner et al., 2008). Hence, the OQ and ACTRE are flexible tools that may be used in the wide range of practice settings where psychosocial issues are relevant.

Time	Mon	Activity Type	Where & people	Tues	Activity Type	Where & people	Wed	Activity Type	Where & people	Thurs	Activity type	Where & people	Sat	Activity type	Where & people
Midnight – 2am	Sleep	Rest	Home alone	Sleep	Rest	Home alone	Sleep	Rest	Home, Alone	Sleep	Rest	Home, alone	Time with mum	Leisure	Mum's home, mum
2- 7am	"	"	"	"	"	"	"	"	"	"	"	"	Sleep	Rest	Home, alone
7am	Nap	Rest	Home alone	No entry	No entry	No entry	Wake, get self and kids ready for school	Productive/ Self-care	Home, kids and sister	Wake, get self and kids ready for school	Productive/ Self-care	Home, kids and sister	"	"	"
9am	Feed kids and go to work	Productive	Home, kids and sister	"	"	"	Light Cleaning	Productive	No entry	Volunteer, school	Productive	Teachers, students	"	"	"
10am	Work	Productive	Library, alone	"	"	"			"	"	"	"	Shower	Self-care	Home
12 noon	Lunch	Self-care	School, teachers	Lunch with friend	Leisure (social)	Friends house, friend	Cook lunch	Productive	No entry	"	"	"	Friend came over	Leisure	Home, friend, sister
1pm	Work	Productive	School, pupils, teachers	"	"	"	Eating, relaxing	Self-care	No entry	"	"	"	Lunch with mum	Leisure/ self-care	Shops, mum, sister
2pm	"	"	"	Shopping	Productive	Friend, shops	Shop	Productive	No entry	"	"	"	"	"	"
3pm	"	"	"	Pick kids up from school	Productive	Friend, kids	Pick kids up from school	Productive	No entry	Pick kids up from school	Productive	Kids	Birthday shopping	Productive	Shops, friend, sister
4pm	Clean	Productive	Home, kids and sister	Clean	Productive	Home, kids, friends	Counselling	Self-care	No entry	Clean	Productive	Home, kids	Pack present	Productive	Home, sister, kids
5pm	Dinner	Productive	"	Work	Productive	Client, friend, kids, sister	Travel	"	"	Shop	Productive	Kids	Organize kids	Productive	Home, kids
6pm	Meet with mum	Leisure (social)	Kids, mum	"	"	"	Dinner	Productive	No entry	Cook, eat	Productive	Kids	"	"	"
7pm	BBQ	Leisure (social)	Home, friends	"	"	"	"	"	"	Kids to bed	Productive	Home, kids	See friend for birthday	Leisure	Kids, sister
8pm	"	"	"	"	"	"	Kids to bed	Productive	No entry	Homework	Productive	Home, alone	Playing with kids	Productive	Mum's home, kids, sister
9pm	Homework	Productive	Home, alone	Dinner	Self-care	Home, Alone	See friend	Leisure (social)	Friends house	Went out for cuppa	Leisure (Self-care)	Friend	Visit friend	Leisure	Out, friends
10pm	"	"	"	Clean	Productive	Home, Alone	"	"	"	"	"	"	"	"	"
11pm	Sleep	Rest	Home, alone	Sleep	Rest	Home, Alone	Cleaning	Productive	No entry	Get ready for bed	Self-care	Home, alone	"	"	"
Rest		10			9			7			7			8	
Productive		10			8			12			14			5	
Self Care		1			1			3			1			2	
Leisure		3			2			2			2			9	
Unspecified		-			4			-			-			-	

Figure 10-1. Stephanie's daily time use log (constructed by occupational therapist, Peter Weymouth).

The Profiles of Occupational Engagement in Persons With Schizophrenia

Another time use–based tool developed by occupational therapists is the Profiles of Occupational Engagement (POES; Bejerholm et al., 2006), which draws on research exploring time use and occupational engagement of men and women diagnosed with schizophrenia (Bejerholm & Eklund, 2004, 2006). The POES was designed not only to gather information about an individual's time use, but also to assess the quality of their occupational engagement, and initial support for its content validity, internal consistency, and clinical utility has been reported (Bejerholm et al., 2006).

The POES is composed of two parts: the first comprises a 24-hour yesterday time-use diary with an interview to support its completion, and the second involves ranking the person's time use in relation to nine dimensions of occupational engagement: daily rhythm of activity and rest, variety and range of occupations, place, social environment, social interaction, interpretation of experiences, extent of meaningful engagement, routines, and what initiates or triggers performance. Underpinning these nine dimensions is the idea that each is important in contributing to well-being. As illustrated in Figure 10-2 for the dimension of place, each of these dimensions is ranked according to one of four categories.

Interdisciplinary interest in time use as a means to understand the relationships between individuals' experiences of health issues and their activity patterns also means that tools to measure time use are being developed by other health care researchers and practitioners. For example, a simplified time budget measure has been designed for use with adults experiencing psychosis (Jolley et al., 2006). It

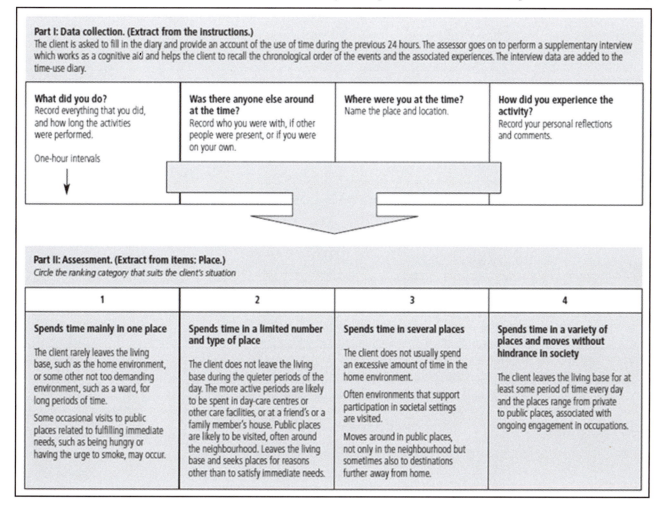

Part I: Data collection. (Extract from the instructions.)
The client is asked to fill in the diary and provide an account of the use of time during the previous 24 hours. The assessor goes on to perform a supplementary interview which works as a cognitive aid and helps the client to recall the chronological order of the events and the associated experiences. The interview data are added to the time-use diary.

What did you do?	**Was there anyone else around at the time?**	**Where were you at the time?**	**How did you experience the activity?**
Record everything that you did, and how long the activities were performed. One-hour intervals	Record who you were with, if other people were present, or if you were on your own.	Name the place and location.	Record your personal reflections and comments.

Part II: Assessment. (Extract from items: Place.)
Circle the ranking category that suits the client's situation

1	2	3	4
Spends time mainly in one place The client rarely leaves the living base, such as the home environment, or some other not too demanding environment, such as a ward, for long periods of time. Some occasional visits to public places related to fulfilling immediate needs, such as being hungry or having the urge to smoke, may occur.	**Spends time in a limited number and type of place** The client does not leave the living base during the quieter periods of the day. The more active periods are likely to be spent in day-care centres or other care facilities, or at a friend's or a family member's house. Public places are likely to be visited, often around the neighbourhood. Leaves the living base and seeks places for reasons other than to satisfy immediate needs.	**Spends time in several places** The client does not usually spend an excessive amount of time in the home environment. Often environments that support participation in societal settings are visited. Moves around in public places, not only in the neighbourhood but sometimes also to destinations further away from home.	**Spends time in a variety of places and moves without hindrance in society** The client leaves the living base for at least some period of time every day and the places range from private to public places, associated with ongoing engagement in occupations.

Figure 10-2. POES assessment process. (From Bejerholm, U., Hansson, L., and Eklund, M., "Profiles of occupational engagement in people with schizophrenia (POES): The development of a new instrument based on time-use diaries," *British Journal of Occupational Therapy, (69)*2, 58-68. Copyright © 2006 by SAGE. Reprinted with permission.)

uses an interview to record activity for four daily blocks of time across the week and rates each block on a scale from 0 (nothing) to 4 (time period filled with varied, demanding, independent activity). Hence, it focuses more on activity levels, rather than on what people are doing or their patterns of participation. Another example is the Social Rhythm Metric, a diary-style self-report tool used to assess the regularity of daily routines, especially the sleep/wake cycle, of persons diagnosed with bipolar disorders, to guide them in developing regular routines in a chronobiological sense as a relapse prevention strategy (Frank et al., 2006). The Social Rhythm Metric records times at which activities were done, the number of people involved, and mood ratings, but again less focus is placed on understanding what the person is doing, experiencing and their patterns of participation. In addition, the recording of daily time use to explore links between activity and mood states, such as depression and anxiety, is a feature of some cognitive interventions.

Few tools have yet been developed to explore or evaluate occupational balance with clients of occupational therapy services. Wagman et al. (2012) suggest that, given occupational balance is subjectively defined, one potential approach to exploring and measuring it might be through the rating of statements related to the different perspectives of occupational balance, as illustrated in Table 10-1.

INTERVENTION RESOURCES

Enabling people whose participation in everyday life is disrupted (whether due to ill-health, disability, or other life circumstances), or to restore or establish meaningful, satisfying patterns of occupational engagement that support health and well-being is a central aim of occupational therapy. In psychosocial practice, identifying, assessing, and understanding time use and patterns of participation are at the core of an occupation-focused practice

TABLE 10-1		
POSSIBLE MEASURES OF EACH OCCUPATIONAL BALANCE PERSPECTIVE		
OCCUPATIONAL BALANCE FROM THE PERSPECTIVE OF OCCUPATIONAL AREAS	OCCUPATIONAL BALANCE FROM THE PERSPECTIVE OF OCCUPATIONS WITH DIFFERENT CHARACTERISTICS	OCCUPATIONAL BALANCE FROM THE PERSPECTIVE OF TIME USE
I am satisfied with my balance between work, leisure activities, restful activities, and sleep.	I have balance between valued, obligatory, and discretionary activities.	I spend sufficient time in physical, mental, social, and restful activities.
I regularly perform activities I regard as leisure.	I have balance between activity and rest.	I spend sufficient time working.
I regularly perform activities I regard as restful.	I have balance between physical, mental, social, and restful activities.	I spend sufficient time doing things with others.
I am satisfied with my sleep.	I have balance between doing things alone and with others.	I spend sufficient time sleeping.
I regularly perform activities I regard as work.	I have balance between challenging and relaxing activities.	I am satisfied with the time I spent on different activities.
From Wagman, P., Håkansson, C., & Björklund, A., "Occupational balance as used in occupational therapy: A concept analysis," *Scandinavian Journal of Occupational Therapy, 19*(4), 322-7. Copyright © 2012 by Informa Healthcare. Reprinted with permission.		

VIGNETTE 10-1

Suppose that the service in which you work has many adult clients with mental health conditions who live in the local community, are unemployed, and report difficulties in finding ways to use their time meaningfully. There are likely to be a range of contributing factors, but applying a knowledge of factors affecting time use and occupational balance, you identify that some of challenges might include lack of occupations that provide time structure, social connections, a sense of contributing or doing something of value to others; limited income and resources to enable participation in leisure or social activities; unwelcoming or exclusionary attitudes in the community; as well as the personal and social impacts of experiencing mental health conditions. Aware that this indicates these clients may not have patterns of occupational engagement that support their well-being, and are at risk of occupational imbalance, you realize that you do not know a lot about what these clients do in their daily lives, or what specific factors they experience as supporting and hindering their finding personally meaningful ways to use their time. Therefore, you offer to facilitate a group and invite these clients to share their time use issues and experiences with each other to better understand their situation and explore possibilities and strategies for meaningful use of time as a group.

since time use gives us access to exploring what people do in daily life.

Many occupation-related interventions address how individuals organize and structure their time use implicitly (Eklund et al., 2009), whether through the ways in which programs are organized to enable occupational engagement that includes structure and routine, or as an outcome of changed occupational engagement (e.g., return to study or work). Examples of specific time-use, focused interventions in occupational therapy literature are rarer. Drawing on Kielhofner's (1977) ideas about temporal adaptation, Neville (1980) described a group program in a short-term inpatient psychiatry setting that focused on exploring individuals'

use of time when living outside the hospital, identifying and supporting plans for change. Another example is a preventative, focused time-use intervention designed to support older workers in preparing for and making the transition to retirement (Cantor, 1981). Such time-use, focused interventions have wide potential applications, because a broad range of clients experience disrupted or restricted patterns of time use and occupational engagement that do not support their well-being.

Vignette 10-1 identifies a set of time-use issues that might be explored and addressed within a group setting; it also argues for designing the group to build peer support and shared knowledge that facilitate clients to self-define meaningful ways to use time and strategies for addressing the difficulties experienced. For example, clients in the vignette might choose to investigate local vocational activity options, or they might decide to develop their own index of valued and accessible local social and recreational options, much as Bryant, McKay, Beresford, and Vacher (2011) described in working with service users to bring about service changes of value to them.

To further guide the development of time-use, focused groups in psychosocial practice contexts like that described in the vignette, Eklund et al. (2009) proposed the following set of 10 general principles:

1. Talking with each participant about his or her individual occupational history

2. Identifying with each person his or her repertoire of occupations (lost, present, or new) and to what extent her or she wishes to engage in them (daily, weekly, or monthly)

3. Identifying each participant's level of engagement and whether he or she experiences being under- or over-occupied, or a sense of balance in his or her occupations, including his or her perceived balance/imbalance between restful, playful and productive occupations

4. Identifying supporting and hindering factors in the social, cultural, and physical environment

5. Framing the optimal use of time with each participant, as a long-term goal, taking into account all of his or her valued, obligatory, and discretionary occupations

6. Identifying short-term goals with each participant for working toward his or her personally defined optimal use of time

7. Supporting each participant to structure daily occupations identified in the short-term goals, into a participation pattern that has a rhythm in synchrony with the light-dark and activity-rest cycles

8. Formulating precise tasks with participants for accomplishment between group meetings

9. Organizing group meetings where participants share experiences, review individual tasks, formulate new goals and strategies, and get feedback and support

10. Offering education about time use and health, as well as information about what is known about the relationship between mental illness and engagement in daily occupations

In comparison, *Action Over Inertia* (AOI; Krupa et al., 2010) offers a time-use intervention designed for working with persons on an individual basis to enable activity engagement and activity patterns that foster and support well-being, quality of life, and health. Initially designed for working collaboratively with community-dwelling individuals experiencing persistent mental illness, this workbook-based intervention is potentially more widely applicable to clients for whom disrupted activity patterns and disengagement from occupations are significant issues. Conceptually, the AOI intervention draws on the Canadian Model of Occupational Performance and Engagement (Townsend & Polatajko, 2007) and a recovery-oriented approach to collaboratively working with living with mental illness, as well as strategies for enabling engagement and change used in occupational therapy, and some educational, cognitive, and behavioral change strategies (Edgelow & Krupa, 2011).

The AOI intervention provides a set of resources readily used for collaborating with individuals to reflect on activity patterns and their impacts on health and well-being, and to promote individuals' understanding of their own activity patterns and activity engagement. Thus, the AOI resources include worksheets for facilitating individuals' exploration and reflection on current activity patterns and engagement, and for planning and supporting immediate and longer-term changes in activity patterns (see Figures 10-3 and 10-4 for examples). There are also materials to guide the provision of information and education about activity patterns and health, and the relationships between mental health issues and occupational engagement. A particular focus of this intervention is on anticipating and addressing the personal and environmental challenges that individuals will inevitably experience in reigniting their activity patterns. For example, people with health conditions may experience associated impairments such as fatigue or pain, limited social networks to support their activity changes, and environmental factors such as limited transportation or a lack of discretionary finances.

Vignette 10-2, together with Figures 10-3 and 10-4, illustrates the use of some of the AOI worksheets in supporting a young woman to explore and reflect on her current activity patterns and engagement.

EVALUATION PROCESSES FOR OUTCOMES

Broadly speaking, time use and occupational balance focused interventions seek to address disrupted activity patterns and disengagement from occupations, and to enable personally satisfying and health-promoting occupational engagement. Time use diaries offer a directly relevant and accessible outcome to evaluate these kinds of interventions in terms that people with lived experience of disrupted activity patterns relate to (Farnworth, 2004). In addition, because time use patterns provide indicators of daily life adaptation, community adjustment, and quality of life, changes in time use patterns might be expected to reflect change in these outcome domains too.

An understanding of the concept of occupational balance highlights the fact that change in personally satisfying and

My current activity patterns

Date: _____ / _____ / _____

Name: _Stephanie_____

Consider each statement and check all that apply

Criteria	✓	Examples
My days are not balanced with time for fun, work, taking care of myself, and rest.		_balanced - not enough rest?_
I have lots of time, but nothing to do.		_it's the opposite for me_
I spend most of my day resting, listening to others or watching television.		_try to rest, always tired but never get to rest_
I do not have a regular routine.		_not tight but some routine_
I don't see many other people during my day or week or do many things with other people.		_I see people every day_
I do not go to many different places to do things during my day or week.		_I go to few places_
I can't think of many things I do that are really enjoyable to me.		_I can think of lots of things, but often don't get to do them_
I get easily upset or overwhelmed when I do activities.	x	_I get easily worked up if things are not working out_
I wish that I could find some things to do that are really enjoyable to me.		_too tired and don't have time_
There are things I would like to do, but there are barriers to why I don't do them, such as lack of money, transportation, or a friend to go with.	x	_don't have time or enegry_

Are you generally satisfied with your daily time use and activities?
Add any other thoughts or ideas here:

I'm not doing all I want to - not satisfied, feel lay, and always tired

Action Over Inertia © CAOT PUBLICATIONS ACE 2010

Figure 10-3. Stephanie's reflection on her current activity patterns, using AOI intervention worksheet. (From Krupa, T., et al., "Action over inertia: Addressing the activity-health needs of individuals with serious mental illness," Ottawa, Canada. Copyright © 2010 by CAOT Publications ACE. Reprinted with permission.)

health-promoting occupational engagement is not solely a matter of more or less time spent in particular occupations. Hence, it is also important to attend to occupational engagement outcomes. Thus, in psychosocial practice, a tool like the POES (Bejerholm et al., 2006) described previously could be used to review and evaluate the extent to which a person is engaged in occupations that are varied, meaningful, socially connected, and occur in varied places.

In addition, engagement in personally meaningful activities is identified by people experiencing ongoing mental ill-health as a key element in recovering and crafting a life beyond illness or disability (Borg & Davidson, 2008; Mezzina et al., 2006). Therefore, the extent to which time use and occupational balance focused interventions support people in their recovery should also be considered an important outcome.

Benefits of my current activities

Date:_____/_____/____

Name: _Stephanie_ _____

Check all of the items that apply to you.

My daily activities give me the opportunity to …	✓	Examples/comments
Develop new skills and knowledge	x	*Volunteering*
Feel as though I am making a valuable contribution to society	x	
Remain physically active and healthy		*not at the moment*
Enjoy beautiful parts of life, such as nature, music, and art	x	*sometimes have time to enjoy nature*
Express my thoughts and feelings	x	*with friends*
Interact with other people socially	x	
Achieve goals and feel as though I have accomplished something	x	*raising kids*
Express values that are personally important to me	x	
Earn a personal income	x	
Interact with important people in my life (family, friends, etc.) and make them feel good	x	*mostly - not all*

Action Over Inertia © CAOT PUBLICATIONS ACE 2010

Figure 10-4. Stephanie's reflection on the benefits of her current activities, using AOI intervention worksheet. (From Krupa, T., et al., "Action over inertia: Addressing the activity-health needs of individuals with serious mental illness," Ottawa, Canada. Copyright © 2010 by CAOT Publications ACE. Reprinted with permission.)

EVIDENCE FOR THE APPROACH

There is substantial research evidence that time allocation and time-use patterns of people experiencing prolonged health conditions and disabilities differ from those of the general populations (Harvey & Pentland, 2010; Pagán, 2013). The time use and occupational imbalance issues faced by people with ongoing mental health issues are also well documented internationally (Edgelow & Krupa, 2011). Hence, there is ample evidence that time use and occupational balance focused interventions are needed in psychosocial practice. There are also well-established practice tools, such as the OQ (Smith et al., 1986), that are

VIGNETTE 10-2. STEPHANIE

Stephanie is in her twenties and lives with family including her sister and two young children. She has casual employment in a school, meaning that her work hours vary from week to week. Waiting for calls about work and uncertainty about when she may be required to work made it difficult to keep things in order in her life, causing her anxiety especially at night. Prior depression and life stressors, as well as her lack of sleep, low levels of energy, and a sense that she was not doing very much led her doctor to recommend Stephanie explore psychosocial interventions with an occupational therapist on an outpatient basis.

Using two of the Action over Inertia intervention worksheets, Stephanie was first supported to reflect on her current activity pattern and how her activities might be affecting her health (see Figures 10-3 and 10-4). These enabled Stephanie to identify that her dissatisfaction with her time use related to often feeling tired, not doing all the things she wanted to, and her regular activities not supporting her to remain physically active and healthy, despite being beneficial to her in other ways. She was then encouraged to complete a time-use log, so that she and the occupational therapist could look together at what she was actually doing, and better understand her sleep and activity patterns.

From her time use log completed for five days (see Figure 10-1), Stephanie identified that she was both doing more than she previously appreciated, and doing activities that she valued and considered productive (parenting and volunteering in particular), but also that few of her activities were physically active. This led to her considering how she might improve her self-care and get in touch with nature again. As a result, she planned to build more physical activity into her leisure by going for walks with friends, and to use the POES (Bejerholm et al., 2006) to review her occupational engagement.

In this way, the occupational therapist used the AOI intervention to work collaboratively with Stephanie to develop greater understanding of her activity patterns, the benefits gained through participating in her current activities, and how to identify ways in which she might change her activity patterns to enhance her sense of satisfaction, health, and well-being through what she does in daily life.

Appreciation is extended to Peter Weymouth, BOT, MAOT (Cand) for this illustration of the use of Action Over Inertia in psychosocial occupational therapy practice.

---

suitable for use in a wide range of practice settings. In comparison, few specific time use, focused interventions have been systematically evaluated (Edgelow & Krupa, 2011; Eklund et al., 2009).

The efficacy and clinical utility of the AOI intervention suggests it is a promising intervention to improve occupational balance and engagement, when used with adults living with mental illness based on evidence from a small-scale, prospective, randomized controlled trial in Ontario, Canada (Edgelow & Krupa, 2011). In this study, occupational therapists employed in five assertive community treatment (ACT) teams worked with 10 individuals using the AOI workbook–based intervention over 12 once-weekly sessions. Outcomes, including time use (collected using time-use diaries), occupational engagement as measured by the POES (Bejerholm et al., 2006), and the Engagement in Meaningful Activities Survey (EMAS) (Goldberg, Brintnell, & Goldberg, 2002) were assessed and compared between baseline and 12 weeks post-test for 18 individuals randomly assigned to receive standard ACT care or ACT care and the AOI intervention. Participants in the AOI intervention increased their occupational balance and commented positively on their experience of the AOI intervention and changes that they had made; however,

no differences in occupational engagement between the groups were detected. While AOI was initially designed and trialled with individuals receiving ACT services, its further use and evaluation in other psychosocial practice settings and as a group-based intervention are recommended (Edgelow & Krupa, 2011). The further articulation of occupational therapy interventions that address time use and occupational imbalance issues and facilitate meaningful, health-sustaining participation in daily life, and the demonstration of their effectiveness are priorities for strengthening of evidence-based, occupational focused psychosocial practice.

CONCLUSION

Time use as a perspective from which to evaluate patterns of occupational participation has a long history within the occupational therapy profession. Advancements in the understanding of time use have highlighted the complexity of time use and its relationship to health and well-being. They have also offered a range of distinct concepts to provide a nuanced understanding of time use and principles and practices to enable health-promoting time use patterns. Recent occupational therapy efforts have been focused on developing and evaluating a range of intervention approaches.

LEARNING ACTIVITIES/ DISCUSSION QUESTIONS

1. What could be the relative strengths and limitations of the time use diaries as tools for gathering information in occupational therapy practice about clients' time use and patterns of participation?

2. In what ways might activity patterns contribute to a sense of well-being?

3. What is meant by the terms *occupational balance* and *occupational imbalance*? Make a list of some of the different ways in which these terms are understood.

4. Think of a client of occupational therapy services with whom you have worked as an occupational therapist or student recently.

    a. Make a list of what you know about how this person's time use and activity patterns, then consider what information-gathering tools might support you and this person to better understand his or her time use and activity patterns.

    b. How might you explore with this person the extent to which he or she has a sense of occupational balance or imbalance in life?

    c. In what ways might an understanding of this client's time use and activity patterns assist you to support his or her engagement in valued occupations and/or to enhance his or her sense of occupational balance?

    d. What information about time use or occupational balance might be useful to promote this client's understanding of his or her own patterns of participation in everyday occupations?

REFERENCES

Backman, C. L. (2004). Occupational balance: Exploring the relationships among daily occupations and their influence on wellbeing. *Canadian Journal of Occupational Therapy, 71*(4), 202-209.

Backman, C. L. (2010). Occupational balance and well-being. In C. H. Christiansen & E. A. Townsend (Eds). *Introduction to occupation: The art and science of living* (2nd ed., pp. 231-249). New Jersey: Prentice-Hall.

Bejerholm, U. (2010). Occupational balance in people with schizophrenia. *Occupational Therapy in Mental Health, 26*(1), 1-17.

Bejerholm, U., & Eklund, M. (2004). Time use and occupational performance among persons with schizophrenia. *Occupational Therapy in Mental Health, 20*(1), 27-47.

Bejerholm, U., & Eklund, M. (2006). Engagement in occupations among men and women with schizophrenia. *Occupational Therapy International, 13*(2), 100-121.

Bejerholm, U., Hansson, L., & Eklund, M. (2006). Profiles of occupational engagement in people with schizophrenia (POES): The development of a new instrument based on time-use diaries. *British Journal of Occupational Therapy, 69*(2), 58-68.

Borg, M., & Davidson, L. (2008). The nature of recovery as lived in everyday experience. *Journal of Mental Health, 17*(2), 129-140.

Brown, C. E. (2014). Ecological Models in Occupational Therapy. In B. A. B. Schell, et al. (Eds.), *Willard and Spackman's occupational therapy* (12th ed., pp. 494-504). Philadelphia: Lippincott, Williams & Wilkins.

Bryant, W., McKay, E., Beresford, P., & Vacher, G. (2011). An occupational perspective on participatory action research. In F. Kronenberg, N. Pollard, & D. Sakellariou (Eds.), Occupational therapies without borders: Volume 2: Towards an ecology of occupation-based practices (pp. 367-374). Edinburgh: Churchill Livingstone Elsevier.

Cantor, S. G. (1981). Occupational therapists as members of pre-retirement resource teams. *American Journal of Occupational Therapy, 35*, 638-643.

Christiansen, C. H. (1996). Three perspectives on balance in occupation. In R. Zemke, & F. Clark (Eds.), *Occupational science: The evolving discipline* (pp. 431-451). Philadelphia, F. A. Davis.

Christiansen, C. H. (2005). Time use and patterns of occupation. In C. H. Christiansen, C. M. Baum, & J. Bass-Haugen (Eds.), *Occupational therapy: Performance, participation, and well-being* (3rd ed., pp. 70-91). Thorofare, NJ: SLACK Incorporated.

Christiansen, C., Backman, C., Little, B. R., & Nguyen, A. (1998). Occupations and wellbeing: A study of personal projects. *American Journal of Occupational Therapy, 52*(1), 91-100.

Christiansen, C. H., & Matuska, K. M. (2006). Lifestyle balance: A review of concepts and research. *Journal of Occupational Science, 13*(1), 49-61.

Clark, F. (1997). Reflections on the human as an occupational being: Biological need, tempo and temporality. *Journal of Occupational Science: Australia, 4*(3), 86-92.

Edgelow, M., & Krupa, T. (2011). Randomized controlled pilot study of an occupational time-use intervention for people with serious mental illness. *American Journal of Occupational Therapy, 65*, 267-276.

Eklund, M., Erlandsson, L., & Leufstadius, C. (2010). Time use in relation to valued and satisfying occupations among people with persistent mental illness: exploring occupational balance. *Journal of Occupational Science, 17*(4), 231-238.

Eklund, M., & Leufstadius, C. (2007). Occupational factors and aspects of health and wellbeing in individuals with persistent mental illness living in the community. *Canadian Journal of Occupational Therapy, 74*, 303-313.

Eklund, M., Leufstadius, C., & Bejerholm, U. (2009). Time use among people with psychiatric disabilities: Implications for practice. *Psychiatric Rehabilitation Journal, 32*(3), 177-191.

Farnworth, L. (2003). 2003 Sylvia Docker lecture: Time use, tempo and temporality: Occupational therapy's core business or someone else's business. *Australian Occupational Therapy Journal, 50,* 116-126.

Farnworth, L. (2004). Time use and disability. In M. Molineux (Ed.). *Occupation for occupational therapists,* (pp. 46-65). Oxford: Blackwell Publishing.

Farnworth, L., & Fossey, E. (2003). Occupational terminology interactive dialogue: Explaining the concepts of time use, tempo and temporality. *Journal of Occupational Science, 10*(3), 150-153.

Fisher, A. G. (1994). Functional assessment and occupation: Critical issues for occupational therapy. *New Zealand Journal of Occupational Therapy, 45*(2), 13-19.

Forhan, M., & Backman, C. L. (2010). Exploring occupational balance in adults with rheumatoid arthritis. *OTJR: Occupation, Participation & Health, 30, 133-141.*

Fossey, E. M. (2009). *Participating as resisting: Everyday life stories of people experiencing mental health issues.* (PhD thesis, The University of Melbourne, Melbourne, Australia).

Frank, E., Gonzalez, J. M., & Fagiolini, A. (2006). The importance of routine for preventing recurrence in bipolar disorder. *American Journal of Psychiatry, 163(6),* 981-985.

Furst, G., Gerber, L., Smith, C., Fisher, S., & Shulman, B. (1987). A program for improving energy conservation behaviors in adults with rheumatoid arthritis. *American Journal of Occupational Therapy, 41,* 102-111.

Goldberg, B., Brintnell, E., & Goldberg, J. (2002). The relationship between engagement in meaningful activities and quality of life in persons disabled by mental illness. *Occupational Therapy in Mental Health, 18*(2), 17-44.

Håkansson, C., Dahlin-Ivanoff, S., & Sonn, U. (2006). Achieving balance in everyday life. *Journal of Occupational Science, 13*(1), 74-82.

Håkansson, C., & Matuska, K. M. (2010). How life balance is perceived by Swedish women recovering from a stress-related disorder: A validation of the life balance model. *Journal of Occupational Science, 17*(2), 112-119.

Hammel, J., Magasi, S., Heinemann, A., Whiteneck, G., Bogner, J., & Rodriguez, E. (2008). What does participation mean? An insider perspective from people with disabilities. *Disability and Rehabilitation, 30*(19), 1445-1460.

Hammell, K. W. (2009). Self-care, productivity, and leisure, or dimensions of occupational experience? *Canadian Journal of Occupational Therapy, 76*(2), 107-114.

Haertl, K. (2010) Study guide – Occupational balance and wellbeing. In C. H. Christiansen, & E. A. Townsend (Eds). *Introduction to occupation: The art and science of living* (2nd ed., pp. 245-247). Upper Saddle River, New Jersey: Prentice-Hall.

Harvey, A. S., & Pentland, W. (2010). What do people do? In C. H. Christiansen & E. A. Townsend (Eds.). *Introduction to occupation: The art and science of living.* (2nd ed., pp. 101-133). NJ: Prentice-Hall.

Harvey, C., Fossey, E., Jackson, H., & Shimitras, L. (2006). Time use of people living with schizophrenia in a North London: Predictors of participation in occupations and their implications for improving social inclusion. *Journal of Mental Health, 15*(1), 43-55.

Illman, S., Spence, S., O'Campo, P., & Kirsh, B. (2013). Exploring the occupations of homeless adults living with mental illnesses in Toronto. *Canadian Journal of Occupational Therapy, 80*(4), 215-223.

Jolley, S., Garety, P. A., Ellett, L., Kuipers, E., Freeman, D., Bebbington, P. E., Fowler, D. G., & Dunn, G. (2006). A validation of a new measure of activity in psychosis. *Schizophrenia Research, 85,* 288-295.

Jonsson, H. (2008). A new direction in the conceptualization and categorization of occupation. *Journal of Occupational Science, 15*(1), 3-8.

Jonsson, H. (2010). Occupational transitions: Work to retirement. In C. H. Christiansen & E. A. Townsend (Eds). *Introduction to occupation: The art and science of living* (2nd ed., pp. 211-230). Upper Saddle River, New Jersey: Prentice-Hall.

Jonsson, H., & Persson, D. (2006). Towards an experiential model of occupational balance: An alternative perspective on flow theory analysis. *Journal of Occupational Science, 13*(1), 62-73.

Kielhofner, G. (1977). Temporal adaptation: A conceptual framework for occupational therapy. *American Journal of Occupational Therapy, 31*(4), 235-242.

Kielhofner, G. (2008). (Ed.) *A model of human occupation: Theory and application* (4th ed.). Baltimore, MD: Lippincott, Williams & Wilkins.

Kielhofner, G., Forsyth, K., Suman, M. Kramer, J., Nakamura-Thomas, H., Yamada, T.,...Henry, A. (2008). Self-reports: Eliciting client's perspectives. In: G. Kielhofner (Ed.), *Model of human occupation: Theory and application* (4th ed., pp. 237-261). Baltimore, MD: Lippincott, Williams & Wilkins.

Krupa, T., Edgelow, M., Chen, S., Mieras, C., Almas, A., Perry, A., ... Bransfield, M. (2010). *Action over inertia: Addressing the activity-health needs of individuals with serious mental illness.* Ottawa, ON: CAOT Publications ACE.

Krupa, T., McLean, H., Eastbrook, S., Bonham, A., & Baksh, L. (2003) Daily time use as a measure of community adjustment for persons served by assertive community treatment teams. *American Journal of Occupational Therapy, 57*(5), 558-565.

Larson, E. A. (2004). The times of our lives: The experience of temporality in occupation. *Canadian Journal of Occupational Therapy, 71*(1), 24-35.

Larson, E., & von Eye, A. (2010). Beyond flow: Temporality and participation in everyday activities. *American Journal of Occupational Therapy, 64*(1), 152-163.

Legault, E., & Rebeiro, K. L. (2001). Occupation as means to mental health: A single-case study. *American Journal of Occupational Therapy, 55*(1), 90-96.

Liedberg, G. M., Hesselstrand, M. E., & Henriksson, C. M. (2004). Time use and activity patterns in women with long-term pain. *Scandinavian Journal of Occupational Therapy, 11*(1), 26-35.

Matuska, K. M., & Christiansen, C. H. (2008). A proposed model of lifestyle balance. *Journal of Occupational Science, 15*(1), 9-19.

Matuska, K. M., & Erickson, B. (2008). Lifestyle balance: how it is described and experienced by women with multiple sclerosis. *Journal of Occupational Science, 15*(1), 20-26.

McNulty, M. C., Crowe, T. K., Kroening, C., VanLeit, B., & Good, R. (2009). Time use of women with children living in an emergency shelter for survivors of domestic violence. *OTJR: Occupation, Participation & Health, 29*(4), 183-190.

Meyer, A. (1922/1977). The philosophy of occupational therapy. *American Journal of Occupational Therapy, 31*(10), 639-642.

Mezzina, R., Borg, M., Marin, I., Sells, D., Topor, A., & Davidson, L. (2006). From participation to citizenship: How to regain a role, a status, and a life in the process of recovery. *American Journal of Psychiatric Rehabilitation, 9*, 39-61.

Minato, M., & Zemke, R. (2004). Occupational choices of people with schizophrenia living in the community. *Journal of Occupational Science, 11*, 31-39.

Neville, A. (1980). Temporal adaptation: application with short-term psychiatric patients. *American Journal of Occupational Therapy, 34*, 328-331.

Pagán, R. (2013). Time allocation of disabled individuals. *Social Science & Medicine, 84*, 80-93. http://dx.doi.org/10.1016/j.socscimed.2013.02.014.

Pentland, W. E., & McColl, M. A. (1999). Application of time use research to the study of life with a disability. In W. E. Pentland, A. S. Harvey, M. P. Lawton, & M. A. McColl (Eds.), *Time use research in the social sciences* (pp. 169-188). New York: Kluwer Academic/Plenum Publishers.

Polatajko, H. J., Backman, C., Baptiste, S., Davis, J., Eftekar, P.,...Harvey, A. (2007). Human occupation in context. In E. A. Townsend & H. J. Polatajko (Eds.), *Enabling occupation II: Advancing an occupational therapy vision for health, wellbeing and justice through occupation* (pp. 37-61). Ottawa, ON: CAOT Publications ACE.

Scanlan, J. N., Bundy, A. C., & Matthews, L. R. (2011). Promoting wellbeing in young unemployed adults: The importance of identifying meaningful patterns of time use. *Australian Occupational Therapy Journal, 58*, 111-119.

Smith, N., Kielhofner, G., & Watts, J. (1986). The relationship between volition, activity pattern and life satisfaction in the elderly. *American Journal of Occupational Therapy, 40*, 278-283.

Stamm, T., Lovelock, L., Stew, G., Nell, V., Smolen, J., Machold, K., Jonsson, H., & Sadlo, G. (2009). I have a disease but I am not ill: A narrative study of occupational balance in people with rheumatoid arthritis. *OTJR: Occupation, Participation & Health, 29*(1), 32-39.

Thompson, J. A., & Bunderson, J. S. (2001). Work-nonwork conflict and the phenomenology of time: Beyond the balance metaphor. *Work and Occupations, 28*(1), 17-39.

Townsend, E. A., & Polatajko, H. J. (Eds.), *Enabling occupation II: Advancing an occupational therapy vision for health, wellbeing and justice through occupation*. Ottawa, ON: CAOT Publications ACE.

Wagman, P., Håkansson, C., & Björklund, A. (2012). Occupational balance as used in occupational therapy: A concept analysis. *Scandinavian Journal of Occupational Therapy, 19*(4), 322-7.

Whiteford, G. E. (2009). Problematizing life balance: Difference, diversity and disadvantage. In K. M. Matuska & C. H. Christiansen (Eds.), *Life balance: Multidisciplinary theories and research* (pp. 23-32). Thorofare, NJ: SLACK Incorporated.

Wilcock, A. A. (2006). *An occupational perspective of health.* Thorofare, NJ: SLACK Incorporated.

Yanos, P. T., West, M. L., & Smith, S. M. (2010). Coping, productive time use, and negative mood among adults with severe mental illness: A daily diary study. *Schizophrenia Research, 124*, 54-59.

Person-Level Models and Frameworks

In Section IV, several well-established practice models that focus on person-level aspects of occupation in psychosocial practice are presented. In addition to providing an overview of the core assumptions and processes of change, the chapters discuss occupational therapy intervention approaches flowing from these models, relevant tools and practices, and, where available, the supporting evidence-base. Chapter 11 focuses on the behavioral models underlying learning and occupation. Chapter 12 focuses on cognitive-behavioral models that provide an understanding of how thought processes influence and can be influenced to enable occupation. Chapter 13 focuses on expression and occupation, and relates to psychodynamic theory and practice. The chapter highlights that, following years of declining interest, there has been a renewed interest in psychodynamic approaches in recent years. Finally, the chapter on coping and occupation describes the relevance of coping to human occupation and the ways that occupational therapists can facilitate positive coping processes.

Each of these models is well grounded in basic knowledge and theory, evolving largely within the field of psychology. Several of these models were prominent in the historical evolution of psychosocial occupational therapy and this is described more fully in Chapter 2. With the resurgence of interest in occupation-focused practice within the profession, efforts have been made to integrate these models and their application into a more holistic approach to influence human occupation. The titles of the chapters have been purposely developed to capture the key processes by which these models influence occupation. So, for example, Chapter 11 is titled "Learning and Occupation," to capture the idea that behavioral models, in their essence, provide a way of understanding how occupational therapists can enable people to develop essential skills and competencies associated with their day-to-day occupations.

The section focuses only on a few of the most widely applied person-level models relevant to psychosocial practice. Other person-level models, such as cognitive disabilities/remediation and sensory models, can provide a valuable perspective from which to view the occupational issues, but they are not included here only because the underlying mechanisms of performance and of treatment approaches are qualitatively distinct. For example, the cognitive-behavioral model and related approaches presented in this text are oriented to changing the negative thoughts and beliefs (psychological functions) that interfere with positive and adaptive occupational behaviors, whereas cognitive remedial models are oriented to correcting, modifying, or accommodating (neuro-behavioral) deficits in important cognitive processes such as attention, memory, and executive functioning. The exclusion of these models from this book is in no way meant to diminish their importance; indeed a holistic view of human occupation will recognize that all of these person-level factors can be operating simultaneously and in a dynamic fashion.

Learning and Occupation

Bonnie Kirsh, PhD, OT Reg (Ont)

To train an animal, you ignore behaviors you don't want, and reinforce behaviors you do. I learned this from Amy Sutherland's wonderful book, What Shamu Taught Me About Life, Love, and Marriage, *which applies the techniques of exotic animal training to human behavior...The same principle applies when training yourself to eat right, stay active, finish your email, or complete any other desirable behavior. Break the challenge into tiny steps, then take one step each day, following the step immediately with a reward of some kind. If you repeat the same behavior-plus-reward...the behavior becomes a pattern, and you'll be able to sustain it with very little effort.* (Martha Beck, 2009. Reprinted with permission.)

OBJECTIVES

The objectives of this chapter are as follows:
- » Define the basic principles underlying behavioral approaches to learning.
- » Describe theorists' contributions across disciplines to the development of these principles.
- » Explain developments and adaptations to learning theory over time.
- » Consider how occupational therapists can apply these principles in their work.

Krupa, T., Kirsh, B., Pitts, D., & Fossey, E. *Bruce & Borg's Psychosocial Frames of Reference: Theories, Models, and Approaches for Occupation-Based Practice, Fourth Edition* (pp 177-189).
© 2016 SLACK Incorporated.

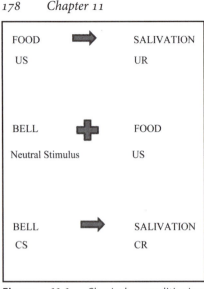

Figure 11-1. Classical conditioning: Unconditioned and conditioned stimuli and responses.

THE VIEW OF HEALTH/DISORDER FROM A LEARNING PERSPECTIVE

Occupational therapy is concerned with helping people develop the skills they need to carry out their everyday roles within a broad range of community contexts, including living, learning, working, and social environments. A learning approach based on behavioral principles is commonly used to help people develop skills and gain mastery in these activities of everyday living. Within a behavioral or learning framework, health is seen to be a state of congruence between the skills that one has, and the occupational demands and roles that are to be fulfilled within context, so that one can live meaningfully according to his or her values and goals. While there is never perfect harmony between these two sides of the equation, occupational therapists who use a behavioral approach emphasize that learning is possible and people can acquire the competencies they need to adapt to the occupational demands of their environments when environmental conditions and behavioral consequences are thoughtfully organized.

Within this framework, disorder is seen as maladaptive behavior that has been learned with the result being unsatisfactory occupational participation and functioning. The behaviorist view explains that disorder results from reinforcement or conditioning that did not meet an individual's needs, was not socially acceptable, or there was lack of learning behavioral cues. The result—problematic and disruptive behaviors or lack of skills—produces ineffective adaptation.

MAIN COMPONENTS/CONCEPTS

Key components of learning theory based on behavioral principles include classical conditioning, operant conditioning, reinforcement, and observational learning.

Classical Conditioning

Ivan Pavlov is the founder of classical conditioning and his dog salivation experiments, conducted in the early 1900s, are still relevant today. Pavlov paired a neutral stimulus—a bell—with a stimulus that would reliably produce the desired response of salivation—food. This pairing was presented to the dogs a number of times and eventually, the bell sound alone was enough to cause the dogs to salivate. In this experiment, the neutral object (bell) that was unrelated to the desired response (salivation) elicited the response because it was associated with a stimulus (food) that already produces that response. This type of learning is known as classical conditioning.

Analyzing this experiment further provides us with the language and concepts needed to apply the theory to occupational therapy practice situations. Pavlov named the salivation that was elicited by the food as the *unconditioned response* because it naturally occurred—it was an unlearned, automatic behavior. For similar reasons, he named the food the *unconditioned stimulus*—it naturally invited the salivary response, or the unconditioned response. The bell is referred to as the *conditioned stimulus* because it produced the salivation only after learning occurred. When salivation occurs in response to the conditioned stimulus, the salivary response is then considered to be a *conditioned response*. This conditioned response is an acquired response—in other words, it is learned behavior (Figure 11-1).

Knowledge of how learning occurs in this way can enable occupational therapists to recognize associations between environmental stimuli and responses in clients that lead to learned behaviors. As an example, one client who was being seen by a community occupational therapist had reported that, on several occasions, she had heard a loud bang as she rode the elevator in her building, causing her heart to race. Here, the stimulus (the bang) and response (heart racing) are unconditioned, as they occur naturally. However, because they were associated with the elevator (the neutral stimulus), the client began to feel anxious each time she approached the elevator and it soon became the conditioned stimulus. This sequence of events continued over some time and escalated to the development of agoraphobia, a fear of going out. The client was working with her occupational therapist to overcome this fear.

Operant Conditioning

Another common form of learning is *operant conditioning*, formalized by B. F. Skinner. While classical conditioning positions the learner as a passive recipient of environmental stimuli that are associated with particular responses, operant conditioning sees the learner as more active or instrumental in this process; thus, operant conditioning is also referred to as *instrumental learning*. Within this theory, the consequences of a particular action determine the likelihood that it will be performed in the future, or learned.

Skinner developed the theory through experiments conducted with rats in his "Skinner box," where rats learned to press a lever in the box to get food. At first, pressing the lever was accidental, but soon the rats would go to the lever as soon as they were placed in the box, as doing so led to the consequence of receiving food. This positive reinforcement increased the likelihood that the response would be repeated again. Accordingly, operant conditioning maintains that behavior is learned because it is reinforced.

Reinforcement

Reinforcers can be primary or secondary. *Primary reinforcers* are those that satisfy biological needs, such as the food in Skinner's experiments. *Secondary reinforcers* do not satisfy biological needs, but nevertheless do increase the likelihood of a particular response being repeated; an example is a sticker given to a child for sharing a toy, or an A for a student paper that has been well thought out and researched.

Reinforcers can also be positive or negative. *Positive reinforcement*, or reward, increases the likelihood of a behavior being repeated because it is pleasurable. A smile given in return for a helpful act, an increase in pay for a job well done, or a new dress for successfully shedding weight on a diet are all examples of positive reinforcement. *Negative reinforcement* increases the likelihood of a behavior occurring through the removal of an aversive stimulus. Examples of negative reinforcement are the removal of noise in a workplace to encourage concentration and productivity, or removal of the mess in one's apartment to encourage an organized daily approach to self-care. Both positive and negative reinforcement increase the likelihood of a behavior occurring.

Punishment, on the other hand, reduces the likelihood of a particular behavior. Positive punishment involves the administration of an aversive stimulus, for example, a child who has misbehaved may be required to do chores that he detests, or a person who ruminates about her ex-partner may snap a rubber band on her wrist to stop the rumination. Negative punishment involves the removal of a pleasurable stimulus; for example, a child who angrily throws a toy across the room may have the toy removed to decrease the likelihood of his aggressive act. In both cases—positive and negative—punishment is intended to suppress a particular behavior.

Punishment should be used sparingly. Although it may successfully suppress the unwanted behavior, it does not provide information about what behavior is preferred. Reinforcing a student for helping his peer is preferable to punishing a student for acting aggressively toward a peer, as, in the former case, the student is able to determine what behaviors are to be repeated. While punishing this student may reduce the undesirable behavior for a while, it would not help the student learn desired behaviors. Punishment is also problematic because it can produce other impacts that are undesirable and not related to learning. So for example, expectations of punishment might lead to an increase in fear and anxiety and negatively influence self-esteem. The use of punishment raises many ethical concerns. If punishment is to be used, it must be done with careful consideration and it is best to be combined with reinforcement of desired behavior.

The timing of reinforcement is one of the most important determinants of the effectiveness of a reinforcer's influence on behavior. While *continuous reinforcement*, or reinforcing a behavior every time it occurs, results in faster learning, this situation rarely occurs in the real world. Partial reinforcement, or reinforcing behavior intermittently, is more common. Behavior that is reinforced intermittently is less likely to subside or be extinguished once reinforcement is withdrawn (Karoly, 1975). *Intermittent reinforcement* can be random or based on schedules.

In a *ratio schedule*, reinforcement is based on the number of times the behavior occurs. To encourage a client to participate in a therapeutic group, for example, the leader may respond with "great point!" every third or fourth time the client contributes. With *interval schedules*, reinforcement is based on an interval of time passing. A disruptive young student may be encouraged to increase his concentration in the classroom by providing reinforcement (e.g., a smile or praise) every 10 minutes while he sits and focuses on his work. In general, ratio reinforcement leads to greater responding than does interval reinforcement. For example, paying a worker for each completed project leads to greater productivity than paying by the hour.

In a *fixed schedule*, the reinforcer is provided following a set number of occurrences or time. In *variable schedules* of reinforcement, the reinforcer is applied at different rates or at different times. Putting these terms together, a schedule can be fixed ratio, fixed interval, variable ratio, or variable interval. An often-cited example of a variable ratio schedule of reinforcement is a slot machine, which results in a jackpot after variable occurrences or number of times the participant drops his or her coins into the machine.

Shaping

Shaping refers to the process of reinforcing skills or behaviors that successively approximate the desired behavior until the target behavior or skill is attained. Responses that approach the desired behavior are called *successive approximations* and by making a list of these steps, from the initial state to the final behavior, therapists can make decisions about which ones to reinforce, as well as the appropriate schedule for doing so. An example of shaping can be found in helping a client persist at a work task for the two hours required of him. First, a baseline level of the length of time the client is able to focus on the task is obtained—perhaps it is 20 minutes. Then the gap between the current behavior (working for 20 minutes) and the desired behavior (working for 2 hours) is broken into steps and reinforcers applied—the client may be first be reinforced for persisting in the task for 25 minutes—when this can be achieved consistently, reinforcement is given at the 40-minute mark, and so on until he is able to persist for the full 2 hours.

Chaining

Chaining is similar to shaping in many respects. While shaping involves reinforcing each successive action, chaining involves linking the actions together in a particular order. Simple skills are combined to form more complex ones. Helping a client develop improved hygiene may successfully use this technique. First, he or she may be reinforced for placing worn clothing in the laundry hamper, then for washing the clothes in the machine, and then for completing a full laundry, including the previous steps as well as folding and replacing the clean clothes. Chaining can also occur in reverse order, through a process called *backward chaining*. As an example, the first step in helping a client learn how to bake a cake may be to assist him with the final step, icing the cake, so that he can be reinforced by the final result. From there the client puts the batter in the oven and completes the cake and then finally makes the batter, bakes it, and ices the cake.

Prompt and Fade

Discriminative stimuli refer to signals or events that indicate the availability of positive reinforcement if particular behavioral responses are made. For example, *prompting* involves providing a cue, which may be a verbal one, a physical one such as touch, or a signal, to guide the client to perform a given behavior. *Fading* refers to the gradual cessation of these prompts so that natural, more subtle elements in the environment will come to evoke appropriate behavior without the learner's reliance on artificial prompts (Karoly, 1975).

Extinction

Extinction, not following a behavior with reinforcement, can reduce undesired behavior. In classical conditioning, extinction occurs when a conditioned stimulus is no longer paired with an unconditioned stimulus. For example, if the woman getting on the elevator did so repeatedly in the absence of the loud bang described previously, her response of anxiety and avoidance would eventually be extinguished. In operant conditioning, extinction can occur if the target behavior is no longer reinforced or if the type of reinforcement used is no longer rewarding. For example, a worker who gets little reward from his work may cease to put in extra effort.

Observational Learning

Thus far, it has been highlighted that learning can occur through classical or operant conditioning. Another way for learning to occur is through observation. Albert Bandura's classic studies are most closely associated with what we know about observational learning. In these studies, children were shown films of adults playing with a Bobo doll, either peacefully or aggressively. Those children who witnessed the aggressive play were themselves more than twice as likely to act aggressively toward the doll than the group who observed peaceful play (Bandura, Ross, & Ross, 1961).

The implication of observational learning is that skills and behaviors may be learned through demonstration. It suggests that *modeling* may be an effective method of helping others gain skills and new behaviors. When a model is reinforced for performing a behavior, an individual may be more apt to adopt the behavior. This was the case in Bandura's experiments; when adults played aggressively with the Bobo doll and were rewarded for it, children were more likely to be aggressive toward the doll themselves. This type of learning—*vicarious learning*—occurs when people learn about the consequences of an action by observing others being rewarded or punished for performing the action. The notion that modeling may be an effective strategy for learning is used by occupational therapists when they facilitate groups. For example, a group member who witnesses another group member getting praise for sharing his feelings in a group may be more likely to do the same. Through modeling, members can learn behaviors that they can then replicate in the real world—a group member may demonstrate what to say and how to act in a job interview and another member may then imitate the behavior and get feedback on it. The following principles guide effective modeling:

- A person is more likely to be imitated if he or she is perceived as having high status; consequently, a therapist or peer viewed by clients as having status has a potentially significant impact as a social model.

- A person is more likely to be imitated if the observer can see the similarities between self and the model. Such similarities could relate to age, sex, nationality, socioeconomic position, similar disability, or skill level.

- An individual will more likely imitate behavior perceived as leading to reward (e.g., when the person sees the model receiving a reward). In addition, he or she is more likely to inhibit a response perceived as leading to punishment, as when the model is observed being punished.

- A model that is perceived as warm and caring and has a history of meeting an individual's emotional needs is more likely to be imitated (Murdoch & Barker, 1991, p. 34).

- Hostility, aggression, and moral behavior have all been shown to be highly accessible to learning through modeling.

- To be successfully imitated, the model behavior must be well attended to. Distraction in the learning setting can be expected to decrease imitative learning.

- Many skilled acts, especially those involving fine motor coordination, can be learned only in part through modeling; participation and practice are necessary adjuncts to learning.

- When the individual can give verbal labels or descriptions to the behavior observed, that behavior is more successfully remembered and imitated (Hilgard & Bower, 1975).

From *Psychosocial Frames of Reference: Core for Occupation-Based Practice* (p. 130), by M. A. G. Bruce and B. Borg, 2002, New Jersey: SLACK Incorporated.

Theoretical Assumptions Underlying the Approach

A number of assumptions underlie the behavioral approach to learning. The central premise is that behavior, including occupational behavior, is learned. The approach dictates that humans are causally and environmentally determined entities; they are drive-centered beings and they are moved by cause-and-effect forces (Barris, Kielhofner, & Watts, 1988, p. 72). Occupational therapists using a behavioral framework consider how environmental stimuli become connected to individuals' responses, through pairing or reinforcement, to promote learning of occupational skills and behaviors. As discussed previously, behavior is learned when conditioned by an environmental stimulus through association (classical conditioning), when it is reinforced (operant conditioning), or when it is

observed and reinforced vicariously (observational learning). In this theoretical framework, the emphasis is on observable behavior rather than internal thought processes or emotions; learning is manifested by a change in observable behavior. As adaptive behavior is learned, the ability to participate in desired and meaningful occupations is enhanced.

The behavioral approach also dictates that newly learned behaviors and skills can generalize to environments of choice, that is, the newly acquired behaviors can occur in the environments for which they were intended. In their classic article on generalization, "An Implicit Technology of Generalization," Stokes and Baer (1977) defined generalization as "the occurrence of relevant behavior under different, non-training conditions (i.e., across subjects, settings, people, behaviors, and/or time) without the scheduling of the same events in those conditions" (p. 350). Research results regarding the effectiveness of behavioral interventions with regard to generalizability are inconclusive, and as Osnes and Lieblin (2003), report, "generalization continues to be an elusive entity…the conceptualization continues to be stronger than the empirical base that supports it" (p. 364). The use of homework in a collaborative client-therapist relationship appears to be a useful and efficient therapeutic strategy for addressing generalization within the context of psychosocial practice (Duncombe, 1998). By applying the skills learned in a therapeutic environment to a home or community setting, they may more easily be incorporated into one's occupational repertoire. A collaborative homework model in occupational therapy (Luboshitzky & Gaber, 2000) is proposed under the Practice Approaches later in this chapter.

Other Key Developers/Theorists

In earlier sections of this chapter, we considered the important work of Skinner, Pavlov, and Bandura. This section looks at the contributions of psychiatrist Joseph Wolpe and occupational therapist Ann Cronin Mosey to the theory and practice of learning within a behavioral framework.

Joseph Wolpe applied behavioral principles to the treatment of neurosis, or the tendency for people to be in long-term negative psychological or emotional states. He postulated that neurotic behavior was learned in the presence of fear-producing stimuli. To reverse this learning, he suggested that these individuals needed to learn to produce nonneurotic, relaxed behavior in the presence of the original stimuli. He developed an approach called *reciprocal inhibition* through *systematic desensitization*. The essence of reciprocal inhibition therapy is to promote new, relaxed behaviors "whose repeated exercise gradually weaken the anxiety response habit" (Wolpe, 1961, p. 89) in other words, that inhibit the anxiety. The underlying belief is that if an anxiety-producing stimulus occurs simultaneously with a response that diminishes anxiety (e.g., relaxation), the stimulus may cause less anxiety. Using the systematic desensitization approach, a client constructs a hierarchy of anxiety-producing stimuli, which he or she then experiences—often through imagery first and then in reality—alongside progressive relaxation techniques. In this process the relaxation response inhibits the anxiety response in the presence of these stimuli. In addition, operant conditioning methods of positive and negative reinforcement and extinction are incorporated into this approach.

Referring back to the example of the woman who developed agoraphobia as a conditioned response to the elevator, an occupational therapist might use systematic desensitization to help her learn new responses. The client would create a *fear hierarchy* that lists steps toward her goal of going shopping independently that are progressively more anxiety-provoking—for example, opening the front door, walking down the hall, pressing the elevator button, entering the elevator, leaving the building, walking across the street to the store, and so forth. Once the fear hierarchy is constructed, the client would engage in relaxation training, where she would learn to use relaxation techniques and contrast muscular tension with muscular relaxation. After mastering deep muscle relaxation, the client would be asked to imagine or enact each of the anxiety-provoking steps she listed in the fear hierarchy, while practicing the relaxation skill. In addition, positive reinforcement in the form of praise could be offered at each step. The client would then work through each anxiety-provoking step and inhibit the anxiety response with a competing relaxation response, leading to extinction of the anxiety. With their understanding of occupational demands and analysis, and their ability to work alongside people as they engage in their daily activities, occupational therapists are in a good position to use these learning techniques in context.

Anne Cronin Mosey is a key occupational therapy theorist who delineated the *acquisitional frame of reference* as a conceptual model derived from learning theory. The acquisitional frame of reference is based on principles of operant conditioning to explain the acquisition of skills and competencies that enable individuals to cope and functionally adapt to their environments.

The general goal of an acquisitional frame of reference is to help the individual acquire an adequate repertoire of behavior relative to his or her current life situation or expected environment (Mosey, 1986, p. 444). Mosey points out that this frame of reference is pragmatic and is easily applied to the question, "What does this client need to learn in order to manage her daily affairs?" (p. 445). The concept of the expected environment plays a major part in determining the goals of the change process.

Mosey described the evaluation process in the acquisitional frame of reference as being focused on the client's present interaction in the environment, what he or she is able to do in the here and now. An initial discussion reveals the nature of client interactions in the environment and assessment includes identification of environmental factors that may be responsible for maintaining particular maladaptive behaviors. The client's expected environment is used as the basis for establishing long-term goals. Intervention begins in the area where skill development is considered to be most important or useful to the client at that time. To address areas of concern—activities of daily living, avocational pursuits, and work—the therapist considers that each of these areas are made up of tasks and interpersonal interactions and that manipulation of the nonhuman environment may be required.

Mosey points out that acquisitional frames of reference are suitable for any age group and no particular level of cognitive or verbal skill is required. This frame of reference is suitable for any client who has not developed an adequate repertoire of behavior or who needs to develop new skills to manage daily life.

IMPORTANT EVOLUTIONARY POINTS

Behavioral approaches have been the subject of much debate and criticism, and as a result, they have evolved over time. A common criticism has been the mechanistic nature of its concepts. Many argue that behavior is not solely determined by environmental antecedents and reinforcers. This is a particularly salient concern for occupational therapists who believe in the value of meaningful occupation. Even within a predominantly behavioral approach, occupational therapists recognize that persons engage in activities (responses) because they are meaningful and provide a sense of stimulation and competence (Barris et al., 1988). Therefore, occupational therapists incorporate the choices and desires of individuals in setting goals, selecting reinforcers, and assigning homework.

Another criticism has focused on the fact that this approach emphasizes skill deficits, making it easy to overlook clients' strengths and competencies. Every client has strengths that can be used in learning and it is incumbent upon therapists to help clients capitalize on their resources. Within occupational therapy, there has been a shift from utilizing the early and "pure" form of the approach, which regards people as subjects with behaviors to be modified by the environment, to a newer approach that accommodates the inner strengths and talents people bring. More and more, people are being seen as active agents who can share in the decision making in a collaborative way. Adopting such a competency perspective enables greater respect for possibilities such as self-help groups and community self-education (where people can seek information, develop skills and gain reinforcement from one another; Fawcett, Matthews, & Fletcher, 1980), and the matching of persons and environments. These refinements do not negate the important ideas about learning developed in behavioral approaches, but they do speak to the need to operate from a perspective that highlights the individual as capable, instrumental, and as an active agents.

Ethical concerns have also been levied against behavioral approaches. The issue of behavioral control has been examined, particularly with regard to children and vulnerable individuals who cannot express their wishes. Critics see the use of reinforcers such as food and praise as methods of manipulating individuals and coercing them to conform to society. Behaviorists counter these concerns by saying that all therapy involves some form of control and that a behavioral approach offers more control by offering access to tools of self-control (Schaefer & Martin, 1975). They propose that by making reinforcers explicit, they can be used transparently by people hoping to help with the learning of new skills or by the learner him- or herself. An example these behaviorists might cite is the person who rewards himself with a new article of clothing as he improves his dietary practices and loses weight.

ASSESSMENT

ABC Approach

One way of assessing and understanding behaviors and the conditions or events that influence them is through an antecedent-behavior-consequence (ABC) behavioral analysis. Behavioral analysis is defined as a scientific method designed to discover the functional relation between behavior and the variables that control it (Sulzer-Azaroff & Mayer, 1991, p. 3). An ABC approach is useful in determining why a particular behavior occurs; it enables a clear view of what is taking place in the environment that may trigger a behavior, as well as what happens after the behavior that might maintain it. If there is a target behavior that interferes with occupational functioning, the therapist, observer, or client him- or herself may document what occurs immediately prior to and following instances of the target behavior; this will determine the consistency with which specific antecedent or consequent events relate to the behavior. Consider, for example, the case of a client with a dual diagnosis (an individual with a mental illness and a co-occurring developmental disability) who, on a daily basis, bangs his head against the wall during hospital mealtime as staff try to assist him with feeding the food that is provided. In frustration, staff give up on the meal and feed him chips and pop to stop him from the destructive head-banging behavior. An ABC analysis helps to understand the function of his maladaptive behavior: the antecedent (A)—staff feeding him food he did not like—results in the behavior (B) of head banging, with the consequence (C) of staff providing him with the junk food he loves. It becomes clear that the function of his behavior is to gain access to his preferred foods.

The information gathered in an ABC analysis helps identify the stimulus-response relationships that support the behavior, behaviors that may not be reinforced but should be, skills that need to be learned, and environmental conditions that need modification. Behaviors that interfere with, and those that are necessary for healthy occupational functioning, should be observed and recorded, and considered with other important pieces of information. For example, it would be important to consider how people in the setting are able to participate in choice around food selection as well as whether troublesome behaviors occur in any other context. This record serves as a baseline of occupational behavior from which new behaviors can be measured. Target behaviors to be encouraged or discouraged can then be identified, and interventions to encourage these changes can be put into place. The ABC model has been validated extensively in fundamental and applied research in learning (for example Cantania, 1992).

PRACTICE APPROACHES

The goal of a behavioral approach to learning is to develop new skills or behaviors that are adaptive to one's current role or circumstances. The *target behavior,* as it is called, must be relevant, observable, understandable, measurable, behavioral, and attainable within a reasonable length of time. An operational definition of the target behavior that uses observable and measurable actions and words allows it to be described, measured, and recorded. Once a baseline level of behavior is attained and the target behavior is defined and described, methods for filling the gap—that is, developing the skill or behavior—are put into place. These methods may include some of the components described previously, such as shaping, chaining, role-playing, rehearsal and practice, modeling, and imitation or systematic desensitization.

Some areas in which occupational therapists use behavioral approaches include helping clients develop social skills, independent living skills, vocational skills, stress management skills, and assertiveness skills (Stein & Tallant, 1988). A behavioral approach to social skills training follows.

Social Skills Training

Occupational therapists have long been assisting their clients with learning the social skills needed for everyday living and in doing so, draw on behavioral principles. Social skills training consists of learning activities utilizing behavioral techniques that enable persons to acquire independent living skills for improved functioning in their communities (Kopelowicz, Liberman, & Zarate, 2006). This intervention aims to help individuals learn the skills required to communicate their emotions, wants, and needs so that they may

---

TABLE 11-1

LEARNING-BASED PROCEDURES USED IN SOCIAL SKILLS TRAINING

- Problem identification is done in collaboration with the client in terms of obstacles that are barriers to personal goals in his or her current life.

- Goal setting generates short-term approximations to the client's personal goals with specification of the social behavior that is required for successful attainment of the short-term, incremental goals. The goal-setting endeavor requires the therapist or trainer to elicit from the client detailed descriptions of what communication skills are to be learned, with whom they are to be used, as well as where, and when they will be used.

- Through role plays or behavioral rehearsal, the client demonstrates the verbal, nonverbal, and paralinguistic skills required for successful social interaction in the interpersonal situation set as the goal.

- Positive and corrective feedback is given to the client focused on the quality of the behaviors exhibited in the role play.

- Social modeling is provided with a therapist or a peer demonstrating the desired interpersonal behaviors in a form that can be vicariously learned by the observing client.

- Behavioral practice by the client is repeated until the communication reaches a level of quality tantamount to success in the real-life situation.

- Positive social reinforcement is given contingent on those behavioral skills that showed improvement.

- Homework assignments are given to motivate the client to implement the communication in real-life situations.

- Positive reinforcement and problem solving is provided at the next session based on the client's experience using the skills.

From Kopelowicz, A., Liberman, R. P., and Zarate, R., "Recent advances in social skills training for schizophrenia," *Schizophrenia Bulletin, 32*(Supp. 1), 12 23. Copyright © 2006 by the Oxford University Press. Reprinted with permission.

---

achieve their goals, more fully develop relationships, and fulfill their chosen roles. To carry out social skills training, there must first be an assessment of the client's current and desired social behaviors, and an exploration of how these social behaviors fit into the expectations and demands of the occupational roles of the individual. Then, a task analysis breaks down each situational goal to small components, which increases the likelihood of success during the training sessions and in applying the skills to everyday life. The occupational therapist incorporates principles of operant conditioning; for example, the therapist may use prompting, cueing, instructing, and coaching the client while he or she practices improved social behaviors. Learning of social skills may occur through direct training or vicarious, observational approaches, and steps toward improved social behaviors are positively reinforced when they are demonstrated. Generalization of the skills for use in everyday life occurs when patients are provided with opportunities, encouragement, and reinforcement for practicing the skills in relevant situations (Kopelowicz et al., 2006). As social competence is strengthened through the successful application of social skills in community life, cognitions and

emotions also shift in positive ways with improvements in self-efficacy, self-esteem, self-confidence, empowerment, optimism, and mood (Kopelowicz et al., 2006). The main features of social skills training are described in Table 11-1.

Social skills training is now being combined with other evidence-based interventions to maximize its effectiveness. For example, social skills training combined with supported employment have shown promising results in improving social and vocational outcomes for people with severe mental illness. Kopelowicz et al. (2006) describe a workplace fundamentals module that was designed to improve the job tenure, success, and satisfaction of persons with mental illness entering the workplace by demonstrating how to (1) anticipate job stressors, (2) use stress management techniques, (3) identify and overcome stigmatizing attitudes, (4) solicit performance feedback and assistance from one's supervisor or employer, and (5) start conversations and relationships with coworkers. They cite four studies that have been conducted with this module supplementing supported employment, with improved job tenure reported in most, and some evidence that job satisfaction also is increased. This approach is a good fit with occupational therapy, where occupational behaviors are not considered only in a detached and discrete way, but rather within the broader context of daily occupations.

Collaborative Therapeutic Homework

Homework has been used effectively by occupational therapists to enable clients to practice and incorporate newly learned skills into their lives. Luboshitzky and Gaber (2000) documented a collaborative homework approach that enables practitioners to enhance generalization and transfer of learning while using client-centered guidelines for practice in occupational therapy. They recommend a six-step sequence suggested by Shelton (1979):

1. A careful identification of client problems (based on the client's self-observation and the therapist's evaluation); identify the target problems and therapeutic objectives

2. A precise definition of therapeutic objectives in behavioral terms

3. A contractual agreement between the client and therapist to work toward these objectives

4. A rank ordering of the therapeutic interventions so that the first objective pursued will make the most difference to the client and is, in the judgment of the therapist, technically the most feasible to pursue

5. Selection of skills and methods of skill training acceptable to the client and effective for working toward the first behavioral objective

6. Systematic skill training using homework assignments as integral parts of behavioral skill building; the format for homework includes one or more of the following instructions: a do statement, a quantity statement, a record statement, a bring statement, and a contingency statement

During the first session, a problem list is generated, and the problems are assigned priorities as targets for intervention. At the end of each session, the therapist assigns a precise, written set of homework instructions for the client to complete between that session and the next. In the next session, homework, as completed, is reviewed by the therapist and client and another assignment is given. The client is expected to play an increasingly active role in determining homework assignments as the sessions progress (Corsini & Wedding, 1989). Before the last session, clients are invited to write their own treatment summary and review. An example using this approach is described in Vignette 11-1.

EXAMPLES OF TOOLS AND INSTRUMENTS DEVELOPED

To enable the ABC approach to behavioral analysis discussed previously, an ABC checklist may be used. Many instruments exist that enable the ABCs to be objectively documented, and include the setting, time, and frequency behaviors occur; what happened just before the behavior itself; and the consequences of the behavior (Stuart, 2013; Sulzer-Azaroff & Mayer, 1977). The US National Center for Learning Disabilities offers one online (Stuart, 2013).

The evaluation of baseline behavior is necessary to know the starting point for the intervention, and the gap that needs to be filled. Data for baseline assessment can be gathered through various means. Detailed interviewing and exploration of specific examples can offer the client's perspective on his or her behavior in particular circumstances, but often this is insufficient. Observation during naturalistic conditions (e.g., in the workplace or school setting), simulations (e.g., role-play of giving negative feedback), or imagery review (e.g., visualization of a recent social encounter) can offer important information about behaviors under particular circumstances. With client permission, information may also be obtained from others (e.g., parents, employers, teachers, partners). Information from records such as health or school records may also be useful. These methods may offer information about responses in particular circumstances. If observational methods are being used, baseline measurements should continue until a stable pattern of behavior is observed.

Additional occupational therapy evaluations that are consistent with this approach include the Kohlman Evaluation of Living Skills, the Milwaukee Evaluation of Daily Living Skills, the Comprehensive Occupational Therapy Evaluation (all of which are detailed in Hemphill-Pearson, 1999).

EVIDENCE FOR THE APPROACH

Before occupational therapists can say that their intervention using this learning approach has been effective, they should consider the following questions: Will the skills and behaviors trained in the structured therapy settings be maintained? Will the client use these skills in a variety of non-training settings in the absence of his or her therapist? Will the client be able to call on skills similar, but

VIGNETTE 11-1. SHARON

Sharon is a 40-year-old single woman who came to be seen by the occupational therapist when she was referred to the psychiatry day unit of a general hospital. She had been living in her own apartment and was unemployed and supported by a government disability pension. She has been living with a diagnosis of schizophrenia for many years and she has had repeated hospitalizations. She came to the day unit in response to deterioration in her emotional state, manifested by excessive tension, personal neglect, and difficulties in maintaining her independent functioning at home.

Occupational performance evaluation: Open-ended and semi-structured interviews were used to obtain initial information concerning Sharon's functional difficulties in daily life tasks. Sharon's personal and oral hygiene were neglected. She described difficulties in cleaning her apartment, in organizing her closets, and in sorting bills, documents, and papers. Although she strongly emphasized her desire to develop close and significant interpersonal relationships, she found it difficult to initiate dates with friends and complained of social isolation and feelings of loneliness. She identified an interest in intellectual activities such as listening to lectures on various topics, watching films, and reading, but she almost never did any of these activities and avoided going out of the house.

Identifying performance assets and impairments: Observation of functional performance, open-ended interview, and structured assessment were used to determine the underlying components interfering with occupational performance.

Cognition: Sharon demonstrated a relatively high intellectual level and answered directly, fluently, and spontaneously to questions asked. She was easily distracted and demonstrated difficulties in concentrating and organizing her thoughts. She exhibited an ability to learn new tasks by repetition, starting with two or three steps at a time, but required assistance in organization, planning, and problem solving. She was responsive to cueing; able to retain information, apply it to subsequent tasks that looked different and improved the efficiency of her cognitive operation within structured and organized environments. Short- and long-term memory and orientation were intact. Difficulties in her process skills were observed especially in the areas of using knowledge (choosing and inquiring), temporal organization (initiating and sequencing), and the use of space and objects (gathering and organizing).

Emotional and psychological components: Sharon felt anxious and depressed. She was preoccupied with her self-hygiene, home-management disorganization, and slowness. She manifested a negative self-image and a pervasive sense of incompetence, hopelessness, and helplessness. She had difficulty making social contacts due to a poor ability to initiate verbal interactions and to listen and understand another's point of view. As a result of her negative attitude toward others, she was ignored and rejected by many clients.

Establishing goals: Together the occupational therapist and Sharon set the following goals:

- Improving independent participation in home management tasks
- Developing knowledge and participation in self-care activities
- Beginning participation in one or two leisure activities
- Improving and developing active participation in social and interpersonal tasks

Occupational Therapy Process

During the first month, various skill acquisition techniques were used in one-to-one and group occupational therapy sessions. However, these methods failed her at home, where they mattered most for her. Incorporating therapeutic homework assignments was offered to her. A framework of one-to-one therapy, three times a week for 30 minutes per session, was initiated. A detailed explanation about how homework assignments might help her in achieving her goals was given and she agreed.

Home management: Cleaning and arranging her apartment was identified as the most important area in which to start. A list of chores that were connected with the upkeep of her apartment was prepared. She was asked to divide the chores into two categories, cleaning and straightening up, and to grade them according to level of difficulty. Task analysis and systematic repetitive graded activity methods were used. In the one-to-one therapeutic sessions with Sharon, the occupational therapist helped her identify the materials, tools, and equipment needed for the tasks and to analyze the task demands by breaking down each chore into discrete, sequential substeps. Her homework assignments included performing the task by following the sequential steps and evaluating her performance according to the pace of performance, satisfaction during and after performance, and results (on a 1 to 10 scale). Problem-solving strategies

(continued)

were used to develop stepwise solutions for complex tasks. For example, Sharon had particular difficulty in sorting out and organizing her papers, documents, and bills. Several options were offered and discussed within the therapeutic session. Classification and sorting tasks (of tools, materials, and papers) were practiced at the clinic, after which she was able to sort and file her documents in different folders at home while evaluating her performance. Educational experiences were used to increase her money management abilities and skills, while remaining sensitive to the many restraints posed by her limited income. The occupational therapist suggested she use an income/expenses chart and to detail prices of every item she bought in addition to calculating change after each purchase. She also learned how to create a weekly personal budget so that she could afford to attend a set of webinars online that caught her interest.

Self-care: Skill preparation assignments using role-play and modeling techniques were used to increase her ability to receive necessary information about medical and dental facilities in the community. This helped Sharon in homework assignments, which included making phone calls to check out prices and set up an appointment for public health dental care, and in comparing prices in three different stores of various items she needed. Her participation in a social skills training group within the day unit helped her to develop more satisfying communication skills. She was able to ask for advice and help from other clients and friends regarding her wardrobe, haircut style, and makeup.

Leisure: Reading newspapers was offered to her as a source of information about entertainment options in her environment. Interpersonal homework assignments were used when she called a friend and arranged to go out to a movie and a lecture at the university together. When monitoring her satisfaction, she graded these activities most satisfying (10 on a 1 to 10 scale) because it was "interesting, enjoyable and not expensive." She had some unpleasant dialogues with family members with whom she tried to reestablish contact. A review of brief excerpts of these dialogues helped her to reveal communication patterns and errors (e.g., talking too much, ignoring nonverbal clues, communicating her needs in a non-direct and unspecified manner, lack of self-assertion).

General guidelines: Each session began with Sharon's detailed description of her homework performance as well as difficulties, thoughts and feeling regarding the tasks. Reinforcement was given to her whenever she applied the task correctly and successfully coped with disturbed thoughts and feelings. Difficulties were supportively addressed and discussed. Sequential graded methods combined with social learning principles provided learning experiences while in parallel, opportunities for repetition and frequent practice were offered through homework assignments. Self-monitoring techniques helped her in identifying her assets and limitations; in evaluating the consequences of task performance and social behaviors; and in monitoring changes in her own behavior, feelings, and thoughts. After 5 months, there was an overall improvement in her appearance: she was clean, dressed in fashionable clothes, looked pleasant, with no body odor, and was taking care of her teeth. The last meeting took place in her apartment, which was clean and orderly. She was connected to a peer support worker with the aim of helping her with her transition to the community and to maintain the skills she had developed. She and the peer support worker met weekly. In a follow-up meeting 6 months later, she was observed to have maintained her appearance and her teeth were restored and shining white. She continued to carry out her household chores, although not on a regular basis. She joined a mental health community support group in which her psychosocial and emotional needs were addressed. On occasion, she went to movies and lectures and felt that her life was more meaningful than ever.

Adapted from "Collaborative Therapeutic Homework Model in Occupational Therapy," by D. Luboshitzky and L. B. Gaber, *Occupational Therapy in Mental Health, 15*(1), 43-60. Copyright © 2000 by Taylor & Francis (http://informaworld.com).

not identical to, those specifically targeted in therapy when appropriate (Hayes, 1993)? For example, will clients trained in social skills through role-playing a conversation with a friend they meet on the street be able to conduct a conversation with someone they meet at a party?

With regard to the efficacy of the approach, studies have been conducted across different health conditions and occupational contexts. For example, Kopelowicz et al. (2006) report on the results of reviews that have critically evaluated the evidence of the effects of social skills training on individuals with serious mental disorders. With regard to the question, "Do individuals learn and retain the skills?" Kopelowicz et al. (2006) report that the reviews cite over 50 studies that document the significant and substantial improvements in participants' knowledge and behaviors as the result of training. The reviews indicate that people retain their improvements for up to 2 years, the maximum duration measured. The studies included in the review articles were conducted in diverse treatment settings (inpatient, outpatient, partial/day hospitals, residential care and community-based, social and vocational programs); by diverse practitioners (psychiatrists, psychologists, social workers, nursing staff, occupational and recreational therapists, mental health counselors, residential managers, and paraprofessional staff), and they cover a broad range of skills (community living, getting and keeping a job, preparation for discharge from inpatient treatment, illness management, smoking cessation, HIV risk reduction, recreational activities, conversation, social assertiveness, and relationship skills). Despite these promising outcomes, results have been mostly discouraging for transferring skills to participants' environments when it comes to the question "Do individuals transfer their learning and perform the skills in their natural environments?" It appears that the more alike the training and natural environments, the more likely the behaviors will be used in everyday life. Recent studies suggest that using the skills in the living environment receiving the appropriate rewards in that environment, increases the likelihood of skill transfer to everyday life settings (Kopelowicz et al., 2006).

Likewise, studies of social skills training with other populations have reported some positive results. A systematic review of social skills groups with children, adolescents, and young adults with autism spectrum disorder suggested that overall social competence can be improved by these interventions. However, it was not clear that such training has an impact on specific social abilities, such as emotional recognition, that are commonly problematic with this population (Reichow, Steiner, & Volkmar, 2012). For people with acquired brain injury, the study of the efficacy of social skills training is relatively new, although the potential relevance of the approach has been identified. A study examined the outcomes for people with acquired brain injury of a structured social skills training intervention that was combined with efforts to remediate social perceptions and provide individual sessions to address psychological issues such as depression and low self-esteem (McDonald et al., 2008). Such multi-element social interventions are becoming increasingly common, given the complex nature of social interactions and disabilities in social relations. The study did demonstrate some modest positive changes in the direct measure of social behaviors, but no effect on broader social functioning and participation. The study participants were largely marginalized from social opportunities such as employment, and therefore likely had a limited range of occupational contexts within which to practice these skills. Taken together, these studies demonstrate the promise of social skills training using behavioral approaches across a range of populations, but also point out the complexity of integrating the approach in a manner that will have the greatest possible impact on occupational and social participation.

CONCLUSION

This chapter has outlined the key concepts and applications of a learning approach to occupational engagement. Behavioral principles underlie this approach and have been modified and adapted by occupational therapists to incorporate the profession's foundational principles of client-centeredness, empowerment, and meaningful occupation. When used in a manner consistent with these principles, the behavioral approach can assist clients to learn skills for everyday living through a graded approach in which tasks and environmental conditions are structured to provide opportunities for internal and external reinforcement.

LEARNING ACTIVITIES/ DISCUSSION QUESTIONS

1. Identify a behavior in your life that you would like to change. Conduct an ABC analysis to identify the stimulus-response relationships that support the behavior.

2. Provide an argument for or against punishment and the conditions under which it should or should not be used.

3. How might you use systematic desensitization to help your client attend his office party that he is so anxious about that he wants to feign sickness?

4. As an occupational therapist, how would you teach your 19-year-old client how to do his own laundry, using a behavioral approach. Identify the target behavior, schedules of reinforcement, and how you might use shaping as an approach.

REFERENCES

Bandura, A., Ross, D., & Ross, S. A. (1961). Transmission of aggression through imitation of aggressive models. *Journal of Abnormal and Social Psychology, 63*, 575-582.

Barris, R., Kielhofner, G., & Watts, J. H. (1988). *Bodies of knowledge in psychosocial practice.* Thorofare, NJ: SLACK Incorporated.

Beck, M. (2009). How to be richly rewarded. *Creating Your Right Life.* Retrieved from www.marthabeck.com/2009/06/how-to-be-richly-rewarded

Bruce, M. A. G., & Borg, B. (2002). *Psychosocial frames of reference: Core for occupation-based practice* (p. 130). Thorofare, NJ: SLACK Incorporated.

Cantania, A. C. (1992). *Learning* (3rd ed.). Englewood Cliffs, NJ: Prentice-Hall.

Corsini, R. J., & Wedding, D. (1989). *Current psychotherapies* (4th ed.). Itasca, IL: F. E. Peacock Publishers, Inc.

Duncombe, L. W. (1998). Cognitive behavioral model in mental health. In N. Katz (Ed.), *Cognition and occupation in rehabilitation* (pp. 165-192). Bethesda, MD: American Occupational Therapy Association.

Fawcett, S. B., Mathews, & R. M., & Fletcher, R. K. (1980). Some promising directions for behavioral community technology. *Journal of Applied Behavior Analysis 13*(3), 505-518

Hayes, S. C. (1993). Analytic goals and the varieties of scientific contextualism. In S. C. Hayes, L. J. Hayes, H. W. Reese, & T. R. Sarbin (Eds.), *Varieties of scientific contextualism* (pp. 11-27). Reno, NV: Context Press.

Hemphill-Pearson, B. (1999). *Assessments in occupational therapy mental health*. Thorofare, NJ: SLACK Incorporated.

Hilgard, E. R., & Bower, G. H. (1975). *Theories of learning*. Englewood Cliffs, NJ: Prentice-Hall.

Karoly, P. (1975). Operant methods. In F. H. Kanfer & A. P. Goldstein (Eds.), *Helping people change: A textbook of methods and materials*. New York: Pergamon.

Kopelowicz, A., Liberman, R. P., & Zarate, R. (2006). Recent advances in social skills training for schizophrenia. *Schizophrenia Bulletin, 32*(Supp. 1), 12-23.

Luboshitzky, D., & Gaber, B. (2000). Collaborative therapeutic homework model in occupational therapy. *Occupational Therapy in Mental Health, 15*(1), 43-60.

McDonald, S., Tate, R., Togher, L., Bornhofen, C., Long, E. & Gertler, P. (2008). Social skills treatment for people with severe, chronic acquired brain injuries: A multicenter trial. *Archives of Physical and Medicine and Rehabilitation, 89*, 1648-1659.

Mosey, A. C. (1986). *Psychosocial components of occupational therapy*. New York: Raven Press.

Murdoch, D., & Barker B. (1991). *Basic behavior therapy*. Bodmin, Cornwall: Wiley-Black.

Osnes, P. G., & Lieblein, T. (2003). An explicit technology of generalization. *Behavior Analyst Today, 3*(4), 364-374.

Reichow B., Steiner A.M., Volkmar F. (2012). Social skills groups for people aged 6 to 21 years with autism spectrum disorders (ASD). Cochrane Library, DOI: 10.1002/14651858. CD008511.pub2

Schaefer, H. H., & Martin, P. L. (1975). *Behavior therapy* (2nd ed.). New York: McGraw-Hill.

Shelton, J. L. (1979). Instigation therapy: Using therapeutic homework to promote treatment gains. In A. P. Goldstein & F. H. Kanfer (Eds.), *Maximizing treatment gains: Transfer enhancement in psychotherapy* (pp. 225-245). New York: Academic Press.

Stein, F., & Tallant, B. K. (1988). Applying the group process to psychiatric occupational therapy part 1: Historical and current use. *Occupational Therapy in Mental Health, 8*(3), 9-28.

Stokes, T. F., & Baer, D. M. (1977). An implicit technology of generalization. *Journal of Applied Behavior Analysis, 10*(2), 349-367.

Stuart, A. (2013). Antecedent behavior consequence (ABC) chart. Retrieved from www.ncld. org/learning-disability-resources/checklists-worksheets/antecendent-behavior-consequence-abc-chart.

Sulzer-Azaroff, B., & Mayer, R. G. (1977). *Applying behavior-analysis procedures with children and youth*. New York: Holt, Rinehart & Winston.

Sulzer-Azaroff, B., & Mayer, R. G. (1991). *Behavior analysis for lasting change*. Fort Worth, TX: Harcourt Brace.

Wolpe, J. (1961). The systematic desensitization treatment of neuroses. *Journal of Nervous and Mental Disease, 132*, 189-203.

Processes of Thought and Occupation

Bonnie Kirsh, PhD, OT Reg (Ont)

Everything can be taken from a man but one thing: the last of the human freedoms—to choose one's attitude in any given set of circumstances. (Viktor E. Frankl, 1905-1997: Austrian psychiatrist, *Man's Search for Meaning*)

What you believe you experience. (J. Krishnamurti, *Commentaries on Living, Volume 1, p. 88*)

Our life is what our thoughts make it. (Marcus Aurelius Antoninus, *Meditations*, Book IV)

OBJECTIVES

The objectives of this chapter are as follows:

- » Describe the core tenets of cognitive behavioral therapy (CBT).
- » Identify the major contributors to CBT.
- » Detail the process and outcomes of CBT applied to practice.
- » Describe the alignment of CBT with occupational therapy principles and the application of CBT principles to occupational therapy practice.

Krupa, T., Kirsh, B., Pitts, D., & Fossey, E. *Bruce & Borg's Psychosocial Frames of Reference: Theories, Models, and Approaches for Occupation-Based Practice, Fourth Edition* (pp 191-210).
© 2016 SLACK Incorporated.

An Introduction to Cognitive Behavioral Therapy

The behavioral approach, outlined in the previous chapter of this book, conceptualizes human behavior as a response to environmental stimuli, but the absence of human control and volition within this model was seen to be insufficient to explain human behavior. Many theorists took issue with the stimulus-response conditioning approaches of behaviorists, arguing that they are too passive and simplistic. These theorists promoted a shift in focus from environmental antecedents and behavioral consequences toward cognitive factors, and specifically processes of thought, promoting the notion that what people think, believe, expect, remember, and attend to influence how they behave (O'Leary & Wilson, 1987). People's conscious thoughts, wishes, and ideals have been increasingly considered important contributors to behaviors. These factors became incorporated into new models, forming the basis of cognitive and cognitive behavioral therapies.

Cognitive approaches to therapy concern themselves with cognitive structures and thought processes, such as beliefs, thinking styles, problem-solving styles, and coping styles (Meichenbaum, 1977). They aim to correct faulty conceptions and self-signals (Beck, 1976) as a means of alleviating psychosocial distress and changing behavior. These approaches may be viewed as existing on a continuum from purely cognitive to a combination of cognitive-behavioral.

In many ways, cognitive and cognitive-behavioral approaches are a good match with occupational therapy principles and practice because of the emphasis on client perceptions and meanings, and a belief in the individual to exercise control. Occupational therapy theory and cognitive-behavioral theory both value cognitive awareness and the person's ability to problem solve. Both recommend a collaborative relationship between client and practitioner, and both integrate activity or tasks into the intervention process.

The View of Health/Disorder

Within a cognitive framework, healthy thinking is the focus. People are seen as capable of creating and guiding their own lives through formulating their thoughts that influence their behaviors and emotions. They engage in activities that provide feedback for healthy thinking, and for experiencing pleasure in their lives. Rational, healthy thoughts enable people to act in ways that are compatible with life satisfaction and positive social interaction (Barris, Kielhofner, & Watts, 1988, p. 92). Disorder, on the other hand, is seen as faulty thinking patterns resulting from dysfunctional thought processes. When people process information in such a way that their thoughts do not align with existing evidence or logic, the result is psychological disturbance that is characterized by irrational beliefs. This can have a significant impact on occupational performance and experience, the focus of occupational therapy.

Main Component/Concepts

Within cognitive approaches, three levels of cognition have been identified and targeted for intervention: full consciousness, automatic thoughts, and schemas (Clark et al., 1999). Consciousness is a state in which rational decisions are made with full awareness. Automatic thoughts are the more autonomous, often private cognitions that flow rapidly during everyday thinking and may not be carefully assessed for accuracy or relevance (Wright, 2006). There has been considerable attention directed to understanding the nature of automatic thought processes associated with particular health conditions. For example, in depression, automatic thoughts typically center on themes of negativity, low self-esteem, and ineffectiveness. In anxiety disorders, automatic thoughts often include overestimates of risk in situations and underestimates of ability to cope (Wright, Beck, & Thase, 2003). Cognitive schemas are fundamental rules or templates for information processing that are shaped by developmental influences and other life experiences. As individuals process information from the environment, they interpret it based on schemas that they have developed. This interpretation then influences self-worth and behavioral coping strategies (Wright, 2006). In depression, schemas are usually concerned with loss, worthlessness, defeat, and deprivation.

The aim of cognitive behavioral approaches is to alter cognitions and cognitive processes at any or all of the three levels described above to facilitate behavioral and emotional changes. The general term for this treatment approach is *cognitive restructuring*. Specifically, cognitive restructuring involves helping individuals recognize errors in thinking and eliciting rational alternative thoughts, and reappraising beliefs about themselves and the world (Thrasher, Lovell, Noshirvani, & Livanou, 1996). Therapists encourage individuals to monitor their daily thoughts—often daily thought diaries are used—and then evaluate them through reasoning, Socratic questioning, collecting evidence for and against each thought, and delineating pros and cons of their way of thinking (Marks, Lovell, Noshirvani, Livanou, & Thrasher, 1998).

In cognitive restructuring, individuals learn to replace negative beliefs and self-statements with positive ones. Two commonly used techniques are self-talk, which involves creating a new internal dialogue characterized by positive self-statements; and cognitive rehearsal, which involves

TABLE 12-1

TYPES OF CBT HOMEWORK

ASSIGNMENT	EXAMPLE
Self-monitoring	Rating moods in relation to activities
Behavioral activation	Scheduling periods of exercise or participation in formerly pleasurable tasks to offset inactivity and increase access to reinforcement
Behavioral symptom management strategies	Practicing use of techniques such as progressive muscle relaxation, thought stopping, or sleep hygiene to improve specific symptoms
Cognitive assignments	Planned practice using the Daily Record of Dysfunctional Thoughts, Examine the Evidence, or Pros and Cons techniques
Schema assessment	Review of cognitive assignments to identify common themes, writing a brief autobiography or filling out the Dysfunctional Attitude Scale (Beevers et al., 2007)

Reprinted with permission from Thase, M. E., and Callan, J. A., "The Role of Homework in Cognitive Behavior Therapy of Depression," *Journal of Psychotherapy Integration, 16*(2), 171. Copyright © 2006 by the American Psychological Association.

imagining positive interactions or experiences. As positive, rational thoughts replace negative, irrational ones, new behaviors can be experienced and coping skills are developed. For example, negative self-statements (such as "If I do that I will fail") may lead to avoiding particular situations, but when such negative statements are replaced with more positive ones (such as "It will be difficult but I can do it"), an individual may actually confront an anxiety-provoking situation, learn to cope with it, and develop new thoughts around it. A two-way relationship between cognition and behavior is established in which cognitive processes influence behavior, and behavioral change influences cognitions.

Cognitive approaches not only aim to change dysfunctional thinking, they also aim to broaden individuals' knowledge (so that new thinking is possible), strengthen the application of knowledge in skill-building, and improve the ability to problem solve. To this end, psychoeducation is a commonly used approach. It aims to broaden and deepen one's knowledge base and prepare clients to respond to life's daily challenges through increasing awareness, improving functional skills and teaching problem-solving strategies. In doing so, new perspectives are gained and thoughts about oneself are changed from incapable to capable.

Homework assignments are frequently used with cognitive and cognitive-behavioral approaches, to supplement skills learned in sessions with the therapist. Homework is used to disconfirm dysfunctional thinking patterns

and to develop more functional responses (Neimeyer & Feixas, 1990) and has been shown to increase the efficacy of CBT. For example, a study examining the relationship between treatment outcome and the extent to which cocaine-dependent individuals completed CBT homework assignments reports that participants who completed more homework assignments demonstrated significantly greater increases in the quantity and quality of their coping skills and used significantly less cocaine during treatment and through a one year follow-up (Carroll, Nich, & Ball, 2005). These data suggest that the extent to which participants are willing to complete extra session assignments may be an important mediator of response to CBT. For examples of CBT homework, see Table 12-1.

The environment is an important domain in cognitive behavioral approaches, and there is a need for careful assessment of antecedent events or stimuli that may act as triggers to negative thoughts or behaviors. For example, researchers have determined a number of situations in which substance use is more likely to occur for people struggling with substance abuse disorders (Marlatt, 1996). While these situations, which may involve an interaction with someone else or reactions to nonpersonal environmental events, are seen to pose a general risk, it is the individual's appraisal of the situations that determines the actual risk for the individual (Myers, Martin, Rohsenow, & Monti, 1996). CBT can be useful in helping clients modify beliefs about these environmental situations as a means of trying to cope with these situations.

UNDERLYING THEORETICAL ASSUMPTIONS

The cognitive-behavioral frame of reference takes the position that a person's cognitive function and beliefs mediate or influence behaviors. Specifically, the approach is based on a number of assumptions with regard to person/cognition, environment/context, and activity/occupation. Table 12-2 summarizes these assumptions within the broad domains of person, environment, and occupation.

KEY DEVELOPERS/THEORISTS

Key theorists who contributed to the development of CBT and practice are Aaron Beck, Albert Bandura, Albert Ellis, and Donald Meichenbaum.

Aaron Beck's early writings focused primarily on pathology in information processing styles in people with depression or anxiety, but he also incorporated behavioral methods to activate, reverse helplessness, and counter avoidance among these people. Beck's initial formulation of the cognitive theory of depression identifies a negative cognitive triad, which includes a negative view of the self, the world, and the future (Beck, 1970). Beck proposed that the negative cognitive pattern leads to other symptoms of depression. For example, a negative view of self or world results in a depressed mood or sadness, whereas a negative view of the future leads to the loss of motivation, a sense of hopelessness, and pessimism (Beck, 1970). Beck noted that cognitions involving low self-esteem, deprivation, self-criticism, and suicidal wishes were common in depression.

Beck also introduced the notion of cognitive errors (Box 12-1), which emerged from his finding that depressed patients distorted reality in a systematic manner that resulted in bias against themselves. He described a number of cognitive errors commonly made in depression, including arbitrary inference, or drawing a specific conclusion in the absence of evidence or when the evidence is contrary to the conclusion; selective abstraction, or focusing on a detail out of context while ignoring more salient features of the situation; overgeneralization, or drawing a conclusion on the basis of one or more isolated incidents; and magnification/minimization, or exaggerating or minimizing the significance or magnitude of an event. Beck subsequently added personalization, or a tendency to relate external events to oneself, and dichotomous thinking, or a black-and-white way of thinking that places experience in one of two categories. Beck acknowledged that most individuals show such cognitive errors but what characterizes the distortion in depression is the systematic negative bias against the self (Clark et al., 1999).

The notion of schemas, mentioned briefly in an earlier part of this chapter, was originated by Beck, who defined them as cognitive structures "for screening, coding and evaluating stimuli that impinges on the organism" (Beck, 1967/1970, p. 283). Beck postulated that in depression, idiosyncratic schemas involving themes of personal deficiency, self-blame, and negative expectations dominate the thinking process. Beck believed that activation of the schemas leads to negative automatic thoughts and cognitive errors and is the mechanism by which depression develops. Although Beck's focus was on depression, he expanded his approach to anxiety and in the years that followed, Beck's work inspired a perspective on human cognition, emotion, and behavior that has wide application to a host of psychological conditions.

Bandura was discussed in another chapter for his contribution to learning theory, specifically observational learning. However, by the 1970s, Bandura was becoming aware that a key element was missing, not only from the prevalent learning theories of the day, but also from his own social learning theory. In 1977, with the publication of *Self-Efficacy: Toward a Unifying Theory of Behavioral Change*, he identified the important piece of that missing element—self-beliefs. According to Bandura (1995) self-efficacy is "the belief in one's capabilities to organize and execute the courses of action required to manage prospective situations" (p. 2). In other words, self-efficacy is a person's belief in his or her ability to succeed in a particular situation. The basic principle behind self-efficacy theory is that individuals are more likely to engage in activities for which they have high self-efficacy and less likely to engage in those they do not. In Bandura's view of human behavior, the beliefs that people have about themselves are critical elements in the exercise of control and personal agency—these beliefs are determinants of how people think, behave, and feel. Bandura's work emphasized that cognition plays a critical role in people's capability to construct reality, self-regulate, encode information, and perform behaviors.

Albert Ellis developed rational emotive therapy in the 1950s, which proposed that people become unhappy and develop self-defeating habits because of unrealistic or faulty beliefs. These unrealistic beliefs usually originate from one of three core ideas: (1) I must perform well to be approved of by others who are perceived as significant; (2) you must treat me fairly—if not, then it is horrible and I cannot bear it; and (3) conditions must be my way and if not, I cannot stand to live in such a terrible and awful world. In Ellis' view, these irrational thoughts lead to psychological distress.

Ellis developed the ABC theory of personality, which was later expanded to the ABCDE model, to explain the relationship among thoughts, feelings, and behavior. In this model, A is the activating event; B is the belief system, which may be rational or irrational; C refers to emotional

TABLE 12-2

PEO ASSUMPTIONS UNDERLYING CBT

PERSON AND COGNITION

1. When you change thoughts and beliefs or enhance knowledge, you affect behavior and occupational performance.

2. People make decisions regarding their behavior based in part on what they expect will be the outcome.

3. A person's emotions and feelings are interdependent with what he or she knows and believes.

4. The person develops as a result of the interaction of the cognitive system, behaviors learned, and the social and physical environments.

5. Being willing to explore one's environment and try out new behaviors depends in part on one's belief that it is safe to make mistakes.

6. People have internalized "rules for living," life themes, and styles of problem solving of which they may or may not be aware, but nevertheless characterize how they approach life's tasks.

7. Cognitive change is a gradual process; changing one's knowledge base and one's attitudes toward the self takes time.

8. The client benefits from psychoeducational programs that integrate educational procedures and skill building with psychological techniques.

9. When an individual learns new cognitive strategies to respond to the present, he or she is preparing to confront and solve future problems.

10. People are unlikely to participate in experiences in which they feel incapable.

11. Increasing one's beliefs about being capable increases one's capability and willingness to initiate tasks and risk change.

12. Beliefs about being capable and in control are more likely to increase when one experiences one's self successfully and is given responsibility for one's own learning.

13. One's thoughts are not always in conscious awareness; making thoughts aware makes them more amenable to change.

14. Learning is facilitated by practice in multiple and varied contexts.

ENVIRONMENT/CONTEXT

15. A learning format or context in which the person identifies the self as a learner is one that promotes exploration, openness to new experience, and a mindset toward enhancing knowledge and skills.

16. A learning context promotes the idea of life as a life-long learning process.

17. Cognitive function is influenced by the arrangement of the learning environment, which can facilitate cognitive development and stimulate problem solving.

18. The client can benefit from a structured intervention setting that controls distractions and provides repeated opportunities for skill practice and problem solving.

ACTIVITY/OCCUPATION

19. Therapeutic occupation is that which facilitates learning.

20. Practice in real-life contexts is a powerful accompaniment to learning in an analog or clinical setting.

21. Cognitive developmental theory can be applied when designing tasks to modify the complexity of the experience and to promote successful learning.

22. The therapeutic tasks used during educational experiences consider the learner's cognitive knowledge, level of cognitive function, and personal interests.

23. Goals that present a moderate challenge help hold the client's interest and facilitate participation in an intervention.

24. Intervention does not eliminate pathology but provides cognitive, affective, and behavioral learning experiences to teach skills, strategies, and methods of coping.

25. Intervention is more effective when specific techniques and skills are learned (e.g., when tasks and psychoeducational experiences are used) than when only verbal methods are used.

BOX 12-1. FIFTEEN COMMON COGNITIVE ERRORS

1. *Filtering*—Taking negative details and magnifying them, while filtering out all positive aspects of a situation

2. *Polarized thinking*—Thinking of things as black or white, good or bad, perfect or failures, with no middle ground

3. *Overgeneralization*—Jumping to a general conclusion based on a single incident or piece of evidence; expecting something bad to happen over and over again if one bad thing occurs

4. *Mind reading*—Thinking that you know, without any external proof, what people are feeling and why they act the way they do; believing yourself able to discern how people are feeling about you

5. *Catastrophizing*—Expecting disaster; hearing about a problem and then automatically considering the possible negative consequences (e.g., "What if tragedy strikes?" "What if it happens to me?")

6. *Personalization*—Thinking that everything people do or say is some kind of reaction to you; comparing yourself to others, trying to determine who's smarter or better looking

7. *Control fallacies*—Feeling externally controlled as helpless or a victim of fate or feeling internally controlled, responsible for the pain and happiness of everyone around you

8. *Fallacy of fairness*—Feeling resentful because you think you know what is fair, even though other people do not agree

9. *Blaming*—Holding other people responsible for your pain or blaming yourself for every problem

10. *Shoulds*—Having a list of ironclad rules about how you and other people "should" act; becoming angry at people who break the rules and feeling guilty if you violate the rules

11. *Emotional reasoning*—Believing that what you feel must be true, automatically (e.g., if you feel stupid and boring, then you must be stupid and boring)

12. *Fallacy of change*—Expecting that other people will change to suit you if you pressure them enough; having to change people because your hopes for happiness seem to depend on them

13. *Global labeling*—Generalizing one or two qualities into a negative global judgment

14. *Being right*—Proving that your opinions and actions are correct on a continual basis; thinking that being wrong is unthinkable; going to any lengths to prove that you are correct

15. *Heaven's reward fallacy*—Expecting all sacrifice and self-denial to pay off, as if there were someone keeping score, and feeling disappointed and even bitter when the reward does not come

Adapted from Beck, A.T. (1976). *Cognitive therapy and the emotional disorders.* New York: Meridian.

consequences (such as anxiety) created by B; D is the disputation or rational challenges to B, which may eliminate disturbing Cs; and E is the new effects or "a more rational philosophy" (Ellis, 1973). According to Ellis, it is not A that causes C but rather B, the beliefs and meanings attributed to the event, that is the causative factor. Rational emotive therapy focuses on the influence of the belief system on emotions and behavior.

Rational emotive therapy is an active therapy, with the therapist taking a challenging and directive stance. A number of strategies may be used to change irrational beliefs and promote rational self-talk: (1) client self-monitoring of thoughts; (2) reframing of situations to view them from a more positive angle; (3) therapist modeling of rational thinking; (4) use of straightforward feedback, challenge, and confrontation of client thoughts and beliefs; and (5) use of homework assignments and practice sessions in which new rational self-statements and behaviors are performed (Barris et al., 1988, p. 94). All of these approaches aim to replace self-defeating thoughts with more positive ones.

Donald Meichenbaum is best known for stress inoculation training, an approach that helps individuals cope with the aftermath of exposure to stressful events and that is used on a preventative basis to inoculate individuals to future and ongoing stressors. This form of CBT aims to empower individuals to expand their repertoire of coping skills and to use existing ones. It uses a three phase intervention. In the first conceptualization phase, a collaborative relationship is established between the client and the therapist. Clients are educated about the role of the appraisal processes with regard to stress, and that they may be—perhaps unknowingly—exacerbating the level of stress they experience. Stresses and threats are reframed as problems to be solved and stressors are broken down with short-, intermediate-, and long-term coping goals in mind. The second phase of stress inoculation training focuses on skills acquisition and rehearsal that follows naturally from the initial conceptualization phase. Coping skills are learned and practiced and may include emotional self-regulation, self-soothing and acceptance, relaxation training, self-instructional training, cognitive restructuring, problem-solving, interpersonal communication skills training, attention diversion procedures, using social support systems, and fostering meaning-related activities. The final phase of application and follow-through provides opportunities for clients to apply the coping skills across increasing levels of stressors. Techniques such as imagery and behavioral rehearsal, modeling, role-playing, and graded in vivo exposure are used in the form of personal experiments.

IMPORTANT EVOLUTIONARY POINTS

While CBT was originally thought to be suitable primarily for people with depression and anxiety, it has since been applied increasingly to people experiencing a range of health conditions. It is being used widely, for example, with individuals who have difficulty adjusting to significant physical illnesses and disabilities, and when these physical illnesses are accompanied by depression and anxiety. Specific CBT strategies have even been developed for people who experience psychosis (e.g., with a diagnosis of schizophrenia), a health condition where the primary impairment is a disorder in thought. In this situation, where an individual may be absolutely convinced that his or her thoughts are true (even when to other people they seem very irrational), CBT has been applied with the intent of reducing the distress experienced in response to these thoughts and to increase coping options (Smith, Nathan, Juniper, Kingsep, & Lim, 2003).

Research over the past decade has shown that CBT helps people with schizophrenia spectrum disorders reduce positive and negative symptoms (Drury, Birchwood, Cochrane, & Macmillan, 1996; Haddock et al., 1998; Kingdon & Turkington, 1991; Sensky et al., 2000; Tarrier et al., 2001). Tarrier (2005) reviewed the evidence from 20 controlled trials of CBT in schizophrenia in which 739 patients were included and concluded that there is evidence that CBT reduces persistent positive symptoms in patients with chronic disease and may have modest effects in speeding recovery in acutely ill patients. However many questions still need to be answered about the efficacy of CBT with schizophrenia. Critiques of research methods in many of the studies have been issued, calling for replications and further research. For example, in an article debating the issue, Turkington and McKenna (2003) pointed out that of the 13 trials of CBT in schizophrenia included in a Cochrane meta-analysis (Cormac, Jones, & Campbell, 2002), only four used a control intervention and were carried out under blind conditions. The two largest studies (Lewis et al., 2002; Sensky et al., 2000) showed no significant advantage for CBT over the control intervention.

CBT has been used with individuals with psychosis, not only to address symptoms, but also to help people move forward with their recovery and realize their potential in domains such as work. It is this application that has greater relevance to occupational therapy. Lysaker et al. (2005) developed an intervention that was an adjunct to a work therapy program which had, as its overarching purpose, helping participants identify and correct dysfunctional beliefs about work. The intervention was aimed at helping people with schizophrenia change dysfunctional beliefs about themselves. In this randomized, controlled trial, participants in the intervention group worked significantly more weeks than those in the standard support group and the intervention group also maintained baseline levels of hope and self-esteem, whereas the control group did not. The authors surmise that these improvements relate to the increased ability of intervention group participants to problem solve and avoid making negative self-attributions.

Cognitive behavioral approaches are being delivered to individuals across the lifespan. Lopez and Mermelstein (1995) administered a cognitive behavioral intervention program to participants at a geriatric rehabilitation unit of a large metropolitan medical center. Patients with elevated depression and anxiety scores participated in a program based on CBT principles and were compared to a control group who scored within normal limits on the depression and anxiety measures. The intervention program relied heavily on a broad-based, cognitive-behavioral, and coping skills/problem-solving framework. Interventions included (1) making graphs of progress and goals and having team members reinforce the participant's progress, (2) encouraging patients to seek information about their conditions and to talk more openly and realistically about their diseases and disabilities, (3) relaxation training where appropriate, (4) helping patients in making social comparisons and in perspective taking, and (5) increasing patients' pleasant activities (e.g., getting them involved in unit social activities and events). The overall therapeutic approach was active and focused on goals. Cognitive restructuring was useful in helping patients to realign their expectations and to increase their confidence. Findings indicated that, compared with patients who were psychologically healthier at admission, participants in this program achieved comparably low levels of distress by discharge, except for anxiety. In addition, both groups achieved their rehabilitation goals to similar degrees. A side benefit of the program identified by the authors was that this approach enabled staff to become advocates, helping patients identify problems and areas of strength on which to build from admission onward. This was an improvement over the previous, and more common

BOX 12-2. FUNCTIONAL ASSESSMENT: ABCs

ANTECEDENTS (WHAT HAPPENED BEFORE?)	BEHAVIORS (WHAT DID YOU DO?)	SHORT-TERM CONSEQUENCES (WHAT WAS THE RESULT 1 SECOND AND 1 HOUR FOLLOWING BEHAVIOR?)	LONG-TERM CONSEQUENCES (WHAT WERE THE LASTING RESULTS?)

Reprinted with permission from Cully, J., & Teten, A. (2008). *A therapist's guide to brief cognitive behavioral therapy.* Department of Veterans Affairs South Central MIRECC, Houston. Retrieved from www.mirecc.va.gov/visn16/docs/therapists_guide_to_brief_cbtmanual.pdf.

approach, of having problem patients referred for psychological treatment while passive, often depressed patients were overlooked.

Perhaps one of the most significant advances in the area of CBT is its adaptation to online formats that enable self-help and easy delivery. A number of specific Internet-based CBT programs have been developed and evaluated. Beating the Blues is a program aimed at "people feeling stressed, depressed, anxious or just down in the dumps" (Beating the Blues, 2006). The course is made up of eight online sessions that help people understand the link between thoughts, feelings, and behaviors, and which teach coping strategies. The effects of this tool on emotional distress in employees with stress-related absenteeism were evaluated through a randomized controlled trial in which 48 public sector employees were randomized equally to Beating the Blues plus conventional care, or conventional care alone. At the end of treatment and 1 month later, adjusted mean depression scores and adjusted mean negative attributional style scores were significantly lower in the intervention group. One month post-treatment, adjusted mean anxiety scores were also significantly lower in the intervention group. The study concludes that this online CBT tool may accelerate psychological recovery in employees with recent stress-related absenteeism (Grime, 2004). Another online program from Australia, called MoodGYM, is designed to prevent depression in young people. Using flashed diagrams and online exercises, MoodGYM teaches the principles of CBT to work through such issues as stress and relationship break-ups, and also teaches relaxation and meditation techniques. Scientific trials evaluating MoodGYM have shown that using two or more modules is linked to significant reductions in depression and anxiety symptoms. The

trials also found that these benefits last after 12 months (MoodGYM, n.d.). These tools are showing great promise; indeed a review of eight studies of supported Internet- or computer-based CBT, six of which were randomized controlled trials, indicate that these programs are potentially more effective than usual care (Høifødt, Strøm, Kolstrup, Eisemann, & Waterloo, 2011).

ASSESSMENT

As part of the assessment process, the individual's perceptions, thoughts, attitudes, values, and beliefs are solicited. An ABC assessment (Box 12-2) is commonly carried out in which antecedents, behaviors, and consequences are documented. This assessment can point out the interactions between situations, thoughts, emotions, and day-to-day behavior.

CBT AND PRACTICE APPROACHES IN OCCUPATIONAL THERAPY

CBT is one of a range of strategies that can be used in addressing the focus of concern in occupational therapy; that is, occupational performance and experience. For complex occupational problems, CBT may be combined with other approaches so that the range of factors—for example, skill deficits, social and family influences, environmental barriers, and other factors—may be addressed. While not the exclusive intervention for complex occupational problems, CBT holds an important place in occupational therapy. Occupational therapy offers an opportunity to test the validity of negative assumptions through involvement in activities that are pleasurable and that promote a sense of self-efficacy. Activities are used to refute clients' automatic thoughts and help change behavior. For example, a client working on broadening his social activities with the help of his occupational therapist may attend a social club, and through this experience may replace negative thoughts such as, "I won't know anyone and no one will want to talk to me," with more positive ones such as, "I can talk to people I don't know and enjoy it." In CBT, changes are made through homework, practicing, and experiencing—that is, "doing"—the unique domain of the profession. With expertise in occupational and task analysis combined with knowledge of cognitive principles, occupational therapists are able to help clients schedule and perform specific activities related to problem areas. They help clients to monitor daily activities and pay attention to the degree of pleasure and accomplishment each activity yields. As awareness increases, clients can gradually increase participation in meaningful and pleasurable activities and feel rewarded by them. To help clients connect their beliefs to their engagement in activity, they can be asked to predict how much pleasure or mastery they will achieve with scheduled activities, then compare their predictions with actual results. At the same time, clients can anticipate obstacles, problem-solve their way around them, and develop contingency plans. A weekly review of the pleasurable activities in which the client engaged can disconfirm negatively biased recall such as, "My week was terrible." Occupational therapists are skilled in grading tasks and assignments according to the client's ability to perform; graded activities that target the needs and interests of the individual enable clients to act on their environments and at the same time monitor thoughts that influence feelings and behaviors. The therapist can help the client experience success by helping break down large, unrealistic goals into smaller, more manageable pieces. With success, negative thoughts such as "I can't do anything well" can be examined and replaced.

Occupational therapists have been using cognitive behavioral principles in their work for some time. In 1987, Mary Johnston published an article titled "Occupational therapists and the teaching of cognitive behavioral skills," in which she reviewed established and longstanding occupational therapy interventions such as communication skills training, assertiveness training, problem solving and management of depression. In the area of communication skills, she explains that the cognitive skills needed to converse more effectively include looking at units of interaction and examining assumptions and beliefs about what has taken place. Recognizing faulty beliefs regarding these interactions is an important step that can then be followed by replacing them with new and more constructive ones. In addition to examining underlying beliefs and assumptions, behavioral skills, such as beginning and ending conversations, using gestures and nonverbal communication, and adjusting tone of voice, are important to learn. Similarly, assertiveness training can be broken into cognitive skills and behavioral skills. Cognitive skills include recognizing the differences between aggression, assertion and passivity, recognizing personal rights and the rights of others, and reducing cognitive and affective obstacles to acting assertively. Examining such beliefs as "If I say no, I won't be liked" can be examined so that they can be replaced with thoughts that enable more control and assertive behavior. Assertiveness training also includes behavioral skills such as role playing and homework assignments aimed at helping people express how they feel and what they want.

Occupational therapists have found that cognitive behavioral approaches provide a solid foundation for resolving the emotional and physiological symptoms of post-traumatic stress disorder (PTSD) because this frame of reference articulates how beliefs about events and behavioral, emotional, and cognitive consequences evolve after traumatic events (Bruce & Borg, 1993). Its concepts of cognitive restructuring, assertiveness training, and stress inoculation training are effective in reducing anxiety and gaining mastery over trauma (Bruce & Borg, 1993; Meichenbaum, 1994; Stein & Cutler, 1998). Creative visualization can be used for behavioral rehearsal, practicing alternative solutions to problems, or to create safe places to use to elicit a relaxation response in times of high stress (Meichenbaum, 1994; Parham & Fazio, 1997; Stein & Cutler, 1998).

Davis (1999) describes how occupational therapists can use this approach to help children who are victims of trauma, and to facilitate mastery over the trauma. In this case, occupational therapists can help a child acquire functional skills that enhance the ability to recognize feelings, eliminate cognitive distortions about the event, problem solve, and identify more rational options for coping. The occupational therapist can begin eliciting irrational beliefs about the event and help to replace them with more rational beliefs. In doing so, guilt and anxiety about the event may be reduced, enabling the child to move forward in his or her occupational roles. Stress management skills and assertive communication skills could be incorporated to enable the child to communicate feelings and needs in an effective manner. In addition, occupational therapists can help survivors of PTSD learn to handle anger and internalized rage, which is vital to recovery from trauma. Meichenbaum's stress inoculation training has been used successfully to teach survivors and their families to manage these powerful and often overwhelming feelings (Meichenbaum, 1994).

Psychoeducation is an important cognitive behavioral strategy that is often used by occupational therapists (Padilla, 2002). A basic assumption of psychoeducation is that information can enhance understanding of the illness, identify needed treatment resources, and the supportive services available (Greenberg et al., 1988). This strategy has been shown to increase clients' awareness of their illness and treatment (Pekkala & Merinder, 2001), to increase daily living skills and adaptive capacities, and create more productive alliances among clients, families, and mental health professionals, making treatment more efficient and cost-effective (Dixon, Adams, & Lucksted, 2000). Occupational therapists bring a unique focus to psychoeducational strategies because they combine skill building, information, and activity to empower clients to make healthy choices in their lives. Davis (1999) suggests that for children suffering PTSD, psychoeducation can be used to teach them and their families signs and symptoms and help them recognize how to gain mastery over intense feelings. She suggests that occupational therapists can act as resource guides and provide children and families with books, websites, handouts, and articles on PTSD to help them learn about the disorder and to teach basic problem solving and stress management. Other occupational therapy interventions that incorporate psychoeducation have been documented within acute mental health units (Cowls & Hale, 2005; Eaton, 2002) and in community settings where practical tasks help clients with severe and persistent mental illnesses optimize community functioning (Crist, 1986).

Addressing adolescents with obsessive compulsive disorders, Söchting and Third (2011) demonstrated how occupational therapists can incorporate CBT into a group format. The group protocol included four main components. In the first, psychoeducation, obsessions, and compulsions were defined, and a model of their connection was outlined and illustrated with patients' own examples. Second, the concept of cultivating *mindful detachment* (March & Mulle, 1998) was introduced and practiced using Schwartz's idea of *relabeling*. Relabeling teaches patients that their obsessions are not ordinary thoughts but rather the symptoms of obsessive-compulsive disorder and, therefore, must be relabeled and referred to as what they are, namely obsessions. Clients are encouraged to distance themselves from these obsessions and view them as bizarre "messages" that "do not belong to me." The third component involves building a master treatment plan in the form of an *exposure hierarchy* to guide a systematic approach to the exposure and response prevention exercises to be practiced both in the group sessions and between them. In each session, the group first reviews homework together, and then breaks out for individual exposure and response prevention as planned by the facilitators ahead of time, with the group reconvening at the end of the session to review the session and receive homework assignments. Last, the concept of *refocusing* as developed by Schwartz (1996) is integrated as a way of increasing tolerance for response prevention. The aim of refocusing on an alternative behavior is to facilitate response prevention. The facilitators strive to work with the established interests of the patients, as this increases

compliance and motivation. Outcome evaluations of this approach show that self-report measures at pre-, post-, and 12-month follow-up suggested clinical improvements for five of the seven patients.

Another example of CBT incorporated into occupational therapy practice can be found in the work of Yakobina, Yakobina, and Tallant (1997), who applied the approach to the treatment of dysthymic women. Here, the occupational therapist helps the client in three ways: (1) to alter a negative view of self in which the woman sees herself as worthless, incompetent, and undesirable; (2) to change the negative interpretation of her life experiences; that is, a perception that the world is a difficult, demanding, and self-defeating place where she can only expect failure and punishment; and (3) to counteract a negative view of the future in which the depressed individual expects continued hardship, suffering, and failure (Andreasen & Black, 1995; Kaplan, Sadock, & Grebb, 1994). The initial step in enabling a client to achieve these goals is to help her increase her awareness of the negative thoughts she uses. This may be done by discussing how thoughts affect behavior, by teaching her how to identify and record her negative automatic thoughts, and by introducing her to the concept that she can control her thoughts and thereby change her behavior. The second step involves helping the client analyze, dispute, and critique her negative cognitions through discussion. The occupational therapist attempts to refute the client's automatic thoughts through the use of activities that will reinforce more appropriate thoughts and help to change the client's behavior (Bruce & Borg, 1993). In so doing, she may be able to assess her daily functioning more realistically. Mastering activities that are meaningful and pleasurable enables the client to test the validity of her negative assumptions (Andreasen & Black, 1995). Activities provide cognitive, affective, and behavioral learning experiences to teach skills, strategies, and methods of coping. With this goal in mind, the occupational therapist, together with the client, must initially select activities that will maximize success, but activities can be graded so that dealing with failures in a way that does not employ faulty thinking can become a skill.

While the examples provided thus far use CBT principles that are directed at particular diagnostic groups, these principles can also be used to address functional limitations or behaviors across diagnostic groups, and they can underlie health promotion as well as treatment programs. For example, Herning, Cook, and Schneider (2005) describe a group CBT intervention that focuses on helping older adults identify and change negative or unrealistic thoughts about exercise so that they can more effectively maintain their exercise behavior. In this program, participants are asked to keep a log of their thoughts about exercise, the situations in which the thoughts occurred, and their subsequent behavior. The authors provide the example of a participant exercising at home in front of a window who may think, "I am so relaxed, I am actually enjoying my exercise while viewing all the beauty of spring." At the beginning of each group session, participants share their thought logs with the group and through the group discussion, and in doing so, gain a broad picture of how unrealistic thoughts may stand in the way of exercise. They then practice generating alternative thoughts and develop a plan of action to use these new thoughts to guide new behaviors. Herning et al. (2005) point out that some older adults may, for example, believe that they should be able to exercise for longer periods than their stamina allows. Participants learn to recognize these negative thoughts, put them in context, and think of other, more realistic thoughts such as "Yes, I would like to exercise longer. However, I am making progress. Last week I could only exercise for 5 minutes." After participants become familiar with basic CBT concepts, group sessions focus on setting short- and long-term goals and eliminating barriers to goal achievement. Here, participants are able to share problem-solving strategies (e.g., scheduling to maximize energy), share information (e.g., free local walking groups), and learn from one another.

Cognitive approaches are being applied across numerous contexts, including the workplace. Gardner, Avolio, Luthans, May, and Walumba (2005) employed a cognitive intervention to determine whether it is effective in helping employees modify their appraisal of stressful situations and lower the effects of stress. The cognitive intervention was compared with a traditional stress management training program that emphasized behavioral coping skills. The cognitive groups received teaching and practice in the cognitive model, identification of negative automatic thoughts, thought challenging, beliefs and attitudes, positive self-talk, distraction, and relaxation using imagery. Both the cognitive and the behavioral intervention were found to reduce symptom ratings at the 3 month follow-up but improvement at follow-up was greater for participants who attended the cognitive intervention.

Finally, there is a growing body of literature pointing to the health benefits of mindfulness, which draws on CBT principles (Baer, 2003; Grossman, Niemann, Schmidt, & Walach, 2004). Mindful awareness is the ability to consciously observe one's habitual thoughts and actions that are transferred to daily activities (Stroh-Gingrich, 2012). Being mindful increases engagement with the present moment and allows for a clearer understanding of how thoughts, feelings and emotions influence health and quality of life (McCorquodale, 2013). In her paper on occupational engagement as it relates to mindfulness, Elliot (2011) states that mindfulness is "a means by which to 'wake up,' more fully and openly participate in the surrounding world, and assume responsibility for one's choices" (p. 368). Occupational therapists are beginning to incorporate mindfulness meditation in their practices—for example, Stroh-Gingrich (2012) describes its application to help people living with persistent pain. Drawing on her experience, she reports how engagement in mindfulness meditation that had a focus on self-observation of thoughts, feelings, judgments, and sensations allowed her to see her persistent pain objectively and observe other sensations in her body, without holding onto the pain. Once she developed this skill, she applied the same principles to her everyday life to learn how to manage her health and engage more fully in meaningful occupations. A specific example of how CBT approaches can be incorporated into occupational therapy practice is provided in Box 12-3.

Examples of Tools and Instruments Developed

Advancement of CBT strategies has relied on measures to assess irrational beliefs and other cognitively related constructs. One commonly used measure is the Automatic Thoughts Questionnaire (Hollon & Kendall, 1980), which was developed to assess spontaneous negative self-statements and intrusive cognitions experienced by depressed persons. The questionnaire lists 30 items, each of which is a negative thought. The respondent is to rate how often the thought has surfaced in the past week on a scale from one (not at all) to five (all the time). This questionnaire is an inventory of an individual's negative cognitions and addresses issues such as low self-esteem, hopelessness, negative self-concept, and negative expectations. Good concurrent validity has been reported and Automatic Thought Questionnaire scores are correlated in the moderate-to-high range with such measures of depression as the Beck Depression Inventory and the Depression scale of the Minnesota Multiphasic Personality Inventory (e.g., Bisno, Thompson, Breckenridge, & Gallagher, 1985; Dobson & Breiter, 1983; Dobson & Shaw, 1986; Eaves & Rush, 1984; Harrell & Ryon, 1983).

Thought records enable individuals to document what was going through their minds under particular circumstances when they felt a particular emotion. Completing thought records enables people to identify what antecedents in the environment may be triggers, and helps people identify the thought that may be automatically called up in response. As a result, automatic thoughts become accessible for questioning, evaluation, and cognitive restructuring.

Additional tools include core belief logs that can track day-to-day evidence that suggests a core belief is not 100% true (Beck, 1995) and life review, which involves re-evaluating a core belief's historical underpinnings. In each of these cases, the occupational therapist and client can examine evidence that supports the core belief and reframe the evidence in a more "rational" manner.

Box 12-3. Applying CBT to a Woman With Depression

Joan, age 29 years, was referred to the community mental health team by her family doctor. She had been complaining of ongoing and persistent depressive symptoms and relationship difficulties with her husband. Joan thought her problems had arisen following the birth of her latest baby.

Community Mental Health Team Assessment

An occupational therapist from the community mental health team visited Joan at her home. At the assessment interview, Joan described low mood, increased irritability, difficulty carrying out simple tasks, reduced libido, reduced memory, anhedonia (loss of pleasure), reduced concentration, and reduced energy levels. She was very tearful when talking about her problems. She expressed some fleeting suicidal ideas but had no plans to act on them as she felt she was too much of a coward. She denied that she wanted to harm herself. She felt that she was no longer in control of her life and had no time for herself with the pressures of full-time employment, children, and housework. Her reluctance to take antidepressants was due to being unsure of the benefits.

Background Information

Joan graduated from college with a diploma in Business Studies. She has been married for 7 years. She worked full time as an administrator at a local health center and had just returned to work following maternity leave but felt unable to cope and went on sick leave. Joan was ambitious and regularly took work home to cope with the high demands but still, she was facing the possibility that she could be laid off due to reorganization at work. Joan believed that her colleagues in the administrative team underperformed and she thought she was expected to do additional work to compensate for this. Before the children were born, Joan had been active, and had enjoyed cycling and swimming with friends.

Cognitive-Behavioral Therapy Sessions

In the first CBT session, the occupational therapist assessed the relationship among thoughts, feelings, and behaviors. It was also important to establish a collaborative rapport to maximize engagement in therapy and introduce the CBT model.

Joan described herself as having "always been shy" and lacking in confidence, particularly when getting to know people. She considered herself to be a "terrible mother" and was concerned that her feelings for her husband had lessened. She also thought that her parents did not care about her. Joan told the occupational therapist that she had decided to go on sick leave following an incident at home when she had lost her temper and had used excessive force while trying to bathe her daughter Sarah who was being uncooperative. She was very distressed about her inability to control her daughter's behavior and upset at her own aggressive behavior.

Following Joan's description of her problems, the therapist described the CBT model and explained how it might be helpful to Joan. The therapist and Joan identified the links between thoughts, feelings, and behavior. Joan and her therapist completed a Five Areas of Assessment form that captures a specific situation (Figure 12-1).

During this process, the therapist asked questions that helped Joan identify her thoughts, feelings, and actions. The aim was for Joan to feel understood and to engender a sense of hopefulness that therapy might be helpful. The therapist explained to Joan that she was expected to take work away from sessions and to try things out to see if they might be helpful.

Together, Joan and the occupational therapist discussed Joan's situation and arrived at a formulation of Joan's problems, as follows: Joan's unhelpful thinking may have been activated when her performance at work was scrutinized. Joan believed that she would be exposed as a failure and this fear was applied to other major areas of her life, such as her role as a mother and relationship with her husband. For example, Joan had thought "My boss thinks I am a failure," "I am a rotten mother," and "My husband does not care for me." All her unhelpful thoughts are reinforced by the way she processes information; she has a negative thinking bias and tends to select certain negative aspects and uses this

(continued)

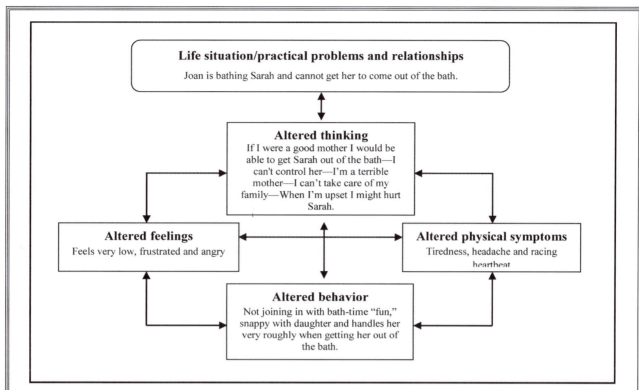

Figure 12-1. Joan's initial five areas of assessment. (Reprinted from Donaghy, M., Nicol, M., and Davidson, K.M. (Eds.), *Cognitive-behavioural Interventions in physiotherapy and occupational therapy*, Edinburgh, New York ButterWorth-Heinemann. Copyright © 2008 with permission from Elsevier Health Sciences.)

to interpret the whole situation. These thoughts link very powerfully to her feeling; a low mood and irritability. When she feels like this she can behave in unhelpful ways such as withdrawing from her daughter and focusing on unpleasant tasks. She avoids pleasure, which increases how badly she feels. The occupational dysfunction resulting from her depression manifested as reduced ability to perform the tasks and activities that are required for her major occupational life roles as wife, mother, and worker.

Session 2

In the second session, Joan discussed some information she had read on depression, on the advice of the occupational therapist. She said she was relieved to find that other people felt the same way. She discussed her roles and daily activities and the occupational therapist noticed that Joan focused only on tasks that needed to be done and spoke little about pleasurable activities, including pleasure time with her children. Joan held the belief that "it's good to be active and get things done" and had very little insight into how having little pleasure had affected her mood, and in turn her ability to get things done, thereby creating a vicious cycle (Figure 12-2).

The occupational therapist asked Joan to keep an activity log as homework, to determine which activities and occupational roles made her happiest.

Sessions 3 to 5: Increasing Pleasurable Activities

Sessions 3, 4, and 5 began by reviewing an activity schedule in which Joan listed her daily activities alongside the level of pleasure (on a scale of 1 to 10) and sense of achievement she derived from each (on a scale from 1 to 10). This helped the occupational therapist and Joan identify pleasurable and valued activities.

Joan's ratings of pleasure and achievement helped her see that there was an overall lack of pleasure in her life and that she had become overly task-oriented with childcare, with little time for herself in the day. It was decided to reintroduce pleasurable activities, broken down into step-by-step action plans. For example, Joan would try to re-establish

(continued)

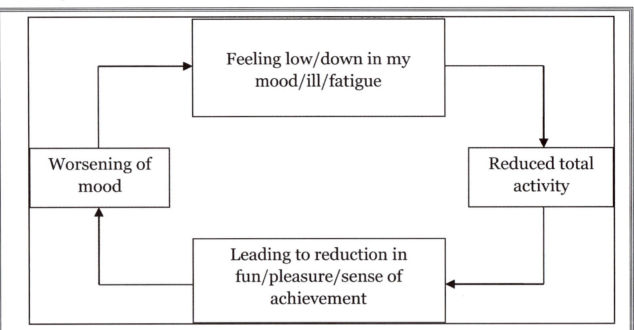

Figure 12-2. Joan's vicious circle of behavior. (Reprinted from Donaghy, M., Nicol, M., and Davidson, K.M. (Eds.), *Cognitive-behavioural Interventions in physiotherapy and occupational therapy*, Edinburgh, New York ButterWorth-Heinemann. Copyright © 2008 with permission from Elsevier Health Sciences.)

cycling with friends at quiet times and build up to using off-road cycling tracks. The work that Joan agreed to carry out between sessions would put these plans into action. The occupational therapist and Joan were able to set some initial goals for therapy:

- Increase awareness of the thoughts Joan has about Sarah, and the impact they have on her depression
- Increase the pleasurable activities in Joan's life

Sessions 6 and 7: Increasing Awareness of Negative Thoughts

Sessions 6 and 7 focused on increasing awareness of negative thoughts. The occupational therapist recommended using a dysfunctional thought record (Greenberger & Padesky, 1995) to focus on increasing Joan's awareness of the impact of her negative thoughts by looking at a specific time when Joan felt particularly low. An example is provided in Table 12-3.

Joan was encouraged to look at specific situations and identify her thoughts, feelings, physical symptoms, and behavior. She was asked to rate her emotions as a percentage (feeling low 90%) and look for negative automatic thoughts. Together, the occupational therapist and Joan identified that Joan was thinking in unhelpful ways that either lowered her mood or made her feel anxious—she tended to focus on the negative in a situation, would mind-read what other people thought of her, would make catastrophic predictions about how her children would "turn out," and would ruminate on personal standards she had set. Looking at the impact of these thoughts identified that she had begun to "withdraw into herself" and that this was also unhelpful.

Session 8: Review of Main Goals of Therapy

The eighth session focused on reviewing Joan's remaining goals in therapy:

- Improving her relationship with her husband
- Exploring her return to work

The occupational therapist and Joan agreed these were long-term goals and split them into short-term and medium-term goals. For example, the goal of improving her relationship with her husband included the short-term goal of planning regular time together apart from the children, and the medium-term goal of exploring images that suggest alternative approaches to their marriage. The goal of return to work included the short-term goal of establishing a routine at home that would enable her return and a medium-term goal of meeting with her boss to establish working

(continued)

TABLE 12-3		
JOAN'S NEGATIVE AUTOMATIC THOUGHTS		
SITUATION	**MOODS**	**AUTOMATIC THOUGHTS (IMAGES)**
At home with Sarah, and she asks if she can have a friend over to visit	*Feel really down* *Panicky and irritable* *90%*	*I can't cope with having her friend over* *The kids never do what I say* *I'm a terrible mother* *They will make a terrible mess in the house* *No one will help me to clean it up*

Reprinted from Donaghy, M., Nicol, M., and Davidson, K. M. (Eds.), *Cognitive-behavioural Interventions in physiotherapy and occupational therapy*, Edinburgh, New York ButterWorth-Heinemann. Copyright © 2008 with permission from Elsevier Health Sciences.

TABLE 12-4			
JOAN CHALLENGING NEGATIVE AUTOMATIC THOUGHTS			
EVIDENCE THAT SUPPORTS THE NEGATIVE AUTOMATIC THOUGHT	**EVIDENCE THAT DOES NOT SUPPORT THE NEGATIVE AUTOMATIC THOUGHT**	**ALTERNATIVE/ BALANCED THOUGHTS**	**RATE MOODS NOW**
I can never get Sarah to do what she is told	*I love Sarah and want her to be happy*	*Feeling low makes it difficult to face the demands Sarah makes but I am a good mother and spending time with her can be fun* *I am making very negative predictions about how the visit would go*	*50%*
She is much cheekier when her friends are over and I don't have the energy to tidy up the terrible mess *I lose my temper and shout at her* *It would be awful if I was upset when a friend visits* *I am too rough with Sarah*	*I want her to have positive memories* *My friends say the same things about their children* *Sarah is excited and happy when her friends visit because they don't visit often*		*40%*

Reprinted from Donaghy, M., Nicol, M., and Davidson, K.M. (Eds.), *Cognitive-behavioural Interventions in physiotherapy and occupational therapy*, Edinburgh, New York ButterWorth-Heinemann. Copyright © 2008 with permission from Elsevier Health Sciences.

terms and conditions. All the while, Joan would need to work on changing the unhelpful thinking patterns that stood in the way of these goals.

Sessions 9 to 12: Challenging Negative Thoughts

In the set of sessions that followed (sessions 9 to 12), Joan began to challenge some of the negative thoughts that contributed to her low mood. She used dysfunctional thought records to guide her in evaluating the evidence for and against negative thoughts. She noticed that evaluating her thoughts, or looking at them in a different way, did make a difference to the way she felt. Table 12-4 documents the process of challenging the negative thoughts that were presented earlier in Table 12-3.

Joan noticed that believing thoughts such as "I am a terrible mother" prevented her from letting her daughter Sarah have positive experiences with her. Joan went on to use thought records to help her identify and challenge negative thoughts related to returning to work. Table 12-5 illustrates this process.

(continued)

TABLE 12-5						
JOAN GATHERING AND CHALLENGING NEGATIVE AUTOMATIC THOUGHTS						
1. SITUATION	2. MOODS	3. AUTOMATIC THOUGHTS (IMAGES)	4. EVIDENCE THAT SUPPORTS THE NEGATIVE AUTOMATIC THOUGHT	5. EVIDENCE THAT DOES NOT SUPPORT THE NEGATIVE AUTOMATIC THOUGHT	6. ALTERNATIVE/ BALANCED THOUGHT	7. RATE MOODS NOW
Feeling undervalued at work and thinking of a conversation with my boss when I made a mistake with the words I used	*Feel really anxious, panicky, and depressed* *Angry with colleagues* *90%*	*Oh no, I've made a mistake* *He'll think I am an idiot who can't speak properly* *If I were good at my job, I would not make mistakes* *I keep remembering a situation when I made a costly mistake with some items ordered for the surgery* *I don't want to make a mistake again*	*I mix my words up a lot* *I always make mistakes* *I made an expensive mistake in the past* *My boss doesn't let me take charge of complex jobs* *My boss doesn't believe my explanation* *He thinks I can't do the job* *I feel like a wee girl in the headmaster's room getting a row* *I don't like being in a situation when I am not in control of my feelings* *His opinion matters to me* *Everybody is dominant over me*	*I don't always make mistakes* *Some of my work is commended* *My workload is higher than everyone else* *I don't know what my boss is thinking unless I ask him* *It's not the same situation as when I was at school* *My feelings are powerful but I can control them*	*I am making too much of a simple mistake—a slip of speech does not mean I am bad at my job*	*40%*
Reprinted from Donaghy, M., Nicol, M., and Davidson, K.M. (Eds.), *Cognitive-behavioural Interventions in physiotherapy and occupational therapy,* Edinburgh, New York ButterWorth-Heinemann. Copyright © 2008 with permission from Elsevier Health Sciences.						

(continued)

Alternative conclusions to her unhelpful thoughts were obtained through looking at the evidence for and against her thoughts. Beliefs and assumptions such as "If I were good at my job, I would not make mistakes" are replaced with "I am making too much of a simple mistake."

Session 13: Final Session

The final session focused on reviewing Joan's progress in therapy to help her to identify what had been helpful or unhelpful, and what "new life rules" she could develop to help her maintain her progress. Joan came to appreciate the value of keeping a record of her achievements, and having a review day when she stopped to take stock of all the things she has done that were acceptable to her or had given her pleasure. Joan and the occupational therapist documented her new life rules:

- I know I tend to see the negative in everything—it would be helpful to challenge this with my thought records and positive event log.
- To be a good mother, I also need to make time to enjoy myself.
- It is good to be active and get things done, but not to the exclusion of pleasurable time for myself.
- I do not need to rely solely on other people's opinion of my work.

EVALUATION PROCESSES FOR OUTCOMES

Outcomes of CBT interventions have typically been captured through measurement of symptomatology, but there are some examples of evaluation processes that go beyond illness indicators. Davis, Ringer, Strasburger, and Lysaker (2008) describe a participant evaluation of a CBT program for enhancing work function in schizophrenia. The survey included questions regarding how well participants liked the intervention, what program elements CBT participants found beneficial, and what program improvements they would suggest. The researchers compared their level of satisfaction with that of participants in a control group receiving support alone. The CBT intervention was associated with greater participant satisfaction than support alone, particularly the perception of the overall quality of services and assistance with problem solving. During the interviews, CBT participants reported that they found connection with other participants and program staff to be beneficial, as well as assistance with cognitive restructuring, problem-solving, and providing/ receiving work-related feedback. The authors conclude that participant evaluations can function as a source of useful data for evaluation of CBT interventions for persons who have schizophrenia.

EVIDENCE FOR THE APPROACH

CBT outcome studies have concluded that this treatment approach is highly effective for depression and anxiety disorders (Butler & Beck, 2000; Gaffan et al, 1995; Wright et al., 2003). Studies typically show CBT to be as effective as antidepressant medication for the treatment of depression, but there are mixed results regarding the effectiveness of combined treatment (CBT and medication) for depression. The most robust evidence of CBT as an efficacious treatment can be found in large-scale studies of people who had chronic or severe depression; these studies show that combined treatment gives better results than either treatment alone (DeRubeis, Gelfand, Tang, & Simons, 1999; Hollon et al., 2005; Keller et al., 2000). The overall results of studies of patients with depression or anxiety disorders indicate that CBT may be used alone as an effective treatment for these conditions and that for severe or chronic depression, combined therapy with medication is recommended.

CBT also has research support in the treatment of other disorders such as bulimia nervosa and schizophrenia, where it can be used as an adjunct to pharmacotherapy (Rector & Beck, 2001; Turkington, Dudley, Warman, & Beck, 2004; Wright et al., 2003) or to increase the attainment of work goals. CBT has also been shown to reduce the risk for relapse in bipolar disorder (Lam et al., 2003) and to help patients with medical disorders cope with pain and disability (Sensky, 2004). CBT has been found in at least one study to significantly reduce the frequency of subsequent suicide attempts among people who had previously attempted suicide (Brown et al., 2005).

Some research exists on the effectiveness of CBT approaches as applied to occupational therapy. A critical review of the published literature on cognitive-behavioral interventions with people with chronic pain was conducted by the McMaster group on evidence-based practice. Their primary question was, "What is the effectiveness of cognitive-behavioral interventions in improving occupational performance (function) for people with chronic pain?" They included studies of CBT that included at least three of the following modalities: relaxation, stress management, goal setting, self-monitoring/self-talking, assertiveness training, modelling, pacing, or family training. Occupational performance outcomes included participation in daily activities and/or in specific areas of self-care, productivity, and/or leisure; performance components such as physical, psychological, cognitive or pain-related behaviors, and perceptions and environmental components. The results of the systematic review indicate favorable outcomes for cognitive-behavioral interventions compared with control (waitlist or no attention) conditions in the short term (that is, immediately after intervention). The strongest effects were found in the short-term outcomes of pain perception and pain intensity. Weaker effects that favored cognitive-behavioral intervention over control conditions include activity level, depression, and cognition.

CONCLUSION

This chapter has outlined the core tenets of CBT and has demonstrated their application to occupational therapy practice. Evidence of positive outcomes associated with CBT, and the strong alignment of its principles with occupational therapy principles, makes this approach an appealing one for occupational therapists. Although the field has taken up the approach across a variety of populations, the manifold ways in which CBT principles can be incorporated into everyday occupational therapy practice are yet to be elucidated and tested.

LEARNING ACTIVITIES/ DISCUSSION QUESTIONS

1. Identify one cognitive error you use in your daily life and how it affects your (1) affect, (2) behavior, and (3) occupational performance.

2. You and your client are discussing her goal of working at a paid job, when she states, "I will never be able to do this; I fail at everything." What are some strategies you can draw on to help her think differently about her potential for work?

3. Discuss how mindfulness can be used in occupational therapy to enhance occupational performance and experience.

4. Discuss how activity can be incorporated into a cognitive behavioral approach.

REFERENCES

Andreasen, N. C., & Black, D. W. (1995). *Introductory textbook of psychiatry* (2nd ed.). Washington, DC: American Psychiatric Publishing Incorporated.

Baer, R. A. (2003). Mindfulness training as a clinical intervention: A conceptual and empirical review. *Clinical Psychology: Science and Practice, 10*(2), 125-143.

Bandura, A. (1995). Self-efficacy in changing societies. Cambridge, U.K.: Cambridge.

Barris, R., Kielhofner, G., & Watts, J. H. (1988). *Bodies of knowledge in psychosocial practice.* Thorofare, NJ: SLACK Incorporated.

Beating the blues. (2006). Retrieved from www.beatingtheblues.co.uk/patients/.

Beck, A. T. (1970). *Depression: Causes and treatment.* Philadelphia: University of Pennsylvania Press. (Original work published 1967.)

Beck, A. T. (1976). *Cognitive therapy and the emotional disorders.* New York: Meridian.

Beck, J. S. (1995). *Cognitive therapy: Basics and beyond.* New York: Guilford Press.

Bisno, B., Thompson, L. W., Breckenridge, J., & Gallagher, D. (1985). Cognitive variables and the prediction of outcome following an intervention for controlling depression. *Cognitive Therapy and Research, 9,* 527-538.

Brown, G. K., Ten Have, T., Henriques, G. R., Xie, S. X., Hollander, J. E., & Beck, A. T. (2005). Cognitive therapy for the prevention of suicide attempts: A randomized controlled trial. *Journal of the American Medical Association, 294,* 563-570.

Bruce, M. A., & Borg, B. (1993). *Psychosocial occupational therapy: Frames of reference for intervention.* Thorofare, NJ: SLACK Incorporated.

Butler, A. C., & Beck, J. S. (2000). Cognitive therapy outcomes: A review of meta-analyses. *Journal of the Norwegian Psychological Association, 37,* 1-9.

Carroll, K. M., Nich, C., & Ball, S. A. (2005). Practice makes progress? Homework assignments and outcome in treatment of cocaine dependence. *Journal of Consulting and Clinical Psychology, 73*(4), 749-755.

Clark, D. A., Beck, A. T., & Alford, B. A. (1999). *Scientific foundations of cognitive theory and therapy of depression.* New York: Wiley.

Cormac, I., Jones, C., & Campbell, C. (2002). Cognitive behavior therapy for schizophrenia (Cochrane Review). *Cochrane Library*, issue 2. Oxford: Update Software.

Cowls, J., & Hale, S. (2005). It's the activity that counts: What clients value in psycho-educational groups. *The Canadian Journal of Occupational Therapy, 72*(3), 176-182.

Crist, P. H. (1986). Community living skills: A psychoeducational community based program. *Occupational Therapy in Mental Health, 6*(2), 51-64.

Cully, J. & Teten, A. (2008). *A therapist's guide to brief cognitive behavioral therapy.* Department of Veterans Affairs South Central MIRECC, Houston. Retrieved from www.mirecc.va.gov/visn16/docs/therapists_guide_to_brief_cbtmanual.pdf.

Davis, J. (1999). Effects of trauma on children: Occupational therapy to support recovery. *Occupational Therapy International, 6*(2), 126-142.

Davis, L. W., Ringer, J. M., Strasburger, A. M., & Lysaker, P. H. (2008). Participant evaluation of a CBT program for enhancing work function in schizophrenia. *Psychiatric Rehabilitation Journal, 32*(1), 55.

DeRubeis, R. J., Gelfand, L. A., Tang, T. Z., & Simons, A. D. (1999). Medications versus cognitive behavior therapy for severely depressed outpatients: Mega-analysis of four randomized comparisons. *American Journal of Psychiatry, 156*, 1007-1013.

Dixon, L., Adams, C., & Lucksted, A. (2000). Update on family psychoeducation for schizophrenia. *Schizophrenia Bulletin, 26*(1), 5-20.

Dobson, K. S., & Breiter, H. J. (1983). Cognitive assessment of depression: Reliability and validity of three measures. *Journal of Abnormal Psychology, 92*, 107-109.

Dobson, K. S., & Shaw, B. F. (1986). Cognitive assessment with major depressive disorders. *Cognitive Therapy and Research, 10*, 13-29.

Donaghy, M., Nicol, M., & Davidson, K. (2008). *Cognitive-behavioral interventions in physiotherapy and occupational therapy.* Edinburgh, New York: ButterWorth-Heinemann.

Drury, V., Birchwood, M., Cochrane, R., & Macmillan, F. (1996). Cognitive therapy and recovery from acute psychosis: a controlled trial. *British Journal of Psychiatry, 169*(5) 593-607.

Eaton, P. (2002). Psychoeducation in acute mental health settings: Is there a role for occupational therapists? *The British Journal of Occupational Therapy, 65*(7), 321-326.

Eaves, G., & Rush, A. J. (1984). Cognitive patterns in symptomatic and remitted unipolar major depression. *Journal of Abnormal Psychology, 93*, 31-40.

Elliot, M. (2011). Being mindful about mindfulness: An invitation to extend occupational engagement into the growing mindfulness discourse. *Journal of Occupational Science, 18*(4), 366-376.

Ellis, A. (1973). Rational-emotive therapy. In R. Corsini (Ed.), *Current psychotherapies.* Itasca, IL: F. E. Peacock Publishers.

Gaffan, E. A., Tsaousis, I., & Kemp-Wheeler, S. M. (1995). Researcher allegiance and meta-analysis: The case for cognitive therapy for depression. *Journal of Consulting and Clinical Psychology, 63*, 966-980.

Gardner, W. L., Avolio, B. J., Luthans, F., May, D. R., & Walumba, F. O. (2005). Can you see the real me? A self-based model of authentic leader and follower development. *The Leadership Quarterly, 16*, 343-372.

Greenberg, L., Fine, S., Cohen, C., Larson, K., Michaelson-Baily, A., Rubinton, P., & Glick, I. (1988). An interdisciplinary psychoeducation program for schizophrenic patients and their families in an acute care setting. *Hospital and Community Psychiatry, 39*, 277-282.

Greenberger, D., & Padesky, C. A. (1995). *Mind over mood: a cognitive therapy treatment manual for clients.* New York: Guilford Press.

Grime, P. R. (2004). Computerized cognitive behavioral therapy at work: a randomized controlled trial in employees with recent stress-related absenteeism. *Occupational Medicine, 54*(5), 353-359.

Grossman, P., Niemann, L., Schmidt, S., & Walach, H. (2004). Mindfulness-based stress reduction and health benefits: A meta-analysis. *Journal of Psychosomatic Research, 57*(1), 35-43.

Haddock, G., Tarrier, N., Spaulding, W., Yusupoff, L., Kinney, C., & McCarthy, E. (1998). Individual cognitive-behavior therapy in the treatment of hallucinations and delusions: A review. *Clinical Psychology Review, 18*(7): 821-838.

Harrell, T. H., & Ryon, N. B. (1983). Cognitive-behavioral assessment of depression: Clinical validation of the automatic thoughts questionnaire. *Journal of Consulting and Clinical Psychology, 51*, 721-725.

Herning, M. M., Cook, J. H., & Schneider, J. K. (2005). Cognitive behavioral therapy to promote exercise behavior in older adults: Implications for physical therapists. *Journal of Geriatric Physical Therapy, 28*(2), 34-38.

Høifødt, R. S., Strøm, C., Kolstrup, N., Eisemann, M., & Waterloo, K. (2011). Effectiveness of cognitive behavioral therapy in primary health care: a review. *Family Practice, 28*(5), 489-504.

Hollon, S. D., Jarrett, R. B., Nierenberg, A. A., Thase, M. E., Trivedi, M., & Rush, A. J. (2005). Psychotherapy and medication in the treatment of adult and geriatric depression: Which monotherapy or combined treatment? *Journal of Clinical Psychiatry, 66*, 455-486.

Hollon, S. D., & Kendall, P. C. (1980). Cognitive self-statements in depression: Development of an automatic thoughts questionnaire. *Cognitive Therapy and Research, 4*, 383-395.

Johnston, M. T. (1987). Occupational therapists and the teaching of cognitive behavioral skills. *Occupational Therapy in Mental Health, 7*(3), 69-81.

Kaplan, H. I., Sadock, B. J., & Grebb, J. A. (1994). *Kaplan and Sadock's synopsis of psychiatry: Behavioral sciences/clinical psychiatry* (7th ed.). Baltimore, MD: Lippincott, Williams & Wilkins.

Keller, M. B., McCullough, J. P., Klein, D. N., Arnow, B., Dunner, D. L., Gelenberg, A. J., & Zajecka, J. (2000). A comparison of nefazodone, the cognitive behavioral analysis system of psychotherapy, and their combination for the treatment of chronic depression. *New England Journal of Medicine, 342*, 1462-1470.

Kingdon, D. G., & Turkington, D. (1991). The use of cognitive behavior therapy with anormalizing rationale in schizophrenia. Preliminary report. *Journal of Mental and Nervous Disease, 179*(4), 207-211.

Lam, D. H., Watkins, E. R., Hayward, P., Bright, J., Wright, K., Kerr, N., ... Sham, P. (2003). A randomized controlled study of cognitive therapy for relapse prevention for bipolar affective disorder: Outcome of the first year. *Archives of General Psychiatry, 60*, 145-152.

Lewis, S., Tarrier, N., Haddock, G., Bentall, R., Kinderman, P., Kingdon, D., ... Dunn, G. (2002). Randomised controlled trial of cognitive-behavioral therapy in early schizophrenia: acute-phase outcomes. *British Journal of Psychiatry, 181*(Suppl. 43), 91-97.

Lopez, M. A., & Mermelstein, R. J. (1995). A cognitive-behavioral program to improve geriatric rehabilitation outcome. *The Gerontologist, 35*(5), 696-700.

Lysaker, P. H., Carcione, A., Dimaggio, G., Johannesen, J. K., Nicolo, G., Procacci, M., & Semerari, A. (2005). Metacognition amidst narratives of self and illness in schizophrenia: Associations with insight, neurocognition, symptom and function. *Acta Psychiatrica Scandinavica, 112*, 64-71.

March, J. S., & Mulle, K. (1998). *OCD in children and adolescents: A cognitive-behavioral treatment manual.* New York: Guilford Press.

Marks, I., Lovell, K., Noshirvani, H., Livanou, M., & Thrasher, S. (1998). Treatment of posttraumatic stress disorder by exposure and/or cognitive restructuring: A controlled study. *Archives of General Psychiatry, 55*(4), 317-325.

Marlatt, G. A. (1996). Taxonomy of high-risk situations for alcohol relapse: Evolution and development of a cognitive-behavioral model. *Addiction, 91*(Suppl.), 37-49.

McCorquodale, L. (2013). Mindfulness in the life of an occupational therapist: The 'being' behind the 'doing.' *Occupational Therapy Now, 15*(3), 14-16.

Meichenbaum, D. (1977). *Cognitive-behavior modification: An integrative approach.* New York, NY: Plenum Press.

Meichenbaum, D. (1994). *A clinical handbook/practical therapist manual for assessing and treating adults with post-traumatic stress disorder (PTSD).* Waterloo, ON: Institute Press.

MoodGYM. (n.d.). *MoodGYM frequently asked questions.* Retrieved from https://moodgym.anu.edu.au/welcome/faq#what.

Myers, M. G., Martin, R. A., Rohsenow, D. J., & Monti, P. M. (1996). The relapse situation appraisal questionnaire: Initial psychometric characteristics and validation. *Psychology of Addictive Behaviors, 10*(4), 237-247.

Neimeyer, R., & Feixas, G. (1990). The role of homework and skill acquisition in the outcome of group cognitive therapy for depression. *Behavior Therapy, 21*, 281-292.

O'Leary, K. D., & Wilson, G. T. (1987). *Behavior therapy: Application and outcome.* Englewood Cliffs, NJ: Prentice-Hall.

Padilla, R. (2002). Teaching approaches and occupational therapy psychoeducation. *Occupational Therapy in Mental Health, 17*(3), 81-95.

Parham, L. D., & Fazio, L. S. (1997). *Play in occupational therapy for children.* St. Louis, MO: Mosby.

Pekkala, E., & Merinder, L. (2001). Psychoeducation for schizophrenia (Cochrane Review). In *The Cochrane Library, 3.* Oxford: Update Software.

Rector, N. A., & Beck, A. T. (2001). Cognitive behavioral therapy for schizophrenia: An empirical review. *Journal of Nervous and Mental Disease, 189*, 278-287.

Schwartz, D. L. (1996). Analog imagery in mental model reasoning: Depictive models. *Cognitive Psychology, 30*(6), 154-219.

Sensky, T. (2004). Cognitive-behavior therapy for patients with physical illnesses. In J. H. Wright (Ed.), *Cognitive-behavior therapy* (pp. 83-121). Washington, DC: American Psychiatric Publishing.

Sensky, T., Turkington, D., Kingdon, D., Scott, J. L., Scott, J., Siddle, R., O'Carroll, M., & Barnes, T. R. (2000). A randomized controlled trial of cognitive-behavioral therapy for persistent symptoms in schizophrenia resistant to medication. *Archives of General Psychiatry, 57*(2), 165-172.

Smith, L., Nathan, P., Juniper, U., Kingsep, P., & Lim, L. (2003). *Cognitive behavioral therapy for psychotic symptoms: A therapist's manual.* Perth, Australia: Centre for Clinical Interventions.

Söchting, I., & Third, B. (2011). Behavioral group treatment for obsessive-compulsive disorder in adolescence: A pilot study. *International Journal of Group Psychotherapy, 61*(1), 84-97.

Stein, F., & Cutler, S. K. (1998). *Psychosocial occupational therapy: A holistic approach.* San Diego, CA: Singular Publishing Group.

Stroh-Gingrich, B. (2012). Occupational therapy and mindfulness meditation: An intervention for persistent pain. *Occupational Therapy Now, 14*(5), 21-22.

Tarrier, N. (2005). Cognitive behavior therapy for schizophrenia—A review of development, evidence and implementation. *Psychotherapy and Psychosomatics, 74*(3), 136-144.

Tarrier, N., Kinney, C., McCarthy, E., Wittkowski, A., Yusupoff, L., Gledhill, A., Morris, J., & Humphreys, L. (2001). Are some types of psychotic symptoms more responsive to cognitive-behavior therapy. *Behavioral and Cognitive Psychotherapy, 29*(1), 45-55.

Thase, M. E., & Callan, J. A. (2006). The role of homework in cognitive behavior therapy of depression. *Journal of Psychotherapy Integration, 16*(2), 162-177.

Thrasher, S.M., Lovell, K., Noshirvani, H., & Livanou, M. (1996). Cognitive restructuring in the treatment of post-traumatic stress disorder: Two single cases. *Clinical Psychology and Psychotherapy, 3*, 137-148.

Turkington, D., Dudley, R., Warman, D., & Beck, A. T. (2004). Cognitive-behavior therapy for schizophrenia: A review. *Journal of Psychiatric Practice, 10*, 5-16.

Turkington, D., & McKenna, P. (2003). Is cognitive-behavioral therapy a worthwhile treatment for psychosis? *British Journal of Psychiatry, 182*, 477-479.

Wright, J. H. (2006). Cognitive behavior therapy: Basic principles and recent advances. *FOCUS, 4*(2), 173-178.

Wright, J. H., Beck, A. T., & Thase, M. E. (2003). Cognitive therapy. In R. E. Hales, S. C. Yudofsky, & J. A. Talbott (Eds.), *Textbook of Clinical Psychiatry* (4th ed., pp. 1245-1284). Washington, DC: American Psychiatric Publishing.

Yakobina, S., Yakobina, S., & Tallant, B. K. (1997). I came, I thought, I conquered: Cognitive behavior approach applied in occupational therapy for the treatment of depressed (dysthymic) females. *Occupational Therapy in Mental Health, 13*(4), 59-73.

13

Expression and Occupation (Psychodynamic Perspectives)

Deborah Pitts, PhD, OTR/L, BCMH, CPRP and
Erin McIntyre, OTD

I have never doubted the existence of the unconscious; in fact it was quite a relief when I realised during my first experience of analysis, at the age of 23, that my dreams, thoughts and feelings were a language that I had not yet learnt to understand, but that were available to me as a guide to my internal life. Perhaps it is this investment in one's own internal life that is the most daunting and fulfilling in working within a psychoanalytic framework with clients. (Nicholls, 2013, p. 32 as cited in Nicholls, Piergrossi, Gibertoni, & Daniel, 2013, p. 4)

In my role as an academic staff member I had a 2-hour "debrief" session scheduled with a group of under-graduate occupational therapy students... Many of the students raised the same concern: that of managing their relationships with the client. They said they wanted to be respectful, show concern (be client centred) and not over-step 'boundaries'... When I suggested to the students that boundaries protect the patient from the therapist's less helpful intensions the students seem confused. They could not imagine that their goodwill and positively stated goal of enabling clients to achieve independence was not sufficient to establish a good therapeutic relationship. What they seemed to deny was that in any relationship there are many conflicted and unconscious layers of interaction. (Nicholls et al., 2013, p. 16)

OBJECTIVES

The objectives of this chapter are as follows:

» Identify and define key psychodynamic components and concepts.

» Differentiate between classical and contemporary psychodynamic theoretical perspectives.

» Define key psychodynamic concepts that can inform aspects of occupational therapy practice.

(continued)

Krupa, T., Kirsh, B., Pitts, D., & Fossey, E. *Bruce & Borg's*
Psychosocial Frames of Reference: Theories, Models, and Approaches for
Occupation-Based Practice, Fourth Edition (pp 211-226).
© 2016 SLACK Incorporated.

> » Identify and describe strengths and criticisms regarding a psychodynamic approach to occupational therapy practice.
> » Identify and describe implications for psychodynamic theory for therapeutic use of self and supervision in occupational therapy.
> » Identify and describe occupational therapy interventions informed by psychodynamic concepts.

BACKGROUND

The psychodynamic perspective in occupational therapy is best understood as providing an explanation for how mental processes, including perceptions, thoughts, and feelings that are in conscious awareness, as well as those that are not, influence one's selection of, participation in, and satisfaction with occupation. As a developmental model, it asserts that as we grow and mature, we create relationships with our human and nonhuman environment. In these relationships, we satisfy our basic needs and the need to use our unique talents, skills, and interests to engage socially with others and to ultimately find purpose in life. In the psychodynamic perspective, therapeutic activity is selected to enhance interpersonal communication, facilitate healthy emotional experiences, enhance self-awareness and self-acceptance, and to enable the identification and pursuit of one's skills and interests.

Psychodynamic perspectives emerged in occupational therapy as early as the 1930s (Gordon, 2002; Reilly, 1969), reached their peak between the 1950s and 1970s (Bruce & Borg, 2002) and have recently re-emerged internationally (Atkinson & Wells, 2000; Eklund, 2000; Nicholls et al., 2013). Bruce and Borg (2002) note that for occupational therapy, the psychodynamic framework is one in which psychological constructs are believed to account for one's occupational and social behavior. They argue that the enduring contribution of a psychodynamic framework has been that it alerts occupational therapists to attend to the emotional and affective part of the person.

Critiques of the psychodynamic perspective within occupational therapy have argued that it runs counter in fundamental ways to our founding philosophy regarding occupational engagement (Kielhofner & Burke, 1977; Reilly, 1969). Reilly (1969) argued in her analysis of "psychiatric occupational therapy" that the more central psychodynamic approaches became to the substance of treatment, the more peripheral became the practice of occupational therapy. She went on to acknowledge that psychodynamic theory revealed many of the strengths and weaknesses of occupational therapy (p. 19).

These criticisms have been countered by contemporary occupational therapists. Eklund (2000), for example, critiques the view espoused by Reilly et al., noting that it rests primarily on applications of what is called "classical" as opposed to contemporary "relational" psychodynamic theories to occupational therapy practice. Atkinson and Wells (2000) argue that the strength of the psychodynamic perspective for occupational therapy practice is that it provides a means of understanding an individual's inner states and his or her relationship to occupational engagement. Nicholls (2007), in her arguments, calls for a renewed psychodynamic discourse in occupational therapy and emphasizes that "perhaps the most profound loss in our current discourse has been an appreciation of the unconscious, and the effect it can have on the actions and choices of individuals and within society" (p. 56).

KEY COMPONENTS/CONCEPTS

Since Freud's initial articulation of his psychoanalytic perspective, and through the various developments of psychodynamic theory, Shedler (2006) argues that a consensus regarding central ideas or tenets common to all psychodynamic theories has emerged. These tenets are understood to be "intertwined and overlapping" (p. 12). It is also well recognized that much of what counts as psychodynamic theory has been infused into contemporary down-on-the-ground ideas about human psychology, as well as most psychotherapeutic approaches. This way of thinking about the human psyche has given a vocabulary and the license to talk about and understand ourselves in a way that we now take for granted. Not only do we have words to describe our "inner life," we also have a better understanding of how this inner life develops and differentiates into the "self." A full accounting of these tenets is not possible in this text, and the reader is encouraged to pursue additional reading and study to obtain a thorough understanding of psychodynamic theory.

Unconscious Mental Life

A central component of Freud's theory was that the mind consists of unconscious processes that influence human behavior. Shedler (2006) emphasizes that some important memory, perceptual, judgmental, affective, and motivational processes are not accessible to conscious thought. He notes that this principle is not unique to psychodynamic theory, but has also been demonstrated by cognitive science. He clarifies, however, that psychodynamic theory takes the view that:

> …it is not just that we do not fully know our own minds, but that there are things we seem not to *want* to know. There are things that are threatening or dissonant or make us feel vulnerable in some way, so we tend to look away. (p. 12)

The Mind in Conflict

Another central understanding upon which psychodynamic theory rests is the "universal recognition that inner dissonance is part of the human condition" (Shedler, 2006, p. 18). These inner conflicts may be conscious or not, result in feelings of anxiety, and may be expressed as psychological symptoms. Shedler (2006) clarifies that these inner conflicts are often experienced in our human efforts to establish intimate relationships and/or when we experience feelings of anger. Freudian classical theory identifies this tension as occurring between the different parts of the human psyche—the id, ego, and superego (see next section). Shedler (2006) emphasizes that psychoanalysis as a therapeutic approach provides a particular interpretative lens for such conflict, as well as a therapeutic means for coming to understand that conflict.

The Past Is Alive in the Present

Psychodynamic theory acknowledges the broadly agreed on psychological notion that humans come to "view the present through the lens of past experience" (Shedler, 2006, p. 19). This understanding emphasizes the developmental nature of human emotional and interpersonal experiences. Freudian classical theory proposed specific stages of development that occurred in infancy and childhood. Disruptions or incomplete development in these childhood developmental states, Freud believed, created emotional and interpersonal difficulties in adulthood. A key context for these early development experiences is our relationships with our key caregivers early in life.

Transference

Transference "refers specifically to the activation of pre-existing expectations, templates, scripts, fears, and desires in the context of the therapy relationship, with the patient viewing the therapist through the lens of early important relationships" (Shedler, 2006, p. 23). Countertransference represents an aspect of the transference experience, and generally refers to feelings that the therapist has toward the person—patient or client. Gabbard (2001) acknowledges

that countertransference is well accepted across all types of therapy approaches as being "a useful source of information about the patient" (p. 984). He also clarifies that views regarding countertransference have evolved over time, and contemporary perspectives are coming to view it as "jointly created," where "the patient draws the therapist into playing a role that reflects the patient's internal world, but the specific dimensions of that role are colored by the therapist's own personality" (p. 984).

In psychodynamic oriented therapy, this transference process is seen as critical to helping the person come to understand how his or her early psychological development is affecting his or her current emotional and interpersonal experiences. During therapy, practitioners will reflect on how the person is responding to him or her emotionally, and encourage the person to consider how his or her reaction to the therapist is similar to early important relationships. Sensitivity to this process of transference is seen as an important therapeutic skill that mental health practitioners must develop and continue to hone. It often begins with the young clinician engaging in his or her own psychodynamic oriented psychotherapy, and continues with experienced clinicians engaging in ongoing supervision and/or consultation throughout their career.

Defending

Given the notion that aspects of the mind are unconscious and in conflict, psychodynamic theory acknowledges that the mind may defend against the dissonance. Shedler (2006) emphasizes that "any thought or feeling can be used to defend against any other" (p. 29). He acknowledges that most basic psychological texts provide taxonomies of *defense mechanisms*, but argues that understanding defense in this way is both mechanistic and sees defenses as discrete events. For him, this is problematic and suggests that a more useful framing of defense is as a verb—defending. These "ways of defending" (p. 31) become patterned and habitual parts of our personality and character.

By coming to be more aware or conscious of these automatic thoughts and feelings through the supported reflection process that is therapy, it is believed we gain more control of our actions. Psychodynamic theory also argues that some defense processes, which emerge within the therapeutic relationship, can block the shared reflection between the person and therapist; this is referred to as *resistance*. This resistance, according to the theory, may be represented in behaviors on the part of the person that therapists may find irritating or annoying, (e.g., arriving late, missing appointments). As with the transference process, therapists must be sensitive to such defensive processes. Again, ongoing supervision and/or consultation can be very helpful in strengthening the therapists' awareness of their own thoughts, feelings, and actions in response to these defensive processes.

Psychological Causation

Psychodynamic theory accepts that psychological symptoms (e.g., disrupted thoughts and feelings) are neither "random nor meaningless," rather they "serve psychological functions, and occur in a psychological context" (Shedler, 2006, p. 35). *Psychic determinism* is the term that describes this phenomenon. However, Shedler (2006) recommends the term *psychic continuity*, as "it reminds us that there is a continuity from one thought to the next, and that thoughts and feelings are chained in meaningful associative sequences" (p. 42). The theory acknowledges that the meaning of these psychological symptoms is complex and layered. Further, that it takes significant effort and emotional risk to identify and make evident the connections between our thoughts, feelings, and perceptions.

Psychodynamic-oriented therapy uses a process known as *free association* as one way to begin the identification of those unconscious thoughts, feelings, and perceptions. This process involves creating a safe "psychological" space within the therapy relationship and encouraging the person to say "whatever comes to mind." It requires the person to avoid the common practice of editing ones thoughts, and is often facilitated via narratively and phenomenologically informed queries on the part of the therapist, (e.g., "Can you say more about that?" "What comes to mind?" "Where do your thoughts go from there?"; Shedler, 2006).

KEY DEVELOPERS AND IMPORTANT EVOLUTIONARY POINTS

Efforts to identify the important evolutionary points in the development of psychodynamic theory differentiate between what is referred to as the classical or Freudian psychoanalytic theory prominent during the early to mid-20th century and contemporary relational developments that emerged in the late 20th and early 21st century (Eagle, 2011b). Influences on contemporary relational developments include the development of attachment theory, recent advances in neuroscience and cognitive research, the post-modern paradigm shift with questions about power and authority, and responses to critiques regarding sex and sexuality, as well as race, ethnicity, and culture (Eagle, 2011b; Westen, Gabbard, & Ortigo, 2008). This section will provide a brief review of the key developments in psychodynamic theory from Freud's models of the mind to the contemporary relational theories.

Freud's Models of the Mind

Freud's earliest model of the mind, known as the *topographic model*, proposed that mental events are organized into layers of consciousness. These layers include the *conscious*, or what we are immediately aware of; the *preconscious*, or thoughts that we are not currently aware of but can readily bring to mind; and the *unconscious*, or thoughts that are actively kept unconscious by repression because of their content. Symptoms, according to Freud, emerged when the unconscious thought was transformed into "psychologically meaningful mental products" (Westen et al., 2008, p. 63).

In addition to his early thinking about consciousness, Freud was interested in human motivation. He theorized a *drive theory* of motivation, also referred to a *dynamic viewpoint* (Barris, Kielhofner, & Watts, 1988). This viewpoint theorizes that mental activity is stimulated by forces or energy—the biologically based libidinal and aggressive drives. These forces, he believed, followed natural laws. That is, that "a psychological motive to which energy has been attached can be consciously or unconsciously suppressed, but it cannot be destroyed" (Westen et al., 2008, p. 63). This is the origin of the now commonplace idea of a "Freudian slip." The psychological motive had to be expressed somehow and may emerge in a "form no longer under conscious control, as a symptom, a dream, a joke, a slip of the tongue, [or] behavior" (p. 63). It is Freud's drive theory of motivation, in particular, that has been criticized by occupational therapy scholars (Kielhofner & Burke, 1977; Reilly, 1969) as being particularly problematic for understanding motives for occupational engagement. Drawing on Adolf Meyer's early articulation of a philosophy of occupational therapy (1922), they argue that the notion that humans engage in occupation to reduce tension runs counter to the belief in intrinsic motivation as a primary motivator for occupational engagement.

Freud's *developmental model*, also referred to as the *genetic viewpoint* (Barris et al., 1988), proposed a psychosexual stage model of libidinal development. He conceptualized that while a person is pleasure seeking by nature, the objects and activities that would be experienced as especially satisfying would change as the individual matured. He related these directly to the physical development of the child, especially in the first three stages. Freud theorized that faulty psychosexual development at any of the stages would be evident in the inappropriate predominance in later life of the erotogenic zones (i.e., body areas that are sensitive and provide a sense of pleasure; Barris et al., 1988). It has been well documented that this particular model, in comparison to Freud's other theories regarding human emotional and interpersonal processes, is the most highly criticized, and aspects of the developmental model are seen as no longer central to contemporary psychoanalytic thinking (Westen et al., 2008).

The following briefly summarizes the model:

- For the newborn infant to about the age of 2 years, the oral region is the focus of pleasure (i.e., erotogenic zone), and the child is in the *oral stage*. For these children, activities that stimulate the mouth, such as those involved in sucking at their mother's breast or one's own fingers, or biting are favored. According to Freud, the mother is the most important person-object at this stage.

- For the child about age 1 to 3 years, the anal region is especially sensitive. At this *anal stage*, activities associated with excreting, particularly in terms of mastering control over excrements, will be satisfying. At this stage, the child tries to gain a sense of autonomy and control over the environment.

- When the child is 3 to 5 years of age, he or she is in the third stage of development—the *early genital* or *phallic stage*. Boys see themselves like Dad (or other significant males), and girls see themselves like Mom and begin to imitate their behaviors in a process termed *identification*. Children in this stage also take large strides in a process known as *separation-individuation* in which the child begins emotional separation from the parent.

- From about age 5 years to puberty, the child is in the *latency stage*. No new body area assumes special significance, and energy is channeled into developing or enhancing performance skills and forming peer friendships.

- From puberty through adolescence, referred to as the *late genital stage*, the genital area is again experienced as especially pleasure related. The development task is focused on the young person becoming capable of mature relatedness to others.

Freud's *structural model* is where he introduced the psychological constructs of id, ego, and superego, theorizing that mental activity can be best understood by their functions or purposes. In his structural model, his "understanding of conflict shifted from conflict between consciousness and the unconscious to conflict between desires and the dictates of conscience or reality" (Westen et al., 2008, p. 65). Westen et al., (2008) express concern that Freud's structural model is still emphasized as central to psychodynamic approaches in contemporary textbooks, stating that this "is unfortunate, given that even the most stalwart advocates of the structural model have now suggested that it has outlived its usefulness" (p. 65). The usefulness of the model, they argue, is in its theorizing of a mind in conflict. The model is briefly summarized in the following:

- The *id* is that portion of the mind or psyche that was unable to differentiate between reality and fantasy and that wanted immediate gratification. The id is present at birth and houses the instincts, including those related to survival. The id experiences intolerable tension when biological needs are not satisfied, and pleasure when those needs are met and tension is released.

- The *ego* refers to that portion of the mind or psyche that can relate functionally with the outside world. The ego also strives to satisfy, or bring pleasure, but unlike the id, it is able to realistically assess the outside world. Anxiety is the signal to the ego of impending displeasure and alerts the ego to action. The ego is the structure that must balance the demands of desired, reality, and morality.

- The *superego* is that portion of the mind or psyche that functions as the moral agent. The superego is the conscience, an inner voice that influences actions by evoking guilt, where we have displeased others, and pride when we do what is perceived as right or approved of. It is influenced by parental training and contains ideals for action (Barris et al., 1988; Westen et al., 2008).

Early criticisms of Freud's models came from two prominent analysts—Alfred Adler and Carl Jung, as well as later neo-Freudians Karen Horney, Erich Fromm, and Harry Stack Sullivan. They rejected Freud's view of the libido as the primary motivational force in human life, and placed much greater emphasis on understanding behavior within a cultural and interpersonal context (Barris et al., 1988; Westen et al., 2008).

Ego Psychology

Ego psychology emerged after Freud's death and represented a significant shift in psychoanalytic theory, and theorized that the ego was the biologically based "executive branch" of the mind that functioned by helping us to adapt and have coherence, identity, and organization. Key theorists and their theoretical contribution in ego psychology include Anna Freud's "ego defense mechanisms," Heinz Hartmann's "conflict-free ego sphere," and Eric Erikson's "psychosocial model of development" (Westen et al., 2008).

Drawing on Hartmann, these theories believed that infants have innate capacity for adaptation. This capacity developed into ego functions distinct from libidinal drives, and could be nurtured in what Hartmann called an "average expectable environment." From Anna Freud, ego psychology argued for unconscious ego defenses that could ward off anxiety to protect the self from harm and unwanted impulses. Finally, ego development was understood as being shaped by culture and the social environment, and matured through the resolution of crises at each stage of life throughout the lifespan (Westen et al., 2008). Erickson's well-disseminated theory of psychosocial development served as the framework for ego psychology.

Self-Psychology

Kohut's *self-psychology* is identified as being another key psychological theory in the psychodynamic tradition. However, scholars disagree on whether it is best understood as part of the relational turn in psychodynamic theory development (Eagle, 2011b; Westen et al., 2008); therefore for purposes of this review, it will be briefly addressed outside that frame. Self-psychology emphasizes the need for "ambitions, ideals and the need for self-esteem" as key sources of human motivation (Westen et al., 2008, p. 68). Development of a strong sense of self, Kohut theorized, is when mentally healthy caregivers—who themselves have a strong sense of self—respond empathically when their children need them. Kohut describes this process of empathy as "mirroring," the absence of which in early development results in psychological and behavioral problems. In the psychotherapeutic relationship, it is the therapist's empathic "mirroring" that is theorized as influencing change in the person's sense of self. The development of empathy is seen as an important professional skill for occupational therapists and critical to the effective and meaningful therapeutic use of self (Cara & Stephenson, 2013).

Object Relations and Relational Theories

Westen et al. (2008) argue that theories associated with what is referred to as the "relational turn" in psychoanalytic theory represent the most significant development since Freud, and identified object relations and contemporary relational theories as key theories within this perspective. Broadly, these approaches are focused on "enduring patterns of interpersonal functioning in intimate relationships and the cognitive and emotional processes that mediate those patterns" (p. 67), known as "object relations." These theories countered earlier psychoanalytic thinking, and argued that humans are motivated by the desire for human contact and relatedness, not sexual/sensual pleasure. W. R. D. Fairbairn is credited with introducing *object relations theory*, theorizing that the "libido is object seeking and not pleasure seeking" (Westen et al., 2008, p. 68). Since its introduction, various theorists have contributed to the development of this perspective. Winnicott and Bowlby's perspectives are reviewed here given their identification is important to occupational therapy practice (Nicholls, Piergrossi, Gibertoni, & Daniels, 2013).

Winnicott's concepts of a "facilitating environment" and "transitional objects and transitional space" have been identified as particularly important to occupational therapy practice (Nicholls et al., 2013). From a developmental perspective, the "facilitating" or "holding" environment is critical to development of the self. It is provided by the primary nurturer of an infant, and includes the nurturer being able to "resonate with the baby's wants and needs,"

as well as providing "a nondemanding presence when the infant is not making demands or experiencing needs" (Greenberg & Mitchell, 1983, p. 193). Failure on the part of the nurturer to effectively sense and respond results in psychological and behavioral problems as the infant grows through childhood, adolescence, and adulthood. In the psychotherapeutic relationship, a holding environment refers to a therapeutic ambiance or setting that permits the person to experience safety, thereby facilitating psychotherapeutic work. Thus, the occupational therapist and the relationship established with the client can be viewed as critical components of the holding environment.

Winnicott's theory of transitional phenomena acknowledges that humans—children and adults—relate to inanimate objects and rely on them to serve psychological functions also provided by persons (Eagle, 2011b). Nicholls et al. (2013) emphasize that for Winnicott, these objects had "the paradoxical function of linking the child to the mother and at the same time providing distance from her" (p. 58). An additional aspect of Winnicott's developmental theory was his fundamental belief in the importance of play—"it is play that is the universal…playing facilitates growth and therefore health" (Winnicott, 1971, p. 41). Play is what children do with the transitional objects and provides what Winnicott called a "potential space" for linking inner and outer reality (Nicholls et al., 2013). Given the explicit use of materials, objects, and creative activities in occupational therapy, it is this aspect of Winnicott's work that Nicholls and colleagues find most useful for occupational therapy.

Bowlby, in his collaboration with Ainsworth, is credited with introducing *attachment theory*. This theory emphasized the biological human need and desire to form attachments with caregivers, and the use of this person as a "secure base" for exploration and self-enhancement. Attachment theory emphasizes the importance of regular and reliable contact with caregivers who are sensitive to the child's needs. Again, when such is not provided or available, psychological and behavioral problems can develop (Eagle, 2011b; Nicholls et al., 2013), and change comes by providing a "secure base" within therapeutic relationships. A significant body of work has developed around attachment theory that extends beyond Bowlby and Ainsworth's work, for example, Una McCluskey's work on the dynamics of attachment in adult life (Nicholls et al., 2013). The reader is again encouraged to explore the breadth of that literature to get a more thorough understanding of this perspective. Neurobiological and infant brain research has provided empirical validation of attachment theory, and pediatric occupational therapists in infant mental health practice have incorporated this research to guide their work (Cara & Holloway, 2013).

The *relational approach* to psychoanalysis, originated by Stephen Mitchell, who "conceptualizes the mind as a fluid, socially constructed product of ever-shifting social interactions" (Eagle, 2011b, p. 134). Primarily a psychodynamic psychotherapy intervention for adults, this approach draws on concepts and research from attachment theory. This perspective includes the notion that both the therapist and the person (i.e., patient/client) influence the therapy relationship, that change comes from what is referred to as a "two-person" approach and includes practices like therapist disclosure when relevant and needed (Eagle, 2011b).

PRACTICE DEVELOPMENTS IN OCCUPATIONAL THERAPY

Early Influences of Psychodynamic Theory in Occupational Therapy

Fidler and Fidler's (1954, 1966) *Occupational Therapy: A Communication Process in Psychiatry* represents the most well-articulated approach informed by object relations theory. Gail Fidler, the occupational therapist, and her husband, a psychoanalyst, collaborated on this text, which served as the sole text for occupational therapists working in mental health for many years. They argued that "as a communication process, occupational therapy is concerned with action, the meaning of action, its use in communicating feelings and thoughts, and the use of such nonverbal communication for the benefit of the patient" (Fidler & Fidler, 1966, p. 19). Situating occupational therapy in relation to psychotherapy of the time, the Fidlers proposed that:

> There are, of course, large areas of similarity and overlap and common theoretic constructs with psychotherapy. However, in occupational therapy the psychodynamics of activities are considered as catalytic agents giving impetus to the development of relationships and catalytic experiences, which are used by the therapist and patient collaboratively to alter and eliminate pathology. On the basis of this concept, then, the nature of the process rather than the end product is of primary importance. By process we refer to the stimuli of the real and symbolic meaning of an object or activity, the intrapsychic responses of the patient to such stimuli, the pervading influence that such feeling, thinking, and acting has on interpersonal relationships, and the collaborative efforts and communication between patient and therapist. The finished product, or what is made, in occupational therapy then has significance only as it reflects or symbolizes the process. (p. 118)

This approach to occupational therapy emerged prior to deinstitutionalization and during a time in which long stay admissions to psychiatric hospitals was common. As a result, the occupational therapist had the opportunity to work with patients over extended periods. This is one of the questions regarding its application in contemporary occupational therapy practice, where health systems are more oriented to achieving desired outcomes combined with reducing the need for formal health services.

Case studies in the Fidler and Fidler (1966) *Occupational Therapy: A Communication Process in Psychiatry*, provides rich descriptions of this practice. The reader is encouraged to read these in the original to get a good sense of how this practice approach was implemented. Fidler, the occupational therapist, over the course of her career continued to argue and provide occupational therapy practice resources for understanding "how objects, materials, and the activities themselves could express meaning linked to one's inner world and could communicate significance without using words" (Nicholls et al., 2013, p. 89). Contemporary applications of Fidler's work have influenced Nicholls and colleagues as they propose a "re-awakening of psychoanalytic thinking in occupational therapy" (p. 87), Eklund (2000) in her application of object relations theory to occupational therapy, and Cole's (2011) inclusion of a psychoanalytic approach to group work in occupational therapy are informed partially by Fidler's "task-oriented" group approach.

Another early application of the psychodynamic perspective in occupational therapy was the use of art media such as clay, paints, and collage as a tool for encouraging expression and potentially accessing unconscious material. This was reflected in the use of what were termed *"projective" assessment batteries*. Many of these assessment batteries included tasks that were structured (having inherent guides as to how they were to be executed) and unstructured (lacking external guides and encouraging creative problem solving) thereby allowing the person to exhibit his or her preferred style through a variety of means (Azima & Azima, 1959; O'Kane, 1968; Williams & Bloomer, 1987). Another focus in these types of assessment batteries was self- and body image, and included a request for a human figure drawing, often for an image of the self (Azima & Azima, 1959; Hemphill, 1982; O'Kane, 1968; Shoemyen, 1970; Williams & Bloomer, 1987). Dialogue was sometimes used to assist the drawer to describe his or her feelings about the drawing, but the therapist might also interpret or make inference about the drawer based on what was depicted in the drawing and/or how the task was approached. One of the most well-known examples of this was the Azima Battery (Azima & Azima, 1959), which included having the person complete a paper and pencil drawing of a man or woman, make an object out of clay, and finger paint. This assessment was designed to help the occupational therapist assess the behavior and psychological constructs of mood, drives, ego organization, and object relations.

While the Fidlers are credited with the earliest articulation of psychodynamic-informed occupational therapy, Anne Cronin Mosey's (1971) *Three Frames of Reference for Mental Health* also articulated an *analytic frame of reference* for occupational therapy in mental health based on psychodynamic perspectives (Stein & Cutler, 1998). This frame of reference emphasized how lack of insight into one's unconscious processes affected occupational functioning. Occupational therapy evaluation and treatment utilized projective techniques to uncover unconscious processes and used unstructured media and transference relationship between patient and therapist to facilitate insight (Stein & Cutler, 1998). Mosey, a student of Gail Fidler, like other important occupational therapy thinkers of her time, argued that practitioners needed to practice from explicit frames of reference, and provided guidance for selecting and developing expertise in such frames of references for mental health (Stein & Cutler, 1998). Like the Fidler text, *Three Frames of Reference for Mental Health* served as the basic mental health text for North American-based occupational therapists of early 1970s.

Contemporary Influence of Psychodynamic Theory in Occupational Therapy

Contemporary applications of the psychodynamic perspective in occupational therapy are for the most part informed by the relational turn in psychodynamic theory (Eagle, 2011b) and have developed mostly in Europe, including Italy and Scandinavia, and the United Kingdom. Applications that will be considered in this section include the therapeutic use of self in occupational therapy practice (Nicholls et al., 2013), clinical supervision (Daniel & Blair, 2002a, 2002b), and occupational therapy interventions, in particular the use of creative expressive modalities (Atkinson & Wells, 2000; Eklund, 1996, 2000; Nicholls et al., 2013).

Psychodynamic Perspectives on Therapeutic Use of Self in Occupational Therapy

Nicholls (2013) describes the *use of self* as "a sensitive receptive capacity that therapists are able to develop towards clients" (p. 18). She acknowledges Fidler and Fidler's (1966) early articulation of this in their 1963 text *Occupational Therapy as a Communication Process*, in which they emphasized the importance of the occupational therapist's relationship with the patient/client, as well as the activity itself. Drawing on object relations theory of the time, Fidler and

Fidler explicitly argued that the relationship itself could be used as a "legitimate therapeutic agent" (Nicholls, 2013, p. 19).

The application of psychodynamic perspectives to the understanding of *therapeutic use of self* in occupational therapy rests on its—meaning, occupational therapy's—fundamentally relational nature, and the expectation that beliefs, thoughts, and feelings emerge for both the practitioner as well as the patient/client in their work together. It assumes that the beliefs, thoughts, and feelings that do emerge profoundly shape the nature and quality of the interpersonal interactions that both the therapist and the patient/client take, within a particular occupational therapy visit or session, as well as across the care relationship itself. Nicholls (2013) argues that the *psychoanalytic* (she and her colleagues preferred this term over *psychodynamic*) perspective provides a unique lens for understanding this process because of its fundamental belief in the unconscious and its influence on human experience.

The particular interpersonal processes drawn from the psychodynamic perspective that have been identified as informing the therapist's experience and understanding of their therapeutic use of self are *transference, projection,* and *containment*. Transference again refers to the process of the person unconsciously redirecting their feelings from past developmental relationships to current relationships, including the therapeutic relationship. Projection refers to a defensive response in which a person unconsciously rejects his or her own unacceptable attributes by ascribing them to others. Containment, drawn from the work of Wilfred Bion, describes the process of "how clients' verbal and non-verbal communication is taken in by the occupational therapist and held (contained) until patients can tolerate understanding it for themselves" (Nicholls, 2013, p. 17).

For the psychodynamic perspective to be useful in guiding practice, the occupational therapy practitioner must engage in an intentional, deeply reflective process in which he or she seeks to understand the meaning of both the patients/clients and their own actions. The psychodynamic perspective suggests that this process can be facilitated by therapists themselves having "been able to explore difficult and painful areas in their past and present life" (Nicholls, 2013, p. 18), most often through their own engagement in psychodynamic-oriented psychotherapy. Psychodynamic-informed supervision is also seen as important to the intentional reflection process and is considered in the next section.

Psychodynamic Perspectives on Clinical Supervision in Occupational Therapy

An understanding of psychodynamic approaches can offer a unique perspective into the supervisory process for occupational therapists. The psychodynamic perspective of clinical supervision stems from several important

---

VIGNETTE 13-1. EMOTION AND THE THERAPEUTIC PROCESS

An experienced occupational therapist came to supervision with some pictures that a 22-year-old woman with an eating disorder had painted. From the start of the supervisory session, the pair were absorbed in the visual material and excited by forming ideas as to how this activity could be developed. The supervisor was monitoring the therapist's behavior and began to realize that they were possibly caught up in enacting something from the therapy session itself (parallel process). The supervisor drew attention to what was happening to them and wondered if there was anything about their behavior and feelings that was familiar to the supervisee. The supervisee recalled how he had been "lit up" by the woman's work and excitedly drawn to helping her come up with more ideas that she could develop.

They began to think about what their actions and feelings were, setting them in context and considering whether their heightened activity was communicating something from the person herself. The supervisor realized that he had been out of his usual pattern and he, too, had been drawn to focusing on the artwork within the session, wanting to offer ideas as to how the paintings could be developed. He realized that he had lost sight of the person behind the work. Here was a young lady who had difficulty eating and perhaps one way that she dealt with her condition was to distract others from seeing her problem. In the supervisory session, both the supervisor and supervisee could recognize that they were "hungry" to come up with ideas and that the therapy session too had been "filled up" with ideas that the occupational therapist rather frantically wanted her to "digest."

The defensive activity being enacted needed to be understood. The energy and excitement within both the therapy and supervision sessions had to be managed in a way that did not overwhelm and that could be returned in a more digestible way to the person.

From *Psychoanalytic Thinking in Occupational Therapy,* by L. Nicholls et al., Oxford, UK. Copyright © 2013 by John Wiley & Sons, Ltd. Reprinted with permission.

---

concepts, which integrate psychodynamic theories in the arena of supervisory experiences and relationships. These concepts include the importance of creating safe spaces for open reflection, the acceptance of feelings and emotions as part of the supervisory process, and the importance of transference/counter transference and creativity as part of the supervisory relationship (Daniel & Blair, 2002a, 2002b). It is also argued that it may be helpful to view clinical supervision as a separate process from managerial supervision as these present with markedly different expectations and environments for supervisory relationships to develop.

A key theme in supervision grounded in psychodynamic ideas is that of allowing for the unconscious process to be addressed to empower both supervisor and supervisee to become aware of how their feelings play an important role in their work both with clients and in the supervisory context. This perspective is developed from the ideas of the psychoanalyst Winnicott, who argued that feelings (subjective) are a key part of an individual's "internal road to poetic truth whereby creativity and feelings can create a deeper understanding from a personal perspective" (Daniel & Blair, 2002a, p. 238; 2002b).

Alternatively, another approach commonly used in clinical supervision is one that follows a more objective and practical process and doesn't emphasize the potential impact of acknowledging one's feelings and unconscious as part of the supervisory experience (Daniel & Blair, 2002a). Daniel and Blair argue that understanding the connection between both of these styles of supervision—feeling (subjective) and doing (objective)—and how they may affect daily work is vital to a productive supervision processes (2002a).

The psychodynamic concept of providing containment within supervision, that is, a safe and secure environment to explore potentially difficult emotions, can help to facilitate opportunities to analyze how both past and present emotional experiences may influence current practice and therapeutic relationships. As described by Daniel and Blair (2002b), "in supervision, the supervisor (like a parent) provides a secure base from which the supervisee can explore their subjective experiences, and where painful and intolerable feelings can be thought about without becoming overwhelming" (p. 3). Because this approach can evoke intense emotions and expose potential vulnerabilities, establishing boundaries within the supervisor-supervisee relationship is key to its continued success. Vignette 13-1 offers just such an example, demonstrating the potential for the supervisor-supervisee relationship to be mutually reflective, growth promoting, and facilitative of the therapeutic process.

Reflective practice and peer supervision are two additional ways of enhancing the supervisory experience. Daniel (2013) emphasizes that "to be reflective the therapist has to have a capacity to take in the outer information, to ponder on the process and consider alternative possibilities" (p. 228). Reflective practice is intended to be a lens for learning from experience in a creative and non-judgmental way. It is important that this process is not split into the concepts of "what went well or not so well, and how it could be improved" (p. 227). Peer supervision has been suggested as a means to support occupational therapists to build skills, confidence, and manage anxiety in a reflective and non-judgmental way (Daniel, 2013).

Within the occupational therapy profession, there are a variety of views and opinions about how clinical supervision should be facilitated and structured. Criticisms of the psychodynamic approach to supervision are based in the idea that supervision should be an objective process that doesn't include exploration of the personal, emotional, or unconscious experiences, and focuses instead on the skills and professional development of the supervisee (Daniel & Blair, 2002b).

Psychodynamic and/or Psychoanalytic Occupational Therapy

As noted previously, contemporary perspectives on psychodynamic and/or psychoanalytic occupational therapy interventions have emerged internationally. Eklund (1996, 2000) encouraged occupational therapists to revisit contemporary perspectives on object relations theory for occupational therapy as practiced, challenging early criticism. To review, this model is based on the assumption that participation in occupations in a social context can influence an individual's well-being and that object relations theories are aligned with this thinking by acknowledging the importance of present and past object relations.

In occupational therapy practice, interventions can provide opportunities to explore object relations in a transitional space in two distinct ways. The materials used in occupational therapy can serve as "transitional objects," facilitating communication and a transitional space, and interactions can provide helpful experiences of contact with others. Eklund (2000) suggests that initially the importance should be placed upon the individual being able to "go on being" without attending to any demands of "doing" (pp. 16-17). In time, the occupational therapist can then confront the individual with more difficult aspects of identity and growth and create further opportunities for doing to support this growth. It is also acknowledged that interventions based on objects relations theory can take a significant amount of time and will vary depending on the level of dysfunction. There are methods that occupational therapists use that can assist with gathering information about a person's object relations. Eklund (2000) describes the three main ways that occupational therapists accomplish this as, observation of an individual interacting with others, interview, and expressive nonverbal techniques such as the use of creative activities (i.e., painting, clay modelling).

The aim of occupational therapy interventions based in object relations is to allow for opportunities for individuals to interact with others, which can have an effect on internalized object relations that may be affecting an individual's occupational performance. Eklund (2000) proposes that:

> The occupational therapy setting can serve as an arena for transitional experiences, the occupational therapist can be the patient's partner in mutual play, and the objects involved in different types of occupations can serve as transitional objects. A process of externalization and internalization can take place. Unbearable internalized experiences can be externalized in occupational therapy situations, in relating to materials, physical objects, and persons. Occupational therapy interventions lead to new experiences being internalized, preferably with a more tolerable content. (p. 18)

Specific applications in occupational therapy that have been described in the literature will be considered here and include Gunnarsson's *Tree Theme Method* (Gunnarsson, 2008; Gunnarsson & Björklund, 2013; Gunnarsson et al., 2006), Nicholls et al.'s (2013) Relational Model of Occupational Therapy (MOVI), and Atkinson and Wells' (2000) Creative Therapies.

The Tree Theme Method

Birgitta Gunnarsson, a student of Eklund, has recently proposed a psychodynamic occupational therapy approach she calls *The Tree Theme Method* (TTM) (Gunnarsson, 2008; Gunnarsson & Björklund, 2013; Gunnarsson, Jansson, & Eklund, 2006). The TTM was developed based on the idea that creative activities can serve as a means for clients to engage in self-exploration and development, and as a process to help reveal potentially difficult inner emotions. The focus of the use of creativity in this method is on the interaction of doing, being, and becoming, drawing upon the ideas of Winnicott who proposed that "an individual can find him/herself by doing things and being creative" (Gunnarsson, 2008, p. 19). Gunnarsson goes on to emphasize that:

> When a client participates in a purposeful creative activity, like painting a picture (doing) and reflecting on it afterwards (being), the verbal conversation that follows between the client and the occupational therapist can promote a development of the client's self-image (becoming) and how they relate to their environment. (p. 19)

The TTM uses the activity of painting pictures of trees and verbally telling one's life story to support positive changes in daily life. Gunnarsson (2008) clarifies that the "tree is an ancient symbol humans used in different cultures to symbolize themselves and their life situations" (p. 20), is an early motif in children's drawings, and has been used in mental health assessment and treatment. The painted pictures of trees are intended to represent specific meaningful periods in one's life. For the story-telling component of this intervention, she draws on the broad literature that supports story-telling as an important human experience, and more specifically on "occupational story-telling and story-making" in occupational therapy (Clark, 1993; Clark, Ennevor, & Richardson, 1996; Mattingly, 1991).

The TTM is a brief intervention that consists of a total of five sessions. The first four sessions include three components—progressive relaxation directed by the therapist, the painting of trees to represent their childhood, adolescence and adulthood while working in silence, and finally a mutual dialogue between therapist and the client to elicit the occupational story-telling. The fifth, and final session, involves occupational story-making and begins with a mutually reflective review of the previous paintings and story-telling between the client and the therapist. This session concludes with a final tree drawing that symbolizes the future and expresses their own expectations for the future, with an accompanying dialogue about the future (Gunnarsson, 2008, p. 26). The therapeutic relationship between the occupational therapist and the client is key to support a dynamic process in which the client is able to develop new perspectives of self and everyday life.

Gunnarsson, Jansson, Petersson, and Eklund (2011) studied, using focus group methodology, a small group of experienced occupational therapists implementing TTM. These therapists found the approach provided structure to the initiating therapy, but thought that life experience and self-knowledge was critical to success with TTM. The occupational therapists in the study emphasized the importance of the client's narrative in the process of reconstructing one's life through the TTM. It was found that some therapists felt that the five sessions allocated in the TTM were too short and didn't allow enough time to develop the therapeutic relationship sufficiently. The therapists thought it was important for the clients to come to the sessions with a degree of interest, curiosity, and motivation in the process of the TTM for it to be successful. There was some difficulty experienced by therapists with clients who were unable to engage in symbolization, and it was suggested that this might be more difficult for clients who have cognitive disabilities. In these instances, the therapist had to adjust to provide a coaching role and focus on giving concrete instruction and support. The study also found that for the occupational therapists, approaching the therapeutic frames of reference with a degree of flexibility was important for the success of the intervention for the client.

Gunnarsson and Björklund (2013), using a longitudinal quantitative design, found that clients experienced positive significant changes in the sense of coherence as measured by the Sense of Coherence scale and satisfaction with occupational performance as measured by Satisfaction With Daily Occupations. This study also showed that the positive changes gained were sustainable

3 years post-intervention, and concluded that TTM may be beneficial to the individual's well-being and participation in activities.

Relational Model of Occupational Therapy

The "Modello Vivaio" (MOVI), developed by Julie Cunningham Piergrossi, Carolina de Sena Gibertoni, and Elisabeth de Verdiere in Italy, is a relational model of occupational therapy practice rooted in psychoanalytic theory (Piergrossi & Gibertoni, 2013). Piergrossi and Gibertoni identify MOVI as a unique model in that it is currently the only occupational therapy practice model that focuses on understanding the unconscious process between the client, the activity, and the occupational therapist. MOVI calls attention to the importance of emotions and their dynamic role in the relationship between the patient, therapist, and "doing." Within the MOVI model, it is believed that the concept of transference, meaning the "unconscious links with other relationships in the patient's or therapist's lives, either past or present" is activated by the doing (p. 107). In this way, MOVI emphasizes the therapist as an active and important part of the therapeutic process. The MOVI model consists of the following seven dynamic elements, which are all connected to the significance of emotions within the therapeutic relationship:

1. *Evaluation.* The building of a relationship is a key factor of the evaluation process as it sets a platform from which to build trust and hope with each patient. The MOVI evaluation can be used with persons across all ages and areas of practice. The evaluation process relies on skilled observation of both external and internal histories and experiences. There are four main activities used during the evaluation—creation of a human figure with clay, a structured task, a free painting, and a magazine collage. The therapist's role in the evaluation stage is to be open to how to help someone, guided not by the therapist's preconceived notions of what help they believe the individual needs, but by creating a space whereby the patient and therapist work collaboratively through a state of "not knowing" to identify what is important to the patient (Nicholls et al., 2013, p. 110).

2. *The interactive process.* Play and choice are key elements of MOVI sessions. Nicholls et al. (2013) emphasize the importance of concepts developed from research with infants as a way of explaining and understanding the connection between emotions and relationships on cognitive development and functioning. The MOVI model asserts that the therapeutic relationship holds similarities to the relationship between infants and their mother or father in that, "The therapists are present and accept the patient's self-agency but they are not

---

VIGNETTE 13-2. PLAY AND THE THERAPEUTIC RELATIONSHIP

At 94 years of age, Giovanna is elegant, well dressed and groomed, and very sociable. She especially likes being with others, and enjoys dinner in the residence where she lives. When a recent fall left her with a very painful shoulder injury, she was told by the doctor to stop using her right shoulder for a certain time. "That's impossible for me," Giovanna explained. "I need my right hand to get dressed and put on my make-up. Otherwise, I can't go to dinner. I lift my right arm with my left one and use it to comb my hair." The occupational therapist was called because the pain was not diminishing at all and Giovanna was becoming angry and depressed, complaining about the doctor, refusing to cooperate, and not accepting a helper in her apartment.

The MOVI-trained therapist began by sitting down and having a chat with her client and completely avoided giving suggestions. She listened and contained Giovanna's pain and fear of losing the ability to "make herself look good." For what the therapist began to understand was that Giovanna's true "play" activity was not just going to dinner; it was dressing well, applying her make-up perfectly, combing her naturally curly hair in a way only she knew how to do. Their first occupational therapy activity was to fashion three different, very elegant slings for her arm of various colors and materials to match her outfits. It was a fun activity full of memories and lots of looking in the mirror to get just the right "look." And as they "played" together, the therapist was also able to talk to her about specific things to do that would help her shoulder to heal faster. These were simple but necessary ideas that would help Giovanna to give her shoulder more rest and that she would be able to understand and accept, such as temporary visits to the hairdresser and learning how to put on a minimum amount of make-up using her left arm and hand.

From *Psychoanalytic Thinking in Occupational Therapy*, by L. Nicholls et al., Oxford, UK. Copyright © 2013 by John Wiley & Sons, Ltd. Reprinted with permission.

---

passive: they interact and add something of their own in an evolving process in which both people proceed and neither remains still" (Nicholls et al., 2013, p. 112). It is expected that therapists will adopt some of their patient's emotional pain, and MOVI necessitates a deeper understanding of the place this pain may hold in the evaluation process.

3. *The setting: space and time.* In the MOVI setting, the concept of providing a sense of containment (described earlier in the chapter) is key to providing a safe space for therapeutic work to take place. The idea of "container" as described in the MOVI model is based in the work of British psychoanalyst Wilfred Bion, who explained that:

> At the beginning of life babies do not yet have a thinking apparatus to be able to make sense of the many different sensory experiences that strike them from within and without. They are only able to evacuate the sensations into the mother, whose primary function is that of containing them, making sense of them, and finding a response to what the child is feeling. (cited in Nicholls et al., 2013, p. 114)

In the MOVI setting, the occupational therapists provide this sense of containment, and the set time allocated for the sessions allows for a sense of stability and consistency.

4. *Choice and play.* Play and creativity are essential elements of the relationship and interactions between therapist and patient. The therapist is present to nurture and encourage creativity, choice, and play and do things with the patient. In MOVI, the concept of providing genuine choice is explored. This concept relates to the idea that a therapist cannot predict what a choice (of the patient) may be and must have an open mind about what choices the patient may make. This relates again to the importance of the potential for emotional growth within the therapeutic process. Furthermore, a genuine choice is described as "the invention of something new" and unpredictable, which the therapist is ready to welcome into the therapeutic setting (Nicholls et al., 2013, pp. 116-117). A brief example of the application of play and choice within a therapeutic relationship guided by the MOVI approach is provided in Vignette 13-2.

5. *Materials and transformations.* All of the work done in the MOVI model includes the use of materials and the experience of transformation. The simultaneous transformation of the materials by both body and mind allow for the creation of a story. This bringing together of emotions and unconscious thoughts with a variety of tangible materials then creates a space for transforming the patient's inner world within the therapeutic space shared with the therapist.

6. *Sensory experience and thought.* MOVI highlights the importance of sensory experiences in the therapeutic

process. The MOVI model describes that although we all experience sensory stimuli, our reactions and the way we make sense of these stimuli are unique and different for each individual (Nicholls et al., 2013). These experiences may be particularly relevant for autistic individuals as the experiences are often the only way of connecting and intervening therapeutically. It is through sensory activities and experiences that the therapist is often more able to connect with and understand the inner world of a child with autism.

7. *The nonhuman environment.* MOVI values the aspects of the nonhuman environment that can influence the thoughts, feelings, and emotions of an individual. Nicholls et al. (2013) describe occupational therapists as "specialists" of the nonhuman environment (p. 124). MOVI is intended to provide a means to better understand the link between human and nonhuman objects within a psychodynamic framework, and how to use the objects in the nonhuman environment to stimulate a transformation of emotional content as part of the therapeutic relationship.

MOVI is a model that grew out Piergrossi, Gibertoni, and de Verdiere's work with children with serious emotional and behavioral disorders, and draws directly from the work of the Fidlers and Azimas described earlier. Given the nature of this intervention, it is best understood as long term and requiring extended relationships between therapist and client. As will be noted later, this makes this approach challenging to implement in many contemporary mental health practice contexts. Piergrossi and Gibertoni have used interpretative phenomenological analysis to capture rich data that have helped them to articulate the MOVI process (Nicholls et al., 2013); however, no patient/client outcome research was found regarding MOVI.

Creative Therapies

Atkinson and Wells (2000), in their *Creative Therapies: A Psychodynamic Approach Within Occupational Therapy*, introduce their perspective on psychodynamic-oriented practice in occupational therapy using creative modalities. They hope to "raise the understanding and credibility of working in this way, offering theory to support the use of creative therapy as a truly rich and versatile intervention" (p. 3). Creative therapies comprise one area of psychosocial occupational therapy practice. They encompass an approach that helps the individual to explore and express conscious and unconscious feelings. Through this, the individual works toward resolution of interpersonal and intrapersonal conflict, thus affecting change. The process involves self-exploration, self-discovery, self-determination, and self-help. Creativity is the core element and exists on four levels: (1) the activities used all offer the potential for creativity, (2) creativity is fundamental within the style of the therapist,

(3) creativity exists within each individual involved in the creative therapy process, and (4) creativity is inherent within the therapeutic process of dynamic change (p. 4).

In their articulation of the psychodynamic theories that inform their thinking about *creative therapies*, they draw heavily on classical psychodynamic theories, as well as existential-humanistic perspectives (i.e., Rogerian approaches). There appears to be less attention to the contemporary relational approaches despite their acknowledgement that the therapeutic relationship is a key ingredient. The key principles of the creative therapy process are the following:

- The individual operates within a unique personal, physical, social, and cultural environment
- The unconscious has an important role to play in present conflicts
- Individuals are capable of choice, are responsible for themselves, and have the potential for their own development
- Both therapist and client are active within the creative therapy process (Atkinson & Wells, 2000, p. 4)

They propose a structure comprising seven dimensions or processes of creative working: environment, membership, working relationships, working processes, the Underneath, making therapeutic sense, and effectiveness, and they provide explanations for each of these within the context of group therapy. They emphasize that the outcome of therapy using the creative therapies approach is not on the development of specific artistic or creative skills (i.e., sculpting) nor the creation of a particular creative object (i.e., a clay pot), but rather change within the person him- or herself.

Atkinson and Wells (2000) acknowledge the importance of research to support intervention development, but do not provide any empirical evidence specifically regarding their approach to psychodynamic oriented occupational therapy. Rather they provide an initial description of the theoretical influences on their thinking, the role of the therapist and the use of different types of media within the creative therapies approach.

Challenges to Implementing Psychodynamic-Oriented Occupational Therapy

Limitations to implementing psychodynamic-oriented occupational therapy have been identified. Eklund (2000) acknowledges the difficulties that arise given the current focus on short admissions, at least for inpatient settings, as well as the pressure to measure functional and behavioral outcomes.

Additional limitations to implementing psychodynamic perspectives in occupational therapy include the limited understanding of this model by most occupational therapy clinicians. Despite psychodynamic ideas being well infused into our sociocultural discourse, occupational therapists who want to use this approach must engage in supervised and focused learning from others with psychodynamic expertise. The work of practitioners described above has been informed to a significant degree by their sustained relationship with the psychoanalytically oriented psychotherapy world. UK-based therapists, for instance, have participated in training opportunities offered by the Tavistock Institute (www.tavinstitute.org). This institute has served as a one of the theoretical centers of psychoanalytic thinking in the United Kingdom for many decades.

Conclusion

The psychodynamic perspective that was introduced in its most articulated manner by Fidler and Fidler (1966) and Azima and Azima (1959) has reemerged. This renewed interest for psychodynamic-oriented occupational therapy is informed by what is referred to as the relational turn in psychodynamic theory (Eagle, 2011a; Westen et al., 2008). A key argument for reawakening psychodynamic thinking in occupational therapy is its capacity for engaging us in what Nicholls (2013) calls "wonder and delight" in the unconscious (p. 15). In addition, proponents of this perspective emphasize that it supports the use of creative expressive modalities within occupational therapy interventions, and offers a powerful lens for reflecting on, and understanding, our therapeutic use of self. While there are very real limitations to its implementation in many mental health practice settings, including both financial and length-of-stay challenges, as well as demand for additional learning and supervision on the part of the therapist, Eklund (2000) argues that this model can serve as a lens to understand occupational problems.

Learning Activities/ Discussion Questions

1. Organize a discussion group to consider the following questions:

   a. How can psychodynamic approaches be used in occupational therapy practice in today's mental health services?

   b. How can a psychodynamic framework be helpful in areas of practice outside of mental health?

   c. How can a psychodynamic framework be included in the current emphasis on integrated behavioral health care approaches?

2. Explore the literature to learn how the creative activity of journaling has been used from a psychodynamic perspective.

3. Thinking of clients you have worked with in the past, consider if counter-transference occurred in the relationship. How was this experienced and expressed (Table 13-1)?

References

Atkinson, K., & Wells, C. (2000). *Creative therapies: A psychodynamic approach within occupational therapy.* Cheltenham, UK: Nelson Thomas.

Azima, H., & Azima, F. (1959). Outline of a dynamic theory of occupational therapy. *American Journal of Occupational Therapy, 8*(5), 215-221.

Barris, R., Kielhofner, G., & Watts, J. H. (1988). *Bodies of knowledge in psychosocial practice.* Thorofare, NJ: SLACK Incorporated.

Bruce, M. A. G., & Borg, B. (2002). *Psychodynamic frame of reference—Person, perspective and meaning psychosocial frames of reference: Core for occupation-based treatment* (pp. 69-119). Thorofare, NJ: SLACK Incorporated.

Cara, E., & Holloway, E. (2013). Mental health of infants: Attachment theory through the lifespan. In E. Cara & A. MacRae (Eds.), *Psychosocial occupational therapy: An evolving practice* (pp. 343-383). United States: Delmar Cengage Learning.

Cara, E., & Stephenson, P. (2013). The use of psychosocial methods and interpersonal strategies in mental health. In E. Cara & A. MacRae (Eds.), *Psychosocial occupational therapy: An evolving practice*, (3rd ed., pp. 643-670). United States: Delmar Cengage Learning.

Clark, F. (1993). Occupation embedded in a real life: Interweaving occupational science and occupational therapy. *The American Journal of Occupational Therapy, 47*(12), 1067-1078. doi: 10.5014/ajot.47.12.1067.

Clark, F., Ennevor, B. L., & Richardson, P. L. (1996). A grounded theory of techniques for occupational storytelling and occupational story making. In R. Zemke & F. Clark (Eds.), *Occupational science: The evolving discipline* (pp. 373-392). Philadelphia, PA: F. A. Davis Company.

Cole, M. B. (2011). *Group dynamics in occupational therapy: The theoretical basis and practice application of group treatment.* Thorofare, NJ: SLACK Incorporated.

Daniel, M. (2013). The relational space of supervision. In L. Nicholls, J. C. Piergrossi, C. d. S. Gibertoni, & M. Daniel (Eds.), *Psychoanalytic thinking in occupational therapy: Symbolic, relational, and transformative* (pp. 222-238). London: Wiley-Blackwell.

TABLE 13-1
DIVERGENCES AND CONVERGENCES BETWEEN CLASSICAL AND CONTEMPORARY PSYCHOANALYSIS

	DIVERGENCES		CONVERGENCES
	Classical Theory	*Contemporary*	
Conceptions of mind	Reality testing emerges out of child coming to understand that need gratification requires thinking and planning	Reality testing is an inborn capacity	Primary function of psychological defenses is to keep anxiety-laden, threatening material from being fully consciously experienced and threatening to the self Anxiety-arousing potential of certain mental contents partly attributable to association with early parental negative reactions such as disapproval, punishment, failure to validate, and anxiety
	Unconscious and conscious is dichotomous	Unconscious and conscious is on a continuum	
	Unconscious IS unconscious by virtue of defense	Unconscious IS unconscious because it is acquired nonverbally early in life	
Nature and origin of object relations	Primary human motive is drive reduction	See humans as inherently object seeking and emphasize need for support as motive for object relations	Endorse central idea that the object serves vital function of regulating tension and affect states and supporting intact ego functioning
Conceptions of psychopathology	Inner conflicts between anxiety-laden wishes and desires and the defenses that emerge are central to psychopathology	Contemporary theories reject the classical theory notion, but depending on theory have different formulations	Identify the role of active, highly emotional clinging to early objects in psychopathology Acknowledge the central role of poor affect and tension regulation in psychopathology Emphasize the role of anxiety and defense in restricting the individual's range of awareness and richness of experience
Conceptions of treatment	Focuses on "uncovering and discovering, gaining self-knowledge, and owning what was disowned" (Eagle, 2011a, p. 273)	Focuses on "constructing persuasive narratives, creating new meanings, and taking new perspectives" (Eagle, 2011a, p. 273)	Expansion of persons' range of experience, and enhanced capacity to relate effectively to others, acknowledgement of importance of therapeutic alliance

Adapted from Eagle, M. N., *Divergence and Convergences from Classical to Contemporary Psychoanalysis: A Critique and Integration*, New York. Copyright © 2011 by Routledge Taylor & Francis Group.

Daniel, M., & Blair, S. (2002a). A psychodynamic approach to clinical supervision: 1. *British Journal of Therapy and Rehabilitation, 9*(6), 237-240.

Daniel, M., & Blair, S. (2002b). A psychodynamic approach to clinical supervision: 2. *British Journal of Therapy and Rehabilitation, 9*(7), 274-277.

Eagle, M. N. (2011a). *Divergence and convergences from classical to contemporary psychoanalysis: A critique and integration* (pp. 249-314). New York: Routledge Taylor & Francis Group.

Eagle, M. N. (2011b). *From classical to contemporary psycho-analysis: A critique and integration.* New York: Routledge Taylor & Francis Group.

Eklund, M. (1996). Working relationship, participation and outcome in a psychiatric day care unit based on occupational therapy. *Scandinavian Journal of Occupational Therapy, 3*(3), 106-113. doi:10.3109/11038129609106693.

Eklund, M. (2000). Applying object relations theory to psychosocial occupational therapy: Empirical and theoretical considerations. *Occupational Therapy in Mental Health, 15*(1), 1-26.

Fidler, G. S., & Fidler, J. W. (1954). *Introduction of psychiatric occupational therapy.* New York: McMillan.

Fidler, G. S., & Fidler, J. W. (1966). *Occupational therapy: A communication process in psychiatry.* New York: The Macmillan Company.

Gabbard, G. O. (2001). A contemporary psychoanalytic model of countertransference. *Journal of Clinical Psychology, 57*(8), 983-991. doi: 10.1002/jclp.1065.

Gordon, D. M. (2002). Therapeutics and science in the history of occupational therapy. Dissertation. Division of Occupational Science and Occupational Therapy. University of Southern California.

Greenberg, J. R., & Mitchell, S. A. (1983). *Object relations in psychoanalytic theory.* Cambridge, MA: Harvard University Press.

Gunnarsson, B. (2008). The Tree Theme Method. Lund, Sweden: Department of Health Sciences, Division of Occupational Therapy and Gerontology, Lund University.

Gunnarsson, B., & Björklund, A. (2013). Sustainable enhancement in clients who perceive the tree theme method as a positive intervention in psychosocial occupational therapy. *Australian Occupational Therapy Journal, 60*(3), 154-160. doi: 10.1111/1440-1630.12034.

Gunnarsson, B., Jansson, J.-A., & Eklund, M. (2006). The tree theme method in psychosocial occupational therapy: A case study. *Scandinavian Journal of Occupational Therapy, 13*(4), 229-240. doi:10.1080/11038120600772908.

Gunnarsson, B., Jansson, J.-A., Petersson, K., & Eklund, M. (2011). Occupational therapists' perception of the tree theme method as an intervention in psychosocial occupational therapy. *Occupational Therapy in Mental Health, 27*(1), 36-49.

Hemphill, B. (1982). *Training manual for the BH battery.* Thorofare, NJ: SLACK Incorporated.

Kielhofner, G., & Burke, J. (1977). Occupational therapy after 60 years: An account of changing identity and knowledge. *American Journal of Occupational Therapy, 31*(10), 675-689.

Mattingly, C. (1991). The narrative nature of clinical reasoning. *American Journal of Occupational Therapy, 45*(11), 998-1005.

Meyer, A. (1922). The philosophy of occupation therapy. *Archives of Occupational Therapy, 1*(1), 1-10.

Mosey, A. C. (1971). *Three frames of reference for mental health.* Thorofare, NJ: Charles Slack.

Nicholls, L. (2007). A psychoanalytic discourse in occupational therapy. In J. Creek & A. Lawson-Porter (Eds.), *Contemporary issues in occupational therapy: Reasoning and reflection* (pp. 55-86). West Sussex, UK: John Wiley & Sons.

Nicholls, L. (2013). The 'therapeutic use of self' in occupational therapy. In L. Nicholls, J. C. Piergrossi, C. d. S. Gibertoni & M. Daniel (Eds.), *Psychoanalytic thinking in occupational therapy: Symbolic, relational and transformative* (pp. 15-31). Oxford, UK: Wiley-Blackwell.

Nicholls, L., Piergrossi, J. C., Gibertoni, C., & Daniel, M. (2013). *Psychoanalytic thinking in occupational therapy.* Oxford, UK: Wiley-Blackwell.

O'Kane, C. (1968). *The development of a projective technique for use in psychiatric occupational therapy.* Buffalo, NY: University of New York at Buffalo.

Piergrossi, J. C., & Gibertoni, C. d. S. (2013). MOVI: A relational model in occupational therapy. In L. Nicholls, J. C. Piergrossi, C. d. S. Gibertoni & M. Daniel (Eds.), *Psychoanalytic thinking in occupational therapy: Symbolic, relational and transformative* (pp. 105-127). London: Wiley-Blackwell.

Reilly, M. (1969). Psychiatric occupational therapy at the crossroads again. Unpublished. Department of Occupational Therapy. University of Southern California.

Shedler, J. (2006). That was then, this is now: An introduction to contemporary psychodynamic theory. Retrieved from www.jonathanshedler.com/PDFs/Shedler%20(2006)%20That%20was%20then,%20this%20is%20now%20R9.pdf

Shoemyen, C. (1970). Occupational therapy orientation and evaluation. *American Journal of Occupational Therapy, 24,* 276-279.

Stein, F., & Cutler, S. K. (1998). *Theoretical models underlying the clinical practice of psychosocial occupational therapy psychosocial occupational therapy: A holistic approach.* San Diego, CA: Singular Publishing Group, Inc.

Westen, D., Gabbard, G. O., & Ortigo, K. M. (2008). Psychoanalytic approaches to personality. In O. P. John, R. W. Robins, & L. A. Pervin (Eds.), *Handbook of personality: Theory and research* (3rd ed., pp. 61-113). New York: The Guilford Press.

Williams, S., & Bloomer, J. (1987). *Bay area functional performance evaluation* (2nd ed.). Palo Alto, CA: Consulting Psychologist Press.

Winnicott, D. W. (1971). *Playing: A theoretical statement playing and reality* (pp. 38-52). London, UK: Tavistock/Routledge.

Coping and Occupation

Terry Krupa, PhD, OT Reg (Ont), FCAOT

Everything can change in a heartbeat; it can slip away in an instant. Everything you trust, and treasure, whatever brings you comfort, comes at a terrible cost. Health is temporary; money disappears. Safety is nothing but an illusion. So when the moment comes, and everything you depend upon changes, or perhaps someone you love disappears, or no longer loves you, must disaster follow? Or will you somehow adapt? (Overton, 2012)

Outcast on a cold star, unable to feel anything but an awful helpless numbness. I look down into the warm, earthy world. Into a nest of lovers' beds, baby cribs, meal tables, all the solid commerce of life in this earth, and feel apart, enclosed in a wall of glass. (Plath, 1982)

OBJECTIVES

The objectives of this chapter are as follows:
  » Define coping as it relates to occupation and occupational therapy practice.
  » Review theoretical ideas about coping.
  » Identify key elements of coping.
  » Describe occupational therapy practices focused on enabling coping.
  » Describe intervention approaches specific to suicide prevention.

Krupa, T., Kirsh, B., Pitts, D., & Fossey, E. *Bruce & Borg's Psychosocial Frames of Reference: Theories, Models, and Approaches for Occupation-Based Practice, Fourth Edition* (pp 227-241).
© 2016 SLACK Incorporated.

BACKGROUND

Coping refers to the processes people use to manage demands and expectations, particularly when those demands are experienced as having some potential to overwhelm their adaptive capacities. Although people are faced with meeting demands and challenges on a daily basis, the concept of coping is typically used to refer to those situations where there is some threat of a mismatch between an individual's capacities and internal and external resources and the demands they are facing.

Coping is distinct from, but very related to, the concept of "adaptation." Coping is often characterized as managing in relatively immediate circumstances and over the short term. Adaptation typically refers to processes that are continual, focused on the longer term, and sustainable over time. Being able to successfully cope with circumstances in the short term is important for long-term adaptation, but not all coping activities that are positive on the short term are beneficial for longer-term adaptation. For example, a young person starting a career might cope with challenges related to interacting with authority figures in his or her new job by avoiding work-related social functions. Yet, avoiding social interactions might not serve this person well as a strategy for long-term personal and workplace expectations for achievement and growth on the job.

The idea of coping to "manage" daily life demands involves human emotional and psychological functioning as much as it does functional performance. In everyday conversation for example, if we say, "I'm not sure I can cope," we may be suggesting that we feel at risk for being psychologically and emotionally overwhelmed. This link between emotion and coping is an important one. When people are emotionally overwhelmed they can become unable to use the personal capacities and resources they might have available to them to manage particularly challenging daily life circumstances.

VIEW OF HEALTH AND DISORDER

Facing challenges in meeting the demands of daily life is a universal experience and subsequently coping is fundamental to human health and well-being. Daily life demands that challenge coping are often referred to as stressors. While all people are generally familiar with the experience of having had to cope in difficult situations, and with a range of stressors, the opening quote by Margaret Overton highlights that circumstances that challenge human adaptation are a fundamental part of the human condition.

The idea of disorder in coping suggests that either people are unable to use the resources and capacities they have available to them to effectively deal with these stressors, they have an impairment of internal and external resources available to cope with challenges, or their coping actions are problematic and maladaptive. Ultimately a significant problem in coping means that an individual is less able to respond effectively to the immediate situation, and is then at risk for longer-term adaptation. At its worst, problems in coping can become so severe as to overwhelm an individual's ability to respond effectively to daily life expectations in an all-encompassing way.

Just as *coping* is the term used to refer to the actions taken to respond to life's stressors, the concept of *resilient* is used to refer to people who demonstrate patterns of effective coping, even under the most trying circumstances. Consistent with our definition of coping, Scaffa and colleagues (2010) highlight that resilience has two dimensions: a pattern of emotional and psychological equilibrium, and effective behavioral responses.

Occupational therapists are typically concerned with coping and resilience as it applies to the populations of people they work with—particularly people with persistent and significant health conditions and disability. Yet these concepts have relevance at a broader societal level, with suggestions that societies themselves can be considered at risk in these areas. The United Nations Development Program (2011), for example, reports that the world is likely to experience dramatic and dangerous events, such as pervasive economic uncertainty and natural or human-made disasters, that challenge the capacities of entire populations to cope economically, psychologically, and socially. In this way, enhancing coping and resilience becomes understood as an important element of population level approaches to human health and well-being. Occupational therapy associations internationally have developed position papers or reports about the potential role of occupational therapists in disaster relief. For example, the American Association of Occupational Therapists has published a report of occupational therapy contributions to disaster relief across the phases of preparation, response, and recovery (Yamkovenko, 2008).

THEORETICAL ASSUMPTIONS

Assumptions about coping have developed with the evolution of related theory over the past few decades. The following are some key assumptions:

- Coping is a response to events or situations that place demands on individuals in specific contexts. While some events or situations are universally considered to be highly likely to be stressful and potentially overwhelming, the actual experience of any challenging event or situation will be highly individual.

- The personal relevance and meaning of specific events or situations will influence the extent to which the demands placed on an individual are experienced as stressful and potentially overwhelming.

- People possess many personal *attributes* that influence their ability to cope. These attributes include, for example, competencies such as attitudes, knowledge and skills, personality qualities, past experiences, health, personal fitness, and social position. While we might think of some people as relatively hardy, in that they possess a robust range of personal attributes that put them in a good position to cope, personal attributes are dynamic and coping capacities do change.

- Resources, external to individuals but accessible to them, can support the ability to cope in stressful situations. Resources are wide ranging but can include people, money, and services. Like personal attributes, access to resources can be relatively stable, but still subject to change.

- Some behaviors and strategies that help an individual to successfully negotiate the demands of a particular demanding situation or event can be effective in the short term, but harmful to coping in the long term if they are used routinely to the detriment of developing other coping responses. For example, using substances such as alcohol to negotiate the interpersonal demands of a work-related social event might help an individual in the short term, but be detrimental to developing effective social skills.

- Even though coping processes are adaptive, particular types of stress experiences can be harmful to human physical health as well as emotional health. Lovallo (1997) offers the examples of the high rates of sudden deaths due to heart attacks associated with uncontrollable exposure to extremely stressful situations such as major earthquakes and the outbreak of war.

- The potential benefits of coping can exceed those associated with effectively managing a specific demanding situation. Coping can, for example, put people in a better position to manage future stressors and demands, or contribute to the accomplishment of greater goals and achievements. In this way, the coping process is assumed to be fundamental to personal growth and well-being.

Key Theoretical Developments

Stress, Health, and Well-Being

Seyle is widely considered to be the "father" of current understandings of the relationship between stressors, stress responses and health, and well-being. He described short- and long-term human responses to life's stressors through his general adaptation syndrome (Seyle, 1950). The general adaptation syndrome outlines a three-stage response to stressors: (1) an alarm response where the body prepares for dealing with stress, either through "flight or fight"; (2) a stage of adaptation to the demands presented by the stressor; and (3) a stage of exhaustion, and vulnerability to health decline if the stress response is prolonged. Seyle differentiated between different forms of stress, including "distress," which referred to demands that were harmful or threatening to well-being, and "eustress," which referred to life demands that were opportunities and positive challenges (Seyle, 1975).

Life Events and Demands as Stress

Another line of inquiry into stress and coping has focused on the events or circumstances that are experienced as taxing to human coping resources. Holmes and Rahe (1967), for example, developed a rating scale of 43 life events that are generally considered to be challenging to people based on the level of change and adjustment they required (e.g., marriage, loss of a loved one, divorce). Major illness and injury ranks among the top 10 stressful life events on this scale.

Although it can be useful to think about the relative stress associated with common life events, identifying and ranking these events is not without problems. Identifying life events that are decontextualized from the person experiencing the event and broader social conditions tells us little about their actual potential to be stressful. Dohrenwend (2000), for example, has offered several characteristics of events that will contribute to how they are experienced, such as the extent to which the event is predictable, the source of the occurrence of the event (external forces accountable or person accountable), and the magnitude of the event in affecting a person's usual activities.

A distinction has been made between stressors that are relatively discrete events or circumstances requiring adaptation over relatively brief periods, and chronic strains that suggest persistent or ongoing demands for coping and adaptation (Avison & Turner, 1988). For example, coping and adaptation that occurs in the context of significant health conditions or disability can be considered an experience of chronic strain (Thoits, 1995). Acute stressors and chronic strain are often connected; for example, major stressful events can lead to shifts in life's demands that place ongoing strains on a person. So, a major accident resulting in a significant disability is a major life event leading to considerable stress, but the ongoing impact on daily life of the disability experience is likely to produce daily strains.

Psychobiological Processes of Stress

It is now well established that both life event stressors and chronic strains can have a negative impact on physical and mental health (see for example, Thoits, 1995), with most of the research in this area focusing on negative events and strains. Theories of physiological regulation suggest that humans have a complex system of controls to maintain homeostasis, or a state of equilibrium, in the face of threats to well-being. It appears that the physiological processes that respond to stressors that are psychologically and emotionally taxing and negative (such as loss of jobs, loss of loved ones, compromised health) may be somewhat distinct from those responses to physical demands or threats and to events that are emotionally positive (such as having a baby, marriage, taking on a new job). Specifically the prolonged release of cortisol in stressful life circumstances has been associated with a range of problematic health conditions (Lovallo, 1997).

COPING PROCESSES AND STRATEGIES

Much of the recent stress-related theory has focused on the processes of coping, highlighting that people are not passive recipients of life events and strains, but rather are active agents in determining how these are experienced and controlled. People have a range of coping resources, both internal personal resources and external social and material resources that can be engaged to respond effectively to stressful events and circumstances (Pearlin & Schooler, 1978). These ideas are important to occupational therapists because they suggest that people can be enabled to manage their responses to stress both to promote their health and well-being and to facilitate positive occupational performance and experience.

Lazarus and Folkman (1984) identified that people use a range of strategies to cope with psychological and emotionally taxing events. Appraisal-focused strategies are oriented to shifting the meaning or the assumptions that an event or situation holds to make it less overwhelming. Problem-focused strategies are those that use problem-solving processes to identify problems at hand and possibilities for action, weighing alternatives and to move forward to implement selected actions. Emotion-focused coping strategies are oriented to managing the difficult emotions that emerge in stressful situations. People typically use all of these coping strategies in their daily lives, although problem-solving coping is generally considered a particularly adaptive response in that it suggests an assertive response to adversity and an attitude of control and personal power.

The idea that people have coping resources available to them, also suggests that occupational therapists can expect to see great variability in how people cope and their coping effectiveness. For example, research on gendered roles and social relations suggests that there may be differences in how men and women cope. Studies have shown, for example, that consistent with socialization theories, women are more likely to use emotion-focused coping and access social supports as coping strategies, compared to men who are more likely to use problem-focused coping (Ptacek, Smith, & Zanus, 1992). Variations in available coping resources may also be seen as a result of differences in individual psychological and emotional resources. For example, people with high internal locus of control and sense of self-efficacy may have the psychological resources that will help them to appraise demanding situations as within their capacities and to demonstrate the resilience required for ongoing coping in the face of illness or disability (see for example, Stuart & Yuen, 2011).

Similarly, people in disadvantaged social and economic situations will likely have fewer and perhaps less robust social resources and means available to them to manage stressful life circumstances. In addition they may experience daily lives characterized by more complex stressors and strains (Thoits, 1995). Hobfall and colleagues (1994) have argued for the development of conceptualizations of coping that go beyond a narrow focus on cognitive appraisals and perceptions to take into account the extent to which social support and material resources mediate individuals' ability to manage significant life stressors and strains.

Current theories related to coping and stress have highlighted the extent to which coping can be conceptualized as a dynamic and positive human response. Schwarzer and Taubert (2002) describe contemporary conceptualizations of positive coping as attending to both the role of meaning in relation to stressful events and also the temporal aspects of coping. The meaning associated with stressful life circumstances may, for example, influence the extent and nature of coping efforts. In this way coping efforts may be stronger when connected to future goals and fulfillment. Temporal conceptualizations of coping highlight that coping should be appreciated as an ongoing process that can be preventative and anticipatory, occurring before stressful events, occurring while stressful life circumstances are experienced, and in response to stressful life events.

DIATHESIS-STRESS MODELS

In an effort to understand the precursors to mental disorders, researchers have considered the fact that people are not equally inclined to experience episodes of acute mental distress or symptoms of mental illness in relation to similar stressors of daily living. The notion of *diathesis* suggests that some people have a vulnerability, or a predisposition, to daily life stressors that leaves them more likely to experience such symptoms. This vulnerability can emerge from a range of sources—genetic, biological, neurophysiological processes, and cognitive structures and processes, to name a few (Ingram & Luxton, 2005). Negative health outcomes linked to the diathesis-stress have been associated with a wide range of mental illnesses such as schizophrenia (Jones & Fernyhough, 2007) and depression (Patten, 2013), but it has also been suggested in a number of other health-related

VIGNETTE 14-1. WINSTON

At 44 years of age, Winston is employed as a relief, residential counselor in a group home for seniors with developmental disabilities. Winston is adamant that no one at work is aware that he has a diagnosis of schizophrenia. He is committed to his job and proud of his expertise as a community worker. The symptoms associated with his illness are well controlled and rarely interfere with his work performance. He typically works alone, or with only one other employee, minimizing the social pressures for sharing personal information that may lead to disclosure of his illness.

His place of employment is a 45-minute drive from his local community. Winston takes a cautious attitude toward stress at work and its potential for exacerbating the symptoms of his schizophrenia. He values the considerable training, the demands, and responsibilities associated with his job, and he emphasizes that not all aspects of the job, which he experiences as stressful, provoke an episode of his mental disorder.

Winston is highly susceptible to feelings of anxiety that escalate into paranoid thoughts. He recognizes that environments that are characterized by poverty trigger memories that evoke intense feelings of physical and psychological vulnerability and present him with a view of himself that is not easily reconciled with a self-image of competence and well-being. Winston and his occupational therapist have worked collaboratively to identify stressors that may threaten his health and well-being and his capacity to cope. The following summarizes some of this work.

POTENTIAL STRESSORS	COPING BEHAVIORS AND STRATEGIES
Potential for disclosure of mental illness on the job: Winston is concerned that despite his very good job performance his employers and coworkers will treat him differently if they know about his illness.	Maintaining social networks distinct from employment social networks Receiving mental health treatments from a primary care site rather than the local mental health service Developing awareness of his rights as an employee related to disclosure
Responding to early signs of mental illness, specifically sleep disruptions, social withdrawal, depression	Following a personal plan for dealing with warning signs including attending to sleep hygiene, medical appointments to review treatments, increasing appointments with health providers to monitor status, reducing work responsibilities, and participating in a stress management group
Maintaining job while managing early signs of illness	Working in a relief position provides Winston with flexibility to refuse shifts. Provides his employer with some sense of anticipated length of time off from work
Exacerbation of symptoms when in environments of poverty, social disadvantage	Avoids poverty environments, planning of outings with residents to avoid these environments, and maintains housing in a quiet residential neighborhood
Dealing with self-doubt, threats to self-concept	Serving as a peer "role model" for other people with mental illness who are marginalized from important social roles

conditions, such as work-related disabilities and chronic pain (Caruso, 2013; Dersh, Polatin, & Gatchel, 2002). This vulnerability is magnified by the fact that people who experience these vulnerabilities can have more complex and stressful daily lives. So, people with mental illnesses or chronic health conditions are more likely to experience poverty, isolation, and other conditions of social disadvantage and these conditions will bring more stress to daily life roles and activities. This means that vulnerability always needs to be understood within context. Winston, in Vignette 14-1, is living with a diagnosis of schizophrenia, a mental illness that is considered to leave individuals vulnerable to experiencing symptoms of acute illness in response to stress. Indeed, the vignette demonstrates how this happens to him within particular environmental contexts. Yet, Winston's experience with mental illness also engages him in dealing with complex social relations in his occupational roles, and these are likely quite complex, increasing his experience of stress. For example, Winston is faced with actively hiding his mental illness on the job for fear of the ramifications to his employment. The vignette highlights that "hiding the illness" actually requires a fair bit of emotional and social skill.

Diathesis-stress models of health and well-being are important for occupational therapists who work with people with a broad range of health conditions and disability in the context of managing their daily lives. The model provides a way of understanding sensitivity to stress in daily life circumstances. The knowledge base behind diathesis-stress models is, however, continually evolving and showing that the relationship between vulnerability and stress is not a simple one. Indeed, health care and other service providers who are concerned about sensitivity to stress can be prone to holding people back from important life roles and activities. This is a reminder to therapists of the importance of a thorough understanding of person, environment, and occupation in relation to coping and stress and of the intervention practice available to support participation in the demands of daily activities.

COPING THEORY AND OCCUPATIONAL THERAPY

Coping theory and best practice related to coping is highly relevant to occupational therapy service delivery. Occupational therapists routinely work with individuals who, in the context of disability, have their coping capacities compromised. This extends to families and social networks that may find their own internal and external coping resources are exceeded. Since, at its core, occupational therapy is directed at optimizing occupational engagement so that people can imagine possibilities for themselves and experience themselves as effectively influencing their environments, the profession is well suited to enabling coping.

There has been limited direct attention to coping theory in the occupational therapy scholarship. Fine, in her 1989 Eleanor Clarke Slagle lecture, offers the possibility that occupational therapists have historically been more oriented to assessing and addressing performance of occupation as it manifests observably, rather than of clients' view of themselves, their situations, their adaptive style, and their patterns of self-regulation. Dawson and Trueman (2010) conducted a survey of knowledge and practice related to several psychosocial factors, including coping, among Canadian occupational therapists working in the area of traumatic brain injury. Their findings suggested that while therapists were generally knowledgeable about these factors, they tended to integrate them into practice in an implicit way rather than addressing coping directly and

explicitly. Prudhomme White and Mulligan (2009) suggest that occupational therapy research has the potential to contribute to theory related to stress and stress responses by studying the self-regulation of stress responses in the context of occupation by including psycho-biological measures of such markers as cortisol levels.

OCCUPATIONAL THERAPY PRACTICE

Occupational therapy scholarship has many examples of applications of coping theory to practice, but again these have not been integrated into an overarching conceptualization of coping and occupation. Applications of coping in occupational therapy practice can generally be placed into the four following broad organizing categories:

1. Using occupation as a means to enable coping efforts: The meaning and value associated with occupation is believed to encourage active coping efforts by people who experience occupational disruptions. For example, Aegler and Satink's (2009) study of the experiences of persons with chronic pain found that participants' need to participate in important occupations could outweigh the pain and engaged them in coping strategies to enable their performance.

2. Active coping in the context of limitations on occupations as a means to personal empowerment: Health conditions, disability, and other significant personal disruption can impose limitations on capacities and leave people feeling overwhelmed and lacking control. Taking a stance of active coping in occupation can lead to increased personal empowerment. For example, McLean and Coutts (2011) discuss how learning strategies to cope with migraine headaches can enhance feelings of self-efficacy and control.

3. Enabling positive coping styles in relation to occupational engagement: Theories of coping have identified several coping styles that can be particularly effective. For example, Crooks and colleagues (2011) examined the problem-focused coping strategies used by university academics with multiple sclerosis to maintain their employment and well-being.

4. Coping strategies can be identified that are relevant to specific health and occupational situations, and enabled to promote positive occupational experiences: To be effective, coping strategies need to be considered in relation to the specific circumstances and context. For example, studies by occupational therapists have identified the types of coping strategies used by people with aphasia (Nätterlund, 2010), mothers of children with disabilities (Helitzer, Cunningham-Sabo, VanLeit, & Crowe, 2002), people coping with traumatic re-enactment (Cowls & Galloway, 2009), and teachers experiencing stress (Austin, Shah, & Muncer,

2005). Occupational therapists have also advanced the understanding of coping strategies, such as spirituality as a coping strategy for people with serious mental illness (Smith & Suto 2012). Interestingly, occupational therapy scholarship has also been directed to the coping strategies used by occupational therapists and occupational therapy students in practice (Bivins, 2001; Sweeney, Nichols, & Cormack, 1993).

Consistent with best practices in the field, occupational therapy practice that is directed to strengthening coping in relation to occupation is guided by the following principles:

- The focus of all intervention approaches is on enabling individuals to feel *empowered* and in control in the face of situations that are particularly challenging and experienced as threatening to the self. Miller (2000) refers to this as "maximizing client power resources."

- Intervention approaches are *sensitive to the specific contexts* of coping. While occupational therapists will work to strengthen the coping capacities of individuals in a general way, outcome-focused practice requires a focused approach.

- Practice is sensitive to the *personal meanings and values* associated with the threats to integrity and well-being that present when individual coping capacities and resources are challenged.

- Good practice is characterized by recognizing and *actively enabling the personal capacities and resources* of the individual. This not only serves to keep the individual firmly in control, it also can serve to promote personal growth and opportunities, or what Fine (1989) referred to as "transforming adversity into possibilities."

As with all occupational therapy, an understanding of the sociocultural and developmental elements influencing coping must ground all practice. Developmentally, the need to cope with stressors in daily life occurs across the life span, but the nature of and context for stressors will vary considerably, as will the factors that will most enable adaptive coping. The coping capacities of young children, for example, will be enhanced in the context of a supportive and stable nuclear family. For adolescents, one must take into account the fact that coping may be challenged by instability in the formation of identity and values and the considerable influence of peers. For older adults, coping occurs in the context of multiple losses, transitions, and changes in personal abilities.

OCCUPATIONAL THERAPY ASSESSMENT OF COPING

There are many useful standardized, psychometrically sound assessments of coping available to assist with the development of a comprehensive and collaborative intervention plan. Assessments relevant to coping are often self-report and can focus on understanding: the presence of life circumstances and events typically considered demanding and stressful in an individual's life, personal stress responses to demanding events and situations, coping styles and dispositions, and coping processes used by the individual.

Eliciting information about demands, stressors, and coping is typically accomplished by occupational therapists through detailed narratives of living with occupational disruptions. This interview style of eliciting stressful events is consistent with current evidence that has suggested there are measurement errors associated with self-report checklists. For example, Monroe (2008) highlights how individuals completing self-report checklists may attribute different meanings than intended to the measurement items. For example, he cites the case of a woman who did not identify her husband's recent heart attack (typically considered a major stressful life event) because his health behaviors had changed for the better, and another case of individuals checking stressful life events to not appear that they have a boring life.

Specific assessments have been developed for children and youth; for example, the Coping Strategies Inventory (Tobin, 2001) has children or adolescents rank their responses to a specified stressful event. In addition, questionnaires and surveys have been developed to understand coping in response to very specific life circumstances, such as coping with pain, the Coping With Chronic Pain Inventory (Romano, Jensen, & Turner, 2003)—often used by multidisciplinary pain management teams—or coping with the burden of caregiving, such as the Carers Assessment of Managing Index (Nolan, Keady, & Grant, 1995), which assesses the use of particular coping strategies in response to specific caregiving situations.

The Stress Management Questionnaire, developed by occupational therapist Stein (2002), engages individuals to consider, in an integrated and occupation-focused manner, the situations that produce stress, the nature of their stress responses, and the problems and coping activities that are used to manage these stressors. The tool has been designed to enhance collaborative planning and to follow outcomes associated with therapy.

OCCUPATIONAL THERAPY PRACTICES THAT ENABLE COPING

Occupational therapy practices that enable coping will overlap considerably with practice frameworks and approaches that have been covered in some detail in other chapters of this book. For example, coping is enhanced with individual self-awareness and the development of psychological defense responses that promote self-acceptance

VIGNETTE 14-2. MICHAEL

Michael was 35 years old when he was seriously injured in the line of duty as a firefighter. When the accident occurred, he was the primary income earner for his family. The injury occurred only a few months following the birth of his third child. As a result of the injury, Michael experienced burn-related scarring on his face and arms, and a spinal cord injury that resulted in paraplegia. Michael received many months of assertive treatment, rehabilitation, and disability management services. The time immediately following the accident was a bleak period for Michael and his family. Initially highly motivated to participate in treatments, he became despondent when he realized that his recovery would not lead to returning to his occupations as he knew them.

With the support of his service providers, who helped him envision new meaningful possibilities, Michael reengaged fully in his rehabilitation. The year following the injury saw many life changes for Michael and his family. They moved to new, accessible housing. With childcare assistance from his in-laws, Michael's wife started a part-time business from home. Michael returned to work in his city's fire department, but in a new job that saw him responsible for community relations and training.

and adaptive ways of interacting in daily life. In this way, coping will be enhanced by practice strategies outlined in the chapter focusing on psychodynamic frames of reference. Similarly, coping-focused practice will likely integrate practices associated with strengthening cognitive and behavioral responses and personal meanings that will promote positive adaptation. These aspects of coping have all been considered in other chapters in this book.

What conceptual frameworks that focus on coping specifically add to this therapeutic mix is their focus on *promoting personal control and power* and *maintaining relationships with people, activities and the future that are characterized by hope and possibilities*, even in the face of circumstances that are threatening, unpredictable, and potentially life altering.

In this chapter, practice strategies are organized with respect to three broadly defined conditions that are understood to evoke stress, challenge coping, and threaten the functional stability of individuals and ultimately positive adaptation. These three conditions are (1) coping in response to disability or persistent illness, (2) coping in the face of vulnerability to stress, and (3) coping in crisis circumstances. Within this latter condition, specific attention is directed to suicide prevention, a particularly important type of crisis experience.

Enabling Coping in Response to Disability or Persistent Illness

Vignette 14-2 introduces Michael, a man who experienced injury that occurred while he was performing the dangerous duties of a job he loved. Although the stressor was an acute and isolated event, it left Michael with significant changes to his body and function, and ultimately the need to evolve coping strategies on the long term, to deal with threats to his identity and body image, role changes,

strains on his relationships, pain, and possibly lifelong health issues. The occupational therapists working with Michael were aware, that like most people who experience life-altering and persistent disability or health conditions, he was at high risk for helplessness, loss of control, and an overall sense of hopelessness.

Occupational therapy assessment related to coping in the context of persistent disability or health conditions begins with consideration of the internal and external strengths that are known to increase coping and adaptation in response to trauma and life-altering events. Michael's occupational therapists observed, for example, that he possessed the following factors that have been connected to resilience in the face of adversity (see for example, Miller, 2000):

- Personal factors such as a positive self-concept and self-efficacy, good self-esteem, a strong sense of meaning and purpose in life, but also a flexible personality style, effective emotional self-regulation, and good problem-solving skills

- Personal resources such as good socioeconomic position, even in the face of reduced financial means; strong family and social relationships that are able and willing to provide a range of practical, emotional, and informational support; an orderly home environment characterized by reciprocity and collaboration

- Community resources, such as a fair and compassionate employer, good quality health and rehabilitation services, and opportunities for training and education

Even where these positive features of resilience are present, in the face of life-altering disability or health difficulties, occupational therapists need to consider how to enable an individual's sustained investment in working through the adversity to engage in meaningful occupations. In the case of Michael, for example, his occupational therapists capitalized on Michael's strong family values and the importance of providing for his family, the altruism that lead him to pursue firefighting as a career, and his moral convictions about how people should live as citizens in the community to encourage him to take supported risks, to withstand difficulties and even failures, and imagine and create new possibilities. These internal personal qualities were complemented by strong and enabling external resources. These included his supportive wife and family, and an understanding employer with formal structures and policies to enable Michael's return to a meaningful job. Persistent disability and health conditions engage individuals in a broad range of disability or illness-related coping tasks. Michael, for example, could be expected to confront tasks related to changes in his relationships with friends, health concerns related to aging with a spinal cord injury, grieving the loss of physical function, and the associated changes in his work roles, and the need to advocate for himself.

Coping theory and research provides occupational therapists an array of possible coping strategies that can be enabled to lead to positive occupational engagement and performance. Working collaboratively, Michael's occupational therapists encourage him to use problem-focused strategies, such as gathering information about the types of fire-fighting jobs that have demands he can reasonably be expected to meet, learning about reasonable accommodations and how they might apply to him, and meeting with his employer to plan and prepare for these possibilities. In his home life, Michael learns about options related to housing accessibility and pursues couples counselling to identify and address changes in his intimate relationship with his wife. With the assistance of his occupational therapist Michael also learns about and uses several emotion-focused coping strategies; he meets with coworkers socially before returning to the workplace in an effort to reduce the impact of embarrassment or anxiety on social exchanges in the workplace, and finds comfort in his religion, which offers him some helpful ways to view his circumstances. Seeking social support is another type of strategy that can be oriented to either providing instrumental or emotional support to meet demands. So, for example, Michael receives practical and emotional support from his friend who has joined him in physical conditioning activities to help him reach an optimal level of fitness.

Enabling Coping in the Context of Vulnerability to Stress

Like Michael, Winston in Vignette 14-1 is dealing with a significant and persistent health-related condition, but his experience includes a vulnerability to stress that sees him prone to acute exacerbations of illness. This vulnerability places Winston in a precarious position where he must balance his personal health and well-being with his efforts to participate in occupations that hold meaning both personally and socially. While Winston's vulnerability is related to his diagnosis of schizophrenia, similar issues related to vulnerability are common for many illnesses and disorders, particularly those that are episodic in nature.

For occupational therapists and other service providers, this vulnerability has the potential to elicit a protective stance and a generalized cautionary stance toward stress that can restrict occupational engagement. While attending to the stress-ill health relationship is good practice, a failure to understand the specific nature of this relationship can lead to a situation where opportunities to enjoy the growth and well-being elements of occupational engagements become restricted. The fallout of this approach is that people like Winston are subject to lives that are occupationally deprived.

The occupational therapist and Winston worked collaboratively to evaluate personal strengths and resources in relation to the specific demands and expectations of occupations he was expected to do, needed to do, and wanted to do. This approach facilitated a detailed understanding of the specific work-related demands that caused Winston harmful distress, and provided information required for problem solving related to coping. They identified, for example, how his emotional stability was compromised in particular types of environments and problem solved how to address this situation at work. Just as important, it considered the many job demands and challenges that Winston could routinely meet or exceed and positively highlighted his considerable knowledge, skills, and experience and contributed to his self-confidence, self-efficacy, and his sustained investment in the work. Winston, for example, was sensitive to the community living needs of the residents, established good working relationships with them, and expertly followed policies and regulations related to their care.

Where vulnerability to stress is present, an important element of practice is assisting individuals with recognizing the signs that sensitivity to stress is heightened, perhaps leaving them particularly susceptible to negative effects. In the case of Winston, for example, he identifies several subtle signs of instability in his mental and emotional state that indicate his ability to deal with stressors is compromised: disrupted sleep patterns; eating less; avoiding social situations, even those he typically enjoyed; and feelings of depression. Occupational therapy intervention practices in the case become directed to two related, but distinct, outcomes. First, practices are directed to avoiding relapse or an acute exacerbation of illness and second, to assisting people to effectively negotiate the important expectations of their occupations. The case vignette of Winston summarizes the many coping strategies developed collaboratively with his service providers.

VIGNETTE 14-3. ELLA

Ania, an occupational therapist working for a community-based service, is conducting a routine home visit to see Ella, a 37-year-old woman diagnosed with multiple sclerosis. On this visit, Ania and Ella had planned to continue with evaluation and planning related to home modifications. Although Ania arrives at the scheduled time, it takes Ella some time to respond to the knocking at her door. When she finally opens the door, Ella is distraught and Ania notices that she appears to have been crying for some time. Ella's appearance is disheveled, and she is wearing her night clothes even though it is 11 am. This is not typical behavior for Ella. Ella is alone in her house. Upon questioning, Ella tells Ania that she did not sleep the previous night despite taking sleeping pills and that she cannot remember the last time she had anything to eat. She states that her husband of 10 years left her very suddenly yesterday afternoon.

Enabling Coping in Crisis

The third vignette featured in this chapter provides an example of an occupational therapist faced with responding in a crisis situation. In the context of service provision in the health or social services, a crisis refers to experiencing an acute emotional upset, sometimes referred to as an emotional disequilibrium that is characterized by the inability to exercise one's typical coping capacities or resources (Aguilera, 1998; Hoff, Brown, & Hoff, 2009). By definition, a crisis experience is not long lasting, but satisfactory resolution of the crisis is important to avoid both the negative immediate outcomes that can occur for the person and communities, but also for longer term outcomes related to the health and well-being of the individual.

In Vignette 14-3, the occupational therapist comes upon her client, Ella, in the course of routine service delivery in the community. Ania, the occupational therapist, is neither expecting, nor prepared to find her client in a crisis situation. This highlights that although occupational therapists may not be working formally as crisis workers, they can find themselves addressing crisis situations, particularly in contemporary practice models in which therapists work solely in community environments.

The first step for occupational therapists is to assess the level of severity of the crisis situation. Features of the situation that are important to consider in the evaluation of severity include (1) how the individual perceives the event and the level of threat it presents; (2) the extent to which an individual is able and willing to use available resources to deal with the situation; (3) the extent to which problem-solving capacities are intact; (4) the level of, and potential for, escalation of emotional instability and despair; and (5) the level of threat of harm to self or others. Guidelines for the triage of level of severity and response interventions have been developed to assist service providers. The following presents a relatively simple, three-level ranking of severity (see for example, Hoff, 1995):

1. Low urgency: The person is likely to mobilize his or her own resources at his or her own pace to address the

situation. An intervention response is required but not necessarily needed immediately. Response should be delivered within the next day.

2. Moderate urgency: Pressure on the individual is present and the threat of escalation of emotional instability is present without intervention. An intervention response should be delivered within the day.

3. High urgency: A life-threatening situation is present and the intervention response must be immediate.

Using these guidelines, Ania evaluates Ella's situation as moderate in urgency. Ania is concerned that in her distress Ella's personal resources will not be mobilized to help her through this situation, and she is concerned that her emotional distress may escalate, and perhaps even have a negative impact on her health, destabilizing her physical condition. Ania evaluates the need to implement an intervention response immediately, expecting that connecting Ella with other supports can occur within the next few hours.

Crisis intervention principles have been developed to assist service providers, including occupational therapists, in the implementation of informed responses. Flannery and Everly (2000), for example, define five principles that can be applied by the occupational therapists working with Ella:

1. *Immediacy*—This first principle reminds therapists that a crisis situation is hazardous and requires some form of immediate attention, even if connecting individuals to other supports is delayed. In Ania's case she recognizes that the focus of her visit to Ella's home needs to shift from home modifications to facilitating a resolution of the crisis state. Ania presents a calm but compassionate demeanor with her client, and discretely arranges for her other home visits that day to be delayed, so that she can attend carefully to Ella's situation. The immediacy of needs related to crisis highlights the importance of the occupational therapist having ready knowledge of the crisis services and resources available in their service environments and community. Ania, for example, is familiar with the mobile crisis services available in her community so that she can readily

access them for assistance. In this vignette, although Ania does not contact the mobile crisis service to provide assistance, she does ensure that Ella is aware of their services and provides her with their contact information.

2. *Understanding*—An informed and sensitive intervention response requires a good understanding of the crisis situation and of the meaning of the situation to the individual and his or her social network. The person's perception of the crisis situation will be closely connected to his or her own response. Therapists need to be particularly aware of situations where individuals are in danger. In this vignette, Ania learns that although there had been strains in their relationship, her husband's actions were experienced as a complete surprise and that the leaving event was filled with anger and hostility. Ania asks directly if there has been any suggestion of violence or threat. Ella provides information that suggests her family was never positive about her marriage; that she feels rejection, guilt, and embarrassment; and is worried now about her financial well-being. With this information, Ania becomes more convinced that Ella's emotional distress is so acute that she is unlikely to use her own problem-solving capacities to reach out to avail herself of supports.

3. *Stabilization*—The occupational therapist can act to create some sense of order in the immediate environment, and thus create conditions that may allow an individual's problem-solving capacities to emerge. Ania, for example, responds in a manner that is likely to spur Ella to actions that are consistent with her automatic, daily routines. She acknowledges Ella's feelings of distress and suggests that Ella take a shower and get dressed, while she makes some tea so that they can take the time to talk. In response to these simple actions, Ella gains some sense of normalcy and control over her immediate situation and is in a better position to use her considerable coping capacities.

4. *Focus on problem solving*—In a crisis situation, even individuals who are very adept at addressing challenges and problems can find their problem-solving capacities compromised. Ella's situation, for example, is highly charged emotionally, and her experience of loss, anxiety, grief, and anger may be so strong as to leave her unable to evaluate her situation and to respond effectively. To enable Ella to use internal and external resources to move ahead, Ania uses focused decision counselling strategies, carefully and sensitively framing questions to stimulate problem solving (Hoff, 1995). Examples of questions might be, "Let's think about the things you have in your schedule today, so you can be free to focus on this," "What have you done so far about this; what have you thought about doing so far?", "Who knows about your relationship with your husband that could be helpful?", "Who else should know about this?", "Are there things you usually do to help you when you are very upset? Would these ideas be helpful now?"

5. *Encourage self-reliance*—Contemporary crisis theory assumes that crises present important opportunities for promoting growth and mastery. Subsequently, crisis intervention is seen as an important opportunity to elicit and support coping mechanisms. In our vignette, Ania ensures that Ella's intact capacities are used. For example, she suggests that Ania call the social worker she has been seeing for couple's counselling to arrange a meeting that day, she supports Ella in calling her sister to engage her assistance, and provides support while she calls her bank to acquire information about her financial situation (an area of particular concern for Ella).

Using practices that align with these principles, the therapist works to move the situation to the point where the individual's coping capacities are spurred toward the resolution of the crisis. Ensuring that follow up is in place to monitor the resolution of the crisis is an important final step. In Ella's case, with the social worker now engaged, an arranged visit to her family doctor, and the elicitation of active family support, Ania felt assured that good follow-up was in place.

Suicide prevention is a particularly important type of crisis intervention. Suicide is the deliberate self-inflicted termination of one's life. It is regarded as existing on one end of a broad continuum of self-destructive or life-threatening behaviors. As the opening quote from the journals of Sylvia Plath (a famous poet who took her own life) so eloquently shows, suicidal feelings can reflect significant and distressing emotional disconnection with the everyday meanings and purpose of life.

While many people who eventually do die by suicide previously exhibited self-destructive behavior, not all self-harming behaviors are associated with efforts to terminate life. For example, people who experience emotional dysregulation may engage in self-cutting behaviors that are not intended to end life. In addition, suicidal intent and actions can be discrete, covert, and intense; the self-destructive potential of forgetting to take one's insulin if diabetic, or drinking alcohol in excess and driving may, for some individuals, represent forms of suicidal intentions and actions.

A wide range of factors have been associated with increased likelihood of attempting suicide, and it is important for occupational therapists to consider these factors to evaluate the potential for suicide and the level of risk. Well-known risk factors associated with suicide are presented in Table 14-1. The Suicide Assessment Five-Step Evaluation Triage for mental health professionals was developed in collaboration between Screening for Mental Health, Inc.

TABLE 14-1

WELL-KNOWN RISK FACTORS FOR SUICIDE

- Family history of suicide
- History of trauma or abuse
- Previous suicide attempt(s)
- History of mental disorders
- Alcohol and substance abuse
- Feelings of hopelessness
- Impulsive or aggressive tendencies
- Major physical illnesses
- Losses, including job loss, financial loss, relationship loss
- Cultural and religious beliefs where suicide is considered as a moral resolution of a personal dilemma
- Local clusters of suicide and exposure to others who have died by suicide including through social media
- Barriers to accessing mental health treatment, including stigma associated with asking for help
- Easy access to lethal methods

---

and the Suicide Prevention Resource Center (n.d.). The five-step process includes and evaluation of the presence of risk factors, and identification of protective factors, such as well-developed coping strategies, good social supports, and responsibility for others. The evaluation includes specific questions about suicidal thoughts, plans, intents, and behaviors. The fourth step involves evaluating the risk as low, medium, or high, and following through with interventions based on this evaluation. For example, a high risk could include the presence of several factors, including a very strong intent with a plan, and few sound protective factors present. In this case, the evaluation would point to an immediate response that includes assertive suicide precautions such as accessing hospital services. A low-risk situation might be one where the individual expresses feelings of hopelessness with vague thoughts of death, but no developed plan or means. This individual would also have some good protective factors, such as responsibility for a beloved pet, or the support of friends and family. In this case referral to the primary physician or connecting the individual to a crisis service could be appropriate. More information about the Suicide Assessment Five-Step Evaluation Triage approach is available online at www.stopasuicide.org, or through the website of the Substance Abuse and Mental Health Administration website.

Occupational therapists need to know the laws and regulations that define their responsibility about the evaluation of risk for suicide and suicide intervention. Ensuring that an individual is safe and receiving the assistance he or she

requires is a first-line intervention whenever potential for suicide is present. This may mean, for example, accompanying an individual to see his or her physician, or staying with an individual until a crisis or an emergency service is organized and implemented.

Given the high prevalence of suicide across a range of populations, it is now widely considered a public health issue. For example, in many countries suicide is the leading cause of death among young people. In response to this, there has been a broad range of advancements in related assessment and intervention approaches. Service providers across the health and social services fields are now being encouraged to consider recognizing and responding to suicidality as basic practice competencies. Certificate training programs have developed to advance this cause. These training programs develop skills in the recognition of suicidality, developing plans for increased safety from suicidal behaviors, and following through with safety commitments. They will also focus on increasing their understanding of how personal beliefs and attitudes related to suicide impact suicide interventions. While training programs will vary in their content and design, a comprehensive program of training would include the following:

- Correcting misguided assumptions that can prevent a therapist from taking action; for example, the assumption that asking an individual about suicide intent directly may actually fuel suicidal thoughts where none existed is a frequently held, but inaccurate and unhelpful, belief.

- Addressing knowledge and skills that can allay personal discomfort around suicide; for example, training can focus on how to dialogue with individuals about suicidal intent, deal with the strong feelings that can accompany suicidality, and explore some of the moral and ethical dilemmas surrounding suicide that interfere with a therapist's ability to respond in a helpful manner.

- Working with individuals with persistent suicide intent or self-injurious behaviors

- Ensuring that the service provider's own needs are met, to support them through difficult therapeutic processes should an individual actually take his or her own life

Occupational therapy values, principles, and practices are well positioned to contribute to the prevention of future crises and suicidality. The profession's focus on highlighting individual personal and environmental strengths and resources, instilling hope, creating meaningful occupational opportunities, and developing mastery and coping skills that can enable an individual to adapt to, and perhaps even welcome, daily life challenges are all examples of intervention principles that may act to reduce the potential for suicidality.

CONCLUSION

This chapter has defined coping as a central psychosocial process in human occupation. The theory related to coping has been growing since the mid-1950s, expanding our understanding of coping as a fundamental human response to life's challenges. To date, occupational therapy scholarship in relation to coping has not been well developed, although there are indications that this is changing. The chapter describes occupational therapy practice in the area of coping, organized into three common practice situations. As a client-centered profession, occupational therapists are in a good position to learn about coping from the people they serve, and to share these insights with others in their practice.

LEARNING ACTIVITIES/ DISCUSSION QUESTIONS

1. Work in groups to discuss your experiences with managing crises. Use the following questions to guide your discussions: Think of a time when you experienced a crisis. Why did you identify this as a crisis? What did you receive from others that helped you through the crisis? Why were these actions helpful? What did you receive from others that were unhelpful? Why were these unhelpful?

2. Participating in the student or occupational therapist role brings many challenges. Identify five significant stressors that you experience in this role. Think about the ways you cope with these stressors. Identify coping strategies you use that are problem based and those that are emotion based. Identify anticipatory coping strategies you use. Think about the ways that your environmental resources contribute to your ability to cope with these challenges.

3. Imagine that you are an occupational therapist conducting a driving evaluation on an elderly gentleman who is showing early signs of dementia. He is very angry and upset about the assessment. Your evaluation suggests that this man is no longer capable of driving safely. Your approach is empathic, and during your discussions about the findings the man becomes increasingly despondent and indicates that he thinks life is no longer worth living. With further discussion, he indicates to you that he plans to go home and drink alcohol and he suggests that he might take some pills.

   a. What is your evaluation of this man's risk for suicide? What specific criteria are you using to make this evaluation?

   b. Investigate the policies and regulations that govern your practice with this man. Given these regulations, describe how you should respond.

4. Form a discussion group with other occupational therapists and consider the following situation:

   You are an occupational therapist working for a community mental health team. The individuals served all have serious mental illness. During a meeting reviewing program evaluation data, it was noted that the employment rates of people served is very low—no more than 10% of those served are employed in any capacity. One of the team members states that this is to be expected, because work will cause individuals served too much stress. What would be the best response in this situation?

5. Conduct a literature search to compare coping among children, adolescents, adults, and older adults.

REFERENCES

Aegler, B., & Satink, T. (2009). Performing occupations under pain: the experience of persons living with chronic pain. *Scandinavian Journal of Occupational Therapy*, 16, 49-56.

Aguilera, D. C. (1998). *Crisis intervention: Theory and methodology*. St. Louis: Mosby.

Austin, V., Shah, S., & Muncer, S. (2005). Teacher stress and coping strategies used to reduce stress. *Occupational Therapy International* 12.2, 63-80.

Avison, W. R., & Turner, R. J. (1988). Stressful life events and depressive symptoms: Disaggregating the effects of acute stressors and chronic strains. *Journal of Health and Social Behavior, 29*, 253-264.

Bivins, M. (2001). Working with adults with enduring mental illness: emotional demands experienced by occupational therapists and the coping strategies they employ. *British Journal of Occupational Therapy, 64*(6), 318.

Caruso, G. M. (2013). Biopsychosocial considerations in unnecessary work disability. *Psychological Injury and Law, 6*(3), 164-182.

Cowls, J., & Galloway, E. (2009). Understanding how traumatic re-enactment impacts the workplace: Assisting clients' successful return to work. *Work, 33*(4), 401-411.

Crooks, V., Stone, S., & Owen, M. (2011). Enabling university teaching for Canadian academics with multiple sclerosis through problem-focused coping. *Canadian Journal of Occupational Therapy* [serial online]. *78*(1), 45-49.

Dawson, D. R., & Trueman, M. (2010). Psychosocial considerations in occupational therapy treatment for adults with acquired brain injury. *Occupational Therapy in Health Care, 24*, 295-307.

Dersh, J., Polatin, P. B., & Gatchel, R. J. (2002). Chronic pain and psychopathology: research findings and theoretical considerations. *Psychosomatic Medicine, 64*, 773-786.

Dohrenwend, B. P. (2000). The role of adversity and stress in psychopathology: Some evidence and its implications for theory and research. *Journal of Health and Social Behavior, 41*, 1-19.

Fine, S. (1989). Resilience and human adaptability: Who rises above adversity? *American Journal of Occupational Therapy, 45*, 493-503.

Flannery, R. B. Jr., & Everly, G. S. Jr. (2000). Crisis intervention: A review. *International Journal of Emergency Mental Health, 2*(2), 119-125.

Helitzer, D., Cunningham-Sabo, L., VanLeit, B., & Crowe, T. (2002). Perceived changes in self-image and coping strategies of mothers of children with disabilities. *OTJR: Occupation, Participation & Health* [serial online]. *22*(1), 25-33.

Hobfall, S. E., Banerjee, P., & Britton, P. (1994). Stress resistant resources and health: A conceptual analysis. In S. Maes, H. Leventhal, & M. Johnston, (Eds). *International review of health psychology*, vol. 3. (pp. 37-63). Oxford, England: John Wiley & Sons, England.

Hoff, L. A. (1995). *People in crisis: Understanding and helping.* San Francisco: Jossey-Bass.

Hoff, L. A., Brown, L., & Hoff, M. R. (2009). *People in crisis: Clinical and diversity perspectives.* New York: Routledge.

Holmes, T. H., & Rahe, R. H. (1967). The social readjustment rating scale. *Journal of Psychosomatic Research, 11*, 213-218.

Ingram, R. E., & Luxton, D. D. (2005). Vulnerability-stress models. In B. L. Hanking & J. R. Z. Abela, (Eds). *Development of psychopathology: A vulnerability-stress perspective.* Thousand Oaks: Sage.

Jones, S. R., & Fernyhough, C. (2007). A new look at the neural diathesis-stress model of schizophrenia: The primacy of social-evaluative and uncontrollable situations. *Schizophrenia Bulletin, 33*, 1171-1177.

Lazarus, R. S. & Folkman, S. (1984). *Stress, appraisals and coping.* New York: Springer.

Lovallo, W. R. (1997). *Stress & health: Biological and psychological interactions.* Thousand Oaks, CA: Sage.

McLean, A., & Coutts, K. (2011). Occupational therapy: Self-management for people with migraines. *OT Now, 13*(5), 5-8.

Miller, J. M. (2000). *Coping with chronic illness*, (3rd ed.). Philadelphia: F. A. Davis.

Monroe, S. (2008). Modern approaches to conceptualizing and measuring human life stress. *Annual Review of Clinical Psychology, 4*, 33-52.

Nätterlund, B. (2010). A new life with aphasia: Everyday activities and social support. *Scandinavian Journal of Occupational Therapy, 17*(2), 117-129.

Nolan, M., Keady, J., & Grant, G. (1995). CAMI: A basis for assessment and support with family carers. *British Journal of Nursing, 4*(14), 822-826.

Overton, M. (2012). *Good in a crisis: A memoir.* Bloomsbury Group.

Patten, S. B. (2013). Major depression epidemiology from a diathesis-stress conceptualization. *BMC Psychiatry, 13*, 1-9.

Pearlin, L. I. & Schooler, C. (1978). The structure of coping. *Journal of Health and Social Behavior, 19*(March), 2-21.

Plath, S. (1982). *The journals of Sylvia Plath.* New York: Random House.

Prudhomme White, B., & Mulligan, S. E. (2009). Applications of psychobiological measures in occupational science and occupational therapy research. *Occupational Therapy Journal of Research, 29*(4), 169-174.

Ptacek, J. T., Smith, R. E., & Zanus, J. (1992). Gender, appraisal and coping: A longitudinal analysis. *Journal of Personality, 60*, 747-770.

Romano, J. M., Jensen, M. P., & Turner, J. A. (2003). The chronic pain coping inventory—42: reliability and validity. *Pain, 104*, 65-73.

Scaffa, M. E., Pizzi, M. A., & Chromiak, S. B. (2010). Promoting mental health and emotional well-being. In M. E. Cassfa, S. M. Reitz, & M. A. Pizzi (Eds). *Occupational therapy in the promotion of health and wellness* (pp. 329-349). Philadelphia: F. A. Davis.

Schwarzer, R., & Taubert, S. (2002). Tenacious goal pursuits and striving toward personal growth: Proactive coping. In E. Frydenberg (Ed.), *Beyond coping: Meeting goals, visions and challenges* (pp. 19-35). London: Oxford University Press.

Screening for Mental Health, Inc. and the Suicide Prevention Resource Center (n.d.). Suicide Assessment Five-Step Evaluation and Triage for mental health professionals. Retrieved from www.integration.samhsa.gov/images/res/SAFE_T.pdf.

Seyle, H. (1950). Stress and the general adaptation syndrome. *British Medical Journal*, 1383-1392.

Seyle, H. (1975). Confusion and controversy in the stress field. *Journal of Human Stress, 1*(2), 37-44.

Smith, S., & Suto, M. J. (2012). Religious and/or spiritual practices: Extending spiritual freedom to people with schizophrenia. *Canadian Journal of Occupational Therapy, 79*(2), 77-85.

Stein, F. (2002). *Stress management questionnaire.* Albany, NY: Delmar Cengage Publishing.

Stein, F., & Cutler, S. (2002). *Psychosocial occupational therapy: A holistic approach* (2nd ed.). San Diego: Singular Publishing Group.

Strauss, J. (1989). Subjective experiences of schizophrenia: Towards a new dynamic psychiatry II. *British Journal of Psychiatry, 15*(2), 179-187.

Stuart, D. E., & Yuen, T. (2011). A systematic review of resilience in the physically ill. *Psychosomatics, 52,* 199-209.

Sweeney, G. M., Nichols, K. A., & Cormack, M. (1993). Job stress in occupational therapy: coping strategies, stress management techniques and recommendations for change. *British Journal of Occupational Therapy, 56*(4), 140-145.

Thoits, P. (1995). Stress, coping and social support processes: Where are we? What next? *Journal of Health and Social Behavior,* Extra Issue, 53-79.

Tobin, D. L. (2001). User manual for the Coping Strategies Inventory. Retrieved from www.ohioupsychology.com/files/images/holroyd_lab/Manual%20Coping%20Strategies%20Inventory.pdf

United Nations Development Program. (2011). Towards human resilience: Sustaining MDG progress in an age of economic uncertainty. New York: United Nations Bureau for Development Policy.

Yamkovenko, S. (2008). Occupational therapy's role in disaster relief. *American Association of Occupational Therapists.* Retrieved from www.aota.org/en/About-Occupational-Therapy/Professionals/MH/Articles/Disaster-Relief.aspx.

section V

Environment-Level Models and Frameworks

The chapters in this section present well-established models and frameworks that focus on population and contextual level factors relevant to psychosocial occupational therapy practice. Occupational therapists have historically focused their practice on working with individuals, largely in health care contexts. Subsequently, population and societal/community level approaches to enable human occupation have not always been well integrated into daily practice. There are a variety of reasons for this; funding limitations, the structure and policies of the practice environment, and education and training needs, to name a few. These restrictions on practice can leave occupational therapists feeling helpless in dealing with broader environmental factors that affect the occupational health of the people they serve. This has perhaps been a most problematic issue in psychosocial practice; societies have generally been slow to acknowledge and address the psychological and social aspects of community life that impact human health and well-being. Fortunately, this state of affairs is changing. There has been a growing body of scholarship and research in this area over the past two decades that has included the development of intervention approaches that can help occupational therapists to both understand and address broader social factors in their daily practice.

In this section, we present a select group of conceptual frameworks and models that suggest intervention approaches to elicit positive change in psychosocial determinants of occupation at the population and broader community levels. Chapter 15 presents models related to health promotion with a particular focus on those who experience mental illnesses and mental health-related disabilities. The chapter highlights how, when we take a step back to consider populations of people with mental illness, we see inequity in their overall health and well-being status and inequities concerning access to health care. Chapter 16 focuses on psychological and social aspects of organizational cultures. With its particular emphasis on workplaces, the chapter highlights the relevance and potential applications of organizational culture to occupational therapy psychosocial practice. Chapter 17 addresses how issues of occupational justice affect human mental health and well-being and are subsequently relevant to psychosocial practice in occupational therapy. The chapter demonstrates how established community development approaches can be used by occupational therapists to advance the ideals of occupational justice.

Health Promotion and Wellness for Persons With Psychiatric Disabilities

Deborah Pitts, PhD, OTR/L, BCMH, CPRP and
Erin McIntyre, OTD

To maintain a sense of well-being, I have had to change my lifestyle and my priorities. My illness taught me (the hard way) the importance of meaningful work, good patterns of rest and sleep, exercise, diet, and self-discipline. (Houghton, 1982, p. 549)

We envision *a future in which people with mental illnesses pursue optimal health, happiness, recovery, and a full and satisfying life in the community via access to a range of effective services, supports, and resources. We* pledge *to promote wellness for people with mental illnesses by taking action to prevent and reduce early mortality by 10 years over the next 10 year time period.* (The Pledge for Wellness [SAMHSA, 2007] http://promoteacceptance.samhsa.gov/10by10/pledge.aspx)

OBJECTIVES

The objectives of this chapter are as follows:

- » Define and articulate elements of health promotion frameworks to support wellness of psychological and social well-being.

- » Describe how health promotion framework are being applied to promote recovery and wellness for persons with disabilities related to mental health.

- » Summarize research findings related to key targets of health promotion interventions (i.e., nutrition and fitness, oral health, sleep hygiene).

- » Identify and describe evidence-based life-style interventions targeting health promotion needs of person with disabilities related to mental health.

Krupa, T., Kirsh, B., Pitts, D., & Fossey, E. *Bruce & Borg's*
Psychosocial Frames of Reference: Theories, Models, and Approaches for
Occupation-Based Practice, Fourth Edition (pp 245-264).
© 2016 SLACK Incorporated.

BACKGROUND

The World Health Organization's Ottawa Charter of Health Promotion (Box 15-1; WHO, 1986) is seen as guiding framework for health promotion efforts worldwide. The Ottawa Charter defines health promotion in the following way:

> Health promotion is a process of enabling people to increase control over, and to improve, their health. To reach a state of complete physical, mental, and social well-being, an individual or group must be able to identify and to realize aspirations, to satisfy needs, and to change or cope with the environment. Health is, therefore, seen as a resource for everyday life, not the objective of living. Health is a positive concept emphasizing social and personal resources, as well as physical capacities. Therefore, health promotion is not just the responsibility of the health sector, but goes beyond healthy lifestyles to well-being. (WHO, 2004, p. 19)

In recent years, health services have experienced a shift from illness-oriented to wellness-oriented perspectives. This has included growing attention to the promotion of mental wellness to foster overall health and well-being of the public. It has also been applied directly within the mental health system to address the needs of persons who experience mental illness, and in particular those labeled with "serious," "persistent," and/or "enduring" mental illness. A significant contribution to this perspective has come from mental health consumers themselves who have emphasized wellness as way of approaching recovery (Copeland, 2001; Swarbrick, 1997). An additional influence toward this shift has been the devastating findings that, in the United States, persons labeled with disabilities related to mental illnesses die 25 years earlier than other Americans, largely due to treatable medical conditions (Manderscheid, 2008), but also because of the marginalized social and economic situations within which they live. This chapter will focus on this latter population, and provide an overview of the current perspectives, targets, and strategies for health and wellness of persons with disabilities related to mental illness.

VIEW OF HEALTH AND DISORDER

Contemporary perspectives on health and wellness for persons with disabilities related to mental illness are informed by and situated within notions about health and wellness for all. The WHO defines health as "a state of complete physical, mental and social well-being and not merely the absence of disease or infirmity" (WHO, 1948). This view is further represented in the *International Classification of Functioning, Disability and Health's* perspective on activity and participation (American Occupational Therapists Association [AOTA], 2013; WHO, 2002).

Wellness applied specifically to people labeled with psychiatric disabilities has been defined "as people's growth toward healthy physical, mental, spiritual lifestyles expressed in healthy environments, and the reduction of co-morbid health conditions and disorders. Health exists within the experience of the psychiatric disability, yet is distinct from the disability" (Hutchinson et al., 2006, p. 245). This definition highlights that we need to see beyond the mental illness and psychiatric disability to consider "whole person" health and well-being.

KEY CONCEPTS

Key concepts for health promotion and wellness have emerged over the last several years.

Determinants of Health

Determinants of health represent the multiple factors that affect the health of individuals and communities, and have been identified as the social and economic environment, the physical environment, and the person's individual characteristics and behaviors (WHO, 2014a). Significant efforts have been undertaken by researchers and policy makers to identify and understand the nature of health determinants to guide health promotion efforts. Over the last two decades, a critical target of these efforts has been what is referred to as the *social determinants of health* (SDH; Braveman & Gottlieb, 2014). The WHO's Commission on the Social Determinants of Health has defined SDH as the "conditions in which people are born, grow, live, work and age" (WHO, 2014b).

Occupational therapy and occupational science researchers and practitioners have taken up the call to focus on SDH (Edwards, 2013). Indeed, there is a close connection between the profession's assumptions about health through occupation and the social determinants of health (Wilcock, 2006). Current efforts that align occupations with ideas about the social determinants of health include occupational justice (Townsend, 2003; Townsend & Whiteford, 2005), and occupational deprivation (Whiteford, 2000). A critical aspect of these perspectives has been the challenge to occupational therapy's traditional approach of targeting our interventions at individuals, rather than at communities and populations (AOTA, 2013; College of Occupational Therapy [COT], 2008; Finlayson & Edwards, 1995; Holmberg & Ringsberg, 2014; Tucker et al., 2014).

Prevention vs. Promotion

Prevention and promotion represent two broad, but linked, perspectives within the fields of public health science

---

BOX 15-1. OTTAWA CHARTER OF HEALTH PROMOTION ACTION STRATEGIES

Build Healthy Public Policy

Health promotion goes beyond health care. It puts health on the agenda of policy-makers in all sectors and at all levels, directing them to be aware of the health consequences of their decisions and to accept their responsibilities for health.

Create Supportive Environments

The inextricable links between people and their environment constitute the basis for a socio-ecological approach to health. Systematic assessment of the health impact of a rapidly changing environment is essential and must be followed by action to ensure positive benefit to the health of the public. The protection of the natural and built environments and the conservation of natural resources must be addressed in any health promotion strategy.

Strengthen Community Action

Health promotion works through concrete and effective community action in setting priorities, making decisions and planning strategies, and implementing them to achieve better health. At the heart of this process is the empowerment of communities, their ownership and control of their own endeavours and destinies.

Develop Personal Skills

Health promotion supports personal and social development through providing information and education for health and enhancing life skills. By so doing, it increases the options available to people to exercise more control over their own health and over their environments and to make choices conducive to health.

Reorient Health Services

The responsibility for health promotion in health services is shared among individuals, community groups, health professionals, health service institutions, and governments. They must work together toward a health care system that contributes to the pursuit of health.

From WHO, 1986 as cited in WHO 2004, p. 23. World Health Organization (WHO). (2004). Promoting mental health: Concepts, emerging evidence, practice. In H. Herrman, S. Sazena, & R. Moodie (Eds.). Geneva, Switzerland: World Health Organization, Department of Mental Health and Substance Abuse in collaboration with the Victorian Health Promotion Foundation and the University of Melbourne. Copyright 2004 by World Health Organization. Reprinted with permission.

---

and practice for addressing health and wellness needs of populations. Disease prevention represents the older of the two concepts (Breslow, 1999), and over time, levels and/or stages of prevention have been defined (Figure 15-1).

In their development of a framework for health promotion services for people labeled with psychiatric disabilities, Hutchinson and colleagues (2006) drew on Cowen's (2000) community psychology perspective that differentiated between primary prevention and wellness enhancement in mental health. While this work focused on the prevention approaches for mental health conditions specifically, Hutchinson and colleagues argued that the distinction between prevention and wellness enhancement was helpful to their thinking regarding overall health outcomes as well. Key concepts of their framework included the following:

- Risk detection-disorder prevention (i.e., primary prevention), Cowen (2000), seeks to prevent serious psychological disorders by mediating impact of specific associated risk factors. Prevention efforts try to "harness 'windows of opportunity'" and are seen as narrow, brief and targeting only those with risk-signs (p. 10). Early intervention psychosis programs that focus on the early detection, support, and treatment during the formative period of health conditions where psychosis is a prevalent feature are an example of such efforts (McFarlane, 2011).

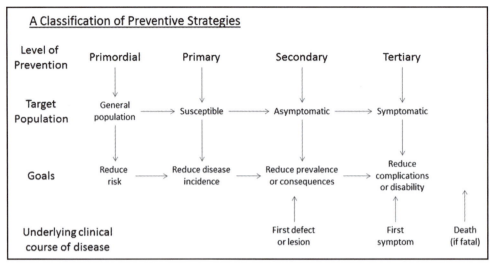

Figure 15-1. Levels of Prevention. (Reprinted with permission from University of Ottawa. (2015). Categories of prevention. Retrieved from www.med.uottawa.ca/sim/data/Prevention_e.htm.)

- Wellness enhancement, on the other hand, seeks to maximize psychological wellness by promoting conditions that serve as protection to "short circuit" trouble and "augment life satisfaction" (Cowen, 2000, p. 10). Unlike prevention efforts, wellness enhancement efforts are targeted at all people and seen as broad, varied, and long term.

The Hutchinson and colleagues framework offers an accounting of potential health promotion outcomes (Table 15-1), and offer a set of guiding principles (Table 15-2) for health promotion efforts targeting the needs of person's labeled with psychiatric disabilities.

THEORETICAL ASSUMPTIONS

Theoretical assumptions underlying health and wellness efforts and the promotion of occupational engagement to influence health and wellness can be drawn from disciplines and professions beyond occupational science and occupational therapy, including public health. These theoretical perspectives inform interventions at both the individual and community level. Those highlighted here include assumptions about how occupation, environmental factors, and behavioral changes influence health and wellness.

Impact of Occupation on Health and Wellness

Occupational therapy is grounded in a deep and profound belief that engagement in occupation promotes health and well-being (Meyer, 1922; Wilcock, 2006), not just of individuals, but of populations. Occupational therapy conceptual practice models provide frameworks for

designing occupation-based interventions and programs to support health and well-being (Reitz, Scaffa, & Pizzi, 2010). The *Model of Human Occupation* and the *Canadian Model of Occupational Performance and Engagement* represent two of the most long standing, well-articulated, and widely disseminated models. Proponents of each of these models have developed a solid body of research, as well as practice tools like assessment and intervention manuals that can be used by occupational therapists to guide their development of interventions to promote health and wellness. To date, however, they have been mostly applied when working with individuals, rather than integrated into population-based interventions. Recent efforts in the profession have tried to address this problem by showing how occupational therapy models can be interpreted to apply to populations to support public health initiatives. For example, in an effort to increase population access to occupational therapy services, Klaiman (2004) from the Canadian Association of Occupational Therapists (CAOT) demonstrated how the Canadian Model of Occupational Therapy aligns with primary health care models. Occupational science (Clark et al., 1991) has also contributed to the design of health and wellness interventions, with Clark et al.'s (1997) Life Style Redesign approach being one of the most well-known.

Impact of Environment on Health and Wellness

Social ecological theories in public health inform the development of population level approaches to health promotion. These theories emphasize the interrelationships among various personal and environmental factors. The assumption that the environment influences health and wellness has its origins in ancient Greek philosophy and medicine (Tountas, 2009). The Lalonde Report is credited

TABLE 15-1

POTENTIAL HEALTH PROMOTION OUTCOMES FOR PERSONS WITH SERIOUS MENTAL ILLNESS

PHYSICAL DIMENSIONS	SELF-DIMENSION
Improved health	Increased self-awareness
Increased energy	Increased self-acceptance
Improved stamina	Increased self-esteem
Improved fitness	Increased inner strength/empowerment
Improved sleep	Improved self-control
Increased physical relaxation	Increased sense of responsibility
Decreased physical pain	Increased capacity to tolerate uncertainty
Reduced somatization	Increased openness
	Increased capacity for self-expression
EMOTIONAL DIMENSIONS	**SOCIAL DIMENSION**
Increased emotional stability	Feeling accepted/supported by others
Increased capacity for mood containment	Improved social skills
Increased capacity for emotional self-regulation	Decreased social isolation
Increased calmness	Increased sense of trust
Decreased fears	Increased capacity for empathy
Decreased social anxiety	Increased tolerance of others
Increased sense of safety/security	
Increased capacity for release of negative feelings	
Decreased impulsivity	
COGNITIVE DIMENSION	**SPIRITUAL DIMENSION**
Decreased negative thinking	Increased hopefulness
Decreased delusional thinking	Increased connectedness
Decreased racing thoughts	Increased sense of meaning/purpose in life
Improved concentration	Sense of spiritual fulfillment
Improved memory	Sense of inner peace
Increased coping behavior	Increased capacity for forgiveness
	OVERALL FUNCTIONING
	Decreased self-destructive behavior
	Improved adaptive behavior
	Improved vocational capacity
	Improved capacity for self-care
	Improved coping capacity
	Increase sense of well-being

Reprinted with permission from Hutchinson, D. S., Gagne, C., Bowers, A., Russinova, Z., Skrinar, G. S., & Anthony, W. A. (2006). A framework for health promotion services for people with psychiatric disabilities. *Psychiatric Rehabilitation Journal*, *29*(4), 241-250. doi: 10.2975/29.2006.241.250.

TABLE 15-2
PRINCIPLES OF HEALTH PROMOTION FOR PEOPLE WITH SERIOUS PSYCHIATRIC DISABILITIES

- Health and access to health care are universal rights of all people.
- Health promotion recognizes the potential for health and wellness for people with psychiatric disabilities.
- Active participation of people with serious psychiatric disabilities in health promotion activities is ideal.
- Health education is the cornerstone of health promotion for people with psychiatric disabilities.
- Health promotion for people with psychiatric disabilities addresses the health characteristics of environments where people live, learn, and work.
- Health promotion is holistic and eclectic in its use of many strategies and pathways.
- Health promotion addresses each individual's resource needs.
- Health promotion interventions must address differences in people's readiness for change.

Reprinted with permission from Hutchinson, D. S., Gagne, C., Bowers, A., Russinova, Z., Skrinar, G. S., & Anthony, W. A. (2006). A framework for health promotion services for people with psychiatric disabilities. *Psychiatric Rehabilitation Journal, 29*(4), 241-250. doi: 10.2975/29.2006.241.250.

as being the first government document to highlight the relationship between the environment to health outcomes and argue the importance of attending to these social and environmental conditions (Lalonde, 1981/1974). As was noted earlier, aspects of the environment that have been identified as influencing health and wellness include the physical, social, and economic environment.

In the early 20th century, improved public health practices around water supply, waste management, etc. had a significant impact on health and safety in industrialized societies. In the 21st century, public health initiatives with similar targets have gone global. In addition, mental health promotion efforts, such as the Mental Hygiene Movement (White, 1923), that influenced the development of occupational therapy emerged at this time and focused on the impact of industrialization and the growth of the urban context on the mental health of the population.

Occupational therapy and occupational science, like many other professions and disciplines, situate our understanding of an individual's health and wellness within the contexts in which they engage. Mary Law's 1991 Muriel Driver Lecture for the Canadian Occupational Therapy Association foregrounded the environment, and set the groundwork for one of the most well-disseminated occupational therapy conceptual practice models, the Person-Environment-Occupation model (Strong et al., 1999). Most comprehensive occupational therapy conceptual practice models include environment as a component of their model, including the Model of Human Occupation (Kielhofner, 2008), Ecology of Human Performance (Dunn, 1994), and the Canadian Model of Occupational Performance and Engagement (Townsend & Polatajko, 2007).

These broad conceptual practice models can provide the occupational therapist with ways to frame their focus on the health and wellness needs and goals of persons labeled with psychiatric disabilities. In addition to these environmentally-focused models, it is critical to draw on others, such as mental health recovery, described in an earlier chapter of this book. Contemporary conceptualizations of recovery highlight the poverty, lack of social support, poor living conditions, and lack of access to adequate health care that serve as external barriers to recovery and wellness for many people labeled with serious mental illnesses and psychiatric disabilities. Public policy initiatives are being promoted that directly target these barriers, including efforts to insure access to health care, the expansion of safe and affordable permanent supported housing, and improving employment outcomes.

Impact of Behavioral Changes on Health and Wellness

Another broad assumption that informs health and wellness efforts is the understanding that behavioral changes and actions taken by the individual can influence his or her health and wellness. The focus here is on the lifestyle practices in which the person engages that either support or place at risk his or her overall health and wellness. From this perspective, individuals are viewed as having self-agency and control in exercising health-related behaviors, and subsequently influencing this self-agency can influence population health. This perspective has been a focus of most health promotion efforts over the past few decades, and has been designed to influence behavior change of individuals at the population level. The most familiar efforts directed to population level individual change are those directed to increasing physical activity, changing dietary habits, and reducing smoking and substance use. This focus on behavior change is not without its critics (Golden & Earp, 2012).

Critics argue that the degree to which we as individuals have control and choice over our daily lives is influenced by social structures (Williams, 1995). Recent efforts in public health and health promotion have proposed what they call a relational approach to balance the understanding of human agency with social structures to strengthen health promotion approaches (Veenstra & Burnett, 2014). Such a perspective emphasizes the "dynamic, recursive, codependent relationships between agency and structure" (Veenstra & Burnett, 2014, p. 3), and calls on those engaged in health promotion activities to attend to the interplay of person-in-context. This idea of agency-structure relationship has been attended to in developing models of mental health recovery (Hopper, 2007; Yanos, Knight, & Roe, 2006). Occupational therapy theorists and occupational scientists drawing on interdisciplinary perspectives have also explored this question. For example, Cutchin, Aldrich, Baillard, and Coppola (2008) describe how actions in occupations are perhaps best understood as relational, "in which the independent notions of structure and agency melt away" (p. 164).

KEY DEVELOPERS AND IMPORTANT EVOLUTIONARY POINTS

Wellness and Health Promotion in the Broader Societal Context

As noted in the introduction to this chapter, the WHO's Ottawa Charter of Health Promotion (1986) has been credited with representing a key evolutionary point in how wellness and health promotion is understood and situated within the broader societal context. Potvin and Jones (2011) note that while the Ottawa Charter significantly influenced health promotion efforts in the western hemisphere, the WHO's 2005 Bangkok Charter extended these ideas to identify the commitments and actions necessary to extend health promotion efforts on a global scale.

Occupational therapy has been concerned with health and wellness in the broader societal context since its founding on the "humanistic ideal of promoting well-being through occupation" (Reitz, 1992, p. 50). Adolf Meyer's foundational accounting of occupational therapy's philosophy fully aligns with health and wellness concepts and beliefs. Despite this early attention to health and wellness, occupational therapy emphasized its curative rather than preventive health focus until the 1960s (Reitz, 1992) when

Reilly, West, and Wiemer called for an explicit focus on health promotion. Reilly's now well-known declaration "that man, through the use of his hands, as they are energized by the mind and will, can influence the state of his own health" (Reilly, 2005/1961, p. 1) served as the mantra for these efforts. More than two decades ago Reitz argued that the profession's real contribution to health and well-being should be at the societal level:

> Strong conviction is held that occupational therapy has the option to elect involvement in prevention and has an obligation to make significant contributions to the promotion of society's health … Prevention in community health care (which is prevention in all health care), more than treatment and rehabilitation, can be the realization of the profession's unique and real value to mankind. (Weimer as cited in Reitz, 1992, p. 52)

West proposed a role for occupational therapists as consultants in the development of programs for the well community, and Weimer (1972) advocated for the role of health advocate and counselor. American Occupational Therapy Association published its first official statement, the "Role of the Occupational Therapist in the Promotion of Health and Prevention of Disabilities," in 1979. It provided a framework for development of health prevention programs by occupational therapists (Reitz, 1992), and continues to do so with recent updates (AOTA, 2013). Similar efforts to explicitly address the link between occupational therapy and health promotion are developing in other countries. For example, a visit to the website of the CAOT will link the reader to a variety of position papers related to the profession's role in a broad range of health promotion efforts from smoking cessation, to reducing obesity, to engaging youth in healthy occupations.

By 1980, occupational therapy was able to capitalize on broader societal health and wellness initiatives like the Ottawa Charter, to strengthen its health and wellness efforts. The *American Journal of Occupational Therapy*'s fall 1986 edition was devoted entirely to the topic of health and wellness. Jaffe and Johnson are key contributors to occupational therapy's participation in health promotion efforts during this period. Their work targeted workplace wellness in particular, with Johnson crafting one of the first occupational therapy texts on health promotion entitled *Wellness: A Context for Living* (Johnson, 1986). She identified three wellness dimensions—the body, the self, and the environment/culture, and argued against a view of "wellness as a 'thing' which one can 'get'":

> Wellness, as a *context for living* (italics added), is a state of being, a place from which to come as we commit ourselves to improving life for all humanity … As a context for living, wellness is not limited to getting something more for me—rather,

it becomes the possibility that my life, my wellness, contributes to you and to your wellness. It is available to all—regardless of whether one is healthy or terminally ill. (p. 14)

Her perspective draws on the pragmatist tradition of the mind-body connection (Meyer, 1922), as well as the contemporary perspective that there is no health without mental health (WHO, 2004).

Beginning in the 1990s and continuing to present day, occupational therapy's promotion of health and wellness in the broader societal context was informed by what has been called the "occupational renaissance" (Whiteford, Townsend, & Hocking, 2000, p. 61). This has been an international effort including the United States' lifestyle redesign approach by Clark and colleagues' (1997); Canada's' critical review of occupation, health, and well-being by Law and colleagues (Law, Steinwender, & Leclair, 1998); and Australia's exploration of the relationship of occupation to health and well-being by Wilcock (2002). A recent effort by the CAOT has led to the development of a national framework and guide for activity-health, called the "Do-Live-Well" Framework (Moll et al., 2014).

Wellness and Health Promotion in the Mental Health Practice Context

The focus on wellness and health promotion for persons labeled with psychiatric disabilities has become a central component of recovery-oriented mental health service systems over the last two decades. Vandiver (2009) argues that a "health promotion" focus aligns well with recent transformational efforts at insuring that mental health systems of care promote wellness and recovery for persons labeled with psychiatric disabilities (Department of Health and Human Services [DHHS], 2005; WHO, 2004, 2007). The United States Surgeon General's 1999 report on mental health (DHHS, 1999) and the President's New Freedom Commission (DHHS, 2003) both had identified the important need to address health outcomes for persons labeled with psychiatric disabilities. In addition, several studies documented higher mortality rates for persons labeled with psychiatric disabilities (Lutterman, Ganju, Schacht, Shaw, & Monihan, 2003), and strategies arguing for the integration of mental health and physical health care services had begun to be identified as important (Bazelon, 2004).

This accumulating evidence sounded the alarm and culminated in the US Department of Health and Human Services' 10 x 10 Campaign (see www.promoteacceptance. samhsa.gov/10by10/default.aspx), which sought to initiate a broad-based, mental health, system-wide effort to increase the life span of persons labeled with psychiatric disabilities by 10 years in 10 years (Center for Mental Health Services, 2007). Specifically this national initiative articulated and defined what they called the "epidemic" of "much

higher rates of cardiovascular disease, diabetes, respiratory disease, and infectious disease (such as HIV/AIDS) than the general population" (p. 1). Further, they identified vulnerability factors for this population contributing to these poorer health outcomes, including the following:

- Higher rates of modifiable risk factors, including smoking, alcohol consumption, poor nutrition/obesity, lack of exercise, unsafe sexual behavior, intravenous drug use, and residence in group care facilities and homeless shelters

- Poverty, homelessness, unemployment, victimization, trauma, and incarceration

- Social isolation/stigma and discrimination

- Side effects from psychiatric medications, including weight gain, diabetes, high cholesterol and abnormal triglyceride levels, insulin resistance, and metabolic syndrome

- Impact of mental illness related symptoms that can mask the symptoms of medical/somatic illnesses

- Lack of coordination between mental health systems and primary care

- Polypharmacy—use of multiple medications with harmful drug interactions (Parks, et al. as cited in CMHS, 2007, pp. 1-2).

Furthermore, the campaign mapped out a National Wellness Action Plan that focused on the following:

- Identification and dissemination of promising practices

- Improvement in financing policies

- Development and implementation of provider training and education

- Development and dissemination of self-management shared decision-making tools

- Ongoing data collection and analysis to measure change

Since the onset of the campaign, wellness and health promotion efforts have become more consistently integrated into most mental health services in the United States. This integration has been strengthened by key features of the 2010 Affordable Care Act, which incorporated health promotion and integrated care approaches.

A key player in the U.S. Substance Abuse and Mental Health Services Administration's (SAMHSA) Wellness efforts has been occupational therapist, Margaret "Peggy" Swarbrick. Dr. Swarbrick's personal experiences inspired her work and passion to advocate for, and create services based on, wellness, recovery and peer support principles. Her work and leadership with the Collaborative Support Programs of New Jersey (CSPNJ) (http://cspnj.org) and the Wellness Institute (www.cspnj.org/#!wellness-institute.c1ie6) provides the base from which she has developed and disseminated a clear perspective on wellness. She believes that:

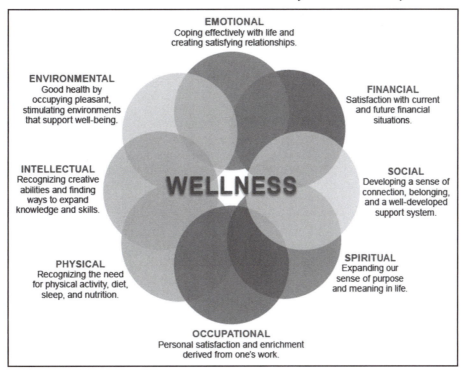

Figure 15-2. Eight Dimensions of Wellness. (Reprinted with permission from Substance Abuse and Mental Health Services Administration. (2015). *The Eight Dimensions of Wellness.* Substance Abuse and Mental Health Services Administration. Retrieved from www.samhsa.gov/wellness-initiative/eight-dimensions-wellness.)

Wellness is a conscious, deliberate process that requires a person to become aware of, and make choices for, a more satisfying lifestyle. A wellness lifestyle includes a self-defined balance of health habits such as adequate sleep and rest, productivity, exercise, participation in meaningful activity, nutrition, productivity, social contact, and supportive relationships. (Swarbrick, 1997, p. 1)

The Eight Dimensions of Wellness model (Figure 15-2), developed in collaboration with her colleagues at the CSPNJ, has come to serve as a key component of SAMHSA's Wellness Initiative. In addition to her perspective on wellness, she has contributed practice innovations including Peer Wellness Coaches (Swarbrick, 2010, 2013; Swarbrick, Murphy, Zechner, Spagnolo, & Gill, 2011) that will be described later in this chapter.

Another key player in contributing to our contemporary perspective on wellness in the mental health practice context is Mary Ellen Copeland, PhD. Dr. Copeland is most known for the development of her Wellness Recovery Action Plan (WRAP) approach. The WRAP approach emerged from Copeland's own lived experience, as well as her work as a mental health provider helping others self-manage their psychiatric symptoms. WRAP has been identified by SAMHSA as an evidence-based practice, supported by good evidence that it can lead to important changes indicative of recovery and well-being. A key element of a

WRAP is the Wellness Toolbox, which includes a rich and full accounting of what the person needs to do and wants to do to maintain wellness (Copeland, 2001). This component of a WRAP is particularly meaningful to occupational therapists, as it aligns well with our notion of occupational engagement as a source of health and wellness. WRAP has become one of the most well disseminated approaches that drew on, and promoted the shift from, illness to wellness for persons labeled with psychiatric disabilities. The Copeland Center for Wellness and Recovery (www.mentalhealthrecovery.com/) now serves as an international resource for the WRAP approach. Many additional resources to support the WRAP approach have been developed and are disseminated by the Copeland Center, including targeted WRAP tools to manage diabetes, weight gain, and pain management, as well as a WRAP App for the iPhone and Android.

Expected Outcomes

In recent years, inclusion of health outcomes measures within existing mental health service system outcome measurement processes has been advocated. For example, in the United States, the *National Association of State Mental Health Program Directors* recommended a set of health and process indicators that should be captured at the individual service level (Parks, Radke, & Mazade, 2008; Box 15-2). For the purposes of this chapter, obesity reduction, smoking

Box 15-2. Recommended Health and Process Indicators for Individual Service Level

Health Indicators

- Personal and family history of diabetes, hypertension, cardiovascular disease
- Weight/height/body mass index (BMI)
- Blood pressure
- Blood glucose or HbAIC
- Lipid profile
- Tobacco use/history
- Substance use/history
- Medication history/current medication list, with dosages
- Social supports

Process Indicators

- Screening and monitoring of health risk and conditions in mental health settings
- Access to, and utilization of, primary care services (medical and dental)

From Parks, J., Radke, A. Q., & Mazade, N. A. (2008). *Measurement of health status for people with serious mental illness* (Vol. 16). Alexandria, VA: National Association of State Mental Health Program Directors. Reprinted with permission.

cessation, oral health, sleep hygiene, and falls prevention, all associated with health outcomes in this population, will be reviewed.

Obesity Reduction

Weight gain secondary to psychiatric medications and sedentary lifestyles has been documented for persons labeled with psychiatric disabilities and are recognized as major risk factors for cardiovascular disease, diabetes, and reduced life expectancy (Bartels & Desilets, 2012). Furthermore, evidence suggests that women with psychiatric disabilities are more likely to be obese than their male counterparts (Robson & Gray, 2007). Robson and Gray (2007) also acknowledge the impact of poor dietary habits of people with psychiatric disabilities on the prevalence of obesity within this population. Studies have shown, for example, that individuals labeled with psychiatric disabilities consume far below the recommended amount of fruits and vegetables and increased amounts of food high in fat and low in fiber (Bartels & Desilets, 2012; Parks et al., 2008; Robson & Gray, 2007). Additionally, research has found that consumption of saturated fats and sugar (e.g., from meat and dairy) are correlated with poor outcomes in schizophrenia (Robson & Gray, 2007).

There is a common misperception that those labelled with psychiatric disabilities are unable or unwilling to make positive changes to their lifestyle and health. Studies have shown that individuals affected by psychiatric disabilities do show an interest in improving their weight and overall health, and many are already working toward these goals (Parks et al., 2008). Research suggests that weight management programs can be useful in promoting weight loss, particularly when they include the following characteristics: lasting 3 months or longer, educational support, activity-based learning, nutritional support, physical activity, as well as motivational and cognitive behavioral components (Bartels & Desilets, 2012; Robson & Gray, 2007). Programs that focus primarily on weight loss are likely to be more successful when an active and joint approach is taken, such as joint monitoring of weight logs and food diaries (Bartels & Desilets, 2012). Parks et al. (2008) suggest that behavioral strategies such as goal setting, problem solving, self-monitoring, and eating slow, further support weight loss.

The attitude and knowledge of mental health professionals about weight management and weight loss is another key factor in the successful implementation of both. A holistic approach to working jointly with those labeled with psychiatric disabilities is paramount in supporting improvements in both physical and mental health of each individual (Parks et al., 2008). It should be emphasized that even a minor reduction in weight (i.e., 5%) can positively impact physical and mental health and well-being, quality of life, and life expectancy (Bartels & Desilets, 2012; Parks et al., 2008).

Smoking Cessation

There is good evidence that rates of smoking in the population are very high in persons labeled with psychiatric disabilities (Kerr, Woods, Knussen, Watson, & Hunter, 2013; Robson & Gray, 2007). For example, the Mental Health Fellowship in Australia (2014) indicates that 40% of the remaining smokers in Australia are people who experience mental illness. High rates of smoking further contribute to their poor physical health and financial hardships. The reasons for these high rates include a complex range of cognitive, behavioral, social, and neurological deficits that are typically associated with many psychiatric disabilities (Robson & Gray, 2007). Research suggests that persons labelled with psychiatric disabilities may experience positive effects from nicotine, such as increases in dopamine, improved attention, and selective processing (Robson & Gray, 2007; Tsai, Porwal, & Webster, 2013). There are also perceived social benefits gained from smoking, such as general feelings of relaxation, pleasure, and increased social contact (Kerr et al., 2013). Historically, smoking has often been encouraged as a cultural component in many mental health services, which has proved a significant barrier to smoking cessation (Tsai et al., 2013). Furthermore, it has been documented that there may be a level of discomfort present in persons labeled with psychiatric disabilities in accessing "mainstream" smoking cessation programs that may be available (Kerr et al., 2013). In occupational therapy, Bejerholm and Eklund's (2004) study of the occupations of people with serious mental illness demonstrated that many use smoking as a kind of "behavioral filler" to fill a void in days filled with passive activity and limited in structured and time-bound activities.

In addition to the many barriers to smoking cessation, the knowledge, attitudes, skills, and beliefs of mental health professionals can often interfere with smoking cessation efforts. A study by Kerr et al. (2013) found that many mental health professionals described being fearful of damaging relationships with those they support by encouraging smoking cessation. Others in the study discussed their lack of confidence in the people they supported to be able to sustain smoking cessation. The results of this study further suggest a lack of knowledge and training of mental health care professionals, which limited the information they were able to share with those they support (Kerr et al., 2013).

Smoking cessation has not historically been routinely addressed or prioritized in mental health services despite the high rates of smoking within the population accessing these services (McKray & Dickerson, 2013). Both persons labeled with psychiatric disabilities and mental health professionals often believe that smoking cessation may cause a worsening of symptoms and overall mental health status; however, there is no strong evidence to support this belief. Occupational therapists in particular may find it difficult to address smoking cessation with individuals for whom smoking constitutes one of the few routine activities in their daily lives. Kerr et al. (2013) suggest that the following characteristics should be considered in interventions for smoking cessation:

> …levels of self-efficacy, motivation, ways of coping with stress and anxiety that bypass the urge to smoke, concerns about deterioration in mental health, knowledge and skills associated with making a cessation attempt (including knowledge of addiction), and an understanding of the link between doses of certain psychotropic medications and smoking/smoking cessation. (p. 11)

Research also demonstrates the importance of considering the effects of smoking cessation on prescribed medications, and ensuring that these are monitored as part of smoking cessation support services (Kerr et al., 2013; Tsai et al., 2013). A study by Tsai et al. (2013) found that certain medications (i.e., bupropion) may be helpful in facilitating sustained abstinence from smoking in persons labeled with schizophrenia. McKay and Dickerson (2013) suggest that the relatively new development of peer-delivered supports for smoking cessation appear to be seen as another helpful approach by persons labeled with psychiatric disabilities, although there is a lack of evidence to support these interventions at present. Kerr et al. (2013) further support the importance of acknowledging the positive impact that peer role models can have on the process of smoking cessation.

Oral Health

Poor oral health affects overall physical health as well as other social and emotional aspects of daily life (Kisley et al., 2011). Poor oral health is associated with diseases such as coronary heart disease, stroke, and respiratory diseases (Kisley et al., 2011). Research has found that persons labeled with psychiatric disabilities are more likely to have oral diseases such as dental caries (tooth decay) and periodontal disease (Almomani, Williams, Catley, & Brown, 2009; Heaton, Mancl, Grembowski, Armfield, & Milgram, 2013; Kisley et al., 2011) than the general population. There are many potential contributors to the poor quality of dental hygiene among those labeled with psychiatric disabilities. These included factors such as motivation, fear, cost, lack of resources, transportation, dental health professionals' attitudes, and knowledge of psychiatric disabilities, as well as the side effects of some psychiatric medications (i.e., dry mouth) (Griffiths et al., 2001; Kisley et al., 2011). Additional factors such as diet, alcohol, substance use, and smoking also contribute to poor oral health.

Kisley et al. (2011) suggest that general screening of oral health is an essential aspect of comprehensive assessments for persons labeled with psychiatric disabilities. The authors suggest the following as basic principles of good oral hygiene:

> …brushing twice a day with a fluoridated tooth-paste; avoidance of sugars in foods or carbonated drinks; healthy eating habits; smoking cessation; and keeping alcohol consumption to a minimum. (p. 191)

Griffiths et al. (2001) further emphasize this point, and discuss the importance of health professionals being trained in basic oral health principles and screening, as well as sharing information and resources with both the individual and their support system. Further research has been done to examine the effects of motivational interviewing on improving oral health education programs for persons labeled with psychiatric disabilities. Almomani et al., (2009) found that the use of motivational interviewing techniques as a component of educational interventions to improve oral health, were associated with improved knowledge and oral hygiene (i.e., reduction in plaque) within this population. Additional support has been given to this approach by Clifton, Tosh, Khokar, Jones, and Wells (2011) who found that motivational interviewing, when combined with educational programs, was the most effective approach in supporting oral health in persons labeled with psychiatric disabilities.

Sleep Hygiene

Sleep disturbances have a negative impact on quality of life and ability to function and are known to also have an impact on the course of many psychiatric disabilities. (Krystal, 2012; Picard, 2012). A study by Hofstetter, Lysaker, and Mayeda (2005) found that poor quality of sleep, which is typical of those labeled with schizophrenia, is directly related to low quality of life and difficulty in coping with stressors. This study suggested the possibility that chronic sleep disturbances may also be related to difficulty in finding positive meaning and the motivation to achieve personal growth. Sleep insufficiency can disrupt a person's life in many different contexts, such as difficulties engaging in activities of daily living, employment, family, and community life. Occupational therapists can address sleep disturbances through holistic assessment of the person, the environment and valued occupations, with the aim of promoting improved sleep to facilitate optimal occupational performance and participation (Picard, 2012).

Research suggests that those labeled with psychiatric disabilities experience a high prevalence of insomnia (Hamera, Brown, & Goetz, 2013; Krystal, 2012). The majority of the research related to sleep disorders for those labeled with psychiatric disabilities focuses primarily on mood disorders, schizophrenia, and alcoholism. In a study looking at sleep disturbances in persons labeled with psychiatric disabilities, Hamera et al. (2013) found that there are distinct sleep disruptions within this population, particularly those who are overweight. The authors suggest that more attention should be brought to screening for conditions such as sleep apnea within this population. This study also supports the importance of limiting daytime naps and adhering to regular bedtime and wake-time routines to promote improved sleep (Hamera et al., 2013).

Sleep deprivation may lead to several negative outcomes such as impairments in cognitive processing, mood, and sensitivity to pain as well as relapse of symptoms (Krystal, 2012). There is clear evidence relating to the negative effect consumption of alcohol can have on the quality and duration of sleep (Krystal & Roth, 2012). Because many individuals use alcohol as a coping strategy for managing insomnia, insomnia is also linked to future alcoholism (Krystal, 2012).

Sleep hygiene is a commonly used approach to change behaviors that are thought to contribute to sleep disturbances. Sleep hygiene refers to:

> …a list of behaviors, environmental conditions, and other sleep related factors that can be adjusted as a stand-alone treatment or component of multimodal treatment for patients with insomnia. (Stepanski & Wyatt, 2003, p. 215)

Although there is limited empirical support for the use of sleep hygiene protocols as the sole treatment approach to support improvements in sleep, there are several key components that are known to be useful. There are also some aspects of sleep hygiene that appear to be more important than others, and research suggests that sleep hygiene techniques are found to be most useful when used in an individualized way and combined with other treatments (Stepanski & Wyatt, 2003).

Stepanski and Wyatt (2003) summarize the key points of sleep hygiene as follows:

- Regular bedtime and wake-time are important factors in a person's daily routine, which promote better quality sleep
- Daytime naps should be avoided as they have a negative impact on the quality of nocturnal sleep
- Consumption of caffeinated beverages prior to bedtime should be limited
- The consumption of alcohol, particularly before bedtime, should be avoided because this is known to negatively affect sleep
- Engaging in exercise several hours prior to bedtime is associated with better quality sleep

- Findings from several studies suggest that raising one's body temperature before bedtime (such as taking a hot bath) can improve sleep quality

In addition to the above sleep hygiene strategies, studies have also shown the positive impact of complementary and alternative therapies on decreasing sleep disturbances. A study by Bosch et al. (2013) found that 3 months of acupuncture treatment was associated with improved sleep quality in individuals with schizophrenia and depression. The acupuncture treatment was found to have the most positive impact on the group with schizophrenia, who also showed a reduction in the reliance on sleep medications following the 12 sessions of acupuncture to aid in improving sleep quality.

Falls Prevention

Research has demonstrated that psychotropic medication increases falls risk in persons labeled with psychiatric disabilities, in particular schizophrenia. Antidepressants and antipsychotics for instance can cause drowsiness, confusion, and balance problems (Ikai et al., 2013; Lee, Mills, & Watts, 2012). In addition, environmental factors, such as lighting, have been found to increase falls risk in inpatient psychiatric units in particular (Lee et al., 2012; Scanlan, Wheatley, & McIntosh, 2012). Outpatient and community-based mental health settings while aware of falls risk, appear to be less likely to have established formal falls prevention programs (Canadian Agency for Drugs and Technologies in Health, 2012).

Lee et al. (2012) studied falls on inpatient psychiatric units and found that falls were most likely to occur when the person was attempting to get up, ambulating, or using the bathroom. These researchers also speculated that staff on mental health units may underestimate falls risk given that most inpatients in mental health units are not medically frail. They also acknowledged that walkers and other assistive devices may not be available. Falls risk assessments of both individuals and the environment are recommended (Lee et al., 2012; Scanlan et al., 2012). While Scanlan, Wheatley, and McIntosh (2012) argued that falls risk assessments available for other populations would be effective, efforts to develop tools specifically for mental health inpatient units are in development. For example, the Edmonson Psychiatric Falls Assessment (EPFRAT; Edmonson, Robinson, & Hughes, 2011) includes weighted ratings related to age, mental status, elimination, medications, diagnosis, ambulation/balance, nutrition, sleep disturbance, and history of falls. Initial testing of the tool found that changes in medication within the past 24 hours and sleep disturbances were most likely to increase risk for falls in an inpatient setting (Edmonson et al., 2011).

PRACTICE DEVELOPMENTS

Key practice developments in the area of health and wellness relevant to occupational therapists include population-level strategies via public health initiatives, organizational-level strategies targeting integration of primary care and behavioral health, and person-level strategies that target lifestyle risk factors, which have been identified as contributing to health problems experienced by persons labeled with psychiatric disabilities.

Public Health Initiatives

Population level health promotion efforts have been strengthened for several decades and disseminated through local and national initiatives across many countries internationally. One example includes the United States' Healthy People initiative, which targets health promotion in the broader societal context. The Healthy People initiative began in 1979 with the Surgeon General's report on health promotion and disease prevention, and has been revisited each decade. The most recent revision is Healthy People 2020 whose vision is "a society in which all people live long, healthy lives" (DHHS, 2000).

Healthy People 2020 has identified the four following foundation health measures that will be used to monitor progress toward goals:

1. General health status

2. Health-related quality of life and well-being

3. Determinants of health (i.e., range of personal, social, economic and environmental factors that influence health status)

4. Health disparities

Note: Health-related quality of life is a multidimensional concept that includes domains related to physical, mental, emotional, and social functioning. It focuses on the effect that health status has on quality of life.

A component of the Healthy People initiative is the National Prevention Strategy (Figure 15-3) This plan outlines the vision, goal, strategic directions, priorities, and resources targeting health promotion (DHHS, 2012). Such initiatives often provide useful resources for down on the ground efforts to promote healthy living that can be incorporated into health and wellness initiatives within mental health services.

Public health initiatives in the broader societal context serve to support public health initiatives targeting particular at-risk populations, for example, the US SAMHSA's 10 x 10 campaign, now known as the Wellness Initiative introduced earlier in this chapter. This public health initiative

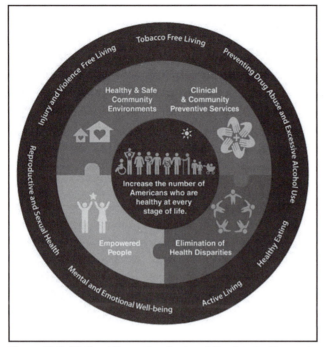

Figure 15-3. "National Prevention Strategy." (Reprinted with permission from National Prevention Council, National Prevention Strategy, Washington, D.C. Copyright 2012 by Department of Health and Human Services.)

targets the health and wellness for people labeled with mental health and substance use conditions in particular. As noted previously, this effort emerged out of growing concern regarding the early mortality rates, and in 2007 SAMHSA hosted the Wellness Summit. An outcome of this summit was the 10 x 10 campaign and a national wellness action plan to improve life expectancy by 10 years in 10 years for people labeled with mental illness. This initiative now hosts an annual National Wellness Week each September around which community- and agency-based wellness promotion efforts can be organized, as well as a resource rich website targeting mental health services that includes wellness tools, webinars, etc.

It is important for occupational therapists to stay abreast of these types of initiatives in their own jurisdiction and be involved in their design and development. They provide an important vehicle to develop, evaluate and disseminate relevant occupational therapy knowledge and practice within newly evolving health-related structures.

Integration of Primary Care and Behavioral Health

Over the last two decades another practice development, influenced by the growing understanding of health risks experienced by persons labeled with psychiatric disabilities is understanding of the need to integrate primary care and behavioral health (Collins, Hewson, Munger, & Wade, 2010;

Koyanagi & Carty, 2004; Mauch & Bartlett, 2013). This has been particularly critical in the United States given the clear disconnect and fragmentation between the mental health delivery system and that part of the health care system targeting physical health needs. This fragmentation has been identified as a contributing factor to the health disparities experienced by persons labeled with psychiatric disabilities (Koyanagi & Carty, 2004).

The Four Quadrant Clinical Integration Model (Mauer, 2003) (see the pictorial version of the model at www.integration.samhsa.gov/clinical-practice/four_quadrant_model.pdf) provides a conceptual framework for primary care and behavioral health care (i.e., mental health) organizations to identify the locus and intensity of care, as well as facilitate decision making and collaboration—who does what, with whom, and where. It was built on a previous model that promoted integration of mental health and substance abuse/addiction services. Each quadrant considers the behavioral health and physical health risk and complexity of the population.

- *Quadrant I* represents the needs of those individuals with low complexity and/or risk with respect to behavioral and physical health complexity/risk. Within this model, services for these individual are most likely to be delivered within the primary care setting, with on-site behavioral health staff. The behavioral health clinician provides consultation to the primary care team, and will engage in triage and assessment, brief treatment, and referrals when behavioral care is indicated. The primary care practitioner provides all biomedical care, including prescribing psychotropic medications.

- *Quadrant II* represents the needs of those individuals with high behavioral health *and* low physical health complexity/risk. Within this model, services for these individuals are most likely to be delivered within what is referred to as the specialty behavioral/mental health service system in coordination with a primary care practitioner or organization. For example, assertive community treatment (ACT) teams represent a well-known full-service, wrap-around *specialty* behavioral health service that has been adopted internationally. The ACT team represents an example of a Quadrant II population and level of care. In this model, in order to promote service integration the ACT team would insure that the ACT clients have access to primary care services. This might be accomplished through a formal inter-organization agreement between an existing ACT team, or the mental health agency that operates the ACT team *and* a local primary care entity.

- *Quadrant III* represents the needs of those individuals with low behavioral health *and* high physical health complexity/risk. Within this model, services for these individuals are most likely to be delivered in the primary care/medical specialty with on-site behavioral staff. The role of the behavioral health clinician here is similar to that identified in *Quadrant I*.

- *Quadrant IV* represents the needs of those individuals with high behavioral health *and* high physical health complexity/risk. Within this model, services for these individuals takes place in both the specialty behavioral health *and* primary care/medical specialty systems. In addition, to behavioral health clinicians, behavioral health case managers *and* the primary care/medical specialty "disease manager" work together to ensure timely and necessary services across the two systems are delivered and coordinated. For example, if an ACT client was hospitalized for medical reasons by the primary care practitioner, the ACT team staff would insure that their client received the behavioral health supports needed during the hospital stay.

This model has been a useful tool in the emergence of integrated behavioral health and primary care services in the United States, especially given the Affordable Care Act.

Lifestyle Interventions

Given the finding that a significant contributing factor to health risks includes the type and level of activity engagement, in particular physical activity, lifestyle interventions have become a critical approach to improving health outcomes for persons labeled with psychiatric disabilities (Bartels & Desilets, 2012). Recently developed lifestyle intervention programs for this population have targeted increased engagement in exercise and improved nutrition knowledge and intake (Bartels et al., 2013; Brown, Goetz, Sciver, Sullivan, & Hamera, 2006; Brown, Goetz, & Hamera 2011; Van Citters et al., 2010). In the United Kingdom, an occupational therapy-lead lifestyle group that focused specifically on the needs of people and included attention to a range of factors including, diet, exercise, and alcohol intake, demonstrated better outcomes in reducing anxiety compared to standard care by a general practitioner (Lambert, Harvey, & Poland, 2007).

Based on a systematic analysis of the evidence for exercise and nutrition interventions targeting persons labeled with psychiatric disabilities, the following key recommendations regarding such interventions have been identified (Bartels & Desilits, 2012):

- Lifestyle health promotion programs of longer duration (3 or more months) consisting of a manualized, combined education- and activity-based approach, and incorporating both nutrition and physical exercise are likely to be the most effective in reducing weight, improving physical fitness, and improving psychological symptoms and overall health.

- Programs that are less likely to be successful include briefer duration interventions; general wellness or health promotion or education-only programs; non-intensive, unstructured, or non-manualized interventions; and programs limited to nutrition only or exercise only (as opposed to combined nutrition and exercise).

- If weight loss is a primary goal, the nutritional component is critical and is more likely to be successful if it incorporates active weight management (i.e., participant and program monitoring of weights and food diaries), as opposed to nutrition education alone.

- If physical fitness is a primary goal, activity-based programs that provide active and intensive exercise and measurement of fitness (e.g., 6-minute walk test or standardized physical activity monitoring) are more likely to be successful, in contrast to programs solely providing education, encouragement, or support for engaging in physical activity

- Evidence-based health promotion consisting of combined physical fitness and nutrition programs should be an integral component of mental health services seeking to provide overall wellness and recovery for persons with serious mental illness

- Lifestyle behaviors (nutrition, physical activity, tobacco use), physical fitness, and weight outcomes, as well as evidence-based program fidelity, should be objectively and reliably measured and monitored both as a component of providing effective health promotion programming and as core indicator of quality mental health services (Bartels & Desilets, 2012).

Occupational therapists have contributed to the development of these interventions. For example the Nutrition and Exercise for Wellness and Recovery (Brown et al., 2011a, 2011b) program developed by occupational therapist and researcher Dr. Cantana Brown and colleagues is now being widely disseminated by the University of Illinois at Chicago's National Research and Training Center on Psychiatric Disability and Co-Occurring Medical Condition (www.cmhsrp.uic.edu/health). As is typical with manualized interventions, the Nutrition and Exercise for Wellness and Recovery includes a Leader Manual and Participant Workbook, and is delivered in eight weekly sessions that facilitate the participants' engagement in an intentional effort at making small lifestyle changes to improve their health. Each session includes weekly goal setting, engagement in a physical activity with the support of other participants, and introduction of guidance on healthy eating and benefits of physical activity. Box 15-3 shows an example from the participant's manual, a modified version of a personal planning document related to weight control. Research of an earlier iteration of the intervention demonstrated that participants who completed the intervention had greater weight loss in comparison to those in the control group (Brown et al., 2011).

BOX 15-3. IDEAS FOR POTENTIAL GOALS

I will drink _____cups of water a day.

I will eat breakfast_____times this week.

I will turn off the television when I eat_____times this week.

I will write out a grocery list before I go to the store this week.

I will portion my snack food in a bowl or baggie instead of eating directly out of the bag/container.

I will tell a friend or family member about what I have accomplished toward being healthy_____times next week.

I will make a plan to exercise with someone else_____times next week.

Selected examples from a worksheet from the Nutrition and Exercise for Wellness and Recovery Participant manual. From Brown, C., Goetz, J., and Bledsoe. C., "Nutrition and exercise for wellness and recovery (NEW-R) leader manual" Copyright © 2011 by UIC Center on Psychiatric Disability and Co-Occurring Medical Conditions, University of Illinois at Chicago. Reprinted with permission.

Peer Providers as Wellness Interveners

A key component of recovery-oriented services has been the full inclusion of peers as service providers (Swarbrick & Schmidt, 2010). Recent innovations in the role of peer specialists in a recovery-oriented mental health service system has been for them to serve as wellness coaches (Swarbrick, 2010, 2013; Swarbrick et al., 2011), peer navigators (Brekke et al., 2013; Kelly et al., 2014), or whole-health specialists (Daniels et al., 2011; Fricks, Powell, & Swarbrick, 2012).

Swarbrick and her colleagues at CSPNJ, a peer-operated agency, collaborated with a local school of allied health to develop a curriculum to prepare peers to become wellness coaches. Curriculum development was informed both by literature and peer review and the findings from family member focus groups. Drawing on contemporary perspectives that distinguish coaching from other forms of counseling or therapy, wellness coaches facilitate goal setting, support to promote progress and accountability, and provide resources to promote wellness and a healthy lifestyle (Swarbrick et al., 2011).

Brekke and colleagues (Brekke et al., 2013) developed the peer navigator intervention that included four components—assessing and planning, coordinated linkages, consumer education, and cognitive-behavioral strategies. This approach drew on existing models for explaining health care utilization rates for vulnerable populations. Adaptations included accounting for the specific factors that may keep persons labeled with psychiatric disabilities from utilizing health services, (i.e., stigma, psychiatric symptoms, and the separation of the physical and mental health services systems). Peer navigators helped their clients to assess their health status, use health services, and address experiences with barriers encountered in accessing and using health services. Further, the peer navigator facilitated their client's actual access and follow-up with health care providers, and provided education regarding health concerns and the health services system. Research demonstrated that the peer navigator intervention improved health outcomes and health care service utilization (Kelly et al., 2014).

SAMHSA's Integrated Behavioral Health initiative known as Whole Health Action Management Support (Fricks et al., 2012) represents another approach to peer-delivered wellness services. This peer-delivered intervention seeks to teach participants the skills needed to better self-manage chronic physical health conditions, and mental illnesses and addictions, to achieve whole health. The Whole Health Action Management intervention consists of a 2-day, 10-session training program focused on 10 health and resiliency factors: stress management, healthy eating, physical activity, restful sleep, service to others, support network, optimism based on positive expectations, cognitive skills to avoid negative thinking, spiritual beliefs and practices, and a sense of meaning and purpose. The whole health perspective that argues for a whole health peer specialist has come to characterize the broad role of peer providers in health and wellness services, especially as efforts for health care reform have evolved in the United States.

CONCLUSION

Public health initiatives have been widely developed internationally to address both the physical and mental health of a population. Health and wellness for persons labeled with psychiatric disabilities has become a central focus of many governments and national behavioral health organizations. The emergence of this as a key element in national public mental health efforts has been strongly influenced by the research identifying reduced morality rates of up to 25 years for persons labeled with psychiatric disabilities in comparison to their peers. Further, evidence that many of the health problems experienced can be improved through lifestyle changes has spurred the development and implementation of health promotion interventions at the individual, program, and community level. Occupational therapists are contributing to the development, dissemination, and evaluation of these lifestyle interventions. In addition to the lifestyle interventions, system change efforts are promoting an integrated approach to behavioral health services. One aspect of this integration is the integration of physical health and mental health services, with the key collaborators in this effort being primary care and specialty mental health services. Occupational therapists' presence in the primary care system is growing and being advocated by national occupational therapy associations.

LEARNING ACTIVITIES/ DISCUSSION QUESTIONS

1. Reflect on your own health and wellness. What intentional practices have you adopted to support your overall health and well-being? What barriers are you experiencing to your enactment of these practices?

2. Reflect on your practice as an occupational therapist. To what degree do you frame your work as an occupational therapist from a health and wellness perspective? To what degree does the organization in which you work foreground health and wellness for its service recipients?

3. How familiar are you with national efforts in your country to promote health and wellness for persons labeled with psychiatric disabilities? Investigate if, and how, your national association is collaborating with other stakeholders in promoting health and wellness for persons labeled with psychiatric disabilities. Identify what you might do locally to promote these collaborations.

4. Reflect on the health and wellness targets and intervention strategies identified in this chapter. Think about the populations of people with mental health issues you know or have worked with. To what degree is the mental health population that you are working with experiencing these health challenges? Which health promotion intervention strategies would make sense in your practice context?

REFERENCES

Almomani, F., Williams, K., Catley, D., & Brown, C. (2009). Effects of an oral health promotion program in people with mental illness. *Journal of Dental Research, 88*(7), 648-52.

American Occupational Therapy Association. (2013). Occupational therapy in the promotion of health and well-being. *American Journal of Occupational Therapy, 67*.

Bartels, S., & Desilets, R. (2012). *Health promotion programs for people with serious mental illness*. (Prepared by the Dartmouth Health Promotion Research Team). Washington, DC: SAMHSA-HRSA Center for Integrated Health Solutions.

Bartels, S. J., Pratt, S. I., Aschbrenner, K. A., Barre, L. K., Jue, K., Wolfe, R. S.,…Mueser, K. T. (2013). Clinically significant improved fitness and weight loss among overweight persons with serious mental illness. *Psychiatric Services, 64*(8), 729-736. doi: 10.1176/appi.ps.003622012

Bazelon. (2004). *How to integrate physical and mental health care for people with serious mental disorders*. Washington, DC: Bazelon Center for Mental Health Law.

Bejerholm, U., & Eklund, M. (2004). Time use and occupational performance among people with schizophrenia. *Occupational Therapy in Mental Health, 20*, 27-45.

Bosch, P., van Luijtelaar, G., van den Noort, M., Lim, S., Egger, J., & Coenen, A. (2013). Sleep ameliorating effects of acupuncture in a psychiatric population. *Evidence-Based Complementary and Alternative Medicine, 2013*, Article ID 969032, 10 p. doi:10.1155/2013/969032

Braveman, P., & Gottlieb, L. (2014). The social determinants of health: It's time to consider the causes of the causes. *Public Health Reports, 129*(2), 19-31.

Brekke, J. S., Siantz, E., Pahwa, R., Kelly, E., Tallne, L., & Fulginiti, A. (2013). Reducing health disparities for people with serious mental illness: Development and feasibility of a peer health navigation intervention. *Best Practices in Mental Health, 9*(1), 62-82.

Breslow, L. (1999). From disease prevention to health promotion. *Journal of American Medicine, 281*(11), 1030-1033.

Brown, C., Goetz, J., & Bledsoe, C. (2011a). *Nutrition and exercise for wellness and recovery (NEW-R) leader manual*. Chicago, IL: UIC Center on Psychiatric Disability and Co-Occurring Medical Conditions.

Brown, C., Goetz, J., & Bledsoe, C. (2011b). Nutrition and exercise for wellness and recovery (NEW-R) participant manual. Chicago, IL: UIC Center on Psychiatric Disability and Co-Occurring Medical Conditions.

Brown, C., Goetz, J., & Hamera, E. (2011). Weight loss intervention for people with serious mental illness: A randomized controlled trial of the RENEW program. *Psychiatric Services, 62*(7), 800-802.

Brown, C., Goetz, J., Sciver, A. V., Sullivan, D., & Hamera, E. (2006). A psychiatric rehabilitation approach to weight loss. *Psychiatric Rehabilitation Journal, 29*(4), 267-273.

Canadian Agency for Drugs and Technology in Health. (2012). Falls prevention strategies in adult outpatient or community-based mental health and/or addiction programs. Canada: Canadian Agency for Drugs and Technologies in Health.

Center for Mental Health Services. (2007). *The 10 by 10 campaign: A national plan to improve life expectancy by 10 years in 10 years for people with mental illness: A report of the 2007 National Wellness Summit*. Rockville, MD: Center for Mental Health Services, Substance Abuse and Mental Health Services Administration.

Clark, F., Azen, S. P., Zemke, R., Jackson, J., Carlson, M., Mandel, D.,...Lipson, L. (1997). Occupational therapy for independent-living older adults: A ramdomized controlled trial. *Journal of American Medicine, 278*(16), 1321-1326.

Clark, F., Parham, E., Carlson, M., Frank, G., Jackson, J., Pierce, D.,& Zemke, R. (1991). Occupational science: Academic innovation in the service of the occupational therapy's future. *American Journal of Occupational Therapy, 45*(4), 300-310.

Clifton, A., Tosh, G., Khokar, W., Jones,H., & Wells, N. (2011). Oral health advice for people with serious mental illness. *Schizophrenia Bulletin, 37*(3), 464-65.

College of Occupational Therapists. (2008). *Health promotion in occupational therapy.* London: College of Occupational Therapists.

Collins, C., Hewson, D. L., Munger, R., & Wade, T. (2010). *Evolving models of behavioral health integration in primary care.* New York: Milbank Memorial Fund.

Copeland, M. E. (2001). Wellness recovery action plan: A system for monitoring, recording and eliminating uncomfortable or dangerous physical symptoms and emotional feelings. In C. Brown (Ed.), *Recovery and wellness: Models of hope and empowerment for people with mental illness* (pp. 127-150). New York: Haworth Press.

Cowen, E. L. (2000). Now that we all know that primary prevention in mental health is great, what is it? *Journal of Community Psychology, 28*(1), 5-16.

Cutchin, M. P., Aldrich, R. M., Bailliard, A. L., & Coppola, S. (2008). Action theories for occupational science: The contributions of Dewey and Bourdieu. *Journal of Occupational Science, 15*(3), 157-165.

Daniels, A. S., Tunner, T. P., Ashenden, P., Bergeson, S., Frisk, L., & Powell, I. (2011). Pillars of Peer Support Services Summitt III: Whole Health Peer Support Services.

Department of Health and Human Services. (1999). *Mental health: A report of the surgeon general.* Rockland, MD: Department of Health and Human Services, U.S. Public Health Services.

Department of Health and Human Services. (2000). Health People 2020: *Understanding and improving health* (2nd ed.). Washington, DC: U.S. Government Printing Office.

Department of Health and Human Services. (2003). *The President's New Freedom Commission on Mental Health Achieving the Promise: Transforming mental health care in America.* Washingston, DC: Department of Health and Human Services.

Department of Health and Human Services. (2005). *Transforming mental health care in America—The Federal Action agenda: First steps.* Washington DC: Department of Health and Human Services.

Department of Health and Human Services. (2012). *National prevention council action plan: Implementing the national prevention strategy.* Washington, DC: National Prevention, Health Promotion, and Public Health Council.

Dunn, W. (1994). The ecology of human performance: A framework for considering the effect of context. *American Journal of Occupational Therapy, 48*(7), 595-607.

Edmonson, D., Robinson, S., & Hughes, L. (2011). Development of the Edmonson PSYCHIATRIC FALL RISK ASSESSMENT TOOL. *Journal of Psychosocial Nursing and Mental Health, 49*(2), 29-36.

Edwards, A. (2013). OT and the social determinants of health—tracking 'the causes of the causes.' *OT News, 4,* 40-41.

Finlayson, M., & Edwards, J. (1995). Integrating the concepts of health promotion and community into occupational therapy practice. *Canadian Occupational Therapy Journal, 62*(2), 70-75S.

Fricks, L., Powell, I., & Swarbrick, P. (2012). *Whole health action management (WHAM) peer support training participant guide.* Washington, DC: SAMHSA-HRSA Center for Integrated Solutions.

Golden, S. D., & Earp, J. A. L. (2012). Social ecological approaches to individuals and their contexts: Twenty years of health education & behavior health promotion interventions. *Health Education & Behavior, 39*(3), 364-372. doi: 10.1177/1090198111418634

Griffiths, J., Jones, V., Leeman, I., Lewis, D., Patel, K., Wilson, K., & Blankenstein, R. (2001). *Oral health care for people with mental health problems: Guidelines and recommendations.* British Society for Disability and Oral Health. Retrieved from https://www.adelaide.edu.au/oral-health-promotion/resources/prof/htm_files/BSDH2000.pdf.

Hamera, E., Brown, C., & Goetz, J. (2013). Objective and subjective sleep disturbances in individuals with psychiatric disabilities. *Issues in Mental Health Nursing, 34* (2), 110-116.

Heaton, L. J., Mancl, L. A., Grembowski, D., Armfield, J. M., & Milgram, P. (2013). Unmet dental need in community-dwelling adults with mental illness: Results from the 2007 Medical Expenditure Panel Survey. *Journal of the American Dental Association, 144*(3), e16-e23.

Hoffstetter, J. R., Lysaker, P. H., & Mayeda, A. R. (2005). Quality of sleep in patients with schizophrenia is associated with quality of life and coping. *BMC Psychiatry* 2005, 5,13 doi:10.1186/1471-244X-5-13.

Holmberg, V., & Ringsberg, K. (2014). Occupational therapists as contributors to health promotion. *Scandinavian Journal of Occupational Therapy, 21,* 82-89.

Hopper, K. (2007). Rethinking social recovery in schizophrenia: What a capabilities approach might offer. *Social Science & Medicine,65*(5), 868-879. doi:10.1016/j.socscimed.2007.04.012

Houghton, J. F. (1982). Maintaing mental health in a turbulent world. *Schizophrenia Bulletin, 8,* 548-552.

Hutchinson, D. S., Gagne, C., Bowers, A., Russinova, Z., Skrinar, G. S., & Anthony, W. A. (2006). A framework for health promotion services for people with psychiatric disabilities. *Psychiatric Rehabilitation Journal, 29*(4), 241-250. doi: 10.2975/29.2006.241.250

Ikai, S., Uchida, H., Suzuki, T., Tsunoda, K., Mimura, M., & Fujii, Y. (2013). Effects of yoga therapy on postural stability in patients with schizophrenia-spectrum disorders: A single-blind randomized controlled trial. *Journal of Psychiatric Research, 47,* 1744-1750.

Johnson, J. A. (1986). *Wellness: A context for living.* Thorofare, NJ: SLACK Incorporated.

Kelly, E., Fulginiti, A., Pahwa, R., Tallen, L., Duann, L., & Brekke, J. S. (2014). A pilot test of a peer navigator intervention for improving the health of individuals with serious mental illness. *Community Mental Health Journal, 50*(4), 435-446.

Kerr, S., Woods, C., Knussen,C., Watson, H., & Hunter, R. (2013). Breaking the habit: a qualitative exploration of barriers and facilitators to smoking cessation in people with enduring mental health problems. *BMC Public Health, 13,* 221. doi:10.1186/1471-2458-13-221.

Kielhofner, G. (2008). *Model of human occupations: Theory and application*, (4th ed.). Baltimore, MD: Lippincott, Williams & Wilkins.

Kisley, S., Quek, L. H., Pais,J., Lalloo, R., Johnson, N.W. & Lawrence, D. (2011). Advanced dental disease in people with severe mental illness: systematic review and meta-analysis. *British Journal of Psychiatry, 199*(3):187-93. doi: 10.1192/bjp.bp.110.081695

Klaiman, D. (2004). Increasing access to occupational therapy in primary health care. *OT Now, 6.*

Koyanagi, C., & Carty, L. (2004). *How to integrate physical and mental health care for people with serious mental disorders.* Washington, DC: Bazelon Center for Mental Health Law.

Krystal, A.D. (2012). Psychiatric disorders and sleep. *Neurologic Clinic, 30,* 1389-1413.

Krystal, A.D.. & Roth, T. M. (2008). Sleep disturbance in psychiatric disorders: Effects of function and quality of life in mood disorders, alcoholism and schizophrenia. *Annals of Clinical Psychiatry, 20*(1), 39-46.

Lalonde, M. (1981/1974). *A new perspective on the health of Canadians: A working document* (Cat. No. H31-1374). Canada: Minister of Supply and Services.

Lambert, R. A., Harvey, I., & Poland, F. (2007). A pragmatic, unblinded randomised controlled trial comparing an occupational therapy-led lifestyle approach and routine GP care for panic disorder treatment in primary care. *Journal of Affective Disorders, 99,* 63-71.

Law, M., Steinwender, S., & Leclair, L. (1998). Occupation, health and well-being. *Canadian Journal of Occupational Therapy, 65*(2), 81-91.

Lee, A., Mills, P. D., & Watts, B. V. (2012). Using root cause analysis to reduce falls with injury in the psychiatric unit. *Science Direct, 34,* 304-311.

Lutterman, T., Ganju, V., Schacht, L., Shaw, R., & Monihan, K. (2003). *Sixteen state study on mental health performance measures.* Rockville, MD: Center for Mental Health Services, Substance Abuse and Mental Health Services Administration.

Manderscheid, R., Druss, B., & Freeman, E. (2008). Data to manage the mortality crisis. *International Journal of Mental Health, 37*(2), 49-68.

Mauch, D., & Bartlett, J. (2013). Integrated behavioral health in public health care contexts: Community health and mental health safety net systems. In M. R. Talen & A. B. Valeras (Eds.), *Integrated behavioral health in primary care: Evaluating the evidence, identifying the essentials.* New York: Springer Science+Business Media.

Mauer, B. J. (2003). *Behavioral health/primary care integration models, competencies, and infrastructure.* Rockville, MD: National Council for Community Behavioral Healthcare.

McFarlane, W. R. (2011). Prevention of the first episode of psychosis. *Psychiatric Clinics of North America, 34*(1), 95-107. doi: 10.1016/j.psc.2010.11.012

McKay, C. E., & Dickerson, F. (2012). Peer supports for tobacco cessation for adults with serious mental illness: A review of the literature. *Journal of Dual Diagnosis, 8*(2), 104-112.

Mental Health Fellowship of Australia (2014). The physical health of people with mental illness. Retrieved from www.mifa.org.au/index.php/media-alias/physical-health-and-wellbeing.

Meyer, A. (1922). The philosophy of occupation therapy. *Archives of Occupational Therapy, 1*(1), 1-10.

Moll, S., Gewurtz, R., Krupa, T., Law, M., Lariviere, N., & Levasseur, M. (2014). Do-live-well: A Canadian framework for promoting occupation, health, and well-being: « Vivez-Bien-Votre Vie » : un cadre de référence canadien pour promouvoir l'occupation, la santé et le bien-être *Canadian Journal of Occupational Therapy,* 0008417414545981, first published on August 21, 2014 as doi:10.1177/0008417414545981.

Parks, J., Radke, A. Q., & Mazade, N. A. (2008). *Measurement of health status for people with serious mental illness* (vol. 16). Alexandria, VA: National Association of State Mental Health Program Directors.

Picard, M. M. (2012). Occupational therapists' role in sleep.. *AOTA Fact Sheet.* American Association of Occupational Therapy. Retrieved from www.aota.org/-/media/Corporate/Files/AboutOT/Professionals/WhatIsOT/HW/Facts/sleep.pdf.

Potvin, L., & Jones, C. M. (2011). Twenty-five years after the Ottawa Charter: The critical role of health promotion for public health. *Canadian Journal of Public Health, 102*(4), 244-248.

Reilly, M. (2005/1961). Occupational therapy can be one of the great ideas of 20th-century medicine. In R. Padilla (Ed.), *A professional legacy: The Eleanor Clarke Slagle lectures in occupational therapy, 1955-2004,* (2nd ed.). Bethesda, MD: AOTA Press.

Reitz, S. M. (1992). A historical review of occupational therapy's role in preventive health and wellness. *American Journal of Occupational Therapy, 46*(1), 50-55.

Reitz, S. M., Scaffa, M. E., & Pizzi, M. A. (2010). Occupational therapy conceptual models for health promotion practice. In M. E. Scaffa, S. M. Reitz & M. A. Pizzi (Eds.), *Occupational therapy in the promotion of health and wellness* (pp. 22-45). Philadelphia: F. A. Davis Company.

Robson, D &Gray R. (2007). Serious mental illness and physical health problems: A discussion paper. *International Journal of Nursing Studies, 44,* 457-466.

Scanlan, J., Wheatley, J., & McIntosh, S. (2012). Characteristics of falls in inpatient psychiatric units. *Australiasian Psychiatry, 20*(4), 305-308.

Stempanski, E. J. & Wyatt, J. K. (2003). Use of sleep hygiene in the treatment of insomnia. *Sleep Medical Review, 7*(3), 215-225.

Strong, S., Rigby, P., Stewart, D., Law, M., Letts, L., & Cooper, B. (1999). Application of the person-environment-occupation model: A practical tool. *Canadian Journal of Occupational Therapy, 66*(3), 122-133.

Swarbrick, M. (1997). A wellness model for clients. *AOTA Mental Health Special Interest Quarterly, 20*, 1-4.

Swarbrick, M. (2010). *Peer wellness coaching supervisor manual.* Freehold, NJ: Collaborative Support Programs of New Jersey, Institute for Wellness and Recovery Initiatives.

Swarbrick, M. (2013). Integrated care: Wellness-oriented peer approaches: A key ingredient for integrated care. *Psychiatric Services, 64*(8), 723-726. doi: 10.1176/appi.ps.201300144

Swarbrick, M., Murphy, A. A., Zechner, M., Spagnolo, A. B., & Gill, K. J. (2011). Wellness coaching: A new role for peers. *Psychiatric Rehabilitation Journal, 34*(4), 328-331.

Swarbrick, M., & Schmidt, L. (2010). *People in recovery as providers of psychiatric rehabilitation: Building on the wisdom of experience.* Linthicum, MD: United States Psychiatric Rehabilitation Association.

Tountas, Y. (2009). The historical origins of the basic concepts of health promotion and education: the role of ancient Greek philosophy and medicine. *Health Promotion International, 24*(2), 185-192.

Townsend, E. (2003). Reflections on power and justice in enabling occupation. *Canadian Journal of Occupational Therapy, 70*(2), 74-87.

Townsend, E. A., & Polatajko, H. J. (2007). *Enabling occupation II: Advancing an occupational therapy vision for health, well-being & justice through occupation.* Ottawa: Canadian Occupational Therapy Association.

Townsend, E., & Whiteford, G. (2005). A participatory occupational justice framework: Population-based processes of practice. In F. Kronenberg, S. S. Algado & N. Pollard (Eds.), *Occupational therapy without borders: Learning from the spirit of survivors.* New York: Elsevier Churchill Livingstone.

Tsai, D. T., Porwal, M. & Webster, A. C. (2013). Interventions for smoking cessation and reduction individuals with schizophrenia (review). *Cochrane Database of Systematic Reviews,* Issue 2. Art. No.: CD007253. DOI: 10.1002/14651858. CD007253.pub3.

Tucker, P., Vanderloo, L. M., Irwin, J. D., Mandich, A. D., & Bossers, A. M. (2014). Exploring the nexus between health promotion and occupational therapy: Synergies and similarities. Explorer le lien entre la promotion de la santé et l'ergothérapie: Synergies et similarités. *Canadian Journal of Occupational Therapy.* doi: 10.1177/0008417414533300

University of Ottawa. (2015). Categories of prevention. Retrieved from www.med.uottawa.ca/sim/data/Prevention_e.htm.

Van Citters, A., Pratt, S., Jue, K., Williams, G., Miller, P., Xie, H., & Bartels, S. (2010). A pilot evaluation of the in shape individualized health promotion intervention for adults with mental illness. *Community Mental Health Journal, 46*(6), 540-552. doi: 10.1007/s10597-009-9272-x

Vandiver, V. L. (2009). *Integrating health promotion and mental health: An introduction to policies, principles and practices.* New York: Oxford University Press.

Veenstra, G., & Burnett, P. J. (2014). Towards a relational health promotion. *Health Promotion International.* doi: 10.1093/heapro/dau068

Weimer, R. (1972). Some concepts of prevention as an aspect of community health. *American Journal of Occupational Therapy. 26*, 1-9.

White, W. A. (1923). *The principles of mental hygiene.* New York: The MacMillan Company.

Whiteford, G. (2000). Occupational deprivation: Global challenge in the new millennium. *The British Journal of Occupational Therapy, 63*(5), 200-204.

Whiteford, G., Townsend, E., & Hocking, C. (2000). Reflections on a renaissance of occupation. *Canadian Journal of Occupational Therapy, 67*(1), 61-69.

Wilcock, A. (2006). *Occupational perspective of health* (2nd ed.). Thorofare, NJ: SLACK Incorporated.

Wilcock, A. A. (2002). Reflections on doing, being and becoming. *Australian Occupational Therapy Journal, 46*(1), 1-11.

Williams, S. J. (1995). Theorising class, health and lifestyles: Can Bourdieu help us? *Sociology of Health & Illness, 17*(5), 577-604. doi: 10.1111/1467-9566.ep10932093

World Health Organization. (1948). Preamble to the Constitution of the World Health Organization as adopted by the International Health Conference, New York, 19-22 June 1946; signed on 22 July 1946 by the representatives of 61 States (Official Records of the World Health Organization, no. 2, p. 100) and entered into force on 7 April 1948.

World Health Organization. (1986). *Ottawa charter for health promotion.* Geneva: World Health Organization.

World Health Organization. (2002). *International Classification of functioning, disability and health.* Geneva, Switzerland: World Health Organization.

World Health Organization. (2004). Promoting mental health: Concepts, emerging evidence, practice. In H. Herrman, S. Sazena, & R. Moodie (Eds.). Geneva, Switzerland: World Health Organization, Department of Mental Health and Substance Abuse in collaboration with the Victorian Health Promotion Foundation and the University of Melbourne.

World Health Organization. (2007). *Mental health: Strengthening mental health promotion.* Geneva, Switzerland: World Health Organization.

World Health Organization. (2014a). Determinants of health. Retrieved from www.who.int/hia/evidence/doh/en/ on September 10, 2014.

World Health Organization. (2014b). Social determinants of health. Retrieved from www.who.int/social_determinants/sdh_definition/en/.

Yanos, P. T., Knight, E. L., & Roe, D. (2006). Recognizing a role for structure and agency: Integrating sociological perspectives into the study of recovery from severe mental illness. In W. R. Avison, J. D. McLeod, & B. A. Pescosolido (Eds.), *Mental health, social mirror.* New York: Springer.

16

Organizational Culture Frameworks Related to Mental Health
Implications and Applications for Occupational Therapy

Rebecca Gewurtz, PhD, OT Reg (Ont) and
Bonnie Kirsh, PhD, OT Reg (Ont)

I think it starts with raising awareness among employers that poor management practices (work overload/treadmill syndrome, lack of direction, lack of recognition/rewards, etc.) can cause or exacerbate a mental health condition. I think many employers see it as strictly a medical event and don't recognize the connection between how people are managed and the prevalence of mental health events.

Executive, Disability Insurance Carrier, Gilbert and Bilsker (2012). *Psychological Health and Safety in the Workplace,* 2013 (the Canadian Standard), p. 24.

OBJECTIVES

The objectives of this chapter are as follows:

» Present an overview of organizational culture frameworks and concepts as they relate to mental health.

» Consider how key concepts from organizational culture frameworks can be applied to psychosocial occupational therapy practice, particularly in the context of the workplace.

» Provide examples of tools and practices used by occupational therapists that are grounded in an organizational culture perspective.

Krupa, T., Kirsh, B., Pitts, D., & Fossey, E. *Bruce & Borg's*
Psychosocial Frames of Reference: Theories, Models, and Approaches for
Occupation-Based Practice, Fourth Edition (pp 265-284).
© 2016 SLACK Incorporated.

BACKGROUND

Occupational therapists are interested in how environmental contexts influence human occupation. Our guiding models such as the Canadian Model of Occupational Performance and Engagement (Polatajko, Townsend, & Craik, 2007) and the Person-Environment-Occupation model (Law et al., 1996) position the environment as a critical component of human functioning and occupational therapy practice. Much literature within occupational therapy has focused on how environments influence occupational performance and engagement, and how environments can be either enabling or disabling (Jongbloed & Crichton, 1990; Law et al., 1996; Letts, Rigby, & Stewart, 2003; Whalley Hammell, 2006). Organizational culture is a specific domain that, although not highly present within the occupational therapy literature, is consistent with the dynamic and complex way that occupational therapists have viewed the relationship between people, their occupations, and environments (Law et al., 1996). It is a critical feature to examine to understand individuals and their occupational experiences within organizations such as modern workplaces.

Occupational therapists who address workplace and employment-related issues have traditionally focused on individuals. They are often called upon to address the needs of an individual experiencing a mental health challenge at work who might be in need of accommodations, or an individual who is preparing to return to work after being on leave. Less common is attention to the organizational culture and organizational features and conditions that affect the mental health of workers (Braveman & Page, 2012). However, a comprehensive approach to workplace mental health and well-being requires attention to organizational factors that affect health and well-being (Shain & Kramer, 2004).

In this chapter, we present organizational culture frameworks related to mental health for integration into the theory and practice of psychosocial occupational therapy. We focus on the impact of organizational culture on the experiences of workers, and how organizational culture can inform the work of occupational therapists. We consider components of organizational culture and suggest how they influence mental health and how they can be used by occupational therapists in practice. We also highlight potential threats and promising developments in the field. Although we most often draw on the workplace as an example, we use the term organization broadly to include any social unit of people that is structured and managed to meet a need or pursue a collective goal (Business Dictionary, n.d.) including for-profit, non-profit, or charitable initiatives, as well as public or private enterprises.

WHAT IS ORGANIZATIONAL CULTURE?

Organizational culture refers to the shared values, beliefs, expectations and daily experiences among members of an organization (Moran & Volkwein, 1992; Spataro, 2005). It emerges through the complex and continuous process of communication and interaction among members (Keyton, 2005), and shapes much of what occurs within an organization by dictating norms, rules, processes, policies, and procedures (Spataro, 2005); leadership and managerial styles (Quick, Macik-Fey, & Cooper, 2007); as well as attitudes and perceptions of members. As articulated by Peterson and Wilson (2002), organizational culture "defines how we act, think and behave, it serves to provide structure that helps make work predictable and stable" (p. 18). Thus, a good understanding of the culture of an organization is critical to examine or modify structures, processes, and behaviors that can affect the health and well-being of all members (Scott, Mannion, Davies, & Marshall, 2003).

Organizational culture encompasses three levels of increasing visibility that have implications for occupational therapists. First, norms and customs are the fundamental level of organizational culture and are often described as the "taken-for-granted" or entrenched and unspoken rules and assumptions that guide an organization (Schein, 1992; Schur, Kruse, & Blanck, 2005). A second level includes qualities such as preferences, goals, principles, and strategies that are more explicitly stated within organizational documents (Keyton, 2005; Schein, 1992; Schur et al., 2005). This level includes, for example, mission statements, vision statements, or values that guide an organization. A third level, the artifacts of organizational culture, consists of the visible and tangible objects, social conventions, routines, or procedures that an outsider would notice (Keyton, 2005; Schein, 1992; Schur et al., 2005). Overall, organizational culture can offer much insight into the way different members are perceived, treated ,and behave.

Why Should We Be Concerned About Organizational Culture?

The mental health of workers has become a pressing issue as workplaces aim to maintain their competitive edge by promoting optimal productivity and innovation, while managing worker absenteeism and employee recruitment and retention. Organizational factors are key to the health, and in particular, the mental health of members (Gilbert & Bilsker, 2012; Kirsh & Gewurtz, 2012; Shain & Kramer, 2004; Wilson, DeJoy, Vandenberg, Richardson, & McGrath, 2004). Indeed, it has been shown that healthy work organizations, characterized by "intentional, systematic, and

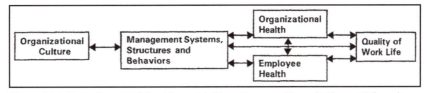

Figure 16-1. The culture-work-health model. (From Peterson, M., and Wilson, J.,"The culture-work-health model and work stress," *American Journal of Health Behavior, 26*, p. 17. Copyright © 2002 by PNG Publications. Reprinted with permission.)

collaborative efforts to maximize employee well-being and productivity by providing well-designed and meaningful jobs, a supportive social-organizational environment, and accessible and equitable opportunities for career and work-life enhancement" (Wilson et al., 2004, p. 567) experience productivity benefits (Kirsh & Gewurtz, 2012; Peterson & Wilson, 2002). By the same token, it is incumbent upon occupational therapists, who have long been involved in promoting health through occupation among people who have experienced, or are at risk for, mental health problems to be concerned with organizational culture as a determinant of occupational performance and engagement, health and well-being. It is from this perspective that we present organizational culture frameworks relevant to mental health, for integration into psychosocial occupational therapy.

ORGANIZATIONAL CULTURE FRAMEWORKS RELEVANT TO HEALTH

Organizational culture frameworks have been developed within the workplace health literature. These frameworks can inform our understanding of the relationship between job and organizational attributes, the health and well-being of workers, as well as work outcomes such as job satisfaction, job performance, retention and turnover, and productivity. In this section, we provide an overview of existing organizational culture frameworks relevant to health, key concepts that are common across such frameworks, and their relevance for psychosocial occupational therapy practice.

The Culture-Work-Health model (Peterson & Wilson, 2002; Figure 16-1) highlights the need to move beyond a focus on individual workers and address the cause of workplace stress through organizational culture. According to this model, organizational culture influences management structures (how people and the work are organized) and behaviors (practices), which in turn impact the health of the organization (success, productivity, innovation, competitiveness, profit), the health of employees (mental and physical), and the quality of work life (moral values, satisfaction, attitudes, and perceptions toward the organization). Organizational health, employee health, and the quality of the work life are inter-related and important

indicators of health and well-being within an organization. By examining group-level perceptions, cultural factors that contribute to unhealthy organizations can be identified and addressed. Rather than focusing on individuals and implementing individual coping strategies, the Culture-Work-Health model highlights the effectiveness of instituting organizational strategies that can improve the overall culture and conditions of the organization. Thus, according to Peterson and Wilson (2002): "[Organizational] culture is the bridge upon which business and health professionals can meet. It is the means by which stress can be mainstreamed into a company's mission and core values" (p. 23).

Another theoretical model of healthy work organization, proposed by Wilson et al. (2004; Figure 16-2), centers on the premise that it should be possible to identify job and organizational characteristics of healthy organizations, and organizations that adopt these characteristics should have healthier and more productive workers. The model was developed based on the available literature on healthy work organizations that has emphasized the importance of job and organization-level actions and attributes that support healthy work organizations. It consists of three distinct domains of work life—job design, organizational climate, and job future. *Job design* emphasizes employees' perceptions of their work, *organizational climate* emphasizes the social and interpersonal environment of the workplace, and *job future* focuses on job security, perceptions of equity and fairness, and opportunities for career development. This model was tested and validated by 1130 employees of a national retailer in the United States and was found to impact psychological work adjustment, and employee health and well-being. The authors highlight the importance of open communication, employee involvement, social support, and recognition and reward in promoting healthy organizations and healthy individuals within organizations.

Another model of organizational health, this one developed by Shain and Kramer (2004) through a review of the research evidence, focuses on the forces acting on the health and productivity of workers (Figure 16-3). The model suggests that both personal health practices and organizational factors contribute equally to the health and productivity of an organization. Personal health practices are typically the focus of research and practice within health promotion. They consist of activities that individuals

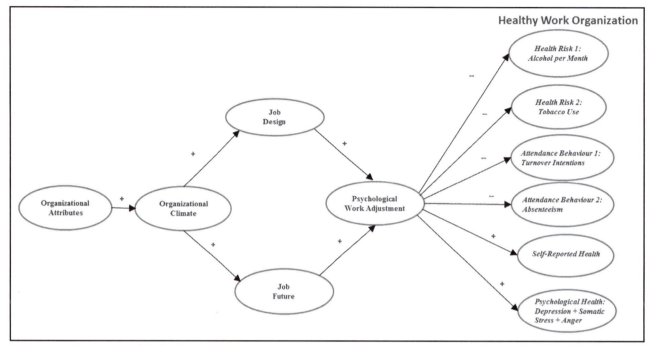

Figure 16-2. Theoretical model of healthy work organization. (From "Work characteristics and employee health and well-being: Test of a model of healthy work organization," by M. G. Wilson, D. M. DeJoy, R. J. Vandenberg, H. A. Richardson, A. L. McGrath, *Journal of Occupational and Organizational Psychology*, *77*, p. 568. Copyright © 2004 by John Wiley and Sons. Reprinted with permission.)

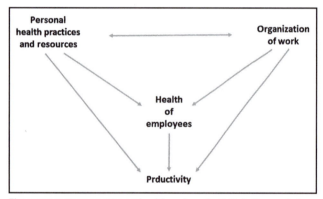

Figure 16-3. Forces acting on health and productivity in the workplace. (From Shain, M., and Kramer, D.M., "Health promotion in the workplace: Framing the concept; reviewing the evidence," *Occupational and Environmental Medicine*, *61*, p. 644. Copyright © 2004 by BMJ Publishing Group Ltd. Reprinted with permission.)

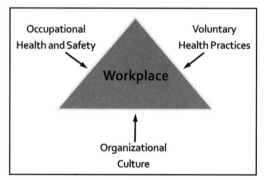

Figure 16-4. The Comprehensive Workplace Health Promotion Model. (From "Comprehensive Workplace Health Promotion—Affecting Mental Health in Workplace," by Health Communication Unit. Retrieved from http://wmhp.cmhaontario.ca/comprehensive-workplace-health-promotion-affecting-mental-health-in-the-workplace. Reprinted with permission.)

can incorporate into their lifestyle such as improving their eating, exercising, sleeping, and their capacity to cope with stress, while reducing smoking and alcohol consumption. Organizational factors, on the other hand, consist of factors related to organizational culture such as work demands, control/autonomy, systems of reward and recognition, and leadership/management practices. According to this model, a comprehensive approach to health promotion that targets both personal health practices and organizational factors together will be most effective for the health and productivity of employees within an organization.

The combined effects of individual and organizational forces forms the basis of the Comprehensive Workplace Health Promotion (CWHP) Model by the Health Communication Unit and the Canadian Mental Health Association, Ontario (Shain & Suurvali, 2001; http://wmhp.cmhaontario.ca/comprehensive-workplace-health-promotion-affecting-mental-health-in-the-workplace#_ftn3; Figure 16-4). The CWHP addresses three important categories: occupational health and safety, voluntary health practices, and organizational culture. According to this model, occupational health and safety is the promotion and maintenance of health and wellness of workers through efforts to reduce workplace injuries, illness, and disability. Voluntary health practices, healthy lifestyles, and personal health practices are used interchangeably to describe the

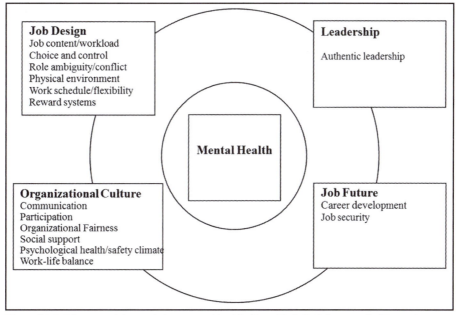

Figure 16-5. A framework for workplace mental health. (From Kirsh, B., & Gewurtz, R., "Promoting mental health within workplaces," *Handbook of Occupational Health and Wellness*, p. 244. Copyright © 2012 by Springer Science+Business Media New York. Reprinted with permission.)

behaviors of individuals that affect health and well-being. Organizational culture, as described throughout this chapter, refers to the underlying values and beliefs that pervade the workplace context and affect the interaction between people, their work, and the organization. The CWHP enables the development of strategies that target these three areas in order to promote workplace health in a comprehensive way.

Drawing on these frameworks and findings from research conducted in the fields of organizational development, health and safety, and mental health, Kirsh and Gewurtz (2012) present a related framework for workplace mental health (Figure 16-5) that delineates key areas of focus for promoting mental health at work. Their framework includes job design, leadership, organizational culture, and job future. Consistent with the Wilson et al. (2004) framework, *job design* refers to work tasks and conditions and how they are perceived and experienced by workers, while *job future* consists of worker expectations for the future within their job and organization. *Organizational culture* is defined broadly as factors that dictate norms, rules, expectations, and actions, and generally refers to the workplace context. *Leadership*, often considered a component of organizational culture, is specifically highlighted given its important contribution to the creation of healthy workplaces. It consists of the overall supervisory/management style, perceptions of justice, and treatment of subordinates.

These frameworks highlight the prominence of organizational culture in the health and mental health of individuals within organizations. In particular, they point to the need to move beyond individual factors and consider

how organizations contribute to the health and well-being of members. Rather than focusing solely on individuals and their behaviors and health practices, there is a need to create and promote healthy organizational conditions that are conducive to health and well-being.

KEY COMPONENTS OF ORGANIZATIONAL CULTURE FRAMEWORKS RELEVANT TO HEALTH

Looking across existing organizational culture frameworks, there are key components that seem particularly important to promoting mental health (Table 16-1) within the practice of occupational therapy. As the following discussion points out, many of these key organizational concepts are related to existing models, theories, and concepts within occupational therapy and occupational science, but a renewed focus that puts organizational culture at the center expands existing approaches. Many of these common components of organizational culture frameworks are grounded in how organizations are able to meet the needs of its members, while still accomplishing organizational goals and objectives.

Organizational Communication

Expectations around communication, including how and when individuals connect, are influenced by organizational culture and can have an important impact on mental

---

TABLE 16-1

KEY COMPONENTS OF ORGANIZATIONAL CULTURE HEALTH FRAMEWORKS

- Organizational communication
- Organizational justice and fairness
- Meaningful participation/ involvement
- Physical environment
- Leadership
- Choice/control

- Work-life balance
- Social relationships
- A culture focused on psychological health and safety
- Flexibility
- Diversity

---

health and well-being among all members of an organization. Communication in the context of the modern workplace occurs in many different forms—face-to-face communication, as well as remote communication formats such as communicating via telephone, digital and social media, mobile devices, etc. Each form of communication places different demands on workers. Employees are often expected to be in constant communication with the workplace, even during their time off work (Quick et al., 2007) and this can lead to challenges related to work-life balance, and work overload. Furthermore, less direct communication styles can affect how connected and supported employees feel in the context of their workplace (Lynch, 2000). Poor communication among organizational members can lead to confusion, anxiety, potential conflicts and misunderstandings, and in some cases, feelings of disconnection and exclusion. Surveys show that poor communication causes increases in workplace stress, absenteeism and turnover (Walters, 2005). In contrast, effective communication that is free from discrimination, harassment and bullying enables trust and cooperation, thereby fostering support and positive work relationships (Gilbert & Bilsker, 2012).

Occupational therapists practicing from an organizational culture perspective should be aware of communication practices and expectations within the organization, as well as individual needs and preferences. They can facilitate the development of effective communication standards within organizations and between members that optimizes mental health and well-being, as well as improved performance. This might be particularly important for managers and supervisors who are required to communicate expectations, work assignments, and feedback to their subordinates. Such standards could ensure that communication between organizational members is clear and respectful, and occurs in predictable ways. However, standards must also be flexible in order to meet diverse needs of individuals. For example, some individuals might prefer regular updates through electronic platforms such as email or instant messenger, while others prefer or require occasional face-to-face contact to allow for both verbal and non-verbal communication.

Meaningful Participation/Involvement

Meaningful participation and involvement among employees is a component of healthy workplaces that can enable workers to bring a diverse set of ideas and perspectives to bear on their organization and can influence how the organization operates (Grawitch, Gottschalk, & Munz, 2006). It can produce positive consequences for both employee well-being and organizational effectiveness (Lawler, 1991; Vandenberg, Richardson, & Eastman, 1999; Wilson et al., 2004). Opportunities for workers to provide feedback on work processes and goals offer them a voice in the workplace and can lead to a sense of empowerment. Workplace-based research by Roebuck (1996) indicates that requests for feedback along with a positive response and action by management can make employees feel that management has made positive efforts toward them and they respond positively in return. The consequences include increased motivation, commitment, and an improved organizational culture that contributes to the well-being of employees and organizations alike. However, despite the multiple positive outcomes for both employees and organizations, employee involvement efforts can also leave employees feeling more manipulated than motivated if their concerns are solicited and then discounted or ignored (McConnell, 1998). Employees need to feel heard and respected, even if all of their ideas and suggestions are not implemented.

These findings suggest that occupational therapists working with organizations can help employers, managers, and supervisors engage members of an organization in providing input and feedback. More importantly, however, occupational therapists can assist organizations to acknowledge, consider, and follow-through with the ideas that have been provided to reap multiple potential benefits. Individuals should feel heard, respected, and engaged in decision-making processes.

Organizational Justice and Fairness

Related to meaningful participation and involvement is the concept of organizational justice, which refers to the extent to which perspectives of all members of an organization are accounted for and how just employees perceive organizational decision-making processes and interpersonal treatment to be (Elovainio, Kivimäki, & Vahtera, 2002; Kivimäki, Elovainio, Vahtera, & Ferrie, 2003; Rhoades & Eisenberger, 2002). Organizational justice is about perceptions of fair treatment, opportunities to influence decisions, and having a valued voice; it has been highlighted as a psychological risk factor in the workplace (Shain, 2001). One study based in Finland shows that low organizational justice is associated with increased risk of sickness absence, increased mental health problems, and poor self-rated health among hospital personnel (Kivimäki et al., 2003; Sutinen, Kivimäki, Elovainio, & Virtanen, 2002). Similarly, drawing on data collected as part of the prospective Whitehall II study of 10,308 mostly white collar British civil servants between 1985 and 1988, Kivimäki et al. (2004) found that low and declining organizational justice was predictive of decreasing health, yet favorable changes in the treatment of employees was associated with reduced health risk. When employees perceive unfair treatment, they are likely to experience a range of negative emotional responses including feelings of anxiety, depression, humiliation, anger, and rejection. According to Shain (2001), these health outcomes can impair performance and lead to increased aggression, substance abuse, and physical illnesses.

These findings highlight the importance of considering how decisions are perceived by employees and ensuring that processes that preserve a sense of justice and fairness are upheld in order to maintain employee morale and support mental health and well-being. It also suggests the role of management style and organizational processes in addressing mental health and well-being in the workplace. Occupational therapists can work with organizations to develop fair and just decision-making processes and standards that include meaningful participation and involvement from stakeholders across the organization, and uphold a sense of justice and fairness among members.

Social Relationships

Many adults spend a large portion of their time at work, and social relationships in the workplace are pertinent to health (Rhoades & Eisenberger, 2002). Much research has demonstrated the benefits of social support in the workplace about enhanced coping and well-being. Social support or helping relationships in the workplace can moderate the experience of stress, work overload, and the associated negative health outcomes through the availability of help and assistance (Dejonge, Jansen, & Vanbreukelen, 1996;

Johnson & Hall, 1988; Karasek & Theorell, 1990; Karasek, Triantis, & Chaudhry, 1982). Furthermore, social support can have a more direct effect by reducing the experience of work strain and reducing the strength of work stressors (Viswesvaran, Sanchez, & Fisher, 1999). In a review of the literature about the health impact of social support in the workplace, Rick, Thomson, Briner, O'Regan, and Daniels (2002) found evidence that workplace support can be an important predictor of psychological health, with low support or deteriorating support leading to increased psychiatric symptoms and increased work stress. These findings highlight the importance of supportive relationships in the workplace as a means of reducing the negative health outcomes associated with organizational problems and creating healthy workplaces.

However, relationships with coworkers and colleagues can also be negative and contribute to increased stress and strain. Negative workplace relationships, which include bullying, harassment, animosity, social conflict, and abusive supervisory styles, are associated with negative work-related and health-related outcomes including increased mental health problems and greater employee turnover (Rick et al., 2002). The requirement of cooperative interactions to complete work tasks can add stress to the workplace (Wong, DeSanctis, & Staudenmayer, 2007). Furthermore, social relationships in the workplace are influenced by other components of organizational culture such as communication styles, opportunities for contact with coworkers, and perceptions of organizational justice.

The influence of social relationships and social support on the health and well-being of workers is particularly relevant given current conditions of precarious employment and short-term, insecure, employment contracts prevalent in many sectors of the labor market (Clarke, Lewchuk, de Wolff, & King, 2007; Crawford, Gutierrez, & Harber, 2005; Lewchuk, Clarke, & de Wolff, 2008; MacEachen, Polzer, & Clarke, 2008). Clarke specifically found that the most vulnerable workers, who were in the greatest need of social support, often have the least access to it because of the precarious nature of their work arrangements. These findings suggest that many current work arrangements could threaten worker health by restricting opportunities to establish positive social relationships at work. In cases of precarious work arrangements or short-term contracts, individuals might need to pay particular attention to ensuring that they have adequate social support outside of the work context.

Occupational therapists have much to contribute to this component of organizational culture. The importance of social relationships in the workplace is consistent with occupational therapy theories about human connections. Rebeiro, Day, Semeniuk, O'Brien, and Wilson (2001) define the concept of belonging as encompassing mutual support, friendship, and being included. Whalley Hammell (2004) highlighted the importance of a sense of belonging and connectedness to the experience of meaning in everyday occupations. Furthermore, the importance of the person-environment-occupation fit in the context of the workplace (Law et al., 1996; Cockburn, Kirsh, Krupa, & Gewurtz, 2004) is particularly relevant to this component of organizational culture. That is, the fit between individual preferences and needs, and workplace demands and expectations can influence health and well-being. If individuals prefer working alone, a culture of collaboration and the expectation of teamwork may lead to stress and threaten well-being. Occupational therapists can encourage reflection and awareness of individual preferences and organizational expectations, as well as ways of fostering supportive relationships and connections in the workplace.

Work-Life Balance

Work-life balance is a component of organizational culture that refers to how workers are able to manage their work and personal lives (Gilbert & Bilsker, 2012). Work-life conflict occurs when the time and energy demands imposed by our many roles, both at work and in our personal lives, become incompatible with one another. Such issues have been addressed more broadly within the occupational therapy and occupational science literature related to occupational or lifestyle balance. In their model of lifestyle balance, Matuska and Christiansen (2008) suggest a person's everyday activities should match his or her desired patterns, and that time spent in activities should enable a person to meet basic needs, have rewarding relationships, feel engaged, challenged and competent, and create meaningful and positive personal identities. From this perspective, issues around work-life balance highlight the need for all people to have a sense of balance across different domains of their lives and the need for organizations to support members in their efforts to achieve this balance.

Although there have always been threats to work-life conflict, modern work organizations are particularly vulnerable. Advances in technology that have allowed for increased flexibility in terms of work hours and working off-site can blur the boundaries between work and personal time. Employees are often expected to be connected to their work at all times and available to work and respond whenever workplace demands present themselves (Harlan & Roberts, 1998; MacEachen et al., 2008). Higgins and Duxbury (2009) conducted extensive research in this area. Drawing on data from 100 Canadian companies with 500+ employees within the private, non-profit, and public sectors, they found that time spent at work has increased over time. Work expectations have also increased and many employees extend their workday in order to meet demand. Work requirements such as travel and overtime do not support a healthy work-life balance. Employees with work-life balance conflicts tend to report high levels of job stress, absenteeism due to fatigue, burnout, stress, depression, and overall poor mental and physical health.

Given our understanding of the need for balance and fit (Law et al., 1996; Matuska & Christiansen, 2008), occupational therapists can contribute to addressing work-life imbalances within organizations. They can help assess and take stock of current threats to work-life balance and help develop healthy policies and practices related to overtime, work demands, flexibility, and time off work. They might develop strategies to reduce burnout within the organization as well as organizational policies and benefit structures that can prevent imbalances from occurring (Gilbert & Bilsker, 2012). Fostering a culture that values personal time, family time and down time, in addition to work commitments and achievements can further strengthen work-life balance.

A Culture Focused on Psychological Health and Safety

Psychological health and safety is a relatively recent development in the organizational culture and workplace health field. The Mental Health Commission of Canada (MHCC), along with researchers in the field, have provided much insight into the concept of psychological health and safety. Through a synthesis of the literature on how workplace factors can contribute to mental health and well-being, Dollard et al. (2012) highlight the importance of management support and commitment to mental health and work stress prevention in the workplace, and a shared commitment to promoting and protecting the mental health and safety of employees by identifying and addressing psychological risk factors. The MHCC has developed resources for organizations wishing to create a culture focused on psychological health and safety, including reports on the legal aspects of creating psychologically safe workplaces (Shain, Arnold, & GermAnn, n.d.), and on addressing workplace stigma (MHCC, 2013). In early 2013, the MHCC, together with the Bureau de normalization du Quebec and the Canadian Standards Association, released and disseminated a voluntary National Standard for Psychological Health and Safety in the Workplace.

Another MHCC initiative, an action guide for employers on psychological health and safety, recommends a six-stage process. Developed by Gilbert and Bilsker (2012), it recommends the following stages: policy, planning, promotion, prevention, process, and persistence. *Policy* includes a clear statement of commitment and endorsement by organizational leadership to enhance psychological health and safety. The *planning* stage consists of the identification of key indicators, selecting actions and specifying objectives related to psychological health and safety that are relevant to the organization. *Promotion* includes actions to promote the psychological health of the workforce within the organization. The focus is on increasing the capacity of employees to manage stress to reduce mental health problems through education and support. *Prevention* includes actions to prevent the occurrence of psychological problems. Primary prevention typically involves identifying and reducing risk factors. Secondary prevention entails identifying and addressing threats to psychological health and safety at a relatively mild or early stage. Tertiary prevention, on the other hand, is focused on reducing distress and dysfunction associated with mental health problems after they have emerged by ensuring prompt access to appropriate treatment, and ensuring effective rehabilitation and return-to-work processes. The *process* stage is focused on evaluating the implementation and outcomes of the actions taken to address psychological health and safety and should include input from across members of the organization as well as short-term and long-term outcomes. And finally, *persistence* is about sustaining organizational efforts in a process of continuous improvement. It includes the creation of an entrenched culture of psychological safety with ongoing leadership commitment and employee involvement.

Building on earlier work, the National Standard on Psychological Health and Safety in the Workplace Provides a framework for psychologically healthy and safe workplaces through the assessment, identification, control, and elimination of risks and hazards in the workplace, followed by the implementation of structures, practices, and a culture that supports and promotes psychological health. The standard includes many of the same steps identified by Gilbert and Bilsker (2012) and positions the focus on psychological health and safety within the organizational climate and culture. It provides clarity about processes and commitments within the organization for ensuring psychological health and well-being. Although voluntary, it highlights the business case for taking action including risk management, cost effectiveness, recruitment and retention, and organizational excellence and sustainability.

Occupational therapists are well positioned to contribute to organizational culture health frameworks. Occupational therapists have a good grasp of the factors that affect psychological health and safety, and can provide consultation to organizations wishing to adopt a culture focused on promoting psychological health and well-being. In addition to helping organizations work through available resources, occupational therapists can assist organizations to identify threats to psychological health within their organizations and adopt policies and procedures that can help mitigate risks.

Physical Environment

Occupational therapists have long been interested in how the physical environment promotes health and enables occupational performance and engagement (Law et al., 1996). When applied to the context of the workplace, the physical environment can affect work-related outcomes

such as productivity and creativity, as well as employee health and well-being. Organizations are realizing the importance of the physical environment in fostering a healthy organizational culture and occupational therapists can provide consultation to help organizations identify the optimal physical design that will best meet their needs.

Generally, environments that are clean, comfortable, aesthetically pleasing, with adequate access to natural lighting have been identified as promoting good mental health and well-being at work (Arwedson, Roos, & Björklund, 2007). However, determining the most effective physical layout of a workplace is quite complex. To promote access to natural lighting while promoting team work and reducing costs, many organizations have moved toward open-plan designs where employees work together in large rooms as opposed to private offices (de Croon, Sluiter, Kuijer, & Frings-Dresen, 2005; Kaarlela-Tuomaala, Helenius, Keskinen, & Hongisto, 2009). However, open-plan designs provide less privacy, increased noise, and can challenge concentration. It is important to consider the fit between the environment, the individual's needs, and the tasks being completed (Cockburn et al., 2004; Law et al., 1996; Vischer, 2007). Open-plan designs might be most helpful when individuals are expected to collaborate or work together, but might be problematic in organizations where individuals work mostly independently on tasks that require high levels of concentration or privacy (Kaarlela-Tuomaala et al., 2009). The physical environment can either support individuals and the tasks being performed (good fit) or hinder them (bad fit). Consideration of the needs of individuals and the specific tasks being performed should guide decisions about the ideal design of the physical environment within an organization.

Flexibility

Some organizations promote a culture of flexibility, where members can choose their hours of work and workspaces, including the option of working from home during evenings and weekends. Such flexibility can be accommodating for workers who are balancing competing responsibilities in their personal and family lives, or have unique scheduling needs (e.g., medication or health care needs), thus promoting improved work-life balance, autonomy, choice, and control (Gilbert & Bilsker, 2012). However, flexible work arrangements often include fluctuating periods of intense demands and pressing deadlines (MacEachen et al., 2008), as well as a lack of investment in health promotion within the organization (Crawford et al., 2005).

These findings highlight that flexibility as an organizational characteristic can have both positive and negative implications. Flexibility in and of itself can promote a culture that is adaptable and accommodating to meet the needs of clients, customers, and workers. However, flexibility is also associated with a lack of commitment to employees and their needs (Crawford et al., 2005; Lewchuk et al., 2008; MacEachen et al., 2008). Rather, the focus becomes meeting organizational demands, and the expectation that employees will work whenever they are needed by the organization (Harlan & Robert, 1998; MacEachen et al., 2008). Thus, flexibility can be associated with fluctuating and unpredictable periods of intense work demands, blurred work-life boundaries, as well as insecure work arrangements.

Occupational therapists can help organizations determine the type of flexibility that might work within their organizations. They can help organizations assess fluctuating work demands and the costs and benefits to adopting flexible work schedules and the option of working remotely. Such assessment would require input from individuals from all levels of the organization. When approached in this way, such discussions can foster a culture of transparency, engagement, and fairness, and promote a sense of control and choice, which are also associated with improved health and well-being.

Leadership

Leadership is an organizational characteristic that has implications for all aspects of organizational culture. The leadership of an organization, including management and supervisory styles, sets the tone for the organization and impacts expectations, priorities and goals. It influences communication styles, how employees are engaged, perceptions of justice and fairness, relationships, balance, safety, and the physical layout. Real growth toward improving organizational culture, or addressing psychological health and safety, requires commitment from the leaders of an organization (Gilbert & Bilsker, 2012). Although there is a clear business case for addressing factors related to organizational culture and building organizations that promote mental health and well-being among its members, organizations are often balancing competing demands and goals (Quick et al., 2007). A healthy organization can lead to improved productivity, creativity, and innovation, and a good leader is able to harness investment in developing and promoting a healthy organization without compromising its organizational goals or targets (Kuoppala, Lamminpaa, Liira, & Vainio, 2008). Thus, good leadership is at the center of a healthy organization (Quick et al., 2007).

There is a vast literature on styles of leadership and qualities of effective leaders, although the focus is not often specific to promoting mental health and well-being within organizations. However, some research discusses "authentic" leaders who are genuine, trustworthy, reliable, compassionate, believable, and can foster healthy work environments by engaging employees in promoting positive behavior (Shirey, 2006). Lohela, Björklund, Vingard, Hagberg, and Jensen (2009) highlight the importance of leadership qualities such as being fair, empowering, and supportive in order to promote health and well-being among organizational members. Thus, according to Quick et al. (2007), "authentic leaders are who they say they are; that is, there is a consistency between their values, their intentions, their beliefs, their spoken words, and their actions and behaviours" (p. 195). Leaders possessing these qualities can energize workers and support workplace mental health.

Attention to leadership issues is particularly important for occupational therapists working in the area of organizational culture. Intervening at the level of the organization, to improve the culture of the organization in a positive way to promote health and well-being among all members requires buy-in and support from the organization's leadership and management (Gilbert & Bilsker, 2012; Quick et al., 2007). Occupational therapists must be prepared to work with leaders to prioritize the importance of mental health and organizational cultures that promote mental health and well-being.

Diversity

A commitment to diversity has often been highlighted as an important component of a healthy and positive organizational culture. Diversity within an organization has been associated with improved creativity, innovation, and performance (Kochan et al., 2003). In terms of its impact on health, respect for diversity and difference has been associated with reduced emotional exhaustion (Ramarajan, Barsade, & Burack, 2008). According to Gilbert and Bilsker (2012) organizational cultures that recognize diversity have clear expectations for courteous communication, and address intolerance, discrimination, harassment, and bullying. Such cultures lead to improved job satisfaction, teamwork, labor relations, and reductions in absenteeism and turnover. In contrast, disrespectful organizational relationships may reduce productivity, lead to increased conflict, and contribute to poor mental health including stress, anxiety, and depression.

Promoting a culture that values diversity requires management endorsement as it can set the tone for the entire organization. Many examples of integrating diversity within the business strategy, vision, targets, and action plans exist (Lengnick-Hall, Gaunt, & Kulkarni, 2008; Schur et al., 2005; Slater, Weigand, & Zwirlein, 2008; Wong, 2008; Zintz, 1997). Practices such as actively recruiting diverse candidates (Schur et al., 2005; Spataro, 2005; Wong, 2008; Zintz, 1997), and promoting organizational values and norms that encourage effective use of diverse perspectives on teams (Chatman, Polzer, Barsade, & Neale, 1998; Kochan et al., 2003) have been successful in increasing creativity, innovation, and productivity. Given these positive outcomes, occupational therapists should promote diversity as a positive component of organizational culture and encourage reflection about how to increase diversity and create space for diverse perspectives.

Choice/Control

Choice and control have been highlighted in the organizational culture literature as being particularly important in terms of considering mental health and well-being of workers. The most commonly cited model pertaining to choice and control is the Karasek model (1979), which suggests that it is the combination of low decision latitude and heavy job demand that leads to mental strain and job dissatisfaction. Job demand within this model refers to workload and comprises the quantity and time pressure of the work, and mental requirements needed for successful completion. Individuals who experience high job demand might report feeling pressured to work fast and difficulty taking time off work. Decision latitude, on the other hand, refers to the ability to make decisions or participate in decision-making at work, exercise discretion and autonomy, and be creative (Vezina, Bourbonnais, Brisson, & Trudel, 2004). Mental strain has been linked to health conditions such as depression, anxiety, apathy, distress, burnout, exhaustion, low self-esteem, drug use, and coronary disease (Leka & Jain, 2010; Vezina et al., 2004). Evidence suggesting that the combination of low decision latitude and high job demands associated with a moderate risk of common mental disorders have been confirmed in subsequent research, including a meta-analysis of studies published between 1994 and 2005 (Standsfeld & Candy, 2006).

Drawing on the Karasek model, occupational therapists can assist organizations to assess perceptions of choice and control among members of an organization and consider ways to increase autonomy and options for employees. For example, they can assist organizations to create opportunities for workers to participate in decision making affecting their work and exercise control over their work conditions including their work schedules, their workloads, and how their work should be completed. Such efforts can have positive effects on mental health and well-being, and contribute to the creation of a positive organizational culture.

THREATS TO A HEALTHY ORGANIZATIONAL CULTURE

In addition to the components of organizational culture that contribute to the mental health and well-being of members, there are also components that can distract from it. These factors typically revolve around security, retention, opportunities for growth, and reward (see Table 16-2). They affect the efforts that members will put forth and their expectations of the response in return.

TABLE 16-2
THREATS TO HEALTHY ORGANIZATIONAL CULTURE
• Job insecurity
• Inadequate reward systems
• Limited opportunities for career advancement

Job Insecurity

Short-term and casual contracts are common work arrangements within the contemporary labor market. Although these arrangements are sometimes desired and sought out by employees at certain stages of their career, they can threaten the development of a healthy organizational culture. Temporary and casual work arrangements can restrict the development of supportive social relationships at work, reduce employee commitment, and put workers in precarious and stressful work situations where they do not have a reliable and predictable source of income, have limited benefits, and have little protection should their contract be terminated. Research among workers has found that job insecurity has adverse effects on self-reported health (Borg, Kristensen, & Burr, 2000; Ferrie, Shipley, Stansfeld, & Marmot, 2002; Lewchuk et al., 2008; McDonough, 2000). Clarke et al. (2007) found that the health effects of insecure employment varied by the reasons for the employment situation. The poorest health outcomes were reported among individuals who were in precarious/insecure employment arrangements, wanted more secure employment but were unable to find any, did not see how they could change their employment situation, and had low expectations that it would change in the near future. These findings suggest that the perception of job security and the amount of choice and control the worker has over his or her job security and work arrangement contributes to the effect it has on his or her health and well-being.

Occupational therapists should attend to issues related to job security in efforts to foster organizational cultures that are supportive of mental health and well-being. This can be accomplished by assisting organizations to reflect on the impact that insecure work arrangements might be having on their workforce and consider ways to improve job security.

Reward Systems

Organizations depend on the contributions of their members. When people contribute, they want to feel appreciated for their efforts, either through acknowledgement, recognition, or pay incentives. A lack of reward can threaten ongoing commitment, the culture of the organization, and the health and well-being of individual members. Siegrist (1996) proposed the "effort/reward imbalance" model based on findings that work situations characterized by high effort and low rewards are associated with poor health outcomes. Within the model, Siegrist further distinguished between extrinsic and intrinsic effort. Extrinsic effort is associated with time pressures, interruptions, competing demands and responsibilities, and increased workload that arises from external sources; intrinsic effort or over-commitment, on the other hand, is an internal attitude or innate drive to push forward and gain esteem or approval. According to this model, reward is primarily measured in terms of salary, esteem/respect, job security, and opportunity for advancement (Siegrist, 2002). The central process or mechanism of action is social reciprocity, the possibility of gaining or earning advantage because of effort expended in the workplace. That is, individuals are more likely to put forth sustained effort when they believe that their efforts will be acknowledged, recognized, and/or rewarded in a meaningful way, leading to some future benefit or advantage. Effort/reward imbalance is associated with increased risk of functional disability from mental health problems and a moderately elevated risk of newly reported psychiatric disorder (Kruper, Singh-Manoux, Siegrist, & Marmot, 2002). Given these findings, occupational therapists can assist organizations in promoting a culture of recognition and reward where individuals feel appreciated and recognized for their efforts and contributions.

Opportunities for Career Advancement

Related to job security and reward systems are opportunities for career advancement. In the absence of opportunities for advancement within an organization, individuals might think that their efforts go unrewarded, unrecognized, and unacknowledged, and that their career trajectories stagnate. Such conditions can lead to an effort/reward imbalance and the associated negative effects on mental health. Individuals can feel unchallenged and unmotivated to exert efforts and make innovative and necessary contributions, thereby also affecting the growth and productivity of the organization (Kaye, 2010). Thus, the lack of opportunity for advancement, growth, and development within an organization can be a threat to a healthy organizational culture and the development of a sense of security and a fair and just system of reward. Occupational therapists working with organizations should attend to this need and ensure opportunities for career advancement.

How Do Occupational Therapists Draw on Organizational Culture Frameworks?

This preceding overview of organizational culture frameworks relevant to health has highlighted concepts that can be incorporated into occupational therapy principles and practices. Occupational therapists have a long history within employment support, return-to-work, and vocational rehabilitation, particularly as it pertains to people with mental health concerns (Braveman & Page, 2012; Kirsh, Cockburn, & Gewurtz, 2005). Despite attention to environmental factors within our theories and models, occupational therapy practice in the realm of work has traditionally focused on individuals rather than organizations. That is, research and practice has tended to focus on individuals returning to work and negotiating workplace accommodations for individuals (Braveman & Page, 2012). Further work has been dedicated to developing programs and services to assist people living with mental illness find and keep jobs (Kirsh et al., 2005). Comparably little attention within occupational therapy has been dedicated to organizational culture and promoting healthy organizational culture. For example, in a review of occupational therapy work-related practices, Braveman (2012) outlines work-related interventions that occupational therapists provide across a wide range of settings and populations with little reference to addressing issues related to protection and promotion of health through the culture of a workplace.

Despite a historic focus on individuals, there is much occupational therapists can contribute to an organizational culture perspective. An important document, *Working Together: Successful Strategies for Return to Work*, was developed by the Institute for Work and Health together with the Ontario Society of Occupational Therapists and the College of Occupational Therapists of Ontario in 2008. The aim of this document was to improve return-to-work success rates through discussion and collaboration among occupational therapists, employers, and other workplace stakeholders. Although six out of the seven strategies outlined in the document pertain to assisting an individual worker back to work, the last strategy is focused on creating a "return-to-work friendly" workplace with a strong commitment to health and safety. This strategy includes a focus on norms and expectations within the organization, a system of social support, and a focus on the culture of the organization. Similarly, a position statement on Return-to-Work and Occupational Therapy released by the Canadian

Association of Occupational Therapists in 2009 includes recommendations directed at addressing organizational culture and promoting healthy workplace cultures that are supportive of the return-to-work process. The recommendations highlight the need for widespread collaboration and communication with multiple stakeholders within the organization. These developments suggest that occupational therapists who are attuned to an organizational culture perspective to promote health and have much to contribute. This perspective shifts attention toward organizational factors that affect mental health and well-being, and encourages further engagement among organizational stakeholders to prevent and address mental health problems among individuals within an organization.

RELEVANT ASSESSMENTS

Grounded in the Person-Environment-Occupation perspective (Law et al., 1996), occupational therapists have used approaches to workplace assessments focused on the interaction between the worker, the workplace, and the work (Cockburn et al., 2004). However, assessments conducted by occupational therapists are typically prompted by the needs of an individual worker who is in the process of returning to work or requesting accommodations. Even when organizational factors are included, assessments have typically revolved around the needs of an individual worker (Fisher, 2012). The notion of assessing components of organizational culture in an effort to prevent mental health problems or improve the mental health of all workers is less common within the profession. However, there is much occupational therapists can contribute by working with organizations to assess components of organizational culture and organizational factors that might be problematic.

Job demands analyses, often used by occupational therapists for rehabilitation goal setting and treatment planning within the return-to-work process (Page, 2012), usually include categories related to the work environment. Despite inclusion of psychological and cognitive factors, they typically prioritize the physical environment and the job demands that affect the working conditions (Innes & Straker, 2002). However, other components of organizational culture, including communication processes, social support, management practices, choice/control, reward systems, and perceptions of fairness/justice, might be captured through a comprehensive workplace assessment involving observation and interviews with key stakeholders (Innes, 2012). Occupational therapists should also consider beliefs, values, and attitudes as part of an assessment of the workplace environment. Such factors can be assessed through observation and discussion with workers, coworkers, supervisors, and management, and should include attention to the perspectives of different stakeholders (Fisher 2012; Scott et al., 2003).

Occupational therapists seeking to assess the culture of an organization might use a variety of tools in order to collect relevant information from multiple stakeholders. There are some good resources available to assist in this process. For example, Guarding Minds @ Work was developed by researchers from the Centre for Applied Research in Mental Health and Addiction (CARMHA) at Simon Fraser University Canada, was commissioned by the Great-West Life Centre for Mental Health in the Workplace. It includes assessment worksheets (typically completed by business owners, managers, or human resource professionals), an employee questionnaire, and an employee survey to assess performance across a number of psychosocial factors at work. These resources are based on extensive national and international research, case law, and legislation. They can be downloaded from the Guarding Minds @ Work website and can be used to promote self-reflection within an organization, and identify areas of concern that require action.

A situational assessment can be used to identify the main issues affecting employees within an organization (CMHA Ontario). A situational assessment includes a review of existing organizational information such as employee surveys, absenteeism reports, exit interview data, and health benefit use data. Following analysis of these data, further information can be collected through focus groups, interviews, audits, surveys of key stakeholder groups, and using a variety of assessment tools. The Health Communication Unit (THCU) at the Centre for Health Promotion at the University of Toronto produced a resource of six different types of situational assessments including current practice surveys, health risk assessments, interest surveys, needs assessments, organizational culture surveys, and workplace audits. In particular, organizational culture surveys can be used to collect information from organizational members (e.g., employees or employers) about all components of the organizational culture. Through a review of the literature, an Internet search, and nominations from the field, the Workplace Health Project team identified 29 recommended situational assessment tools. Tool summaries, ratings, and available online resources are provided in a catalogue on the project website (THCU, 2006).

PRACTICE APPROACHES FOR OCCUPATIONAL THERAPISTS BASED ON ORGANIZATIONAL CULTURE FRAMEWORKS RELEVANT TO HEALTH

Occupational therapists are well positioned to contribute to the field of organizational culture. Building on the Person-Enivronment-Occupation lens, an organizational culture framework allows expansion of traditional workplace assessments to consider the psychosocial aspects of the workplace environment and workplace conditions that affect mental health and well-being. As outlined in Vignette 16-1, such a perspective allows occupational therapists to move beyond working with individual workers, to providing consultation and recommendations that can contribute to the creation of healthy workplaces and work practices that will benefit all workers (Burton, 2010; IWH, OSOT & COTO, 2008). Even within their work with individual workers, occupational therapists can draw on an organizational culture perspective. For example, there is some evidence that although the decision to disclose a mental health problem and request accommodations might revolve around an individual worker, the culture of an organization is an important consideration (Brohan et al., 2012; Gewurtz & Kirsh, 2009; Krupa et al., 2009). Specific concerns with disclosure include unfair treatment by supervisors and coworkers, loss of credibility, gossip and rejection, which can stall career development and reduce opportunities for advancement within the organization. Higher perceived emotional support is associated with higher rates of disclosure of mental health problems to supervisors and coworkers (Rollins, Mueser, Bond, & Becker, 2002). Drawing on an organizational culture perspective, occupational therapists can help individuals navigate their organization and make informed decisions about disclosing their illness and requesting needed accommodations.

While occupational therapists have only begun to address organizational cultures in a systematic way, awareness and creation of work cultures that are health promoting have been at the core of several work initiatives for people with serious mental illness. Two such initiatives—social businesses and supported employment—have been shown to have outcomes that exceed those of traditional vocational programs (MHCC, n.d.) and literature suggests that it is the emphasis on work environments that at least in part, accounts for these differences (Kirsh et al., 2005). These initiatives offer unique examples of how the culture of an organization can be used to create healthy and supportive work organizations for people living with mental illnesses.

Social businesses are commercial ventures that market goods and services to the public and use this economic activity to achieve social outcomes. They have been developed to address the employment and economic disadvantage experienced by people with mental illness (MHCC, n.d.). In these initiatives, social integration and inclusion are emphasized in addition to productivity and economic development. Most social businesses aim to balance sensitivity to the needs and issues facing people with mental illness in business and meeting the business goals of the firm. There is a focus on job accommodations that correlates with workers' needs, such as offering support around managing social conflict, or providing flexibility with respect to time off. Social businesses also offer opportunities for involvement in a range of meaningful roles and responsibilities, including management, entrepreneurial or front-line work,

as well as representation on boards and committees. The decision-making structure is democratic, and promotes a strong sense of ownership through the ranks (MHCC, n.d.).

Supported employment programs typically provide individual placements in competitive employment—that is, community jobs paying at least minimum wage that any person can apply—in accord with client choices and capabilities, without requiring extended prevocational training (Bond et al., 2001). They actively facilitate job acquisition, often sending staff to accompany clients on interviews; and they provide ongoing support once the client is employed (p. 314). Although therapists working within supported employment programs work with individuals through skill training and provision of emotional and instrumental support, they also attend carefully to the workplace culture. In this way, they are able to effectively guide their clients toward healthy work environments and/or modify the workplace environment to enable client success. To this end, providing education or training to employers and coworkers may be necessary. In this model, the therapist works with the organizational setting to help the client establish job accommodations, which can include, but are not limited to, re-arranging work schedules, modifying client duties, or modifying workplace procedures and/or rules (Auerbach & Richardson, 2005; Fabian, Waterworth, & Ripke, 1993) or allowing the presence of a job coach on site (Blitz & Mechanic, 2006). Work cultures that are inclusive of people with diverse skills and abilities are more likely to embrace these opportunities to provide support and accommodations, which can be transformative in the workplace.

Expected Outcomes

Expected outcomes of an organizational culture framework for occupational therapy include improved mental health and well-being among all members, improved recruitment and retention, reduced absenteeism and injury, improved engagement and satisfaction among all members or employees, increased productivity and innovation, and ultimately increased profits/efficiency/effectiveness for the organization. According to a review conducted by Way and MacNeil (2006), characteristics of the work environment including work demands, lack of control, and lack of support account for between 20% and 40% of the variance in job dissatisfaction and employee health and well-being across most studies. Similarly, Stone, Du, and Gershon (2007) surveyed hospital nurses and found that most organizational culture factors were related to occupational health outcomes and measures of burnout, as well as organizational outcomes such as employee turnover. Dollard et al. (2012) studied the experiences of two unrelated samples of Australian nurses working in remote areas across 24 months and found that the individual experience of exhaustion and psychological distress can be predicted

Vignette 16-1. Molly

XYZ is a medium-sized IT company that employs about 250 staff members. The nature of the work that the organization does results in frequent and often unforeseen periods of high demand with tight deadlines. As a result, many employees work long hours, including evenings and weekends, in order to meet the needs of their clients. Many employees have complained of being called into work without notice to deal with a crisis at work and their inability to plan for time off work.

The organization has had difficulty retaining highly qualified staff and several employees have gone on sick leave. This rapid turnover is beginning to affect their client relationships. Therefore, they have contracted Molly, an occupational therapist, to help them identify what they can do to address the problem. Molly uses an organizational culture framework to guide her work.

Assessment

Molly wants to better understand the nature of the problem from the perspective of all stakeholders involved. Why are employees leaving the organization, or going on sick leave? What can the organization do to protect the health of its members? Working with the organization, she conducts a situational assessment.

Analysis of Existing Data

She begins by gathering existing data such as exit surveys, rates of absenteeism, turnover, return to work and accommodation data, short-term and long-term disability rates, and incident reports/worker complaints.

Gathering New Data

Molly also gathers data by surveying current staff and meeting with representatives from all levels of the organization.

Findings

From these data, Molly notices many complaints about intense periods of stress within the organization and how managers communicate with employees. She also notes that many employees have worked during their planned vacation time because of issues that have come up at work. Many employees noted that their efforts during these periods of intense stress or their willingness to complete time sensitive work during their personal time usually went unacknowledged and unrewarded. It was just expected of them as part of their job. Molly further notes that employees were generally disengaged from most decision-making processes within the organization, even those that directly affected their work. This left many employees feeling unheard and unvalued within the organization. Therefore, using an organizational culture perspective relevant to health, Molly identifies several areas of concern around organizational communication, work-life balance, meaningful participation/involvement, organizational justice/fairness, flexibility, choice/control, and systems of reward.

Objectives and Plan

Molly shares the assessment findings and her analysis of the findings with all members of the organization through an email summary and in-person meetings. She facilitates discussions about priorities for intervention and change that might improve the work conditions within the organization. Most of the workers prioritized improved communication standards, work-life balance, organizational justice/fairness, opportunities to be involved in decision making and to have control over their work, and reward/recognition. They recognized that there were client demands that had to be met but felt that there could be more attention to how managers communicated with employees, protecting personal time, employee input on decision making and control over their work, and developing an appropriate bonus structure to reward employees for their efforts in mitigating or fixing issues. When these priorities were shared with the management team, they were able to consider the following reasonable organizational strategies that could be implemented:

(continued)

1. A committee would be formed that will work with an external consultant to develop communication standards for the organization.

2. All managers would complete mandatory training in communication strategies.

3. A committee would be formed to develop standards for contacting employees during their personal time.

4. All managers would attend a course focused on improving staff engagement and facilitating democratic decision making within teams/departments.

5. When possible, staff would be able to determine how to best approach their job tasks and be involved in decision making within their team or department. This would involve managers relinquishing some control over procedures and operations.

6. The management team would consult with staff to develop an appropriate bonus structure that provides reward and recognition.

IMPLEMENT AND EVALUATE

The strategies were implemented. Molly worked with the organization to conduct a follow-up employee survey to evaluate the strategies. This enabled the organization to consider the success of the strategies, and adjust them accordingly.

Six months after the strategies were implemented, Molly found the following through employee opinion surveys and through discussions with representatives from across the organization:

1. Although organizational communication had improved, there remained some areas of concern.

2. Most employees indicated that they were more satisfied with how they were contacted about work issues during their time off and the new process was perceived to be fair across the organization.

3. Employees on some teams noted improvements in the amount of choice/control they had over their work and work hours, and some increase in their involvement in decision making, but this was not consistent across the organization.

4. Employees were somewhat satisfied with the bonus structure but highlighted areas that could be improved.

Once again, Molly shared these findings across the organization and collaborated with the management team to set new objectives for ongoing improvement.

---

by work conditions such as organizational support, communication, participation/involvement, and choice/control. Overall, an organizational culture approach can improve the organizational climate and environment, making for a more satisfying, effective, and competitive organization where individuals within the organization are engaged and committed, and report fewer incidents of poor health and mental health concerns.

Furthermore, an organizational culture approach to addressing mental health and well-being can be one mechanism to reduce stigma toward people with mental illness and mental health problems within the context of the workplace. The impact of stigma on engagement in occupations has been highlighted in the literature. Moll et al. (2013) examined organizational policies and practices that perpetuate stigma for health care workers struggling with mental health issues in a large mental health organization. Silence emerged as a central process that characterized the organizational responses to mental health issues among workers within the organization. The expression of stigma is often grounded in assumptions about people with mental illness that are expressed and endorsed at all levels of an organization (Krupa et al., 2009; Moll et al., 2013). Krupa (2008) encourages occupational therapists to counteract assumptions about people with mental illness that perpetuate stigma in the context of work. Adopting an organizational culture health framework can challenge stigmatizing processes and lead to healthier and more supportive organizational environments.

CONCLUSION

In this chapter, we presented key concepts relevant to adopting an organizational culture framework relevant to health within occupational therapy, and threats to adopting an organizational culture health framework to occupational therapy practice in the context of the workplace. We highlighted how this approach is consistent with occupational therapy theory focused on environments. However, an organizational culture perspective represents a shift from traditional occupational therapy practice in the workplace that has tended to focus on negotiating accommodations or return-to-work processes with individual workers. Organizational culture frameworks for health open new opportunities and challenges for occupational therapists in this sector. Occupational therapists can position themselves as experts in creating healthy and supportive workplace environments focused on promoting mental health and preventing mental health problems in the workplace. Occupational therapists can assess and intervene at the organizational level to promote supportive and healthy organizational cultures.

LEARNING ACTIVITIES/ DISCUSSION QUESTIONS

1. Working in a group, reflect upon the organizational culture within your program or workplace and identify/discuss the following, drawing on the material presented in this chapter:

    a. The organizational factors/characteristics that promote or detract from health and well-being.

    b. The organizational factors that promote or detract from the productivity of individuals within the organization.

    c. Strategies that could improve the organizational culture that might be relevant to your organization.

    d. Anticipated challenges to intervening at the level of the organization.

REFERENCES

Arwedson, I. L., Roos, S., & Björklund, A. (2007). Constituents of healthy workplaces. *Work: A Journal of Prevention, Assessment & Rehabilitation, 28*, 3-11.

Auerbach, S., & Richardson, P. (2005). The long-term work experiences of persons with severe and persistent mental illness. *Psychiatric Rehabilitation Journal, 28*(3), 267–273.

Blitz, L., & Mechanic, D. (2006). Facilitators and barriers to employment among individuals with psychiatric disabilities: A job coach perspective. *Work: A Journal of Prevention, Assessment and Rehabilitation, 26*(4), 407–419.

Bond, G. R., Becker, D. R., Drake, R. E., Rapp, C. A., Meisler, N., Lehman, A. F., Bell, M. D., & Blyler, C. R. (2001). Implementing supported employment as an evidence-based practice. *Psychiatric Services, 52*, 313-322.

Borg, V., Kristensen, T. S., & Burr, H. (2000). Work environment and changes in self-rated health: A five year follow-up study. *Stress Medicine, 6*, 37-47.

Braveman, B. (2012). Work in the modern world: The history and current trends in workers, the workplace, and working. In B. Braveman & J. J. Page (Eds.), *Work: Promoting participation and productivity through occupational therapy* (pp. 2-27). Philadelphia: F. A. Davis Company.

Braveman, B., & Page, J. J. (2012). *Work: Promoting participation and productivity through occupational therapy*. Philadelphia: F. A. Davis Company.

Brohan, E., Henderson, C., Wheat, K., Malcolm, E., Clement, S., Barley, E. A., Slade, M., & Thornicroft, G. (2012). Systematic review of beliefs, behaviours and influencing factors associated with disclosure of a mental health problem in the workplace. *BMC Psychiatry, 12*(11). doi:10.1186/1471-244X-12-11

Burton, J. (2010). *WHO healthy workplace framework and model: Background and supporting literature and practices*. Geneva, Switzerland: World Health Organization.

Business Dictionary. (n.d.). Organization. Retrieved from www.businessdictionary.com/definition/organization.html.

Canadian Association of Occupational Therapists. (2009). *CAOT position statement: Return-to-work and occupational therapy*. Ottawa, ON: CAOT. Retrieved from www.caot.ca/pdfs/positionstate/Return%20to%20Work.pdf.

Chatman, J. (1989). Improving interactional organizational research: A model of person-organization fit. *Academy of Management Review, 14*, 333-349.

Chatman, J. A., Polzer, J. T., Barsade, S. G., & Neale, M. A. (1998). Being different yet feeling similar: The influence of demographic composition and organizational culture on work processes and outcomes. *Administrative Science Quarterly, 43*(3), 749-780.

Clarke, M., Lewchuk, W., de Wolff, A., & King, A. (2007). 'This isn't sustainable': Precarious employment, stress and workers' health. *International Journal of Law and Psychiatry, 30*, 311-326. doi:10.1016/j.ijlp.2007.06.005.

CMHA Ontario. Comprehensive workplace health promotion: Affecting mental health in the workplace: Element 3: Conducting a situational assessment—getting to the root of the problem. Retrieved from http://wmhp.cmhaontario.ca/comprehensive-workplace-health-promotion-affecting-mental-health-in-the-workplace/element-3.

Cockburn, L., Kirsh, B., Krupa, T., & Gewurtz, R. (2004). Mental health and mental illness in the workplace: Occupational therapy solutions for complex problems. *Occupational Therapy NOW, 6*(5), 7-14.

Crawford, L., Gutierrez, G., & Harber, P. (2005). Work environment and occupational health of dental hygienists: A qualitative assessment. *Journal of Occupational and Environmental Medicine, 47*, 623-632. doi: 10.1097/01.jom.0000165744.47044.2b

de Croon, E. M., Sluiter, J. K., Kuijer, P. P. F. M., & Frings-Dresen, M. H. W. (2005). The effect of office concepts on worker health and performance: A systematic review of the literature. *Ergonomics, 48*(2), 119-134. doi: 10.1080/00140130512331319409

Dejonge, J., Jansen, P., & Vanbreukelen, G. (1996). Testing the demand-control-support model among health care professionals: A structural equation model. *Work and Stress, 10*, 209-224.

Dollard, M. F., Opie, T., Lenthall, S., Wakerman, J., Knight, S., Dunn, S.,... MacLeod, M. (2012). Psychosocial safety climate as an antecedent of work characteristics and psychological strain: A multilevel model. *Work & Stress, 26(4)*, 385.

Elovainio, M., Kivimäki, M., & Vahtera, J. (2002). Organizational justice: Evidence of a new psychosocial predictor of health. *American Journal of Public Health, 92*, 105-108.

Fabian, E. S., Waterworth, A. & Ripke, B. (1993). Reasonable accommodations for workers with severe mental illness: Type, frequency and associated outcomes. *Psychological Rehabilitation Journal, 17(2)*, 165-172

Ferrie, J. E., Shipley, M. J., Stansfeld, S. A., & Marmot, M. G. (2002). Effects of chronic job insecurity and change in job security on self reported health, minor psychiatric morbidity, physiological measures, and health related behaviours in British civil servants: The Whitehall II study. *Journal of Epidemiology & Community Health, 56*, 450-454.

Fisher, T. (2012). Psychosocial assessment of the worker. In B. Braveman & J. J. Page (Eds.), *Work: Promoting participation and productivity through occupational therapy* (pp. 246-262). Philadelphia: F. A. Davis Company.

Gewurtz, R., & Kirsh, B. (2009). Disruption, disbelief and resistance: A meta-synthesis of disability in the workplace. *Work: A Journal of Prevention, Assessment, and Rehabilitation, 34(1)*, 33-44. doi: 10.3233/WOR-2009-0900

Gilbert, M., & Bilsker, D. (2012). *Psychological health & safety: An action guide for employers*. Mental Health Commission of Canada and the Centre for Applied Research in Mental Health & Addiction.

Grawitch, M. J., Gottschalk, M., & Munz, D. C. (2006). The path to a healthy workplace: A critical review linking healthy workplace practices, employee well-being, and organizational improvement. *Consulting Psychology Journal: Practice and Research, 58(3)*, 129-147.

Harlan, S. L., & Robert, P. M. (1998). The social construction of disability in organizations: Why employers resist reasonable accommodation. *Work & Occupations, 25*, 397-435.

The Health Communication Unit. (2006). Comprehensive workplace health promotion: Recommended and promising practices for situational assessment tools, version 1.02. Retrieved from www.mentalhealth promotion.net/resources/comprehenisve-workplace-health-promotion.pdf

Higgins, C., & Duxbury L. (2009). Key Findings and recommendations from the 2001 national work-life conflict study. Retrieved from Health Canada at www.hc-sc.gc.ca/ewh-semt/pubs/occup-travail/balancing_six-equilibre_six/index-eng.php.

Innes, E. (2012). Assessing and modifying the workplace. In B. Braveman & J. J. Page (Eds.) *Work: Promoting participation and productivity through occupational therapy* (pp. 325-346). Philadelphia: F. A. Davis Company.

Innes, E., & Straker, L. (2002). Workplace assessments and functional capacity evaluations: Current practices of therapists in Australia. *Work, 18(1)*, 51-66.

Institute for Work & Health, the Ontario Society of Occupational Therapists, & the College of Occupational Therapists of Ontario. (2008). Working together: Successful strategies for return to work. Retrieved from www.iwh.on.ca/working-together.

Jongbloed, L., & Crichton, A. (1990). A new definition of disability: Implications for rehabilitation practice and social policy. *Canadian Journal of Occupational Therapy, 57*, 32-38.

Johnson, J., & Hall, E. (1988). Job strain, workplace social support and cardiovascular disease: Across-sectional study of a random sample of the Swedish male working population. *American Journal of Public Health, 78*, 1336-1342.

Kaarlela-Tuomaala, A., Helenius, R., Keskinen, E., & Hongisto, V. (2009). Effects of acoustic environment on work in private office rooms and open-plan offices—longitudinal study during relocation, *Ergonomics, 52(11)*, 1423-1444. doi: 10.1080/00140130903154579

Karasek, R. (1979). Job demands, job decision latitude, and mental strain: Implications for job redesign. *Administrative Science Quarterly, 24(2)*, 285-308.

Karasek, R., & Theorell, T. (1990). *Healthy work: Stress, productivity, and the reconstruction of working life*. New York: Basic Books.

Karasek, R., Triantis, K., & Chaudhry, S. (1982). Coworker and supervisor support as moderators of associations between task characteristics and mental strain. *Journal of Occupational Behavior, 3*, 181-200.

Kaye, B. (2010). Career development: It's a business imperative. *Leadership Excellence, 27(1)*, 4.

Keyton, J. (2005). *Communication and organizational culture*. Thousand Oaks, CA: Sage Publications, Inc.

Kirsh, B., Cockburn, L., & Gewurtz, R. (2005). Best practice in occupational therapy: Program characteristics that influence vocational outcomes for people with serious mental illnesses. *Canadian Journal of Occupational Therapy, 72(5)*, 265-279.

Kirsh, B., & Gewurtz, R. (2012). Promoting mental health within workplaces. In R. J. Gatchel & I. Z. Schultz (Eds.), *Handbook of occupational health and wellness* (pp. 243-266). New York: Springer.

Kivimäki, M., Elovainio, M., Vahtera, J., & Ferrie, J. E. (2003). Organizational justice and health of employees: Prospective cohort study. *Occupational and Environmental Medicine, 60*, 27-34.

Kivimäki, M., Ferrie, J. E., Head, J., Shipley, M. J., Vahtera, J., & Marmot, M. G. (2004). Organizational justice and change in justice as predictors of employee health: the Whitehall II study. *Journal of Epidemiology and Community Health, 58*, 931-937. doi: 10.1136/jech.2003.019026

Kochan, T., Bezrukova, K., Ely, R., Jackson, S., Joshi, A., Jehn, K.,...Levine, D., Thomas, D. (2003). The effects of diversity on business performance: Report of the diversity research network. *Human Resource Management, 42*, 3-21. DOI: 10.1002/hrm.10061

Krupa, T. (2008). Muriel Driver Memorial Lecture 2008: Part of the solution...or part of the problem? Addressing the stigma of mental illness in our midst. *Canadian Journal of Occupational Therapy, 75*, 198-205.

Krupa, T., Kirsh, B., Cockburn, L., & Gewurtz, R. (2009). Understanding the stigma of mental illness in employment. *Work: A Journal of Prevention, Assessment, and Rehabilitation, 33*(4), 413-425. doi: 10.3233/WOR-2009-0890

Kruper, H., Singh-Manoux, A., Siegrist, J., & Marmot, M. (2002). When reciprocity fails: Effort-reward imbalance in relation to coronary heart disease and health functioning within the Whitehall II study. *Occupational and Environmental Medicine, 59,* 777-784.

Kuoppala, J., Lamminpaa, A., Liira, J., & Vainio, H. (2008). Leadership, job well-being, and health effects—A systematic review and a meta-synthesis. *Journal of Occupational and Environmental Medicine, 50,* 904-915. doi: 10.1097/JOM.ob013e31817e918d

Law, M., Cooper, B., Strong, S., Stewart, D., Rigby, P., & Letts, L. (1996). The Person-Environment-Occupation Model: A transactive approach occupational performance. *Canadian Journal of Occupational Therapy, 63,* 9-23.

Lawler, E. E., III. (1991). Participative management strategies. In J. W. Jones, B. D. Steffy, & D. W. Bray (Eds.), *Applying psychology in business: The handbook for managers and human resource professionals.* Lexington, KY: Lexington Books.

Leka, S., & Jain, A. (2010). Health impact of psychosocial hazards at work: An overview. World Health Organization. Retrieved from http://whqlibdoc.who.int/publications/2010/9789241500272_eng.pdf.

Lengnick-Hall, M. L., Gaunt, P. M., & Kulkarni, M. (2008). Overlooked and underutilized: People with disabilities are an untapped human resource. *Human Resources Management 47*(2), 255-273.

Letts, L., Rigby, P., & Stewart, D. (Eds.). (2003). *Using environments to enable occupational performance* (pp. 17-32). Thorofare, NJ: SLACK Incorporated.

Lewchuk, W., Clarke, M., & de Wolff, A. (2008). Working without commitments: Precarious employment and health. *Work, Employment and Society, 22*(3), 387-406. doi: 10.1177/0950017008093477

Lohela, M., Björklund, C., Vingard, E., Hagberg, J., & Jensen, I. (2009). Does a change in psychosocial work factors lead to a change in employee health? *Journal of Occupational and Environmental Medicine, 51,* 195-203. doi: 10.1097/JOM.ob013e318192bd2c

Lynch, J. J. (2000). *A cry unheard: New insights into the medical consequences of loneliness.* Baltimore, MD: Bancroft Press.

MacEachen, E., Polzer, J., & Clarke, J. (2008). "You are free to set your own hours": Governing worker productivity and health through flexibility and resilience. *Social Science & Medicine, 66,* 1019-1033. doi:10.1016/j.socscimed.2007.11.013

Matuska, K. & Christiansen, C. (2008). A proposed model of lifestyle balance. *Journal of Occupational Science, 15,* 9-19.

Mental Health Commission of Canada. (2013). Opening Minds: Interim report. November 18, 2013. Retrieved from www.mentalhealthcommission.ca.

Mental Health Commission of Canada. (n.d.). The aspiring workforce: Employment and income for people with serious mental illness. Retrieved from www.mentalhealthcommission.ca/English/system/files/private/document/Workplace_MHCC_Aspiring_Workforce_Report_ENG_0_0.pdf.

McConnell, C. R. (1998). Employee involvement: motivation or manipulation? *Health Care Supervision.*, 1998 Mar; 16(3): 69-85.

McDonough, P. (2000). Job insecurity and health. *International Journal of Health Services, 30,* 453-476.

Moll, S., Eakin, J., Franche, R-L., & Strike, C. (2013). When health care workers experience mental ill health: Institutional practices of silence. *Qualitative Health Research, 23,* 167-179. doi:10.1177/1049732312466296

Moran, T. E., & Volkwein, F. J. (1992). The cultural approach to the formation of organizational climate. *Human Relations, 45*(1), 19-47.

Page, P. P. (2012). Physical assessment of the worker. In B. Braveman & J. J. Page (Eds.), *Work: Promoting participation and productivity through occupational therapy* (pp. 263-282). Philadelphia: F. A. Davis Company.

Peterson, M., & Wilson, J. F. (2002). The culture-work-health model and work stress. *American Journal of Health Behavior, 26,* 16-24.

Polatajko, H. J., Townsend, E. A., & Craik, J. (2007). Canadian model of occupational performance and engagement (CMOP-E). In E. A. Townsend & H. J. Polatajko (Eds.), *Enabling occupation II: Advancing an occupational therapy vision of health, well-being & justice through occupation* (p. 23). Ottawa, ON: CAOT Publications ACE.

Quick, J., Macik-Frey, M., & Cooper, C. (2007). Managerial dimensions of organizational health: The healthy leader at work. *Journal of Management Studies, 44*(2), 189-205. doi: 10.1111/j.1467-6486.2007.00684.x

Ramarajan, L., Barsade, S. G., & Burack, O. (2008). The influence of organizational respect on emotional exhaustion in the human services. *Journal of Positive Psychology 3*(1), 4-18.

Rebeiro, K. L., Day, D., Semeniuk, B., O'Brien, M., & Wilson, B. (2001). Northern initiative for social action: An occupation based mental health program. *American Journal of Occupational Therapy, 55,* 493-500.

Rhoades, L., & Eisenberger, R. (2002). Perceived organizational support: A review of the literature. *Journal of Applied Psychology, 87*(4), 698-714.

Rick, J., Thomson, L., Briner, R. B., O'Regan, S., & Daniels, K. (2002). Review of existing supporting knowledge to underpin standards of good practice for key work-related stressors—Phase 1. Research Report #024 HSE Books, Her Majesty's Stationary Office, Norwich, UK. Retrieved from http://hse.gov.uk/research/rrpdf/rr024.pdf.

Roebuck, C. (1996). Constructive feedback: key to higher performance and commitment. *Long Range Planning, 29*(3), 328-336.

Rollins, A. L., Mueser, K. T., Bond, G. R., & Becker, D. R. (2002). Social relationships at work: Does the employment model make a difference? *Psychiatric Rehabilitation Journal, 26,* 51-61.

Schein, E. (1992). *Organizational culture and leadership* (2nd ed). San Francisco: Jossey-Bass.

Schur, L., Kruse, D., & Blanck, P. (2005). Corporate culture and the employment of persons with disabilities. *Behavioral Sciences and the Law, 23*(1), 3-20.

Scott, T., Mannion, R., Davies, H., & Marshall, M. (2003). The quantitative measurement of organizational culture in health care: A review of the available instruments. *Health Service Research. 38*(3), 923-945, doi: 10.1111/1475-6773.00154

Shain, M. (2001). Returning to work after illness or injury: The role of fairness. *Bulletin of Science, Technology & Society, 21*(5), 361-368.

Shain, M., Arnold, I., & GermAnn, K. (n.d.). The Road to Psychological Safety: Legal, scientific and social foundations for a national standard for psychological safety in the workplace. Mental Health Commission of Canada. Retrieved from www.mentalhealthcommission.ca.

Shain, M., & Kramer, D. M. (2004). Health promotion in the workplace: Framing the concept; reviewing the evidence. *Occupational and Environmental Medicine, 61,* 643-648. doi: 10.1136/oem.2004.013193

Shain, M., & Suurvali, H. (2001). Investing in comprehensive workable health promotion. *Centre for Addiction and Mental Health (CAMH).* Retrieved from www.excellence.ca/assets/files/products/investing_in_chwp_(full).pdf.

Shirey, M. (2006). Authentic leaders creating healthy work environments for nursing practice. *American Journal of Critical Care,.15(3),* 256.

Siegrist, J. (1996). Adverse health effects of high-effort/low-reward conditions. *Journal of Occupational Health Psychology, 1*(1), 27-41.

Siegrist, J. (2002). Reducing social inequalities in health: Work-related strategies. *Scandinavian Journal of Public Health, 30,* 49-53.

Slater, S. F., Weigand, R. A., & Zwirlein, T. J. (2008). The business case for commitment to diversity. *Business Horizons, 51,* 201-209.

Spataro, S. E. (2005). Diversity in context: How organizational culture shapes reactions to workers with disabilities and others who are demographically different. *Behavioral Sciences and the Law, 23*(1), 21-38.

Standsfeld, S., & Candy, B. (2006). Psychosocial work environment and mental health—a meta-analytic review. *Scandinavian Journal of Work, Environment & Health. 32,* 443-462.

Stone, P. W., Du, Y., & Gershon, R. R. M. (2007). *Journal of Occupational & Environmental Medicine, 49*(1), 50-58.

Sutinen, R., Kivimäki, M., Elovainio, M., & Virtanen, M. (2002). Organizational fairness and psychological distress in hospital physicians. *Scandinavian Journal of Public Health, 30*(3), 209-215.

Vaananen, A., Kalimo, R., Toppinen-Tanner, S., Mutanen, P., Perio, J. M., Kivimäki, M., & Vahtera, J. (2004). Role clarity, fairness, and organizational climate as predictors of sickness absence: A prospective study in the private sector. *Scandinavian Journal of Public Health, 32,* 426-434. doi: 10.1080/14034940410028136

Vandenberg, R. J., Richardson, H. A., & Eastman, L. J. (1999). The impact of high involvement work processes on organizational effectiveness: A second-order latent variable approach. *Group and Organization Management, 24,* 300-339.

Vandenberghe, C. (1999). Organizational culture, person-culture fit, and turnover: A replication in the health care industry. *Journal of Organizational Behaviour, 20*(2), 175-184.

Vezina, M., Bourbonnais, R., Brisson, C., & Trudel, L. (2004). Workplace prevention and promotion strategies. *Healthcare Papers, 5*(2), 32-44.

Vischer, J. C. (2007). The effects of the physical environment on job performance: Towards a theoretical model of workplace stress. *Stress and Health, 23,* 175-184. doi: 10.1002/smi.1134

Viswesvaran C., Sanchez, J. I., & Fisher, J. (1999). The role of social support in the process of work stress: A meta-analysis. *Journal of Vocational Behaviour, 54*(2), 314-334.

Walters, J. (2005). Workplace communication essentials. *The Officer, 81*(8), 42.

Way, M., & MacNeil, M. (2006). Organizational characteristics and their effect on health. *Nursing Economics, 24*(2), 67-77.

Whalley Hammell, K. (2004). Dimensions of meaning in the occupations of daily life. *Canadian Journal of Occupational Therapy, 71*(5), 296-305.

Whalley Hammell, K. (2006). *Perspectives on disability & rehabilitation: Contesting assumptions, challenging practice.* Edinburgh: Churchill Livingstone.

Wilson, M. G., DeJoy, D. M., Vandenberg, R. J., Richardson, H. A., & McGrath, A. L. (2004). Work characteristics and employee health and well-being: Test of a model of healthy work organization. *Journal of Occupational and Organizational Psychology, 77,* 565-588.

Wong, S. (2008). Diversity: Making space for everyone at NASA/Goddard space flight center using dialogue to break through barriers. *Human Resource Management, 47*(2), 389-399.

Wong, S-S., DeSanctis, G., & Staudenmayer, N. (2007). The relationship between task interdependency and role stress: a revisit of the job demands–control model. *Journal of Management Studies, 44,* 284-303.

Zintz, A. C. (1997). Championing and managing diversity at Ortho Biotech Inc. *National Productivity Review,* 21-28.

SUGGESTED READINGS

Comprehensive Mental Health Promotion: A How-To Guide—Developed by The Health Communication Unit at the Della Lana School of Public Health, University of Toronto, and the Canadian Mental Health Association, Ontario. Retrieved from http://wmhp.cmhaontario.ca/comprehensive-workplace-health-promotion-affecting-mental-health-in-the-workplace.

Guarding Minds @ Work—Commissioned by Great-West Life Centre for Mental Health in the Workplace and developed by researchers from the CARMHA within the Faculty of Health Sciences at Simon Fraser University. Retrieved from www.guardingmindsatwork.ca/info/index.

17

Developing Occupationally Just Communities

Ellie Fossey, PhD, MSc, DipCOT (UK) and
Terry Krupa, PhD, OT Reg (Ont), FCAOT

Every time we would drive up and down the strip… or visit someone in their home [neighbourhood], we had nothing to offer them, because there was nothing happening in their neighbourhood that we could identify unless they belonged to a particular local church. There really was very little for them right in their community area. (Evelyn, occupational therapist, cited in Lauckner, 2005)

How do you look at the needs of the community? I don't know. I guess you just talk with people who are there… You look at the same kind of aspects you'd look at as the individual, I suppose. You look at their basic kind of self-care needs, just on a larger community level. So whether there are larger community leisure needs… you try to be a bit more general as who goes there and what the needs of the population are. (Carla, occupational therapist, cited in Lauckner, 2005)

Never doubt that a small group of thoughtful, committed citizens can change the world. Indeed, it is the only thing that ever has. (Margaret Mead, cited in Wilcock & Townsend, 2014, p. 547)

OBJECTIVES

The objectives of this chapter are as follows:
- » Describe the concept of occupational justice, its development, and key contributors.
- » Link occupational justice to mental health and well-being.
- » Identify ways in which occupational injustices may be understood.
- » Position occupational justice in the arena of social justice.
- » Outline emerging approaches for identifying and addressing occupational injustices.
- » Apply community development strategies to address occupational injustices.

Krupa, T., Kirsh, B., Pitts, D., & Fossey, E. *Bruce & Borg's*
Psychosocial Frames of Reference: Theories, Models, and Approaches for
Occupation-Based Practice, Fourth Edition (pp 285-301).
© 2016 SLACK Incorporated.

BACKGROUND

Occupational justice was an implicit concern in occupational therapy's early history, the profession being founded on the idea that human beings have a need for and right to participate in meaningful and valued occupations. Yet, questions of rights and injustices related to participation in occupations of daily life were not typically part of occupational therapy discussion prior to the mid-1990s. As an emerging concept, *occupational justice* has brought into focus experiences of rights, fairness, equity, and power in people's everyday lives and occupations as issues of direct concern to occupational therapy. It has placed the profession's concern more firmly in the broader social realm. In turn, occupational justice invites occupational therapists to view the occupational issues of people with whom they work within a wider frame that accounts for how social, economic, and cultural conditions impact what they do. In keeping with the opening quotes then, occupational justice represents a vision and a call for actions to bring about change in the everyday world: to work not only with individuals, but also with groups and communities experiencing occupational injustices as a means to promote human health and well-being through empowerment, enhanced participation, inclusion, and meaningful and just opportunities for participation (Wilcock & Townsend, 2014).

What Is Occupational Justice?

Occupational justice and injustice are emerging concepts within the fields of occupational science and occupational therapy. These concepts are concerned with human needs for occupations, and how social, structural, and political factors affect participation in everyday occupations. The idea of occupational justice is founded on the views that:

- humans are occupational beings with inherent needs to engage in occupation (Stadnyk, Townsend, & Wilcock, 2010); and that
- "an occupationally just society would be one in which each person and community could meet their own and others' survival, physical, mental and social development needs through occupation that recognised and encouraged individual and communal strengths" (Wilcock & Townsend, 2014, p. 542).

Moreover, occupationally just conditions in society depend, at least in part, on the fair allocation of resources and opportunities to enable people's participation in occupations that recognize their needs, and on the equitable distribution of associated rights, privileges, and benefits. Infringement of freedom to participate in such occupations is considered unjust. Therefore, broad social conditions and structures within society shape the occupations and ways of life available to people, which mean that some individuals,

groups, or populations are able to meet occupational needs and others are not—this is the basis of occupationally unjust situations (Stadnyk et al., 2010).

Occupational justice is also grounded in an occupational perspective; that is, a way of looking at or thinking about the human doings of individuals and communities, which is contextual, inclusive of the diversity of occupations, connects occupation with health and wellbeing, and recognizes occupations as contributing to being, becoming, and belonging (Njelesani, Tang, Jonsson, & Polatajko, 2012). Occupation-related knowledge about time use, occupational balance/imbalance, meaning in occupation, and the contextual influences on participation, all addressed in earlier chapters in this book, also informs understanding how occupational justice and injustice are experienced.

View of Health and Disorder

Realizing health and well-being from an occupational justice perspective depends on individuals and communities being able to participate in occupations that meet their occupational needs, and on community, social, structural, and political conditions that equitably enable participation. This view is rooted in the ideas linking occupation and health: that humans are occupational beings and that occupation is an essential human need and a determinant of mental, physical, and social health and well-being (Wilcock, 1998, 2006; Wilcock & Townsend, 2014). It also recognizes that broader social conditions and structures in society affect what people do and their health and well-being outcomes unequally.

To describe humans as occupational beings is to posit that occupation is an integral part of a person's being, and that humans need to engage in occupation to flourish (Wilcock, 1993). More specifically, occupation is a biological and social necessity for human survival, development, and thriving, as well as for health (Wilcock, 2006). In her historical research, Wilcock drew on archaeological and anthropological sources to show that human beings address basic needs essential for survival (such as for food and shelter) through engaging in occupations; that occupational engagement allows individuals to develop, exercise and maintain capacities of a biological, social, and cultural nature; and that occupational engagement enables both individual and collective development so that humans and societies can adapt to changing environments over time (Wilcock, 1993, 1998). In turn, since each of these occupational needs is essential to human life and health, societal restrictions to participation in occupations of daily life are matters of occupational injustice (Durocher, Gibson, & Rappolt, 2013; Townsend & Wilcock, 2004).

Occupational justice, then, is thought to contribute to well-being in the sense that occupationally just situations enable people to engage in occupations that meet their survival, physical, mental, and social development

---

TABLE 17-1

KEY SOCIAL DETERMINANTS OF MENTAL HEALTH AND WELL-BEING

- Social inclusion—including social connections through which people feel valued, respected and a sense of belonging or membership; social networks (including family members, friends, acquaintances and colleagues) that provide social support, opportunities for social engagement, meaningful social roles, one-on-one contact, and access to resources.

- Access to economic resources—including access to work and meaningful engagement, access to education, and access to adequate housing and financial resources.

- Freedom from discrimination and violence.

Compiled from Commission on Social Determinants of Health. (2008). *Closing the gap in a generation: health equity through action on the social determinants of health. Final report of the Commission on Social Determinants of Health.* Geneva: World Health Organization; and VicHealth. (2005). Social determinants of mental health. Melbourne, Australia: Author. Retrieved from www.health.vic.gov.au/mentalhealthpromotionresources.htm#determinants.

---

needs and thus contribute positively to their well-being (Hammell, 2008; Wilcock & Townsend, 2014). "What people do" as part of their daily lives influences their experiences of empowerment, hope, personal agency and autonomy, positive interpersonal interactions, and so on. It also has a relationship to the security, prosperity, and stability of society. Occupational injustice is considered to occur "when participation in occupations is barred, confined, restricted, segregated, prohibited, underdeveloped, disrupted, alienated, marginalised, exploited, excluded or otherwise restricted" (Townsend & Wilcock, 2004, p. 77). The social, institutional, economic, and political conditions that give rise to these participation restrictions are often complex and multifaceted, and can become ongoing sources of stress in people's daily lives (Stadnyk et al., 2010). When such conditions impose prolonged restrictions on participation in everyday occupations, they put people at risk for detrimental impacts to their health as individuals and communities. Occupational injustice threatens human dignity and reduces opportunity for individual advancement and self-sufficiency; it also denies society the potential contributions of much of its citizenry and gives rise to social imbalance in opportunity among groups within communities and inequitable control over resources.

The links drawn between occupationally unjust conditions and health align with how social determinants of health and inequities in health are understood (Durocher, Gibson, & Rappolt, 2014). The social determinants of health are factors related to health outcomes, and are described in Chapter 15 focused on health promotion. They are discussed here as they apply to occupational justice. Known health determinants in general include factors that are biological (e.g., related to genes, sex, age), behavioral (e.g., behaviors with known health risks like smoking, alcohol use, unprotected sex), environmental (e.g., toxic waste),

and social in nature (Commission on Social Determinants of Health [CSDH], 2008). Of these, social determinants of health include social and economic conditions shaped by income, power, and access to resources; as well as social characteristics such as sex, race, sexuality, disability, and culture, that are known to differentially affect health outcomes. Furthermore, social determinants of health are thought to be more important than either access to health care or behavioral lifestyle choices in influencing health.

Several social determinants of health are of particular importance for mental health and well-being (Table 17-1). Experiences of these social determinants of mental health may vary for differing populations and communities. Resources and opportunities for meaningful occupation and social roles are influenced by gender, income, culture, and disability, and their interactions. For example, occupational therapists who work in health-related contexts will likely be very well aware of the occupational and participation restrictions that impact people with disabilities, but they will also need to consider that these will be further magnified when disability is also considered through the lens of gender or race. The impacts of lacking these social supports, access to occupation, and meaningful social roles contribute to poorer mental health than in the general population (CSDH, 2008).

Key social determinants of mental health and well-being listed in Table 17-1 underscore the centrality of occupation for connecting people with others and with resources. They also emphasize that enabling social, community, and productive forms of occupational engagement should be a priority when working with individuals, populations, or communities whose mental health is poor, not only to enhance participation but also to improve health outcomes. Hence, an occupational justice approach to health also argues for re-orienting health services toward valuing and giving priority to engagement in meaningful and

TABLE 17-2
PRINCIPLES ON HUMAN RIGHTS IN RELATION TO OCCUPATION AND PARTICIPATION
• People have the right to participate in a range of occupations that enable them to flourish, fulfill their potential, and experience satisfaction in a way that is consistent with their culture and beliefs.
• People have the right to be supported to participate in occupation and, through engaging in occupation, to be included and valued as members of their families, communities, and society.
• People have the right to choose for themselves: to be free of pressure, force, or coercion; in participating in occupations that may threaten safety, survival, or health, and those occupations that are dehumanizing, degrading, or illegal.
• The right to occupation encompasses civic, educative, productive, social, creative, spiritual, and restorative occupations. The expression of the human right to occupation will take different forms in different places because occupations are shaped by the cultural, social, and geographic context.
• At a societal level, the human right to occupation is underpinned by the valuing of each person's diverse contribution to the valued and meaningful occupations of the society, and is ensured by equitable access to participation in occupation, regardless of difference.
• Abuses of the right to occupation may take the form of economic, social, or physical exclusion through attitudinal or physical barriers, or through control of access to necessary knowledge, skills, resources, or venues where occupation takes place.
• Global conditions that threaten the right to occupation include poverty, disease, social discrimination, displacement, natural and man-made disasters, and armed conflict. In addition, the human right to occupation is subject to cultural beliefs and customs, local circumstances, and institutional power and practices.
Reprinted with permission from World Federation of Occupational Therapists. (2006). *Position Statement on Human Rights (CM2006)*. Retrieved from www.wfot.org.

health-enhancing occupations as a right and an essential part of health care (Durocher et al., 2014; Wilcock, 2006; Wilcock & Townsend, 2014).

Key Concepts

Occupational needs—Engagement in occupations fulfills basic human needs essential for survival; to exercise and develop innate capacities of a biological, social, and cultural nature; to adapt to environmental changes; and to flourish as individuals (Wilcock, 1993, 1998). More recently, needs met through occupation have also been described in other ways (Durocher et al., 2013). Notably, they include needs to exercise choice, control, and power in daily life (Townsend & Wilcock, 2004); needs to do, be, become, and belong (Wilcock, 2006); and occupational needs focused not only on looking after oneself but also on contributing to and caring for families and communities (Stadnyk et al., 2010). Participation in a range of occupations is necessary to address these needs. Indeed, the full range of meanings that humans ascribe to their occupations, described in detail in Chapter 5 of this book, may be considered fundamental occupational needs.

Occupational rights—Occupational rights refer to the rights of people to engage and be included in occupations

that they need and want to do, and that contribute positively to their communities and well-being (Hammell, 2008; Townsend, 2012). Deciding whether the occupational rights of an individual or group/community are being violated depends on a comprehensive appreciation of occupational patterns and opportunities. To assist with evaluating occupational rights, four occupational rights have been proposed: the right to meaningful and enriching occupation, the right to develop through participation in occupations that enable health and social inclusion, the right to exercise choice in occupations, and the right to participation in diverse occupations and its benefits (Stadnyk et al., 2010). More broadly, a number of human rights relevant to participation in occupations are stated in the United Nations' (1948) Universal Declaration of Human Rights and the World Federation of Occupational Therapists' *Position Statement on Human Rights* (WFOT, 2006) outlines a set of principles regarding human rights in relation to occupation and participation (Table 17-2).

Considering these principles can help us to evaluate occupational justice and injustice more fully. For example, the vignettes of Frank and Sindu (Vignettes 17-1 and 17-2) present scenarios where the individuals are engaged in some forms of occupation where it would be difficult to say that they are "wanted" or chosen free of constraints. Yet,

VIGNETTE 17-1. FRANK

Frank is a husband and father of two children. He immigrated to Canada as a displaced person in the aftermath of war in his homeland. He supports his family working on the assembly line of a factory. He finds the work repetitive and boring, but he is thankful for the work, and enjoys the financial and social stability that it provides. His life experiences and context did not give him the opportunity for any specific training, so he is not prepared for any other work. He sends money and other resources back to family members living in his country of origin. During his time off from work he enjoys reading, gardening, following world politics, and spending time with his family.

VIGNETTE 17-2. SINDU

Sindu is a husband and father of two children. He immigrated to Canada from his homeland to try and secure a better life for his children. Sindu trained in a regulated health profession in his homeland, but he has been unable to secure the approvals he needs to practice in his new country. He has found the costs related to licensing in his field have affected his family's financial well-being and he has difficulty sorting out all the policies and procedures involved in the licensing process. He is working two jobs to make ends meet and hopes that his employment as a home support worker might give him an edge to secure his license. His working hours have severely limited the time he has to give to his other interests and his family.

using the principles of human rights in relation to occupation and participation, we can evaluate Frank's occupational engagement as more consistent with occupational justice, in that he participates in a range of occupations that provide him meaning, and the opportunity to flourish. Sindu, on the other hand, experiences an occupational life that is seriously constrained in the context of restrictive social structures.

Occupational injustice outcomes—Occupational injustice is an evolving concept, with several forms of occupational injustice so far proposed. The terms outlined in Table 17-3 have somewhat overlapping meanings, so that they are as yet not readily distinguished as distinct categories. They are, however, a useful way to begin thinking and describing the kinds of outcomes that are associated with occupational injustice.

Occupational Justice and Ideas About Social Justice

Broadly speaking, justice is concerned with the ethical, moral, and civic principles that define a just society, such as fairness, equity, trustworthiness, and so on. Philosopher John Rawl's theory of distributive justice has been particularly influential. The theory is complex, but at its core proposes three principles for a just society: equality in basic liberties, equality of opportunity for advancement, and positive discrimination toward the underprivileged to ensure equity (Ife, 2002). Hence, social justice may be defined as justice in the distribution of wealth, opportunities, and privileges within a society (www.oxforddictionaries.com). This implies social justice is concerned with social relations in society, such as the fair and equitable treatment of people, and with the proper and fair distribution or sharing of resources in society (or distributive justice). For instance, policies that seek to redistribute material resources more equitably in a community through taxation, income support, and other forms of welfare assistance may be considered examples of distributive forms of social justice.

Although Rawl's theory of social justice is helpful in our developing understanding of occupational justice, it does have limitations. For example, while there is no doubt that occupational justice is closely tied to the distribution of resources and economic and monetary gains, these are not, in and of themselves, adequate frameworks for conceptualizing the human experiences and issues underlying occupational justice. Distributive justice cannot, for example, adequately account for respect of human differences about occupational needs, potentials, and aspirations, or for the potential of these individual differences to contribute to a flourishing society.

Concepts of social justice that explicitly address power, opportunity, and capability may be particularly useful to consider in relation to occupational justice (Stadnyk et al., 2010). For instance, philosopher Iris Marion Young viewed

TABLE 17-3	
FORMS OF OCCUPATIONAL INJUSTICE	
Occupational deprivation	Arises from prolonged restrictions or denial of access to opportunities and resources to participate in occupations (Townsend & Wilcock, 2004; Wilcock, 2006) produced by restrictive social, economic, environmental, cultural, and political conditions (Whiteford, 2010). Prolonged denial of opportunities to exercise and develop one's physical, mental, and social capacities; and the resulting loss of capacities, knowledge, and skills have detrimental effects on health and well-being (Whiteford, 2010).
Occupational alienation	Describes prolonged experiences of disconnectedness, isolation, emptiness, lack of identity, choice, and meaningfulness in daily life and ways of participating. Wilcock (1998; 2006) drew on a Marxist critique of industrial production as an alienating force, in which people's natural inclinations toward (work) activities and connection with its products/rewards are degraded when power over one's participation is removed. Occupational alienation exacts a toll on well-being through powerlessness over one's ways of living and participating, in which profound meaninglessness and estrangement are experienced (Townsend & Wilcock, 2004).
Occupational marginalization	Occurs when people are not afforded opportunities to participate in particular occupations, or to make their own choices about participation, due to societal expectations about how, when, where, and by whom they may be undertaken. These expectations may operate invisibly, are often because of discrimination on grounds of age, gender, disability, and so on, and serve to marginalize some individuals and groups in society from socially valued forms of occupation (Stadnyk et al., 2010). People experiencing occupational marginalization are therefore likely to have limited access to occupational resources and fewer occupational choices than others in society.
Occupational imbalance	Describes occupational patterns that limit people's expression of interests, values, or use of capacities in a prolonged manner, and therefore pose risks to their health through not gaining the physical, mental, and social benefits of diverse occupations (Wilcock, 2006). Thus, occupational imbalance is conceptualized as a form of occupational injustice when characterized by prolonged disproportionate involvement in particular occupations at the expense of other occupations, or by involvement in occupations with a limited range of these qualities (Backman, 2010; Wilcock, 2006).

justice and injustice as explicitly rooted in unequal power relations, wherein some people are enabled to exercise power to direct their lives and others are subject to exploitation, marginalization, disempowerment, subordination, or violence in everyday life. She further argued that a distributive view of social justice ignores the social structures and practices that contribute to these inequalities, and instead proposed a justice based on opportunity irrespective of difference based on age, sex, social class, culture, race, sexual orientation, or disability (Mullaly, 2002).

The capabilities framework is a theoretical perspective of social justice that may be particularly applicable to occupational justice. The capabilities framework is applicable to a range of human conditions and experiences where the expression of the full potential of people is compromised,

rather than confined exclusively to health contexts. In essence, it focuses on capabilities defined as the freedoms that we experience, value, and that "...not only make our lives richer and more unfettered, but also allows us to be fuller social persons, exercising our own volitions and interacting with—and influencing—the world in which we live" (Sen, 2000, p. 15).

The central concept of *capability* refers to what people are actually able to do and to be, as distinct from what people have or possess. The fundamental idea is that there are central capabilities that derive from basic human dignity and these capabilities must be guaranteed for everybody. Health and well-being are defined as the guarantee of these capabilities; that is, people's effective freedoms to participate in the actions and activities they value, to be and

> ### TABLE 17-4
>
> ## NUSSBAUM'S CENTRAL HUMAN CAPABILITIES
>
> 1. *Life*—Being able to live to the end of a human life of normal length.
>
> 2. *Bodily health*—Being able to have good health, be adequately nourished, and have adequate shelter.
>
> 3. *Bodily integrity*—Being able to move freely from place to place, to be secure against violent assault, and having opportunities and choice in matters of sexual satisfaction and reproduction.
>
> 4. *Senses, imagination, and thought*—Being able to use the senses to imagine, think, and reason—and to do these things in a "truly human" way, to have pleasurable experiences, and to avoid non-beneficial pain.
>
> 5. *Emotions*—Being able to have attachments to things and people outside ourselves; in general, to love, to grieve, to experience longing, gratitude, and justified anger, and not having one's emotional development blighted by fear and anxiety.
>
> 6. *Practical reason*—Being able to form a conception of the good and to engage in critical reflection about the planning of one's life (this entails protection for the liberty of conscience and religious observance).
>
> 7. *Affiliation*—(A) Being able to live with and toward others, to recognize and show concern for other human beings, to engage in various forms of social interaction; to be able to imagine the situation of another. (B) Having the social bases of self-respect and non-humiliation; being able to be treated as a dignified being whose worth is equal to that of others.
>
> 8. *Other species*—Being able to live with concern for, and in relation to, animals, plants, and the world of nature.
>
> 9. *Play*—Being able to laugh, to play, and to enjoy recreational activities.
>
> 10. *Control over one's environment*—(A) Political: Being able to participate effectively in political choices that govern one's life, having the right of political participation, and protections of free speech and association. (B) Material: Being able to hold property, and having property rights on an equal basis with others; having the right to seek employment on an equal basis with others; having the freedom from unwarranted search and seizure; and in work, being able to work as a human being, exercise practical reason, and enter into meaningful relationships of mutual recognition with other workers.
>
> Adapted from Wells, T. (2012). Sen's Capability Approach. *Internet encyclopaedia of philosophy.* Retrieved from www.iep.utm.edu/sen-cap.

become who they want to be, as fundamental entitlements, across the population. Thus, these freedoms are indicators of well-being and quality of life. Conversely, disorder and deprivation occur where the guarantee of these capabilities falls below an acceptable threshold for particular communities and populations.

The major contributors to the capabilities framework are Amartya Sen (2005) whose background is in economics, development, social choice theory, philosophy, and includes a Nobel Prize in Economics, and the well-known philosopher, Martha Nussbaum. In an effort to further the advancement and operationalization of a capabilities approach in practice, Nussbaum (2003, 2011) has proposed 10 fundamental human capabilities, defining these capabilities as "opportunities that people have when, and only when, policy choices put them in a position to function effectively in a wide range of areas that are fundamental to a fully human life." (cited in Townsend, 2012, p. 12.) Nussbaum argues that everyone is entitled to each capability at least to a degree, and that access to

these capabilities is a requirement for human dignity, albeit that lacking any particular capability is not intended to imply a life less human. She also makes a distinction here between choice and deprivation. For example, for someone who chooses not to take up certain capabilities, respecting this choice is an aspect of respecting the person's dignity; whereas if someone lacks access to certain capabilities, this is considered to reflect a failure of society to respect his choice or dignity (Wells, 2012). Nussbaum's list of ten capabilities is briefly summarized in Table 17-4.

In proposing these ten fundamental human capabilities, Nussbaum's intention was to highlight central entitlements in terms of opportunities, resources, and power necessary for people to choose and act, regardless of biological and social differences (Townsend, 2012). Therefore, capabilities and rights are closely linked. Indeed, according to Nussbaum (2003), specific rights should be thought of as secured only when people are put in a position of capability to do and be in that capability area (e.g., a right to work is only secured when individuals are in a position to exercise

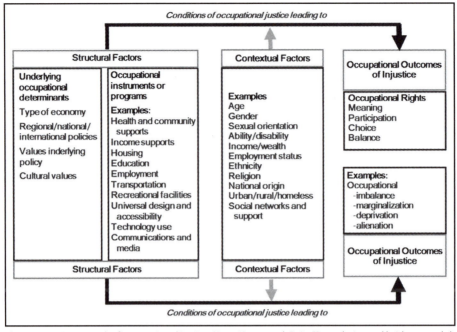

Figure 17-1. Framework of occupational justice. (From Townsend, E. A., "Boundaries and bridges to adult mental health: critical occupational and capabilities perspectives of justice," *Journal of Occupational Science, 19*(1), p. 13. Copyright © 2012 by Taylor & Francis. Reprinted with permission.)

that right), and so society should not be considered just unless these capabilities have been effectively achieved. Nussbaum's list of capabilities also resonates strongly with the central idea of occupational rights, that is, with the entitlement to realize occupational possibilities and to engage in the kind of life that one needs and wants to lead (Townsend, 2012).

Townsend argues that the capabilities approach of Sen and Nussbaum offers a framework within which the exclusion or inclusion from everyday occupations of particular groups or populations may be viewed and investigated as matters of occupational injustice or justice. For instance, to consider the exclusion from everyday occupations of adults experiencing persistent mental health issues in terms of these capabilities, we would need to ask: What is permitted for adults experiencing persistent mental health issues in our communities to do and be? How have their circumstances, familial, social and political, affected their ability to enjoy good health? To protect their bodily integrity? To attain an adequate education? To work on terms of mutual respect and equality with other workers? To participate in politics? To achieve self-respect and a sense of their own worth as persons and citizens? (Adapted from Nussbaum cited in Townsend, 2012, p. 12). Thus, in mental health contexts, adopting a capabilities framework lends itself to focusing on what people can do and be in their day-to-day living as key in their recovering and inclusion (Davidson, Rakfeldt, & Strauss, 2010; Hopper, 2007). These ideas have broader relevance to the general practice of occupational therapy.

The Framework of Occupational Justice

This framework of occupational justice offers an emerging theory of occupational justice and injustice from a critical standpoint (Townsend, 2012). As shown in Figure 17-1, it grounds an understanding of everyday occupations and conditions that lead to occupational justice and injustice in interconnected *structural factors* and *contextual factors* that support or restrict possibilities for doing in everyday life (Stadnyk et al., 2010; Townsend, 2012). It also describes *occupational rights* related to choice, meaning, participation, and balance in occupations and provides examples of *occupational injustice*.

- *Structural factors*: Stadnyk et al. (2010) propose two types of structural factors (occupational determinants and occupational instruments or programs) that create the conditions for occupational justice or occupational injustice. Occupational determinants include economic structures that determine which occupations are remunerated (e.g., paid work) and those deemed of private or social value, which often includes occupations like child-rearing, housework, and volunteering. In addition, the possibilities and limits of occupational engagement within societies and communities are regulated through policies and cultural values. Thus, policies concerning employment conditions, education options, health and welfare provision, as well as cultural traditions, may support or limit the possibilities for occupational justice through the ways in which service systems and programs are organized. To illustrate, an employment policy (occupational determinant) to enable access to jobs for those most disadvantaged in the labor market (e.g., people with disabilities who experience long-term unemployment) may be operationalized through the development of employment support services, job creation schemes, and rehabilitation services (occupational instruments or programs). Depending on their funding priorities, eligibility criteria and other ways in which these programs are organized, they may be more or less successful in creating just employment and working conditions. In addition, these employment initiatives could be supported or hindered by how policies and programs are implemented in other areas (e.g., access to education, transport, and income support).

- *Contextual factors*: Stadnyk et al. (2010) propose that the characteristics of individuals, populations, and communities mediate the effects of structural factors that contribute to occupational justice or occupational injustice. In other words, the structural factors described previously are experienced differently by individuals, populations, and communities with differing characteristics. Importantly, this means that characteristics such as age, sex, race, poverty, disability, geographical location, and so on do create conditions in which people do not experience equal access to opportunities, resources, and services to enable their occupational engagement. Hence, while some people may be afforded opportunities, resources, and services to participate in their occupations consistent with their needs and rights, others are not.

As illustrated, an extensive and complex range of structural and contextual factors may either enable or hinder engagement in the occupations that people need, want, or are expected to do. Thus, Stadnyk et al.'s (2010) *Framework of Occupational Justice* indicates that occupational justice is enabled when these factors are aligned so that occupational rights are respected, and opportunities, resources, and services to participate in their occupations are afforded (Durocher et al., 2013). Conversely, it suggests that where structural and contextual factors lead to circumstances that hinder occupational engagement, then occupational rights are undermined or violated and occupational injustice may be experienced (Durocher et al., 2013). Therefore, this framework highlights that the extent to which people may experience occupationally just or unjust situations depends upon many interrelated factors, the impacts of which will vary in differing occupations of daily life, although it does not explicitly account for whether or not occupational needs are met.

Theoretical Assumptions About Occupational Justice and Injustice

Occupational justice is broadly concerned with ethical, moral, and civic principles related to rights; fairness and equity; and conditions specific to meeting human needs for diverse and meaningful occupation that impact individuals and communities justly or unjustly. Occupational justice is also an emerging concept, so that scholars are continuing to explore and articulate its theoretical roots and assumptions. The most detailed description to date is that of Stadnyk et al. (2010), which outlines a set of four beliefs and four principles about occupational justice.

Stadnyk et al.'s (2010) proposed four beliefs reflect ideas, values, and assumptions about human beings, occupation, and an occupational perspective of health, as articulated by Wilcock (1998, 2006). These beliefs are as follows:

- *Humans are occupational beings*—As described earlier, occupational justice is underpinned by a view of humans as occupational beings with needs to engage in occupations so as to survive, develop, and flourish.

- *Humans participate in occupations as active agents*—In other words, humans are considered to be persons with agency (will and drive) to participate in occupations. So, while, albeit that individuals differ in their capacities, needs, and power to choose and engage in occupations, agency is central to participation and processes of transformation or recovery (Davidson, Rakfeldt, & Strauss, 2010).

- *Occupational participation is interdependent and contextual*—That is, people carry out occupations in specific contexts, including real time and places with particular people and material resources, which may support or hinder their participation. All human doings are also interdependent in the sense that they are "dependent on what other people have done before or are doing around us" (Stadnyk et al., 2010, p. 342), even though this is not always immediately visible to us. For example, an occupation like reading a book might be carried out in different places (e.g., library, commuter train, study, bed); it may also seem solitary but nevertheless depends on having to learn to read, and on those who wrote, published, and produced the book.

- *Occupational participation is a determinant of health and quality of life*—Participation in diverse and meaningful occupations can promote mental, physical, and social health and well-being. Some occupations can also be detrimental to health, as is a lack of occupation (Stadnyk et al., 2010; Wilcock, 2006; Wilcock &

Townsend, 2014). For example, in the case of employment, the nature of the job or working conditions may either promote or undermine health, whereas unemployment is associated with poorer mental and physical health.

Stadnyk et al. (2010) also outlined the following four principles related to rights, responsibilities, empowerment, and enablement of participation:

1. *Empowerment through occupation*—This principle acknowledges that power as a central issue in everyday life, operates unequally so that some people are able to exercise rights to participate in occupations that they need and want to do, and that contribute positively to their communities and well-being, while others are not (Stadnyk et al., 2010). Empowerment is linked to occupational injustice because economic and social policies, laws, and cultural forces can limit the possibilities for exercising power to choose and to participate in occupations of different kinds, resulting in people experiencing diminished power to influence what they do, and how they do everyday occupations. Thus, interventions to promote personal power or agency as means of empowerment through occupation must also take account of power relations in the broader social context of community structures and conditions that may be disempowering, but can also have transformative potential.

2. *Inclusive classification of occupations*—This principle proposes an inclusive classification of occupations on the grounds that some types of occupations have come to be defined as paid work, whereas others are considered private, and so occupations that are not being equally valued economically or socially is a source of occupational injustice. For example, unpaid domestic work, child-rearing, caring, creative pursuits, and volunteering—not infrequently the domain of women, older persons, and those who are underemployed or unemployed—are accorded neither the pay, privileges nor status of employment and often deemed of lesser importance (Stadnyk et al., 2010). This perpetuates occupationally unjust situations that can be especially challenging for those who are marginalized or excluded from paid work and economic self-sufficiency, as often occurs for adults with disabilities, those experiencing persistent mental ill-health, and those seeking resettlement in countries where policies restrict their work options (as in Vignettes 17-1 and 17-2).

3. *Enablement of occupational potential*—Interconnected with the previous principles, the enablement of occupation potential emphasizes the right of all people, irrespective of individual differences, to develop their capacities, knowledge, and skills for participation in occupations. The development of enabling conditions refers to approaches and situations that create the opportunities and resources for individuals, populations, and communities to expand their choices and pursue their occupational potential (Stadnyk et al., 2010).

4. *Diversity, inclusion, and shared advantage in occupation participation*—To enable occupational potential demands respect for differences on grounds of capacities and abilities, but for diverse personal and cultural meanings ascribed to participation. Therefore, an occupationally just community would be inclusive in the sense that individuals are empowered and enabled to engage in occupations that they need and want to do, and to share in the benefits and privileges that accrue from participation.

KEY DEVELOPERS/THEORISTS

Much of the published writing to date exploring the concept of occupational justice reflects the work of three occupational therapy scholars: Professors Ann Wilcock, Elizabeth Townsend, and Gail Whiteford. Wilcock's historical research draws explicitly on a public health perspective of health determinants and risk factors and seeks to understand the relationships between occupation and health. Elaborated in two textbooks on an *Occupational Perspective of Health* (Wilcock, 1998, 2006), her work articulated the nature of human needs for occupation (as outlined previously), and identified that occupational determinants of health outcomes are strongly influenced by sociopolitical and cultural factors. In asserting the inherently occupational nature of human beings, Wilcock also highlighted that restrictions to participation in meaningful, socially valued occupations are detrimental for health and well-being and therefore represent injustice (Durocher et al., 2013; Townsend & Wilcock, 2004). Through a critical ethnography investigating empowerment- and enablement-based practices in psychosocial occupational therapy, Townsend, too, identified many institutional and societal conditions that "overruled" the possibilities for achieving social justice in the everyday lives of occupational therapy clients, be they individuals, families, communities or populations (Townsend, 1998; Townsend & Wilcock, 2004). Their respective research led both to question the adequacy of social justice to identify and address the occupation-related rights to participate in valued occupations of individuals and communities, leading to their subsequent conceptualization of occupational justice (Wilcock & Townsend, 2014).

A growing number of other studies are exploring experiences of occupational injustices. Whiteford (1997, 2005, 2010) sought to investigate the occupational experiences of people who are imprisoned and in refugee camps, and to highlight the occupational injustice arising from participation restrictions imposed by these settings. Several other studies, too, highlight the challenges to participation in everyday occupations faced by people seeking asylum and by refugees and migrants during the processes of resettlement in new countries (e.g., Burchett & Matheson, 2010; Nayar, Hocking, & Wilson, 2007), whereas others have examined occupational justice issues related to domestic violence, working, and disability (Jakobsen, 2004; Smith & Hilton, 2008), conditions of domestic work (Galvaan, 2000), and how everyday technologies can marginalize older adults from participation in leisure (Nilsson & Townsend, 2010).

Several texts have been published by occupational therapy scholars that highlight the breadth of occupational justices experienced by people in many different parts of the world, and the diverse, practical, and inclusive ways in which engagement in everyday occupations can become the means for enabling people to transform their lives in differing local geographic, cultural, and political contexts (Kronenberg, Simó Algado, & Pollard, 2005, 2011; Whiteford & Hocking, 2011). Pollard, Sakellariou, and Kronenberg (2009) further explore the political nature of occupation and tools for raising political awareness of the occupational justice issues present in diverse practice arenas. Collectively, their work provides a rich range of practice wisdom and resources on which to draw to appreciate how occupational justice perspectives may inform occupational therapy practice.

Further specific examples of ways in which occupational therapy scholars are employing social and occupational justice concepts to frame psychosocial occupational therapies include occupational therapists' use of principles of occupational justice to understand problems rooted in societal issues that contribute to challenges encountered in the criminal justice system, and to adopt an occupationally relevant approach to practice within this system (Muñoz et al., 2011; White, Dielman Grass, Hamilton, & Rogers, 2013), and use of the Model of Human Occupation as an analytic tool for understanding and addressing issues framed in terms of oppression and promoting social justice (Abelenda, Kielhofner, Suarez-Balcazar, & Kielhofner, 2005; Kielhofner, de la Heras, & Suarez-Balcazar, 2011).

Expected Outcomes

Occupational justice is not an outcome in itself. Experiences of occupational justice and injustice are also not mutually exclusive since the social, economic, and cultural conditions impacting participation may vary in differing occupations and contexts. Nevertheless, the intent of actions to address occupationally unjust situations is to enable people to transform their lives through diverse, practical, and inclusive ways of engaging in everyday occupations. Occupational justice is a highly relevant lens

for psychosocial occupational therapy practice, given the extent to which individuals, groups, and families with a range of disabilities experience marginalization or exclusion from opportunities and resources to participate in everyday occupations, and the extent to which processes of occupational injustice impact mental health and well-being.

Practice Developments

Occupational Justice and Community Development

There is no fully developed occupational therapy practice framework focused on occupational justice to provide guidelines for psychosocial practices concerned with addressing potential occupational injustices. A promising approach is to connect concerns about occupational injustice to the practice field of community development. While many definitions of community development have been advanced, in this chapter community development is presented as a deliberate process that engages community members in understanding their needs and building the capacities of their communities to meet these needs. The field of community development has developed many approaches and techniques that can be used to enable this process (see Bennett, 1973; Ife, 2002). In this way, it offers promising practices that occupational therapists can use in their work to promote occupational justice both generally and in specific circumstances. The approaches and strategies of community development are typically reflective of a set of core principles, including the following:

- Empowering individuals and groups to influence the issues that affect their own lives and their communities

- Being conscious that some people and groups may need additional support to enable their capacity to address their issues and to participate in actions to influence the conditions of their lives

- Respecting and supporting the right of people and groups to be self-determining, to make their own choices

- Operating from a holistic perspective that recognizes the community is made up of many structures, organizations, entities, activities, groups, and so forth

- Engaging in practices that consider sustainability in harmony with nature and with long-term social equity

Two conceptual frameworks have been developed that link occupational therapy explicitly with community development principles and practices. First, Whiteford and Townsend (2005, 2011) have proposed a conceptual framework known as a Participatory Occupational Justice Framework, which aims to guide making occupational justice explicit in occupational therapy practices with

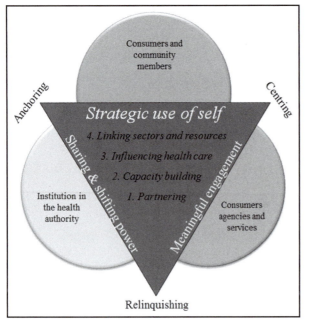

Figure 17-2. Framework for understanding community development from an occupational therapy perspective. (From Lauckner, H. M., Krupa, T., and Paterson, M. L., "Conceptualizing Community Development: Occupational Therapy Practice at The Intersection of Health Services and Community," *Canadian Journal of Occupational Therapy*, 78(4), 260-268. Copyright © 2011 by SAGE Publications. Reprinted with permission.)

individuals and populations. This framework is structured around six interrelated processes intended to enable collaboration in practice and wider system contexts, each of which is accompanied by guiding questions and enablement skills. These processes, identified briefly here, are highly reflective of the principles underlying community development practice.

- Raise conscious awareness of occupational injustices
- Engage collaboratively with partners
- Mediate agreement on a plan
- Strategize resource funding
- Support implementation and continuous evaluation
- Inspire advocacy for sustainability or closure.

Vignettes 17-3 and 17-4 describes two examples of occupational therapists using assertive participatory strategies to engage communities to identify and address specific needs. The vignettes highlight how the participatory processes unleashed the capacities of the communities to give shape to their experiences and needs, and to work toward real solutions. They illustrate the application of some of the early processes of the Participatory Occupational Justice Framework. Moving forward in each case, we could expect to see these communities apply efforts to secure funding for supporting implementation and monitoring regardless of whether intended outcomes were met for all community members.

The second conceptual framework developed by Lauckner and colleagues (2011) explicitly explicates community development from an occupational therapy perspective (Figure 17-2). The framework suggests how occupational therapy practices can evolve from narrowly defined individual and service-based approaches to being more consistent with community development practices. For example, the model suggests how occupational therapists working in the health sector can strategically "use the self" to enable real power sharing with people with lived experience, meaningfully engage with a broad range of potential community partners, and help shift the power dynamics between institutions and the people they serve in a way that will ultimately enable human occupation. Lauckner and colleagues' (2011) work offers case examples of occupational therapists working in community development capacities across a range of practice scenarios.

The field of community development offers many specific approaches that can be applied by occupational therapists to problems of occupational justice. Two such examples are (1) mobilizing community assets, and (2) community economic development.

1. *Mobilizing community assets*: Community researchers Kretzmann and McKnight (1993) argue that traditional approaches to dealing with issues of participation and inclusion in the community have tended to be deficit based; that is, focused on the problems and limitations of individuals and groups and the broader communities in which they reside. Viewing issues from this perspective naturally leads to an expert-driven approach, and privileges expert-driven solutions over enhancing community capacities. Alternatively, a community capacity-building approach would consider these issues from the perspective of identifying and releasing the capacities that potentially exist in both the population of interest and the local community. Vignette 17-5 illustrates how the following four steps of mobilizing community capacities were used to address occupational issues experienced by seniors living in one neighborhood: (1) identifying the community need, (2) identifying the range of skills and resources of the group/population, (3) identifying potential partners in the community, and (4) mobilizing reciprocal connections, formed to bring together the capacities of the community and the group.

2. *Community economic development*: Community economic development approaches focus on building stronger, socioeconomic conditions within a community. The approach can be applied broadly to a community that is economically disadvantaged (e.g., regions experiencing the collapse of single economies, such as fishing, mining, or forestry), or to specific populations of people who are socially and economically marginalized within their communities. People with disabilities, for example, experience

VIGNETTE 17-3. ENABLING INCLUSIVE, DIVERSE, AND MEANINGFUL PLAY

Playgrounds are community spaces designated for children's recreations. Playgrounds are typically designed to engage children of differing ages in recreation. However, since they do not necessarily enable access for all children, regardless of difference in sensory, motor, and cognitive capacities and challenges, some children may have difficulty participating in play within typical playground environments (Shapiro, 2006). This may be framed as an occupationally unjust situation in that some children can play, participate with other children, and enjoy the benefits of playing (e.g., fun, friendship, learning, skill development, confidence-building), while other children's participations are limited or restricted within typical playground environments.

To address this situation, Shapiro (2006) describes a 3-year collaborative project between Beit Issie Shapiro (a community-based organization in Israel that provides educational and therapeutic services to people with developmental disabilities and their families) and the local community to design and build a playground suitable for children with diverse abilities, which would also serve to promote the inclusive participation of children with special needs in society. In its planning stage, a project team of therapists, education staff, community workers, and community members (including user groups, organizations serving populations with differing impairments and needs, people with special needs, parents of children with special needs), were involved in gathering information so as to collaboratively develop playground design principles, user requirements, and a plan of action informed by community needs and knowledge, as well as that of the professionals involved. The resulting design for the outdoor playground takes account of key considerations that included creating safety and stability through a range of environmental features that enable easy spatial orientation; "way finding" and comfort in the playground for children with diverse sensory capacities; considering physical and psychological dimensions of accessibility; creating aesthetically pleasing and attractive, but also durable spaces; promoting social interaction, varied levels of challenge, diverse sensory stimulation, and outlets for emotional expression within the playground (Shapiro, 2006).

Established by Beit Issie Shapiro in 2005, Park Chaverim is Israel's first accessible and inclusive outdoor playground designed to enable all children, whatever their abilities or disabilities, to have opportunities to play and have fun together while raising community awareness about the importance of inclusion. (http://en.beitissie.org.il/about/inclusive-playground)

VIGNETTE 17-4. COLLABORATING WITH MENTAL HEALTH SERVICE USERS TO EXPLORE AND PROMOTE SOCIAL NETWORKING POSSIBILITIES

At a time of mental health service reform to promote social inclusion and service user involvement, occupational therapist Wendy Bryant, together with some mental health service users and other colleagues set up a local forum to promote dialogue, in which different understandings of what the community services were for and perceptions of their power to influence service development were explored (Bryant et al., 2011). These forums gradually developed a focus on the importance of social contact and safe places for social networking, with mental health service users directly involved in developing ideas and taking action to investigate and promote options and resources for social networking in their local community. Examples of the actions undertaken included a project involving taking photographs of how spaces at a valued local resource center were used for informal social contact, information-sharing with peers, and building social networks, following which the group produced a report calling for a safe space for this kind of social networking to be protected in the service redevelopment (Bryant et al., 2011). A further project involved an action group creating a checklist to learn more about places for social and recreational activities valued by service users, which generated valuable information not only about the range of places and activities available, but also what made participation accessible from service users' perspectives (Bryant et al., 2011). Occupational therapy knowledge of occupation and varied methods of enabling participation, power-sharing, and dialogue was a key resource to facilitate the involvement of many different people who used and provided services, and to enable their sharing of experiences and ideas in multiple ways (Bryant et al., 2011).

high rates of unemployment and poverty among the general population; suggesting that forces of exclusion are operating within the community economy. There are many such exclusionary forces at play. For example, to the extent that people with disabilities experience poverty, they may not have the resources they require to access and compete for jobs. To the extent that they have experienced restrictions and even discrimination in educational settings, they may be less able to compete for jobs based on educational preparation. To the extent that the general public assumes that they will not be productive and reliable, they will not be seriously considered for jobs. Community economic development approaches use market-based strategies to create employment opportunities and support access to fulfilling, secure and financially rewarding employment (Lysaght & Krupa, 2009; Krupa, Lagarde, & Carmichael, 2003; Paluch, Fossey, & Harvey, 2012). Unlike traditional vocational rehabilitation approaches that work with individuals with disability to develop their skills and capacities to prepare to enter the workforce, community economic development creates employment-related structures and opportunities. These structures are developed to neutralize these forces of disadvantage and to capitalize on the capacities, and strengths of individuals and groups. Vignettes 17-5 and 17-6 illustrate two such examples of occupational therapists who participated in creating economic structures that created real employment opportunities for people with mental illness while contributing to the social and economic fabric of the broader community.

CONCLUSION

Occupational justice and associated concepts and frameworks, such as social justice and capabilities frameworks, will each resonate with psychosocial occupational therapy, albeit that not all explicitly articulate an occupational perspective. Occupational justice and injustice are interconnected ways in which to think about occupational needs, strengths, and potentials of individuals and communities, as well as rights, fairness, empowerment, and enablement of participation in occupations of daily life. Health from an occupational justice perspective is reflected in the extent to which individuals and communities are able to participate in meaningful and diverse occupations that address their occupational needs, with fair and equitable access to the resources and opportunities for doing so. A

relatively new way of thinking and addressing population-level needs, this chapter suggests that occupational therapists can look to the field of community development to learn about and apply strategies and approaches to occupational justice issues. Given the fact that this is an evolving area of practice, its advancement will depend on growing an evidence base in the coming years.

LEARNING ACTIVITIES/ DISCUSSION QUESTIONS

1. Discuss the following with other occupational therapists: Does the concept of occupational justice contribute something unique and significant to the field of social justice? If yes, what is this uniqueness? If not, why not?

2. Describe how experiences of occupational justice and injustice influence personal mental health and well-being.

3. Think of a client/client group of occupational therapy services, with whom you have worked as an occupational therapist or student recently, whose participation in occupations of daily life was either severely disrupted or restricted due to external factors/circumstances.

   a. Make a list of the external factors or conditions that are contributing to occupational injustice in this situation.

   b. Make a list of some ways in which community resources could be mobilized to address this situation, using the five steps outlined in the chapter.

4. Identify an event/situation reported in the media (local, national or international) that could be viewed as reflecting occupational injustice in some way. Then consider:

   a. What is the nature of the occupational injustice in this event/situation, and why do you think it reflects occupational injustice?

   b. What might be key factors contributing to occupational injustice in this event/situation?

   c. How might a community capacity-building approach be used to identify capacities in the community concerned?

VIGNETTE 17-5. MOBILIZING COMMUNITY CAPACITIES

Aruna is an occupational therapist working for a community health center that serves neighborhoods located in an older district of her city; the area is socioeconomically one of the poorest areas. In her daily work she and her coworkers have noticed that many seniors are significantly under-occupied, isolated, and largely on the fringes of community activities. Aruna and a colleague undertake a focused effort to bring seniors in the area together for discussions centered on the question: "What can we contribute to our community?" Through a facilitated process they come up with several examples of contributions: Offer our knowledge and expertise to young people (e.g., participate in school reading programs; help with school intramural activities; teach skills in gardening, knitting, woodworking), participate in community events (e.g., participate in planning to represent the needs of seniors, volunteer for specific activities), and develop community resources (e.g., oversee a community food garden, develop a local "museum" of historical community artifacts).

Working with the seniors, Aruna and her colleagues created an asset map of local community organizations, services, and structures. Together they then selected, as a start, four activities that could link local senior capacities with local organizations to meet larger community needs. Over the past year, 35 local seniors have been routinely involved in moving these initiatives forward, and more than 50 seniors have participated in some way in at least one initiative.

VIGNETTE 17-6. THREE EXAMPLES OF COMMUNITY ECONOMIC DEVELOPMENT INITIATIVES

1. Staff of a Norwegian community-based mental health day activity program observed that clients were making little progress based on counselling, activity groups, and socialization. The occupational therapist, Birgit Granhaug, led the re-invention of the program into a community bakery and café. The former clients are now workers rather than clients. They are building their employment-related skills in a supportive atmosphere. Membership has doubled over 6 months and the bakery and café have become a cultural and social center in the community.

2. "Cleanable" is an Australian social firm that has provided property management services, including commercial cleaning and parks and garden maintenance, since 2005. This commercial organization is designed as a supportive work environment for people re-entering the workforce and living with disability. This firm uses occupational therapists as consultants for a variety of services.

3. Concerned about occupational deprivation and marginalization from employment opportunities of offenders with mental illness, occupational therapist Tracy Davidson enabled the development of the Free Spirit Affirmative Business. It has provided work through a largely offender-run social business for 14 federal offenders with mental illness. The business produces environmentally friendly products from recycled prison items, and workers contribute part of their proceeds to support local community charities. During an evaluation of the initiative, one offender commented: *"Our initial efforts were meager and half hearted, rife with skepticism and lack of commitment. However, under the leadership of the [occupational therapist], whose vision we were playing out, we began to see success in our efforts. We started to feel better about ourselves and our chances of making this work"* (Davidson, 2010).

REFERENCES

Abelenda, J., Kielhofner, G., Suarez-Balcazar, Y., & Kielhofner, K. (2005). The model of human occupation as a conceptual tool for understanding and addressing occupational apartheid. In F. Kronenberg, S. Simó Algado, & N. Pollard (Eds.), *Occupational therapy without borders. Learning from the spirit of survivors* (pp. 183-196). Edinburgh: Churchill Livingstone/Elsevier.

Backman, C. L. (2010). Occupational balance and well-being. In C. H. Christiansen & E. A. Townsend (Eds.), *Introduction to occupation: The art and science of living* (2nd ed., pp. 231-249). Upper Saddle River, NJ: Prentice-Hall.

Bennett, A. (1973). Professional staff members' contribution to community development. *Journal of the Community Development Society, 4*(1), 58-68.

Burchett, N., & Matheson, R. (2010). The need for belonging: The impact of restrictions on working on the well-being of an asylum seeker. *Journal of Occupational Science, 17*(2), 85-91.

Commission on Social Determinants of Health. (2008). *Closing the gap in a generation: health equity through action on the social determinants of health. Final Report of the Commission on Social Determinants of Health.* Geneva: World Health Organization.

Davidson, L., Rakfeldt, J., & Strauss, J. (2010). *The roots of the recovery movement in psychiatry: Lessons learned.* Chichester: John Wiley & Sons.

Davidson, T. (2010). Free spirit affirmative business: Employment for offenders with mental illness. (Unpublished master's thesis). Queen's University, Kingston, Ontario.

Durocher, E., Gibson, B. E., & Rappolt, S. (2013). Occupational justice: A conceptual review. *Journal of Occupational Science,* DOI:10.1080/14427591.2013.775692

Durocher, E., Gibson, B. E., & Rappolt, S. (2014). Occupational justice: Future directions. *Journal of Occupational Science, 21*(4), 431-442.

Galvaan, R. (2000). The live-in domestic workers' experience of occupational engagement. Unpublished Master's Thesis. University of Cape Town, Cape Town, South Africa.

Galvaan, R. (2011). Occupational choice: The significance of socioeconomic and political factors. In G. E. Whiteford, & C. Hocking (Eds.), *Occupational science: Society, inclusion, participation* (pp. 152-162). Hoboken, NJ: John Wiley & Sons.

Hammell, K. W. (2008). Reflections on...wellbeing and occupational rights. *Canadian Journal of Occupational Therapy, 75*(1), 61-64.

Hopper, K. (2007). Rethinking social recovery in schizophrenia: What a capabilities approach might offer. *Social Science & Medicine, 65,* 868-879.

Ife, J. (2002). *Community development: Community-based alternatives in an age of globalisation* (2nd ed.). French Forrest, NSW: Pearson Education.

Jakobsen, K. (2004). If work doesn't work: How to enable occupational justice. *Journal of Occupational Science, 11*(3), 125-134.

Kielhofner, G., de la Heras, C., & Suarez-Balcazar, Y. (2011). Human occupation as a tool for understanding and promoting social justice. In F. Kronenberg, N. Pollard, D. Sakellariou (Eds.), *Occupational therapies without borders. Vol. 2: Towards an ecology of occupation-based practices* (pp. 269-277). Edinburgh: Churchill Livingstone/Elsevier.

Kretzmann, J., & McKnight, J. (1993). *Building communities from the inside out: A path toward finding and mobilizing a community's assets.* Evanston, IL: Center for Urban Affairs and Policy Research, Northwestern University.

Kronenberg, F., Pollard, N., & Sakellariou, D. (Eds.). (2011). *Occupational therapies without borders, Volume 2: Towards an ecology of occupation-based practices.* Edinburgh: Churchill Livingstone Elsevier.

Kronenberg, F., Simó Algado, S., & Pollard, N. (Eds.). (2005). *Occupational therapies without borders: Learning from the spirit of survivors.* Edinburgh: Churchill Livingstone Elsevier.

Krupa T., Lagarde M. & Carmichael K. (2003). Transforming sheltered workshops into affirmative businesses: An evaluation of outcomes. *Psychiatric Rehabilitation Journal, 26,* 359-67.

Lauckner, H. (2005). Exploring occupational therapists' experiences in community development: Coming to understand our role. (Unpublished doctoral thesis). Queen's University, Kingston, Ontario.

Lauckner, H., Krupa, T., & Paterson, M. (2011). Conceptualizing community development: Occupational therapy practice at the intersection of health services and community. *Canadian Journal of Occupational Therapy, 78*(4), 260-268.

Lysaght, R., & Krupa, T. (2009). Social business: Advancing the viability of a model for economic and occupational justice for people with disabilities. Kingston: Queen's University. Retrieved from http://ccednet-rcdec.ca/en/node/10056.

Mullaly, R. P. (2002). *Challenging oppression: A critical social work approach.* Toronto: Oxford University Press.

Muñoz, J. P., Farnworth, L., Hamilton, T., Prioletti, G., Rogers, S., & White, J. A. (2011). Crossing borders in correctional institutions. In F. Kronenberg, N. Pollard, & D. Sakellariou (2011) (Eds.), *Occupational therapies without borders, Volume 2: Towards an ecology of occupation-based practices* (pp. 235-246). Edinburgh: Churchill Livingstone Elsevier.

Nayar, S., Hocking, C., & Wilson, J. (2007). An occupational perspective of migrant mental health: Indian women's adjustment to living in New Zealand. *British Journal of Occupational Therapy, 70,* 16-23.

Njelesani, J., Tang, A., Jonsson, H., & Polatajko, H. (2012). Articulating an occupational perspective. *Journal of Occupational Science,* DOI:10.1080/14427591.2012.717500.

Nilsson, I., & Townsend, E. (2010). Occupational justice—bridging theory and practice. *Scandinavian Journal of Occupational Therapy, 17,* 57-63.

Nussbaum, M. (2003) Capabilities as fundamental entitlements: Sen and social justice. *Feminist Economics, 9*(2/3), 33-59.

Nussbaum, M. (2011). *Creating capabilities: The human development approach.* Cambridge, MA: Harvard University Press.

Paluch, T., Fossey, E., & Harvey, C. (2012). Social firms: Building cross-sectoral partnerships to create employment and supportive workplaces for people with mental illness. *Work, 43,* 63-75.

Pollard, N., Sakellariou, D., & Kronenberg, F. (Eds.). (2009). *A political practice of occupational therapy.* Edinburgh: Churchill Livingstone Elsevier.

Sen, A. (2000). *Development as freedom.* New York: Anchor.

Sen, A. (2005). Human rights and capabilities. *Journal of Human Development, 6*(2), 151-166.

Shapiro, M. (2006). A model for an adapted playground developed for all children. *The Israel Journal of Occupational Therapy, 15*(4), E137-E147.

Smith, D. L., & Hilton, C. L. (2008). An occupational justice perspective of domestic violence against women with disabilities. *Journal of Occupational Science, 15*(3), 166-172.

Stadnyk, R. L., Townsend, E. A., & Wilcock, A. A. (2010). Occupational justice. In C. H. Christiansen, & E. A. Townsend (Eds), *Introduction to occupation: The art and science of living* (2nd ed., pp. 329-358). Upper Saddle River, NJ: Prentice-Hall.

Townsend, E. (1998). *Good intentions overruled: A critique of empowerment in the routine organisation of mental health services.* Toronto, Canada: University of Toronto Press.

Townsend, E., & Wilcock, A. (2004). Occupational justice and client-centred practice: A dialogue in progress. *Canadian Journal of Occupational Therapy, 71*(2), 75-87.

Townsend, E., & Whiteford, G. (2005). A participatory occupational justice framework: Population-based processes of practice. In F. Kronenberg, S. Simó Algado, & N. Pollard (Eds.), *Occupational therapies without borders: Learning from the spirit of survivors* (p. 110-126). Edinburgh: Churchill Livingstone Elsevier.

Townsend, E. A. (2012). Boundaries and bridges to adult mental health: critical occupational and capabilities perspectives of justice. *Journal of Occupational Science, 19*(1), 8-24.

United Nations. (1948). *Universal declaration of human rights.* Geneva,Switzerland: General Assembly of the United Nations. Retrieved from www.ohchr.org.

VicHealth. (2005). Social determinants of mental health. Melbourne, Australia: Author. Retrieved from www.health.vic.gov.au/mentalhealthpromotion/resources.htm#determinants

Wells, T. (2012). Sen's Capability Approach. *Internet encyclopaedia of philosophy.* Retrieved from www.iep.utm.edu/sen-cap.

White, J. A., Dieleman Grass, C., Hamilton, T. B., & Rogers, S. L. (2013). Occupational therapy in criminal justice. In E. Cara, & A. MacRae (Eds.), *Psychosocial occupational therapy: An evolving practice* (pp. 715-773). Clifton Park, NY: Delmar.

Whiteford, G. (1997). Occupational deprivation and incarceration. *Journal of Occupational Science, 4*(3), 126-130.

Whiteford, G. (2010). Occupational deprivation: understanding limited participation. In C. H. Christiansen, & E. A. Townsend (Eds.), *Introduction to occupation: The art and science of living* (2nd ed., pp. 303-328). Upper Saddle River, NJ: Prentice-Hall.

Whiteford, G., & Townsend, E. (2011). Participatory occupational justice framework (POTJ 2010): Enabling occupational participation and inclusion. In F. Kronenberg, N. Pollard, & D. Sakellariou (2011) (Eds.), *Occupational therapies without borders, Volume 2: Towards an ecology of occupation-based practices* (pp. 65-84). Edinburgh: Churchill Livingstone Elsevier.

Whiteford, G. E. (2005). Understanding the occupational deprivation of refugees: A case study from Kosovo. *Canadian Journal of Occupational Therapy, 72*(2), 78-88.

Whiteford, G. E., & Hocking, C. (Eds.). (2011). *Occupational science: Society, inclusion, participation.* Hoboken, NJ: John Wiley & Sons.

Wilcock, A. (1993). A theory of the human need for occupation. *Journal of Occupational Science, 1*(1), 17-24.

Wilcock A., & Townsend, E. (2014). Occupational justice. In B. A. B. Schell et al. (Eds.), *Willard and Spackman's occupational therapy* (12th ed., pp. 541-552). Philadelphia: Lippincott, Williams & Wilkins.

Wilcock, A. A. (1998). *An occupational perspective of health.* Thorofare, NJ: SLACK Incorporated.

Wilcock, A. A. (2006). *An occupational perspective on health* (2nd ed.). Thorofare, NJ: SLACK Incorporated.

World Federation of Occupational Therapists. (2006). *Position Statement on Human Rights (CM2006).* Retrieved from www.wfot.org.

Financial Disclosures

Dr. Lynn Cockburn has no financial or proprietary interest in the materials presented herein.

Dr. Larry Davidson has no financial or proprietary interest in the materials presented herein.

Dr. Ellie Fossey has no financial or proprietary interest in the materials presented herein.

Dr. Rebecca Gewurtz has no financial or proprietary interest in the materials presented herein.

Dr. Bonnie Kirsh has no financial or proprietary interest in the materials presented herein.

Dr. Terry Krupa has no financial or proprietary interest in the materials presented herein.

Dr. Erin McIntyre has no financial or proprietary interest in the materials presented herein.

Dr. Deborah Pitts has no financial or proprietary interest in the materials presented herein.

Dr. Patricia Rigby has no financial or proprietary interest in the materials presented herein.

Index